Yale Library of Medieval Philosophy

Founded by Norman Kretzmann

GENERAL EDITORS

Eleonore Stump

St. Louis University

John F. Wippel

The Catholic University of America

Scott MacDonald

Cornell University

The Yale Library of Medieval Philosophy is a series of commissioned translations of philosophical texts from the Latin Middle Ages. The series is intended to make available in English complete works of philosophical and historical importance, translated by scholars whose linguistic abilities are complemented by a philosophical understanding of the subject matter. Each translation published in the series will be accompanied by a brief introduction, sparse notes (confined to indispensable explanations and references), and an index.

Previously published

William of Ockham, *Quodlibetal Questions*

Volume 1

Quodlibets 1–4

Translated by Alfred J. Freddoso
and Francis E. Kelley

Volume 2

Quodlibets 5–7

Translated by Alfred J. Freddoso

Francisco Suarez, S.J., *On Efficient Causality*

Metaphysical Disputations 17, 18, and 19

Translated by Alfred J. Freddoso

Thomas Aquinas, *A Commentary on Aristotle's De Anima*

Translated by Robert Pasnau

Walter Burley, *On the Purity of the Art of Logic*

The Shorter and Longer Treatises

Translated by Paul Vincent Spade

John Buridan, *Summulae de Dialectica*

An annotated translation, with a philosophical introduction, by Gyula Klima

VNION ACADÉMIQVE INTERNATIONALE

CORPVS PHILOSOPHORVM MEDII AEVI
ACADEMIARVM CONSOCIATARVM AVSPICIIS ET CONSILIO EDITVM

AVERROIS OPERA
EDITIONI CVRANDAE PRAEEST
GERHARD ENDRESS

SERIES C
AVERROES LATINVS
XXXIII
COMMENTARIVM MAGNVM
IN ARISTOTELIS DE ANIMA LIBROS

IN LINGVAM ANGLICAM VERTIT
PROLEGOMENIS COMMENTARIIS INDICIBVSQVE INSTRVXIT
RICHARD C. TAYLOR
ADIVVANTE THÉRÈSE-ANNE DRVART

Averroes (Ibn Rushd) of Cordoba

Long Commentary on the **De Anima** *of Aristotle*

Translated and with introduction and notes

by Richard C. Taylor

with Thérèse-Anne Druart, subeditor

YALE UNIVERSITY PRESS

New Haven & London

Set in Palatino type by Integrated Composition Systems.
Printed in the United States of America.

ISBN: 978-0-300-11668-7
Library of Congress Control Number: 2007942427

A catalogue record for this book is available from the British Library.

The paper in this book meets the guidelines for permanence
and durability of the Committee on Production Guidelines
for Book Longevity of the Council on Library Resources.

10 9 8 7 6 5 4 3 2 1

For my wife, Carolyn,
in thanks for her support and encouragement

Contents

Preface

This book is the result of a collaborative effort, with Professor Thérèse-Anne Druart generously providing invaluable detailed critique, comment, and advice on every part of the project in the role of subeditor, as indicated on the title page. Her expertise in Arabic philosophy and in medieval and ancient philosophy generally, her thoughtful insight, her patient and sustained commitment to this project, and her personal generosity were essential to the success of this project. Still, final decisions in matters of translation and interpretation have been mine, so I must take responsibility for the final form of this work.

Financial support for this project has come from the National Endowment for the Humanities, from the Institute for Research in the Humanities at the University of Wisconsin at Madison, and from Marquette University. This I gratefully acknowledge, as I also acknowledge with thanks the support of many colleagues in medieval and Arabic philosophy and my colleagues at Marquette University who have encouraged me in the completion of this work and freely shared their expertise, only some of which could be acknowledged in notes. In particular, I want to thank the editors of this series for their continued interest in the completion of this project, which was initiated under the editorship of the late Norman Kretzmann. Finally, I must thank my wife, Carolyn, to whom this book is dedicated. This project is complete only thanks to her support and ceaseless encouragement.

Note on References
and Editorial Method

In the texts and notes which follow, references in curly brackets { } are to the *Long Commentary* (1953) (*Averrois Cordubensis Commentarium Magnum in Aristotelis De Anima Libros*, F. Stuart Crawford [ed.] [Cambridge, MA: Mediaeval Academy of America, 1953]).

Note, however, that in *Long Commentary* Fragments (2005), Sirat and Geoffroy use curly brackets { } to indicate conjectured text where margins have been cut off. My citations of this work follow their usage.

Square brackets [ ] in the translation are used to indicate my additions, clarifying the meaning with referents and assumed phrases made clear.

Angle brackets < > are used to indicate additions to texts noted by editors or translators of works cited.

+ . . . + indicate text bracketed by Crawford indicating missing or faulty Latin text.

In the introduction and the notes to the translation, I refer to the text of Aristotle's *De Anima* as provided in the *Long Commentary on the De Anima* as "the Text." I refer to the text of the commentary of Averroes as "the Comment."

Other primary and secondary sources are indicated by abbreviated references with author and title and year of publication in parentheses ( ). Full source information is found in the bibliography.

Introduction

In 1168–1169, at the age of about forty-two, Abû al-Walîd Muḥammad Ibn Aḥ-mad Ibn Rushd al-Ḥafîd (Averroes), whose grandfather was the famous legal and religious scholar of the same name, had already devoted serious study to Aristotle and the Greek Commentators.[1] This was clearly evidenced in *Short Commentaries* or *Epitomes* (مختصرات *mukhtaṣarât* or جوامع *jawâmiʿ*) on the works of Aristotle, drawing heavily on the understandings of the Greek and Arabic commentators. Yet thanks to Ibn Ṭufayl, the work of Averroes came to be even more focused on the texts and thought of Aristotle, even while he continued his studies and writing on law and theology and also served as *qâḍî* (judge). In this period Ibn Ṭufayl presented Averroes at the court of the Almohad ruler Abû Yaʿqûb Yûsuf, who succeeded his father, ʿAbd al-Muʾmin, champion of the teachings of al-Mahdî Ibn Tûmart (d. ca. 1129–1130) and vanquisher of the Al-moravides. As the story goes, Abû Yaʿqûb Yûsuf raised the question of whether the heavens were eternal or had a temporal beginning, much to the distress of Averroes, who knew well that the issue had important religious ramifications since the Qurʾân was held to have taught the temporal creation of the world. Only after Abû Yaʿqûb Yûsuf had displayed his sophisticated understanding of the issue in discussion with Ibn Ṭufayl did Averroes feel sufficiently at ease to join the discussion and to show his own erudition on this matter. Apparently at the request of Ibn Ṭufayl and with the patronage and support of Abû Yaʿqûb Yûsuf, Averroes, appointed *qâḍî* at Seville in 1169, undertook the task

1. With the exception of the *Middle* and *Long Commentaries* on the *De Anima*, which are discussed below, I follow for the most part the chronologies of Jamâl al-Dîn al-ʿAlawî (1986) and Miguel Cruz Hernández (1997), who benefited from Manuel Alonso's (1947) chronology in *Teología de Averroes*. The most recent account of the works of Averroes is that of Gerhard Endress (1999), which is an inventory of "the present state of critical work on the text of Ibn Rushd" (339) and supplements Wolfson (1931) and (1963). Also see Bouyges (1922) and (1923); Gómez Nogales (1978a); Anawati (1978); and Rosemann (1988). For more recent and current work on Averroes and his thought, consult Daiber (1999) and the bibliographies of Druart and Marmura (1990), (1993), and (1995) and Druart (1997b) and (2001). Druart's most recent versions of her "Brief Bibliographical Guides in Medieval Islamic Philosophy and Theology" are available on the Internet. See Druart (2002), (2004a), and (2006). The most comprehensive bibliography concerning Averroes is part of the Internet Averroes Database, located at the Thomas Institut in Cologne and presented by David Wirmer. See Wirmer, Thomas Institut (2006). The 1998 celebrations in honor of the anniversary of the death of Averroes resulted in a great many new studies of the thought of Averroes; a number of these are still in press.

of clarifying the works of Aristotle by pressing ahead with his explanatory commentaries.[2] The support of Abû Ya'qûb Yûṣuf is generally taken as the commissioning of what we now have as the *Middle Commentaries* (singular تلخيص *talkhîṣ*). The epitomizing *Short Commentaries* were followed by these paraphrasing *Middle Commentaries* until Averroes apparently completed the first of his *Long Commentaries* (singular شرح *sharḥ* or شرح كبير *sharḥ kabîr*) with the *Long Commentary on the De Anima*, probably sometime shortly before 1186.[3] In contrast to his other commentaries, the *Long Commentaries* are neither accounts based on commentators and other sources (*Short Commentaries*) nor paraphrastic summaries of Aristotle's teachings (*Middle Commentaries*). Rather, the *Long Commentaries* contain a complete Arabic version of the text commented (as is the case for Averroes' famous response to al-Ghazâlî in the *Tahâfut al-Tahâfut, The Incoherence of the Incoherence*) and detailed analyses of arguments drawing on the Greek commentators, as well as on thinkers in the Arabic tradition such as al-Fârâbî, Avicenna, Ibn Bâjjah, and others where available. But perhaps what is most remarkable about these *Long Commentaries* is Averroes' efforts in following carefully the text and in providing detailed explanations of the reasoning involved in Aristotle's often terse arguments. In addition

2. The story is recounted in al-Marrâkushî (1949), 242–243. George Hourani translates this account into English in *Decisive Treatise* (1961), 12–13.

3. In her review of Ivry's *Middle Commentary* (2002), Ruth Glasner cites a previously unknown comment by Averroes relevant to the dating of the *Middle* and *Long Commentaries* on the *De Anima*. She translates Averroes' remarks—which, she says, are unique to the Hebrew translation of the *Long Commentary on the Physics* (Paris BNF ms. héb 884, fol. 35b11–16) and not found in the Iunta edition—as follows: "we have the book of animals and we have already completed its commentary according to the signification and we shall further work, if God wills in our life, on its word by word commentary, as we shall try to do, God willing, in the rest of his books. We have not yet had the opportunity to carry out this intention except in the case of the *De anima*, and this book that we start now [the *Physics*]. But we have already laid down commentaries on all his books according to the signification in the three disciplines, logic, natural science, and metaphysics." Glasner (2004), 58–59. The common notion that the first of the *Long Commentaries* was that on the *Posterior Analytics* in 1180 or 1183 seems no longer tenable in the light of this discovery by Glasner. Cf. Cruz Hernández (1997), 59, and al-'Alawî (1986), 102. Much common thinking about the order of the *Long Commentaries*, as well as the other *Commentaries*, needs to be reconsidered, taking into account the material conditions in which Averroes worked and under which his works were revised and transmitted. For the *Long Commentaries*, see the following items under Averroes in the bibliography: *Long Commentary on the Posterior Analytics* (1962), (1984); *Long Commentary on the De Caelo* (2003), (1994); *Long Commentary on the Metaphysics* (1952), (1962), (1984); *Long Commentary on the Physics* (1962); and (for the *De Anima*) *Long Commentary* (1953).

to the *Long Commentary on the De Anima*, during the last dozen or so years of his life Averroes wrote *Long Commentaries* on the following works of Aristotle, though dates are now far from certain: *Posterior Analytics* (?), *Physics* (1186 or later?), the *De Caelo* (1188), and the *Metaphysics* (1190).

The vicissitudes of religion and politics were both unkind and kind to Averroes and his works. In 1184 al-Manṣûr succeeded his father and continued to hold Averroes in high favor throughout the period in which the *Long Commentaries* were completed. Still, although he had served al-Manṣûr's father as *qâḍî* in Seville and grand *qâḍî* in Cordoba, in 1195 Averroes fell into disfavor with al-Manṣûr and was sent into exile to Lucena, near Cordoba. After an apparent rehabilitation from exile shortly thereafter, Averroes went to Marrakesh, where he died in 1198. Various possible reasons for the exile are given, all or some of which may be on the mark. Some understand it to be merely the consequence of court intrigues and jealousies on the account of al-Marrâkushî or perhaps an attempt by al-Manṣûr to curry favor with conservative jurists of the dominant Malikite school.[4] Still, the possibility that it was due in some measure to a reaction to Averroes' Aristotelian positions cannot be ruled out. His Aristotelian views are not limited to his *Commentaries* and philosophical treatises. Each of the works in his 1179–1180 legal and theological trilogy—*Faṣl al-maqâl* (*Decisive Treatise*), *al-Kashf ʿan manâḥij* (*Explanation of the Sorts of Proofs in the Doctrines of Religion*), and the so-called *Ḍamîmah*[5]—reflects an approach to Islamic religion deeply critical of traditional Islamic philosophical theology (*kalâm*) and strongly reflective of his Aristotelian rationalism.[6] These were fol-

4. See Geoffroy (1999), 12; Arnaldez (1998), 28; (2000), 15.

5. As Charles Butterworth points out in his recent translation of the *Decisive Treatise*, also containing this text and a selection from the *Incoherence of the Incoherence*, this short treatise, labelled by some as *Ḍamîmah* (Appendix), is a distinct work on the nature of divine knowledge which properly should be understood to precede the *Decisive Treatise*. Butterworth contends that this should be understood as a preface to the *Decisive Treatise*. See *Decisive Treatise* (2001), xxxixff. As Butterworth notes, this understanding was put forth by Muhsin Mahdi in 1964. See Mahdi (1964), 118.

6. On *kalâm* (Islamic dialectical theology), see Gardet (1971) and (1978). There have been numerous attempts to grasp the overall thought of Averroes since Renan's pioneering account of Averroes and his works (1852). These have worked to understand Averroes in his own cultural, religious, and historical context. Although many have offered valuable and intriguing insights, none—in my view—has yet sufficiently captured Averroes' unified perspective and approach, found throughout his legal, theological, and philosophical works. See, among very recent works, those by Fakhry, de Libera, Geoffroy, Benmakhlouf, Arnaldez, Davidson, Leaman, Cruz Hernández, al-ʿAlawî, and Urvoy cited in the bibliography. Rafael Ramón Guerrero offers an insightful and valuable account of the place of Averroes in the history of the development of views on the relationship of religion and philosophy in the introduction to his *Averroes. Sobre filosofía y*

lowed immediately by his *Ṭahâfut al-Ṭahâfut*, responding to al-Ghazâlî's attack
on the *falâsifah* (philosophers).[7] Whatever the explanation, the brief exile and

---

religión (1998). While admitting for Averroes the superiority which philosophy has in
interpreting the symbolic language of religion (see, for example, 59), Ramón Guerrero
understands Averroes' assertion in the *Ṭahâfut al-Ṭahâfut* (*Incoherence of the Incoherence*
[1930], 584; [1969], 361) that religion based on reason (العقل *al-ʿaql*) alone would be in-
ferior to one based on reason and religious inspiration or revelation (الوحى *al-waḥy*) to
mean that a natural religion based on reason would be lacking in the social function
of binding a community together. Ramón Guerrero (1998), 62–63. In this he cites and
follows Cruz Hernández, who writes, "On the other hand, his philosophical works
present a 'reading' which he believes to be radically uncontaminated by theology, and
in those where Allâh and the Qur'ân appear it is to give thanks to the First for the gift
which he gave to man by means of the intelligence of Aristotle and to apply to him
some of the expressions which the revealed book reserves for the elect. When Ibn Rushd
writes as a Muslim thinker (*Ṭahâfut al-Ṭahâfut, Faṣl, Kashf, Ḍamîma*), he moves on the
plane of a [certain] wisdom. Allâh is the fountain, the Qur'ân is the guide. When he
writes as a man seeking human knowing, reason alone is the fountain, the Aristotelian
Corpus the guide. Perhaps because Ibn Rushd may have been and may have considered
himself to be personally (*íntimamente*) more a believing Muslim, he would also more
freely be able to think himself a rational and philosophical thinker." Cruz Hernández
(1978), 142. Given the dialectical character of the *Ṭahâfut al-Ṭahâfut* (see note 7 below),
what requires explication is the nature of the connection between "religious inspiration"
or revelation and the valuable social function of religion, as well as the precise nature
of that which the term denotes for Averroes. Cf. Taylor (2000b). For a brief account of
the thought of Averroes, see Taylor (2003).

7. I understand the *Faṣl al-maqâl, al-Kashf ʿan manâhij*, the so-called *Damîmah* (*Question
on Divine Knowledge*), and *Ṭahâfût al-Ṭahâfût* (all ca. 1178–1181) for the most part to be
dialectical, non-demonstrative works, while Averroes' philosophical commentaries and
distinctly philosophical treatises are meant by him to be for the most part demonstrative works. His famous statement on this in the *Ṭahâfût al-Ṭahâfût* supports this view:
"All this is the theory of the philosophers on this problem, and in the way we have
stated it here with its proofs, it is a persuasive not a demonstrative statement. It is for
you to inquire about these questions in the places where they are treated in the books
of demonstration, if you are one of the people of complete happiness, and if you are
one of those who learn the arts, the function of which is proof. For the demonstrative
arts are very much like the practical; for just as a man who is not a craftsman cannot
perform the function of craftsmanship, in the same way it is not possible for him who
has not learned the arts of demonstration to perform the function of demonstration,
which is demonstration itself: indeed this is still more necessary for this art than for
any other—and this is not generally acknowledged in the case of this practice only
because it is a mere act—and therefore such a demonstration can proceed only from
one who has learned the art. The kinds of statements, however, are many, some demonstrative, others not, and since non-demonstrative statements can be adduced without

also the condemnation of his works with the attendant orders for their burning were likely detrimental to the availability of Averroes' writings.[8] Nevertheless, today a great many of his works are extant, but some of the most important are found only in Hebrew or Latin translation.[9] Among the extant *Long Commentaries* in Arabic and in translations directly from the Arabic, there are texts of the Arabic and of the medieval Latin-from-Arabic translations of the *Metaphysics* and the *De Caelo*, while the *Physics* is extant only in Hebrew-from-Arabic and medieval Latin-from-Arabic translations, and the *De Anima* only in Latin-from-Arabic translation. The *Posterior Analytics* is extant in Arabic but incomplete, while there is a complete Renaissance Latin translation from Hebrew. These *Long Commentaries* generally represent Averroes' most mature reflections on Aristotle's teachings, as well as his own most mature philosophical views. And it is only in his *Long Commentaries*, particularly in those on the *De Anima* and the *Metaphysics*, that Averroes finally resolves to his satisfaction the much vexing issue of the nature of intellect, the philosophical issue which is the primary focus of this introduction. However, before Averroes' ultimate position can be explicated, his much different earlier views need to be expounded to provide a context for his new position arrived at later in life.

Averroes on Human Intellect Prior to the Long Commentary

Consideration of Averroes' teachings on human intellect for the most part concerns his understanding of the nature of the material intellect, the agent intellect, and the human soul.[10] The Arabic tradition accepted that Aristotle's distinction between active and receptive aspects of intellect in *De Anima* 3.5

---

knowledge of the art, it was thought that this might also be the case with demonstrative statements; but this is a great error. And therefore in the spheres of the demonstrative arts, no other statement is possible but a technical statement which only the student of this art can bring, just as is the case with the art of geometry. Nothing therefore of what we have said in this book is a technical demonstrative proof; they are all non-technical statements, some of them having greater persuasion than others, and it is in this spirit that what we have written here must be understood." *Incoherence of the Incoherence* (1930), 427–428; (1969), 257–258. Translation slightly modified.

8. For a valuable account of the historical, religious, and intellectual context of Averroes, including discussion of his friends, supporters, opponents, and disciples, see Puig (1992).

9. See note 1 for bibliographical works with lists of extant writings. Also see note 3.

10. Averroes writes of six different "intellects" or intellectual powers of the soul: (1) The agent intellect (*intellectus agens* or *intelligentia agens* usually renders العقل الفعّال *al-ʿaql al-faʿʿāl*, though, as indicated in note 20, Averroes does use العقل الفاعل *al-ʿaql al-*

was a distinction between a distinct active, separate, intellectual entity and a receptive human power of understanding. This position, found in Theophrastus, Alexander, Themistius, and others, is in accord with two assertions. First, in *De Anima* 3.5 Aristotle holds that one of these two intellects is immortal (ἀθάνατον) and eternal (ἀΐδιον). Second, in *Generation of Animals* 2.3, 736b27, he holds that the power of reason or intellect is not communicated in semen by physical reproduction but comes from outside (τὸν νοῦν . . . θύραθεν).[11] As Davidson has made clear, Averroes held varying views on the nature of the

---

fāʿil to denote the same entity) is the active intellect of *De Anima* 3.5. Its role is to actualize intelligibles in potency and to provide them to the receptive material intellect. For Averroes and most thinkers of the Arabic tradition, this agent or active intellect is an eternal, separately existing substance. (2) The term "material intellect" (ὑλικὸς νοῦς, *intellectus materialis*, العقل الهيولاني *al-ʿaql al-hayûlânî*) was coined by Alexander of Aphrodisias in his *De Anima*. See Alexander, *De Anima* (1887), 81.24; (1979), 105. This is also called "the potential intellect" (العقل الذى بالقوة *al-ʿaql alladhî bi-l-quwah, intellectus in potentia*). For Averroes in the *Short Commentary* this is an individually existing disposition of the forms of the imagination; in the *Middle Commentary* this also exists "in" or associated with each individual, but as intellect it is above imagination as an inchoate disposition provided by the agent intellect at birth and later actualized by the agent intellect in abstraction as the material intellect receives abstracted intelligibles. In the *Long Commentary*, this is the famous separately existing and unique receptive intellect shared by all human beings. (3) The acquired intellect (*intellectus adeptus*, العقل المستفاد *al-ʿaql al-mustafâd*) is the intellect as realized in the immediate moment of the actualizing reception of intelligibles in act. This is sometimes called "the intellect which is in act" {390}, though that designation can also be used of the agent intellect {484}. (4) The intellect in a positive disposition (*intellectus in habitu*, العقل بالملكة *al-ʿaql bi-l-malakah*) is the state of a human being who has come to be positively disposed by the reception of knowledge and who understands such that this knowledge can be easily recalled at will. It is not merely dispositive as able to be disposed but rather positively disposed with knowledge. (5) The theoretical intellect (*intellectus speculativus*, العقل النظري *al-ʿaql al-naẓarî*) refers to the intellect as containing the intelligibles in act. For the mature Averroes this intellect and its intelligibles exist as eternal in the separate material intellect and also as perishable in their individual perishable human subject. Note that (3), (4), and (5) all exist in the human soul and might be considered moments of the same reality, though Averroes does not use that phraseology. In the mature account of the *Long Commentary*, (1) and (2) are also clearly "in the soul" as well. (6) The passible intellect (*intellectus passibilis*, العقل المنفعل *al-ʿaql al-munfaʿil*) denotes the general power of imagination or cogitation in the perishable individual which provides denuded intentions in the process of abstraction. This is "a kind of reason" {449}, not intellect per se but rather only equivocally in virtue of its contribution to the process leading to intellectual understanding.

11. Aristotle, *Generation of Animals* (1965).

active intellect, initially viewing it as an emanative cause of the forms of the natural world but finally holding in his mature work that generation is due only to natural reproductive powers and the physical influence of the sun and heavens. In his late work the agent intellect persists for the most part only in its nature as a transcendent power essential to the explanation of human thought through its relationship to the receptive human material intellect, a role it also played in Averroes' earlier works.[12]

The major focus of Averroes' reflections on human intellect takes place in the context of his awareness of the incompleteness of Aristotle's account of human intellect. Like his predecessors in the Greek tradition, Averroes was acutely aware that Aristotle never fulfilled his promise at *De Anima* 3.7, 431b17–19: "In every case the mind which is actively thinking is the objects which it thinks. Whether it is possible for it while not existing separate from spatial conditions to think anything that is separate, or not, we must consider later."[13] What is at issue here is simply the most important and fundamental epistemological question of the Aristotelian and Platonic tradition: Is it possible for human beings while existing in extended physical bodies to think intelligible objects which are separate from physical conditions?[14] For Plato in the *Phaedo* as well as in the *Republic* the body is a hindrance to intellectual understanding, which can be attained fully only by the soul's separation from the body. For Aristotle, with his hylemorphic view of human beings as genuine composites of body and soul, the issue was nevertheless similar to that of Plato. If knowledge consists in an identity of knower and known, with the soul be-

---

12. See Davidson (1992), chs. 6 and 8.

13. Aristotle, *De Anima* (1984). This is noted by Alexander Altmann (1965), 49.

14. Curiously enough, the converse of this issue is raised in the *Liber de causis* or *Discourse on the Pure Good*, an Arabic work substantially based on the *Elements of Theology* of Proclus and the *Plotiniana Arabica*. In proposition 6 of the Arabic version (7 in most Latin versions), the author of this work draws upon proposition 171 of Proclus in arguing that intelligences are indivisible substances. He follows the argument of Proclus that the indivisible unity of separate intellectual substances is shown in the complete reversion of that substance upon itself in self-knowledge. But he then adds to the thought of Proclus that an intellectual substance lacks extension, so that when it seeks knowledge of a corporeal thing, it cannot be extended with it but must remain fixed in its state and unaffected. This implies that extended things cannot be known with the identity of knower and known appropriate for separate intellectual substances. See (in the primary sources) *Liber de causis* (1882), 72–73, and Proclus (1963), 148–151. The converse of this is that insofar as human beings are divisible particular entities in bodies, they cannot know separate entities with an identity of knower and known while in the body. This seems to indicate an awareness on the part of the author of the *Liber de causis* of *De Anima* 3.7, 431b17–19. Regarding the *Liber de causis*, see D'Ancona and Taylor (2003).

coming not the apprehended object but the form of the object as Aristotle
teaches explicitly in *De Anima* 3.8 and implicitly in 3.4, how can the understanding of intelligibles in act take place where those intelligibles are separate from
particulars of the world—as in the case of abstraction—or where they are altogether separate from the sublunar world as separate agent intellect or separate cosmic intellect? That is, if human beings are enmattered entities, how
will anything more than sense perception be possible? For Averroes this is the
question of the nature of the material intellect in itself and in its relationship
with individual human beings, a question which dominated his thought and
to which he returned repeatedly with varying solutions from his earliest writings on the soul right up to his final resolution in the *Long Commentary on the
De Anima* and cited in his *Long Commentary on the Metaphysics*, believed to be
the last of his *Long Commentaries.*

Today eight distinct works dealing substantively with the nature of the human
intellect and the material intellect by Averroes survive.[15] On the basis of the
philosophical doctrine set forth in these works they can be grouped into four
categories: initial, middle, transitional, and final positions. The initial period is
that of the *Short Commentary on the De Anima* (ca. 1158–1160?), the *Epistle on the
Possibility of Conjunction*, *Epistle 2 On Conjunction*, and probably *Against the Avicennians on the First Cause*. The middle period is represented in the *Middle Commentary* on the *De Anima* (ca. 1181?). What I call his transitional position is found in
his *Epistle 1 On Conjunction*. And, as already indicated, Averroes' final philosophical position on the human intellect is to be found most complete in the *Long
Commentary on the De Anima* (ca. 1186); this is also reflected in his *Commentary
on the* De Intellectu *of Alexander,* the Arabic text of which has only recently been
published.[16] Also relevant in subsidiary ways are the *Short Commentary on the
Parva Naturalia* (1170) and the *Long Commentary on the Metaphysics* (1190).

Averroes' Initial Position

Averroes' first account on the nature of the intellect in human beings is found
in his *Short Commentary on the De Anima* (ca. 1158–1160), also known as his *Epitome
(مختصر mukhtaṣar*).[17] This is an organized set of notes and arguments on the *De*

15. Elamrani-Jamal (2003), 356–357, like Davidson (1992), 262–264, lists seven works. To
these I add *Against the Avicennians on the First Cause* (1997). If the short commentary on
Ibn Bâjjah's *Treatise on the Conjoining of the Intellect with Man*, attached to the chapter on
the rational faculty in the *Short Commentary*, is counted separately, the number is nine.
See *Short Commentary on the De Anima* (1950), 90–95; (1987), 214–221.

16. See *Commentary on the De Intellectu of Alexander* (2001).

17. Some portions of the account which follows also appear in Taylor (2004b). My
thanks to the volume editors for permission to draw upon that article here.

Anima formed not so much from the direct study of the *De Anima* itself but rather from his study of the Greek commentators and authors of the Arabic tradition, so as "to affirm on the basis of the Commentators' statements on the science of the soul what we hold to concur most with what has been shown in the science of physics and is most suitable with the aim of Aristotle."[18] It is in chapter 8, devoted to the theoretical power (النظري *an-naẓarî*), that Averroes sets forth his position. He locates the issue in the manner in which theoretical intelligibles (المعقولات النظرية *al-maʿqûlât an-naẓariyyah*) are somehow separate intelligibles in act and yet somehow can be received into individual human beings as human intellectual understanding. Insofar as a human being is a receptive subject which moves from not knowing to knowing these intelligibles, in that person there comes to be the ultimate disposition (استعداده الأخير *istiʿdâdi-hi al-akhîr*) of the apprehension and emergence of these intelligibles (72–73; 106–107; 195–196).

The intelligibles which come to be in the soul are forms received from experience of the world into the external and internal senses as intentions (معان *maʿânin*). Their reception into the imagination, however, is distinct from reception into a physical organ since the displacement of a contrary is not necessary in the case of the imagination. What is more, "The imaginative soul is distinguished by the fact that it does not need an organic instrument for its activity" (74; 108; 197). As grounded in the particularity of the changing experience of worldly individuals, the intelligibles are able to come to be only in those human beings who have experienced them in the world. As Davidson phrases it, "intelligible thoughts . . . share two crucial traits with forms of physical objects and forms in the soul at the subintellectual levels of perception, both of which Averroes terms 'material' forms."[19] These traits are that they are consequent

---

18. *Short Commentary on the De Anima* (1950), 3; (1985), 5; (1987), 99. Page references to the text of the *Short Commentary* in the rest of this section will be parenthetical, referring first to the 1950 Arabic edition, then to the 1985 Arabic edition, and finally to the 1987 Spanish translation. Al-ʿAlawî holds that this work does not follow the pattern of the other *Short Commentaries* and calls it "an anomaly." See al-ʿAlawî (1992), 807. He is also strongly critical of the editions of (1950) and (1985). See al-ʿAlawî (1986), 53, n. 8, and (1992), 807–811. On this work also see Druart (1994) and Davidson (1992), 265–272. In the *Long Commentary on the De Anima*, Averroes refers critically to himself when he writes of Ibn Bâjjah, "But what made that man err, and we too for a long time, is that modern thinkers set aside the books of Aristotle and consider the books of the commentators, and chiefly in the case of the soul, in their believing that this book is impossible to understand. This is on account of Avicenna who followed Aristotle only in dialectics, but in other things he erred, and chiefly in the case of metaphysics. This is because he began, as it were, from his own perspective" {470}. For a full outline of the contents of the *Short Commentary*, see Ivry (1997b).

19. Davidson (1992), 266.

upon multiple stages of change and that they are individuated by the subjects into which they are received—that is, they are "multiplied with the multiplication of their subjects and numbered by their enumeration." As such these intelligibles are true (صادقا *ṣâdiqan*) in virtue of a subject external to the soul (the thing in the world causally giving rise to the intelligible) on which the imagined form is completely based (80; 116–117; 203).

This process of the generation of intelligibles in the receptive human power called the material intellect requires an agency whereby what is potentially intelligible (the forms in the world and their intentions in the external and internal sense powers) is transformed into the intelligible in act. For Averroes only what already has the nature of intellectuality and is itself intelligent and intelligible in act can be cause of intelligibility in act—that is, the agent intellect (العقل الفاعل *al-ʿaql al-fâʿil*).[20] "For the material intellect needs necessarily for its existence that there be here an intellect existing in act eternally" (88; 126–127; 212). This separate intellect has the essential actuality not present in the material intellect which by conjoining (اتصال *ittiṣâl*) enables material intellects to be actualized so that individual human beings become knowers.[21] "The agent intellect is more noble than the material (intellect) and . . . in itself exists in act (موجود بالفعل *maujûd bi-l-fiʿl*) as an eternal intellect"—irrespective and independent of our understanding and awareness of it—as intelligible, as form, as agent and as "ultimately form for us" (بآخرة . . . صورة لنا *bi-l-âkhirah . . . ṣurah li-nâ*) (89; 127; 213). This agent intellect actualizes "the disposition which is in the forms of the imagination (فى الصور الخيالية *fî ṣuwar al-khayâlîyah*) for receiving the intelligibles," the "first material intellect" (العقل الهيولانى الأول *al-ʿaql al-hayûlânî l-awwal*).[22] The reason for this identification is simply that human

---

20. In the *Short Commentary* Averroes uses both العقل الفاعل *al-ʿaql al-fâʿil* and الفعّال *al-ʿaql al-faʿʿâl* to denote the agent or active intellect. See *Short Commentary on the De Anima* (1985), 123.13 and 127.4.

21. "As Averroes presents it here, conjunction is not a state which one may hope to achieve only at the end of a life spent striving for knowledge; it is not a total and absolute joining of two separate substances. Rather, it is a state experienced when one has truly understood something, it is possession of a particular truth. The Agent Intellect in this construal is not so much the repository of all ideas, as it is the facilitator or actualizing agent for the comprehension of them all. In joining with the Agent Intellect, the individual intellect becomes part of the eternal intelligible world of ideas, to the extent of those ideas which it has mastered. The ideas are part of the intelligible order of our world, its species and genera, for the intelligibility of which the Agent Intellect is ultimately responsible." Ivry (1997b), 544.

22. فاذا الاستعداد الذي في الصور الخيالية لقبول المعقولات هو العقل الهيولاني الأول. (*Short Commentary on the De Anima* [1950], 86; [1985], 124; [1987], 209). I read الفعل as a typographical error in place of العقل in ibid. (1985). This is in agreement with ibid. (1987).

thinking (as Aristotle held in *De Anima* 3.8) takes place with the existence of images and does not take place in their absence (86; 124; 209). "By this disposition which exists for man in the forms of the imagination, the soul [in man] is distinguished from the imaginative soul in animals" (87; 125; 210). Not identical with the imagination itself, the material intellect is an immaterial disposition of the soul having as subject by which it exists in a human being the forms of the imagination as receptive of intelligibles. These intelligibles, however, must remain unmixed with the forms of the imagination and so are, we might say, linked but adjacent and transcendent to their subject, the forms of the imagination, since (as Aristotle says following Anaxagoras) intellect must remain unmixed in order to know (87; 125; 210).[23]

This doctrine in the *Short Commentary* is to some degree based on the thought of Alexander of Aphrodisias but is more evidently founded on that of Ibn Bâjjah. For Alexander the active intellectual power to which Aristotle referred in *De Anima* 3.5 is a separate intellectual entity responsible for the realization of intellectual understanding in individual human beings. But the receptive power of the soul, which he termed "material intellect," he considered a disposition belonging to each human being to be actualized by the transcendent agent intellect, which Alexander identified with God. Yet on Alexander's view this disposition, though not a body nor in the body as a power, is still intrinsically associated with its subject in such a way that the perishing of the human being and its body also entails the cessation of intellectual activity and the perishing of the individual material intellect.[24]

Ibn Bâjjah's view is related to Alexander's approach of considering the material intellect as a disposition, though his more Platonic views on the nature of intelligibles and the intellect would not allow him to follow Alexander in holding for the perishing of the intellectual part of the soul. For Ibn Bâjjah, all human activities have the end of intellectual perfection on the way to the ultimate end of conjoining with separate intellect. As he puts it,

---

23. As Geoffroy stresses and as will be seen below, Averroes' understanding of cosmology provided him with a model for explicating the relationship between corporeal powers such as imagination or cogitation and the immaterial power of intellect. See Geoffroy and Steel (2001), 71ff. The *Short Commentary on the De Anima* does not in any explicit way draw upon Averroes' cosmological views in expounding his understanding of the relationship of the material intellect and the imagination or forms of the imagination. Geoffroy and Steel point out that Averroes seems to have in mind this cosmological model to explain the transcendence of the material intellect in his *Against the Avicennians on the First Cause* (1997), composed in the same period. See Geoffroy and Steel (2001), 71–73.

24. Alexander, *De Anima* (1887), 90.6–11; (1979), 119. Regarding Alexander's *De Anima* and *De Intellectu*, see Davidson (1992), 30–41.

The philosopher must perform numerous [particular] spiritual acts—but not for their own sake—and perform all the intellectual acts for their own sake: the corporeal acts enable him to exist as a human, the [particular] spiritual acts render him more noble, and the intellectual acts render him divine and virtuous. The man of wisdom is therefore necessarily a man who is virtuous and divine. Of every kind of activity, he takes up the best only. He shares with every class of men the best states that characterize them. But he stands alone as the one who performs the most excellent and noblest of actions. When he achieves the final end—that is, when he understands simple essential intellects, which are mentioned in the *Metaphysics*, *On the Soul*, and *On Sense and the Sensible*—he then becomes one of those intellects. It would be right to call him simply divine. He will be free from the moral sensible qualities, as well as from the high [particular] spiritual qualities: it will be fitting to describe him as a pure divinity.[25]

Transcending the perishable body by its intellectual independence, the material intellect for Ibn Bâjjah is the receptivity fulfilled by the separate agent intellect through a conjoining of an intellectual sort. The agent intellect illuminates the images of things in the imagination in such a way that human understanding of intelligibles comes about "with no mention of an emanation of thoughts directly from the agent intellect."[26] In Ibn Bâjjah's understanding, individual human beings employ the material intellect toward their realization of intellectual perfection in conjoining with the agent intellect and attaining happiness in a unity with it and all human intellects.[27] This is the highest level of the acquired intellect (العقل المستفاد *al-ʿaql al-mustafâd*), which involves "the ultimate science which is the forming of a concept (تصور *taṣaw-wur*) of intellect, i.e. the existence (وجود *wujûd*) of the acquired intellect."[28] This process is begun with the material intellect, which is understood to be a disposition in the soul illuminated by the agent intellect. Ibn Bâjjah, as Hyman puts it, "attempts to avoid Alexander's difficulties by showing that it is corporeal in a secondary sense. This he does by assigning it to the actualized imagination as its underlying subject. Since the actualized imagination is a corporeal form, but not a body or corporeal faculty, the material intellect is corporeal but only in a derivative sense. It follows that the imagination as material intellect possesses the image as its form and that, as a result of thinking, it acquires the intel-

25. Ibn Bâjjah, *The Governance of the Solitary* (1983), 131–132; (1991), 79–80. Translation slightly modified.

26. Davidson (1992), 145.

27. Davidson (1992), 145–146.

28. Alexander Altmann's translation of Ibn Bâjjah, *Letter of Farewell* (1943), section 15, p. 30, in Altmann (1965), 70. Arabic inserted; translation slightly modified.

ligible as a second form."[29] Regarding the intelligible, Ibn Bâjjah writes in his *Treatise on the Conjoining of the Intellect with Man*, "it is a form having as its matter the intermediate spiritual forms of the imagination."[30]

In the *Short Commentary* Averroes does not follow Ibn Bâjjah on the soul's ascent into highest unity but rather is content to make use of his thought on the agent intellect primarily in its epistemological function in the process of human knowing. Yet Averroes' account of the material intellect is clearly that of Ibn Bâjjah, which he calls true (حَقّ *ḥaqq*) and demonstrative (برهانية *burhânîyah*).[31] This view seems also to be found in at least three other works by Averroes. In his *Short Commentary on the Parva Naturalia* he attributes our intellectual understanding to reception of intelligibles from separate intellect into the imaginative soul (النفس الخيالية *an-nafs al-khayâlîyah*).[32] In his *Epistle 2 On Conjunction* he holds that the material intellect is a disposition found in the forms of the imaginative soul, not insofar as they are material (that is, particular) forms, but insofar as they are forms.[33] And in his *Epistle on the Possibility of Conjunction* he writes that "the imaginative forms serve as substrates for the intelligibles with respect to perfection, just as sense is perfected by the imaginative forms."[34] This also appears to be the doctrine expounded in his *Against the Avicennians on the First Cause*.[35] However, in a revised later version of the *Short Commentary*, done after he had embraced his final position on the material intellect, Averroes complains of having been misled by Ibn Bâjjah's account, asserts that the forms of the imagination could not be suitable subjects for the intelligibles because of distor-

29. Hyman (1999), 194.

30. Ibn Bâjjah, *Treatise on the Conjoining of the Intellect with Man* (1942), 13; Spanish, 30; (1968), 160; (1981), 185.

31. *Short Commentary on the De Anima* (1950), 90–91; (1987), 214–216. Cited in Druart (1994), 193. This text is omitted in the 1985 edition.

32. "If all the foregoing is ascertained, it cannot be denied that the separate intelligence endows the imaginative soul with the universal nature (الطبيعة الكلية) that the individual that comes into being possesses, that is to say, with a comprehension of its causes, and the imaginative soul will receive it as a particular (جزئيا) by virtue of the fact that it is in matter. It may receive the individual (شخص) of that which has been comprehended, in reality, or it may receive something similar to it. Just as the intelligence endows one with the universal perfections of the soul and matter receives them as particulars, so here too the intelligence endows the imaginative soul with the final perfection as a universal, and the soul receives it as a particular (يعطى هاهنا الكمال الأخير للقوة المتخيلة كليا ، وتقبله النفس جزئيا)." (*Short Commentary on the Parva Naturalia* [1972], 79.7–12; [1961], 46; [1949], 109–110).

33. *Epistle 2 On Conjunction*. See Geoffroy and Steel (2001), 226.

34. *Epistle on the Possibility of Conjunction* (1982), 28.

35. See *Against the Avicennians on the First Cause* (1997), 112–120, particularly 118.

tions and mixture from a subject with its own nature, and refers readers to "my Long Commentary on the book of Aristotle *On the Soul*" (فى شرحي لكتاب أرسطو في النفس *fî sharḥî li-kitâb Aristû fî n-nafs*).[36]

Averroes' Middle Position

A new position is found in Averroes' *Middle Commentary* on the *De Anima* (تلخيص *talkhîṣ*), a work for which the text and dating have been matters of controversy among scholars in recent years. The date given by both al-'Alawî and Cruz Hernández is 1174,[37] but Alfred L. Ivry, editor of the *Middle Commentary*, has argued that the *Middle Commentary* draws upon the *Long Commentary* (usually dated ca. 1190, but now ca. 1186) and is consequently posterior to the *Long Commentary*.[38] What is more, Herbert Davidson has contended that the *Middle Commentary* contains an excursus of two pages which he interprets as an interpolation by Averroes expressing yet another understanding of the material intellect, one identical to neither that of the *Short Commentary* or the *Long Commentary* nor to the original *Middle Commentary*. Davidson has also asserted that the evidence marshalled by Ivry in various articles is not sufficient to show the priority of the *Long* to the *Middle* and perhaps not sufficient even to show the existence of identical texts in both commentaries. Abdelali Elamrani-Jamal also entered the discussion, holding against the view of Davidson regarding an interpolated excursus and against Ivry on the priority of the *Long Commentary*.[39] The most recent comprehensive account of Averroes on intellect is that of Marc Geoffroy, who sides with Elamrani-Jamal.[40] Since these matters are germane to both the

36. *Short Commentary on the De Anima* (1950), 90; (1985), 128–129; (1987), 213–214. Cf. *Long Commentary* {398}.

37. Al-'Alawî (1986), 85; Cruz Hernández (1997), 58. Alonso (1947), 84, hypothesizes 1173.

38. Cf. p. xvi n. 3 above.

39. Ivry's views on the priority of the *Long Commentary* to the *Middle Commentary* are expounded in Ivry (1990) and on pp. 10–14 of the introduction to his 1994 edition of the *Middle Commentary*. Also see the following: *Middle Commentary* (2002); Ivry (1995), (1997a), (1997b), and (2001). Elamrani-Jamal's views are expounded in Elamrani-Jamal (1997). For Davidson's thesis on the interpolated excursus, see Davidson (1992), 276–282. For his rejection of Ivry's thesis of the priority of the *Long Commentary* to the *Middle Commentary*, see Davidson (1997); Ivry's brief "Response" is in Ivry (1997a). For an understanding by Josep Puig Montada which integrates elements of the accounts of Davidson and Ivry, see note 51 below. I will address these issues and others mentioned there in detail and at greater length elsewhere.

40. Geoffroy, in Geoffroy and Steel (2001), 42–81, follows Elamrani-Jamal in rejecting the interpolated excursus of Davidson and also rejects Ivry's thesis of the priority of the *Long Commentary*. While much of what follows here regarding the arguments of the

dating of the *Long Commentary* and to the understanding of the concerns which led Averroes to his final position in the *Long Commentary*, translated here, a brief consideration of some of these issues concerning the *Middle Commentary* is certainly warranted.

As is made clear in the notes to the present translation, there are at least eighteen Comments in the *Long Commentary* which have portions of text identical with what is found in the *Middle Commentary*. These range from substantial clauses to entire paragraphs of texts. While in some cases it has been necessary to compare closely the Arabic of the *Middle Commentary* with Latin texts of the *Long Commentary*, in a number of cases a direct comparison of the Arabic of the *Middle Commentary* with the extant fragments of the original Arabic of the *Long Commentary* has made it unequivocally evident that the two works contain numerous identical passages.[41] But the close comparison of the texts has also made it apparent that these two works were done by Averroes at different times. While the two works are necessarily close because both are based on the *De Anima*, the philosophical analysis and interpretation of Aristotle's texts is in a large number of cases quite distinct.[42] What also is apparent

---

Middle Commentary and also *Epistle 1 On Conjunction* is in accord with many of the descriptive accounts of Geoffroy, my analysis of the reasons for Averroes' doctrinal changes is distinct.

41. For the identical passages, see the notes to {8–11}, {13}, {14}, {26}, {30}, {40}, {336}, {370}, {372–373}, {517}, {522–528}, {537}, {538}, {540}, and {541}. All Arabic fragments are printed in the notes to the corresponding Latin texts. The comparison of other fragments to corresponding texts of the Arabic of the *Middle Commentary* also shows differences between the works.

42. This is evident in comparing Comment passages of the *Long Commentary* to their corresponding passages in the *Middle Commentary*. *Long Commentary* (LC), Book 1, Comments 17–18: *Middle Commentary* (MC), paragraph 17; LC 1.22: MC 21–22; LC 1.32: MC 34–39; LC 1.33: MC 40; LC 1.44: MC 55–57; LC 1.48: MC 65–66; LC 1.53: MC 70–71; LC 1.55: MC 73; LC 1.60: MC 76; LC 1.63: MC 79–80; LC 1.64: MC 81; LC 1.65: MC 82; LC 1.66: MC 83–84; LC 1.69: MC 87–88; LC 1.77: MC 95–97; LC 1.79: MC 99–100; LC 1.80–1.81: MC 101; LC 1.82: MC 102; LC 1.85: MC 107–108 to page 40, line 1; LC 2.2: MC 115, page 43, lines 6ff.; LC 2.6: MC 117, page 44, lines 12ff.; LC 2.7: MC 118; LC 2.12: MC 124–127; LC 2.13: MC 128; LC 2.14: MC 128, page 48, line 10, to 129, page 48, line 18; LC 2.19–2.20: MC 131, page 49, line 19 to page 50, line 6; LC 2.25: MC 134–135; LC 2.26: MC 136; LC 2.27: MC 137–138, page 52, lines 15ff.; LC 2.28: MC 138, page 52, line 15, to 139, page 53, line 8; LC 2.32–2.33: MC 142–145; LC 2.51: MC 159; LC 2.56: MC 163, page 62, lines 5ff.; LC 2.61: MC 168; LC 3.8: MC 288; LC 3.9: MC 289; LC 3.11: MC 290; LC 3.13: MC 292; LC 3.14: MC 293; LC 3.15: MC 294; LC 3.17: MC 295 to page 116, line 2; LC 3.18–3.19: MC 295, page 116, line 2, to MC 297; LC 3.24: MC 305 to page 119, line 7; LC 3.25: MC 305, page 119, line 7, to MC 307; LC 3.26: MC 308 to page 120, line 5; LC 3.29: MC 308, page 205,

is that although Averroes certainly had the *De Anima Paraphrase* of Themistius at hand while preparing each work, his use of Themistius was not the same in each work. In one work he made use of the *Paraphrase* for some passages, while at the corresponding passages in the other he did not.[43] The works are also distinguished by the use of the texts of the *De Anima*. For the *Long Commentary*, Averroes uses two texts, his main text, one traditionally ascribed to Isḥâq, and a second, alternate translation, while the *Middle Commentary* gives no indication of that alternate translation.[44] What is more, while both works make use of the Arabic *De Anima* attributed to Isḥâq, there are indications that Averroes used different redactions of it when composing each of his works.[45] And, as is made clear below, the doctrines of the material intellect in Averroes' *Middle* and *Long Commentaries* are quite different. The *Middle Commentary* holds for a plurality of individual material intellects and a hardly noticed role for the cogitative power; the *Long Commentary* argues for a single transcendent material intellect for all human beings and for a very robust and detailed teaching on the internal powers of the brain, in particular the cogitative power.

With this evidence it is appropriate to conclude that these two commentaries on the *De Anima* were composed as separate studies at different times by Averroes. This becomes evident by consideration of his use of different redactions of the Isḥâq translation, his differing uses of the *Paraphrase* of Themistius, his differing analyses of passages of the *De Anima*, his differing division of Books 2 and 3, and his differing doctrines of the material intellect and cogitative power.[46] On the basis of the identical texts in both works which I have been

---

lines 5–9; *LC* 3.30: *MC* 309; *LC* 3.31–3.32: *MC* 310 to page 121, line 2; *LC* 3.35: *MC* 311, page 121, lines 10ff.; *LC* 3.36: *MC* 312; *LC* 3.38: *MC* 313, page 122, lines 9ff.; *LC* 3.39: *MC* 314; *LC* 3.41: *MC* 316 to page 124, line 7; *LC* 3.50: *MC* 322, page 126, lines 11ff.; *LC* 3.51: *MC* 323; *LC* 3.57: *MC* 327, page 130, line 11, to *MC* 328; *LC* 3.62: *MC* 332 to page 132, line 21; *LC* 3.66: *MC* 338–339; *LC* 3.68: *MC* 340, page 137, line 5, to *MC* 341.

43. For example, *Long Commentary*, Book 1, Comments 26 and 27 read the *Paraphrase* differently than do *Middle Commentary* paragraphs 27–29. *Middle Commentary* 67–68 uses Themistius, but the corresponding Comment in the *Long Commentary*, 1.49, does not. This is also the case for *Middle Commentary* paragraph 170 to page 65.2, which uses Themistius, while the corresponding passage at *Long Commentary*, 2.63, does not. *Long Commentary* 3.1 uses Themistius, but the corresponding text of the *Middle Commentary*, 276, does not.

44. The text of Isḥâq is extant only in fragments; Averroes' alternate text in his *Long Commentary* is Aristotle, *De Anima* (1954). Regarding the text of Isḥâq, see below, pp. lxxviff.

45. See below, pp. lxxviii–lxxix.

46. While the *Middle Commentary* observes the divisions of the books of the *De Anima* common today, the *Long Commentary* extends Book 2 to our modern *De Anima* 3.3, 429a9, and begins Book 3 with the account of intellect, starting at 3.4, 429a10. Averroes makes no comment on this.

able to identify in 18 of the 325 sections of Comment, it is far from obvious that one can conclude the priority of one work to the other. On the basis of philosophical doctrine, though, as argued below, the *Long Commentary* is more mature than the *Middle Commentary*, as is acknowledged by all parties to recent debate.[47] While Elamrani-Jamal has rightly cautioned that we do not have sufficient information on precisely how Averroes worked on his commentaries to make a firm determination to abandon the traditional dating of the *Middle Commentary* (1174), it is also not unreasonable to hold the priority of the *Middle Commentary* on doctrinal grounds as he too holds.[48] With remarks in a 1997 article Ivry points in the direction of a more subtle understanding of the issue: "Averroes may well have published his *Middle* before the *Long Commentary*, but he did not write it beforehand. This holds true for the bulk of both texts, though it is possible, and even likely, that Averroes made certain revisions in both commentaries, the *Middle* after its initial publication, and the *Long* before its publication. That is, Averroes may well have continued working on his *Long Commentary* after he had published the *Middle Commentary*; the latter based upon a first unpublished draft of the longer and more detailed work."[49]

Given that the *Middle Commentary*'s identical texts—some only short sentences or substantial clauses—are found in only 5.5 percent of the Comments in the *Long Commentary*, it seems plausible that the *Long Commentary* was incomplete at the time of the composition of the *Middle Commentary*. It may well be that Averroes drew upon a common but incomplete work, deciding, while writing these distinct studies of the *De Anima*, to retain some explanations in each but generally to compose each as a separate philosophical study involving separate readings and consultations of the *Paraphrase* of Themistius and separate redactions of the *De Anima* translated by Isḥâq. These considerations, combined with the generally acknowledged maturity of the doctrine of intellect in the *Long Commentary* (to which the 1190 *Long Commentary on the Metaphysics* refers), make it somewhat more reasonable to conclude for the traditional order of the *Middle Commentary* as completed and released or "published" prior to the *Long Commentary*. For the purposes of this introduction, then, I follow the traditional order in the dating of these *Commentaries*. However, due to a recent discovery by Ruth Glasner, I understand the *Long Commentary* as likely completed by circa 1186.[50]

47. Alain de Libera writes, "If one compares the ensemble of Averroes' writings on the soul to the GC [*Long Commentary*], it seems clear to us that it is this last text which preserves the essential and, according to us, the last state of his theory on the soul and on the intellect." *Long Commentary. Book 3* (1998), 17.

48. Elamrani-Jamal (1997), 292.

49. Ivry (1997b), 516.

50. Glasner (2004). See note 3 above. Also see Geoffroy's analysis of this and his understanding of the relationship of the commentaries in Geoffroy (2005), 760–764.

Based on manuscript evidence and the discussion above, it seems possible to speculate that the *Middle Commentary* was completed shortly before the final version of the *Long Commentary*, perhaps as late as circa 1181.[51] I follow Ivry,

---

51. "The codices in which the *Middle Commentary on Aristotle's* De Anima is found contain only two dates for its composition, AH 567/1172 CE and 577/1181, both falling within the period generally attributed to Averroës' middle commentary compositions." *Middle Commentary* (2002), 148, n. 50. Puig (1998), 125, gives 1181 for the *Middle Commentary* and "1187–1190?" for the *Long Commentary*. Endress (1999), 360–361, does not provide dates for the *Short* and *Middle Commentaries* on the *De Anima*. More recently Puig, accepting Davidson's argument for an interpolated excursus (see above, pp. xxviiiff. and n. 39), has suggested that at the time of the original composition of the *Middle Commentary* in 1171, "Averroes did not have access to Themistius' commentary" but did have it when the revised version was completed in 1181. Puig (2002a), 343; (2002b), 32–33. But what Puig proposes is more extreme than Davidson's proposal of a revised version with interpolated excursus since Puig supposes Averroes did not have Themistius for the initial version. While a more detailed examination of this view and that of Davidson cannot be pursued here, two considerations militate against it. First, the extensive use of Themistius by Averroes in the *Middle Commentary*, noted by Ivry (*Middle Commentary* [2002], xv), is documented in his notes and also is sometimes indicated in the notes to the present translation of the *Long Commentary*. That is, Puig's thesis entails that Averroes made a *comprehensive* revision, something not previously proposed or yet established by any study of the *Middle Commentary*. Second, Averroes had access to the *Paraphrase* of Themistius while composing the earlier *Short Commentary*, so its content was not unknown to him when he composed the postulated initial version of the *Middle Commentary*. Nevertheless, the issue of Averroes' methods and habits in revising his works requires much more study, as the following considerations attest. We know that the *Short Commentary on the De Anima* was later emended, as was the *Short Commentary on the Metaphysics*. See Davidson (1992), 235–241 and 265–272. Glasner's study of the *Physics* commentaries leads her to write, "The 'oddities' in the commentaries on the *Physics* can be explained in terms of the first contention, namely, that parts of the middle commentary were written after the long commentary." As she sees it, "the middle commentary [on the *Physics*] was revised and includes passages that are later than the long commentary." Glasner (2004), 60. But not all of Averroes' works show such signs of revision. What is more, just what constitutes a *Short Commentary* as opposed to a *Middle Commentary* is not always clear, as Steven Harvey has indicated. In the case of the *Physics*, Harvey (forthcoming) holds for the conventional order of composition: short, middle, long. A comprehensive study of Averroes' different commentaries also must include consideration of his purpose with each commentary, as suggested by Henri Hugonnard-Roche (1977), 104. As indicated by Elamrani-Jamal (1997), 292, present knowledge of Averroes' revisions and emendations of "published" texts is weak and far from precise. The dating of works which I provide in this introduction should be regarded as tentative and likely to be subject to considerable revision in the light of various projects currently under way.

Elamrani-Jamal, and Geoffroy in declining to accept Davidson's view that the *Middle Commentary*'s excursus following the discussion corresponding to *De Anima* 3.5 is a later interpolation with a distinct understanding of the material intellect. My understanding of the issues allows the *Middle Commentary* to be seen as containing Averroes' middle or second major position on the material intellect.

Recent work by Colette Sirat and Marc Geoffroy with the marginal notes in the Modena manuscript of the *Middle Commentary* confirms the view that some version of the *Long Commentary* was available to Averroes when he composed his *Middle Commentary*. Their study, preliminary to the preparation of an edition of the Arabic fragments of the *Long Commentary*, concludes that (i) a first version of the *Long Commentary* was composed before the *Middle Commentary* and is used in it; (ii) the *Middle Commentary* itself was later used in a revision of the first version of the *Long Commentary*; and (iii) the final version of the *Long Commentary* represented in the Latin translation was completed after the *Middle Commentary*.[52] What is more, as they see it, the earlier versions are distinguished from the final version of the *Long Commentary* by "the absence of the long development on the separated and eternal nature of the material intellect."[53]

The doctrine of the human material intellect in the *Middle Commentary* is fundamentally controlled by the issue of the required unmixed nature of human intellectual understanding.[54] Aristotle required that knowing entail the

52. "To recapitulate, the order of succession which seems to result from our analyses will be the following: Averroes initially wrote a first 'Long Commentary,' Sharh 1; this is the text which he used (and cited) in composing the Middle Commentary; later, he undertook a substantial revision of Sharh 1, for which he also made use of the Middle Commentary: Sharh 1+. In a final period, he resumed work with Sharh 1+ to add there in particular the excursus of [Book 3] Comments 5 and 36, and to take the opportunity to review the rest of the text. In many ways, Sharh 1+ presents only some minor differences with Sharh 2." *Long Commentary* Fragments (2005), 47. "Sharh 2" here denotes the final version as found in the Latin *Long Commentary*.

53. *Long Commentary* Fragments (2005), 48. While it remains to be established whether the early versions of the *Long Commentary* were complete or only partial, Sirat and Geoffroy are certainly right that the *Long Commentary*'s teaching on the material intellect marks a distinct doctrinal change. My account of the reasons for that change is detailed below in this introduction.

54. For Geoffroy's understanding of the metaphysical principle at work here, see note 65 below. The *Long Commentary* contends that the position of Ibn Bâjjah (and implicitly Averroes' own position in the *Short Commentary*) must be rejected because its view that the material intellect is a disposition of the imagination entails that what is mover in the generation of knowledge (the imagination, which provides intentions from the senses required for knowledge) cannot also be what is moved (the imagination as what receives the intelligibles in act). See {398} and Book 3, n. 61.

receptive power be unmixed to be able to think all things (*De Anima*, 429a18–21), not have any character of its own except receptivity (a21–22), be in some way nonexistent before thinking (a24), be free of mixture with body and free of bodily organ (a24–27), and be separable from matter to the extent that its objects are separable (b21–23). Though not explicitly referring to the *Short Commentary*, Averroes now seems to find that his earlier view of the material intellect was too closely tied to the body, with its notion that the images in the imagination, a corporeal power, are the subjects for what is called material intellect. This becomes apparent in the examination of his discussion of *De Anima* 3.4 in the *Middle Commentary*, where he devotes much of paragraphs 277 and 278 to concerns about the unmixed nature of the material intellect, even though there is no mention of it in the precisely corresponding text of Aristotle (*De Anima*, 428a13–18). Now the human material intellect must be

> completely unmixed with any material form. For, this faculty, which is called the material intellect, if it is to think all things—that is, receive the forms of all things—cannot be mixed with any one form; that is, it cannot be mixed with the subject in which it is found, as the other material faculties are.
>
> (278) If the rational faculty were mixed with any form, then one of two things would have to occur: either the form of the subject with which it was mixed would impede the forms this faculty would receive, or it would change them—that is, it would change the form being received. Were this so, the forms of things would not exist in the intellect as they really are— that is, the forms existing in the intellect would be changed into forms different from the actual forms. If, therefore, the nature of the intellect is to receive the forms of things which have retained their natures, it is necessary that it be a faculty unmixed with any form whatsoever.[55]

Aristotle does raise the issue in the next passage of the *De Anima* (429a18–20), which Averroes paraphrases as follows.

> (279) This is what Anaxagoras wanted [to convey] in saying, reportedly, that the intellect has to be unmixed in order to have knowledge, for, if [a form] were to manifest itself in the intellect, it would prevent the appearance of a different form or change it. That is, if any form were to be manifested in this disposition, one of two things would have to occur: either that form would prevent us from knowing a different form which we want to know, since [the intellect's] knowledge of a form is a recep-

---

55. *Middle Commentary* (2002), 109. Note that in all my quotations of Ivry's translation I have changed his rendering of العقل الهيولاني *al-ʿaql al-hayûlânî* from "hylic intellect" to "material intellect."

tion of it; or the [first form] would change the [other form] when it received it.[56]

This stress on the unmixed nature of the material intellect here requires that it not be conceived as something existing in a subject in the manner of a form in a substance or an accident of a substance. That mixture would interfere with the material intellect's ability to grasp the intelligible form itself. As indicated above, the *Short Commentary*'s view is that "The imaginative soul is distinguished by the fact that it does not need an organic instrument for its activity," something which perhaps rightly highlights the nature of imagination as less material than the external senses. Still, the notion that the material intellect could be described as "the disposition which is in the forms of the imagination for receiving intelligibles" appears to have struck Averroes as allowing for an unacceptable mixture with a bodily power.[57] This is because the forms of the imagination would function as potential substrate for intelligibles (that is, as the material intellect) while retaining their own natures.[58] In the *Middle Commentary*, however, Averroes will not permit any such thing and instead provides an unequivocal rejection of his earlier view in the *Short Commentary*.[59]

Averroes is now content only to assert in the *Middle Commentary* that what is called "material intellect" and denotes the ability here and now of human beings to grasp intelligibles as intelligibles in act must not be primarily tied to or in some particular power such as the imagination in the individual corporeal human being. That is, since the very nature of the activity itself which comes about in us is per se intellectual and concerned with intelligibles in act, the activity has to be one of an intellect in the appropriate sense of the term. Yet since we are involved in such activity because we are knowers, we must in the appropriate sense have a capacity for such activity. That capacity qua intellectual is nothing before it thinks per Aristotle, and so the presence of the external agent intellect to the individual human being gives rise to the remote capacity for knowing at the individual's birth.[60] The agent intellect then later joins with the human being to develop this human intellectual capacity into

56. *Middle Commentary* (2002), 109–110.

57. فاذا الاستعداد الذي في الصور الخيالية لقبول المعقولات هو العقل الهيولاني الأول
(*Short Commentary on the De Anima* [1950], 86; [1985], 124; [1987], 209). Cf. note 22 above.

58. That is, they would be receptive subjects for intelligibles and at the same time movers (scil. generative causes supplying content) of knowledge had in the intelligibles. Cf. note 54.

59. *Middle Commentary* (2002), 111–12.

60. Averroes was well aware of Aristotle's assertion of τὸν νοῦν . . . θύραθεν, reason or intellect which enters human beings from outside, at *Generation of Animals* 2.2, 736b27. Aristotle, *Generation of Animals* (1965). See {397}.

actuality by conjoining, and it does so in a twofold way. The remote but natural human capacity for knowing must be affected by the agent intellect such that (1) a receptive disposition comes to be so that intelligibles can be received (this is the material intellect), and (2) those intelligibles must come to be received in their actuality: "one should not believe that the subject of this receptivity is anything other than a disposition to receive the intelligible, and it is not anything in actuality before it is perfected by the intelligible."[61] In both moments the agent intellect is a causal agent. In this way Averroes is able to hold that the capacity called "material intellect" in us is in fact intellectual in its own nature and unmixed insofar as it receives immaterial intelligibles in act. He is also able to maintain that it is a disposition belonging to us, since its presence comes only from the coincidence of a natural albeit inchoate disposition and a relation realized by the agent intellect in the twofold way indicated. He writes,

> It has thus been explained that the material intellect is something composed of the disposition found in us and of an intellect conjoined to this disposition. As conjoined to the disposition, it is a disposed intellect, not an intellect in act; though, as not conjoined to this disposition, it is an intellect in act; while, in itself, this intellect is the Agent Intellect, the existence of which will be shown later. As conjoined to this disposition, it is necessarily an intellect in potentiality which cannot think itself but which can think other than itself (that is, material things), while, as not conjoined to the disposition, it is necessarily an intellect in act which thinks itself and not that which is here (that is, it does not think material things).[62]

This disposition, the material intellect, is essentially a human disposition insofar as it is part of the definition of human beings as rational animals who are able to come to know. Still, it is not fully per se contained in the individual human being insofar as it needs the causal influence of the external agent intellect for the being of the material intellect in the individual. Yet this power of intellect that gives rise to the material intellect does belong essentially to its cause, the agent intellect, which is essentially intellect. Although it is not in full ontological actuality present in the same essential way in the human soul, the agent intellect and its power are operationally and also formally present in the soul as manifested in the material intellect. It is not the agent intellect, simply; it is the lower manifestation of the presence of the agent intellect, which has its own being as a substance apart from its activity of actualizing in a twofold way this disposition, the material intellect. This immaterial disposi-

---

61. *Middle Commentary* (2002), 115.
62. *Middle Commentary* (2002), 111–112.

tion, which makes knowing possible for individual human beings in the reception of intelligibles in act, is related to the soul of the individual as a disposition of the human being. As such it is not merely some pure disposition but a disposition belonging to a human being, an immaterial disposition essentially conjoined with its substance, a human being.[63] In this way Averroes avoids what he calls an absurd position of locating the "material intellect" in the nature of a separately existing intellectual substance—a position absurd for two reasons. First, it would mean that disposition and potentiality, characteristics of material things, would be said to exist in separate, immaterial intellectual substances which are as such fully active in their being. Second, it would mean that our first actuality and perfection as human beings qua rational animals—namely, our capacity for intellectual development called "material intellect"—would be something eternal, while our realization of this capacity would be generable and corruptible, taking place through time. That is to say, the fulfillment of an eternal entity would be through temporal and generated activities, something which is unacceptable because these entities are not in the same genus.[64]

63. *Middle Commentary* (2002), 112: "For, by our position as stated, we are saved from positing something separate in its substance as a certain disposition (مفارقا في جوهره استعدادا ما), positing [instead] that the disposition found in it is not due to its [own] nature but due to its conjunction with a substance which has this disposition essentially (بالذات)—namely, man—while, in positing that something here (هاهنا) is associated incidentally (بنوع من العرض) with this disposition, we are saved from [considering] the intellect in potentiality as a disposition only." Note that I have changed Ivry's "substantively separate" to "separate in its substance." Ivry's explanation of this in "Averroes' Three Commentaries on the *De Anima*" is that "the material intellect, which represents the potentiality for rational thinking, and as such is the first expression of this faculty in an individual, is connected 'incidentally' (*bi'l-'arad*) to the human soul, belonging 'essentially' to the universal Agent Intellect." (1999), 204. For this Ivry mistakenly cites 125.8 of his first edition of the *Middle Commentary*, which in fact has بنوع من العرض, not بالعرض. Geoffroy writes, "The material intellect which thus results from the agent intellect is essentially, insofar as it is intellect, the same thing as it, but considered only under the aspect of reception." Geoffroy and Steel (2001), 67. Davidson (1992), 281, understands this to mean the location of "the disposition, *essentially*, within the human organism, and . . . in an *accidental* fashion, in the incorporeal active intellect." The importance of Averroes' phraseology will become evident below, where I expound the grounds for his movement from the teachings of the *Middle Commentary* to those of his *Long Commentary*. See pp. xlii–xlix, lv–lxvi.

64. *Middle Commentary* (2002), 111. As will be expounded below, the position which Averroes adopts in the *Long Commentary on the De Anima* is essentially the one he here calls absurd: "that there should be a separate substance, the existence of which occurs in disposition and potentiality," وهو أن يكون جوهر مفارق وجوده في الاستعداد والقوة.

As Geoffroy has noted, the doctrine set forth here is related to Averroes' teaching on the nature of the celestial bodies, souls, and intellects.[65] Averroes asserts the existence of three celestial entities—a celestial body, a celestial soul, and a celestial intellect—as distinct celestial substances. The body moves, and the soul, without being composed with the body, impels it through the desire of an intellectual sort for the separate intellect. This intellectual soul is not composed with the celestial body but is a disposition attached or related to the celestial body. That is, the soul is a disposition in the subject so as to make it move, but it is not mixed with the subject as are material composites. At section 280 in the *Middle Commentary* Averroes similarly describes the material intellect on Alexander's view as "nothing other than disposition only—that is, the potential intellect is solely disposition, not something in which disposition exists. Although this disposition is in a subject, since it is not mixed with the subject, the subject does not serve as an intellect in potentiality. This is the opposite of what obtains with other material faculties in which the subject is a substance—either composite (that is, something composed of form and matter) or simple (the first matter)."[66]

By locating the being of the material intellect in an activity by the agent intellect, Averroes in the *Middle Commentary* has avoided the problem of a

---

Ibid. Just prior to this passage in section 281 he writes, "In general, disposition is a distinguishing characteristic of matter, and it is impossible for disposition to be found in one genus and its subject in another—that is, that which is disposed to receive something intelligible must be an intellect." Ibid., 110.

65. Geoffroy and Steel (2001), 64–65, 71ff. Geoffroy (64) calls Averroes' acceptance of the analogy of the material intellect to the intellectual soul of the celestial body "the second great ontological decision" of Averroes. The first ontological decision, he says (48), is Averroes' determination that a body can only have a corporeal form such that it cannot be apprehensive of other forms. This first decision allowed for the complete rejection of Alexander's account and the acceptance of that of Ibn Bâjjah that the material intellect is a disposition of imagined forms. Yet, as I have indicated above, here in the *Middle Commentary*, Averroes came to reject even the notion of the material intellect as a disposition of the forms of the imagination because of the need for a properly immaterial receptive subject for intelligibles in act in each human being. This is the problem, and the cosmological analogy is the proposed solution of the *Middle Commentary*. Geoffroy and Steel also note that Averroes seems to have had the notion of an analogy of human thinking with celestial movement when he wrote *Against the Avicennians on the First Cause* which appears to date from the time of the *Short Commentary*. See Geoffroy and Steel (2001), 71–73, and *Against the Avicennians on the First Cause* (1997). Also see Twetten (1995) and Taylor (1998a). For a detailed discussion of this and related matters with emphasis on the *De Caelo* commentaries by Averroes, see Endress (1995).

66. *Middle Commentary* (2002), 110.

theory which holds for the material intellect to be something which is a mixture as an accidental or substantial composition, as is the case for Ibn Bâjjah's notion of the material intellect being a higher function founded in the forms of the imagination as its subject. Rather, in the *Middle Commentary* the material intellect is a kind of being which results from the conjoining of a power in an individual human being and a power supplied by the agent intellect in a way ontologically prior to the actualizing of the intelligibles by the agent intellect. This power then is an individual power belonging individually to each human being; that is, there is a plurality of material intellects. That it has a reality of its own apart from the agent intellect Averroes makes clear by reference to the human ability to know both forms and privations. Insofar as it knows privations, which are not positive realities, the material intellect must know itself and also have a nature peculiar to it which makes that possible. This indicates that the material intellect has a nature of its own, distinct from the agent intellect, and is not in fact solely potentiality and disposition.[67] Nevertheless, this transcendent and immaterial disposition does not have an existence of its own separate from its subject, the human soul, upon which it depends essentially.

With his account of the material intellect as an unmixed receptive disposition and also as a reality distinct in being from the agent intellect which brings it about in particular individuals, Averroes has established that it is a power in the souls of particular human beings[68] and that the essence of the human intellect "is nothing other than thinking things external to it."[69] He has moved away from Ibn Bâjjah's view that the material intellect is a disposition of the imagination by placing it above and outside imagination so that it can be unmixed and able to receive all intelligibles without distortion by a definite and restricting subject in which it inheres as an accident or a material form might inhere. Rather, the material intellect is a real power associated with a subject

67. See *Middle Commentary* (2002), 119, secs. 306 and 307. In the latter Averroes writes, "This statement of his indicates that [Aristotle] considers the intellect in potentiality to be something other than [pure] potentiality and disposition." Cf. 111 (sec. 283), where he says that "Proof that it is not purely a disposition is had in that we find that the material intellect apprehends this disposition devoid of the forms and apprehends the forms, making it possible thereby to think of privations—that is, by virtue of apprehending its essence devoid of forms. This being the case, necessarily, that which apprehends this disposition and the forms which obtain in it is other than the disposition."

68. "Two functions exist in our soul, one of which is the producing of intelligibles and the other is the receiving of them. By virtue of producing intelligibles, it is called agent, while, by virtue of receiving them, it is called passive, though in itself it is one thing." *Middle Commentary* (2002), 112 (sec. 284).

69. *Middle Commentary* (2002), 115 (sec. 294). Translation slightly modified.

(the individual soul) while not being in it as composed or mixed with its subject. Instead, it is related after the manner of the relationship of an intellectual soul to its eternally moving associated celestial body, with the important difference that the existence of the individual's material intellect is dependent on the individual soul. By distinguishing it from the being of the agent intellect, which has a separate existence of its own, Averroes has allowed the material intellect itself to be a transcendent power realized "in" the soul of each human being, who, by that power, is able to grasp intelligible essences of things of the world of experience by a process of abstraction.

> The intellect . . . judges the image of a thing, and the image grasps the intention from the sense. Therefore, one who does not sense a genus of sensible objects cannot know it, nor can an intelligible [of this genus] ever reach him. Intelligibles are other than images; for, affirmation and denial are other than imagination, and truth and falsity are found only through combining the intelligibles of imaginative things with one another. Even first premises—of which the time of our [intentioned] sensation is not known to us—undoubtedly reach us from sense, even if we do not know when they reach us from it. Therefore, even though these premises are not imaginative, they do not reach us other than with images.[70]

Again, as in the case of the doctrine of the *Short Commentary*, what guarantees the veridical nature of intelligibles as being the intelligibles of the things of the world is their relation to the agent intellect, which made their existence as intelligibles in act possible. In this way all intellectual understanding on the part of human beings is grounded in the one shared agent intellect, which thereby must provide for the unity of intellectual thought and for any intersubjective discourse. Yet each human being has a unique material intellect by which each is able to become actually knowing. What is more, as indicated above, Averroes has avoided the absurd position that the material intellect be a separate substance in its own right apart from individual human beings by making it part of the essence of human beings, even if the rationality of human nature requires the completion of its disposition by the twofold action of the agent intellect. Hence, by that action on the part of the agent intellect, we come to have knowledge by the reception of intelligibles in our own individual souls thanks to this realization and fulfillment of our inborn powers as our now actualized material intellects.

In light of the foregoing account of the unique agent intellect and its causal activity of preforming, preparing, and actualizing the individual material intel-

---

70. *Middle Commentary* (2002), 123 (sec. 314). Translation slightly modified. On the grasp of first intelligibles in al-Fârâbî, see Druart (1997a).

lect, it is not surprising that Averroes employs the *Short Commentary*'s descriptive expression "form for us" in the *Middle Commentary* to characterize generally the relationship of the separately existing agent intellect to the human soul.

> It is clear that, in one respect, this intellect is an agent and, in another, it is form for us (صورة لنا *ṣûrah la-nâ*), since the generation of intelligibles is a product of our will. When we want to think something, we do so, our thinking it being nothing other than, first, bringing the intelligible forth and, second, receiving it. The individual intentions in the imaginative faculty are they that stand in relation to the intellect as potential colors do to light. That is, this intellect renders them actual intelligibles after their having been intelligible in potentiality. It is clear, from the nature of this intellect— which, in one respect, is form for us (صورة لنا *ṣûrah la-nâ*) and, in another, is the agent for the intelligibles—that it is separable and neither generable nor corruptible, for that which acts is always superior to that which is acted upon, and the principle is superior to the matter. The intelligent and intelligible aspects of this intellect are essentially the same thing, since it does not think anything external to its essence. There must be an Agent Intellect here, since that which actualizes the intellect has to be an intellect, the agent endowing only that which resembles what is in its substance.[71]

That is, insofar as the generation of intelligibles must be considered "a product of our will" and insofar as it is we who are thinking, the agent intellect is not outside and separate, acting only as agent or efficient cause. Rather, it is intrinsic as "form for us," such that the agent intellect is "our final form" (الصورة الأخيرة لنا *aṣ-ṣûrah al-akhirah la-nâ*) and is appropriately said to be a formal cause in us in some fashion.[72]

> You ought to know that Themistius and most commentators regard the intellect in us (العقل الذى فينا *al-'aql alladhî fî-nâ*) as composed of the intellect which is in potency and the intellect which is in act, that is, the Agent Intellect. In a certain way it is composite and does not think its essence but thinks what is here, when the imaginative intentions are joined to it. The intelligibles perish due to the passing away of these intentions, forgetting and error thus occurring to [our intellect]. They interpret Aristotle's statement in this manner, as explained in our commentary on his discourse.[73]

71. *Middle Commentary* (2002), 116 (sec. 297). Translation slightly modified.
72. *Middle Commentary* (2002), 116 (sec. 298).
73. *Middle Commentary* (2002), 117 (sec. 299).

Precisely what Averroes has in mind here by this characterization of the agent intellect as "form for us" and "our final form" will become more clear below through consideration of this teaching in the *Long Commentary* and the importance of Averroes' reconsideration of the account of Themistius in the latter's *Paraphrase of the De Anima*.

Averroes' Transitional Position

The position on the material intellect and the nature of intellectual understanding which Averroes reaches in the *Middle Commentary* is in many respects like that found in *Epistle 1 On Conjunction*, as noted by Davidson and Geoffroy.[74] In this work Averroes argues again that "what is called 'material intellect' has only the sole nature of possibility and disposition since it is mixed neither with matter nor any sensible natures. That is why this disposition is not anything existing in a subject."[75] He then goes on to argue that if it were like sensible forms or it were in another subject, it would not have the nature of an intellect which is able to know its own essence when it becomes the intelligibles in the activity of knowing for which its existence was asserted.[76] The nature of the material intellect, then, is like that explained "in *Physics* 8 regarding the first separate power, that this is not divisible by way of the division of bodies nor is it mixed with matter."[77] And earlier in this work he had held that a basic principle of his account here is that the causality of the agent intellect in relation to the material intellect is not merely that of efficient causality common

74. Davidson (1992), 274–275. Geoffroy and Steel (2001) provide an edition of the *De Beatitudine Animae* with extensive studies and notes, as well as French translations of the two Hebrew *Epistles* and the Latin *De Beatitudine Animae*. My account of *Epistle 1 On Conjunction*, the later of the two *Epistles* according to Geoffroy, is based on Geoffroy's French translation. The *De Beatitudine Animae* is a treatise on the perfection and fulfillment of human nature by way of knowledge via conjunction with the separate agent intellect. Wrongly attributed to Averroes and based on those two *Epistles* and an extract from al-Fârâbî's *Principles of the Opinions of the People of the Virtuous City* (كتاب مبادئ آراء أهل المدينة الفاضلة *Kitâb mabâdi' ârâ' ahl al-madînah al-fâdilah*: see al-Fârâbî, *Principles of the Opinions of the People of the Virtuous City* [1985]), this work is a Latin concoction which arose out of the Hebrew philosophical tradition. For more details on this work and its content and origins, see Davidson (1988) and Geoffroy and Steel (2001).

75. Geoffroy and Steel (2001), 204. I render *préparation* as "disposition" here and throughout, understanding it to correspond to استعداد *isti'dâd*, ἐπιτηδειότης.

76. Geoffroy and Steel (2001), 208.

77. Geoffroy and Steel (2001), 210. Averroes also argues here that the material intellect may be an immaterial disposition and a substance since it is not delimited by its relation to body. He may also have in mind that such an immaterial reality is per se one because of its lack of a relation of delimitation and enumeration by body.

to the movement of bodies but also that of formal and final causality. "Separate intellects are forms for [the souls of the spheres] and also their ends, because it is by [the separate intellects] that the being and the activity of [the souls of the spheres] are attained, since [the separate intellects] become the object of a representation on the part [of the celestial souls] and since these strive to assimilate themselves to [the separate intellects]."[78] In this way the separate intellects act as formal and final causes for the celestial souls, which are not in the celestial bodies as in a subject but associated with them as movers in a way unlike what is found in the sublunar realm.[79] In light of these considerations, therefore, Averroes raises a question concerning what will be a central doctrine in his teachings in the *Long Commentary on the De Anima*: What is there to prevent our thinking that some dispositions might be able to exist in the way the celestial souls exist—that is, as attached to celestial bodies but not composed with them as in a subject and also as having their final and formal cause in a way separate from them?[80] What is more, he continues, "it seems, on the issue of this disposition, that it is a substance one in number for all human beings in itself, but many by accident, which is not the case for material forms."[81] Averroes does not pursue the issue of the nature of the material intellect further in this work but is content to leave it aside for a more profound study at another time.

As Geoffroy makes clear in his study of this text and of the development of Averroes' doctrine of the material intellect, the very suggestion of this analysis, the posing of this question and the insinuation of the consequence of a single material intellect for all human beings, is the first anticipation of the *Long Commentary*'s teaching of the material intellect as a separately existing intellectual substance with the nature of receptivity only and as one for all humankind. This is an exciting and valuable discovery which places *Epistle 1 On Conjunction* both after the composition of the *Middle Commentary* and before the final version of the *Long Commentary*.[82] But it remains to consider the question of Averroes himself: What prevents the assertion of this view of the material intellect at this stage in Averroes' thought?

As we have seen, in the *Short Commentary* Averroes was concerned to establish with Ibn Bâjjah that the material intellect is not mixed with the body and

78. Geoffroy and Steel (2001), 200. "Representation" here indicates intellectual understanding on the level of the celestial soul.

79. Substantial discussion of cosmology and intellectual thought among celestial entities is beyond the parameters of this introduction. For a valuable account of relevant cosmological considerations at work here, see Twetten (2007).

80. Geoffroy and Steel (2001), 210.

81. Ibid.

82. Geoffroy and Steel (2001), 48–51, 68–69, 261.

so followed Ibn Bâjjah in holding it to be a disposition of the forms of the imagination. In the *Middle Commentary*, he appears to have been concerned over the implications of the doctrine found in the *Short Commentary*—namely, the notion that the material intellect is a disposition of the forms of the imagination in such a way that it was in them as being in a subject. But even to be in a subject would normally mean being composed with the subject either as an accident or as a material form. Yet such composition would be contrary to the nature of the material intellect as something which must be without matter, unmixed and receptive without distortion of the intelligibles it receives. Hence, the material intellect must have a nature similar to that of the celestial souls, which are only equivocally "in" the celestial bodies. That is, the celestial souls, are associated movers of the celestial bodies but do not exist in the celestial bodies as in a subject with which they are composed. Similarly, the material intellect is not in the human soul after the manner of a composition, but rather it is a disposition associated with the human soul and its intentional powers but necessarily free from composition with the soul. In each of these two works Averroes holds for the existence of material intellects in or associated with powers of individual souls in such a way that there is a plurality of material intellects. The analogy yields the following:

many celestial souls	:	many material intellects
many celestial bodies	:	many human souls
many celestial intellects	:	one agent intellect

How then could he come even to suggest in *Epistle 1 On Conjunction* such a contrary view as the notion of there being one material intellect for all individual human beings? There are several possible ways to consider this.

First, since in the *Middle Commentary* Averroes has come to base his understanding of the human material intellect on the analogy with the celestial soul for the sake of accommodating the unmixed nature of the material intellect, it may be that he has merely extended the analogy further. That is, each of the unique moving celestial bodies has its own unique celestial soul causing its movement through the soul's conceptualization of its unique celestial intellect above it.[83] But in the analogy, the one agent intellect stands in the place of the many unique celestial intellects. Given that there is one agent intellect for all human beings, then analogously there should perhaps be one corresponding material intellect for all human beings. Yet this simple correspondence is hardly an argument of sufficient persuasive force.

---

83. On the issue of Averroes' celestial cosmology and its development, see Endress (1995), particularly 24ff., where the issue of the celestial soul's conceptualization (تصور بالعقل *taṣawwur bi-l-ʿaql*) of its separate intellect is discussed.

Second, the issue of the nature of the causality of the agent intellect in relation to the material intellect may contribute to the argument. Perhaps one of the most vigorously argued issues in *Epistle 1 On Conjunction* is the notion that the agent intellect is only an agent or efficient cause. Averroes attributes this notion to Alexander and asserts that it was also held by al-Fârâbî, who was sorely misled by it.[84] Averroes writes that the understanding of the issue of conjoining with the material intellect is based on two principles, the second of which concerns knowledge of the way in which the separate intellect is the cause that the material intellect becomes an intellect in act. This concerns knowing whether

> it is the cause of it only in the way of the agent and moving cause, as natural movers, such as the light of the sun which is cause of sight in potency and brings it to a state of act; or such as the movement of the sphere and what follows upon it, namely the light and darkness which are cause of warmth and cold. For this movement and what follows upon it are cause of the being of natural existents and bring them from potency to act. And all these natural movers are agent causes and no other sort of cause at all, because they are not causes of the matter, form or end, since every natural body has a determinate matter, a determinate form and a determinate end.[85]

Averroes then goes on to assert that the separate intellect, scil. the agent intellect, may be their cause as form and end as are the celestial intellects for the celestial souls. This takes place insofar as the separate intellects provide the forms and the ends for the celestial souls since the being and activity of the celestial souls are founded on the intellectual representation of the celestial intellect in the celestial soul. That is, the actuality of intellect in the associated separate intellect provides the final cause toward which the celestial soul strives. That striving takes place by the conceptualization of its associated separate intellect in imitation within the limits of its nature. Through this it also achieves its own perfection and end. In this way by final causality the associated separate intellect provides the final and formal cause of the celestial soul which moves the celestial body in perfect motion. On this account, then, the separate intellect is the formal, final, and agent cause of the being and

84. Geoffroy and Steel (2001), 216. Averroes several times discusses al-Fârâbî's change late in life to the view that the human immortality through intellectual conjoining is "an old wives' tale." See Averroes' remarks in *Epistle 1 On Conjunction*, Geoffroy and Steel (2001), 220; *Epistle 2 On Conjunction*, Geoffroy and Steel (2001), 230; and *Long Commentary* {433}. Also see Pines (1978) and (1979); Davidson (1992), 70–73. The source of this in Ibn Bâjjah is identified with precision by Harvey (1992a), 225 n. 56. This issue is discussed at length in Taylor (2005).

85. Geoffroy and Steel (2001), 200.

activity of its associated celestial soul. All this was stated by Averroes to explain by analogy the nature of the relationship of the agent intellect and the material intellect, which are understood to be related as the associated separate intellect is related to its celestial soul. Since he holds that there is one agent intellect for all human beings, then it may well follow in his mind that it is reasonable to assert that there is one material intellect for all human beings. If there is one agent, formal, and final cause for all human beings, the unique agent intellect, then perhaps there must be one effect in which that causality is manifest (a unique material intellect shared by all human beings). This analogical account is more persuasive than the simple correspondence mentioned above, but it is not yet compelling.

Third, is there something about the very nature of intellection at issue here? Theophrastus and other ancient commentators, writes Averroes, thought that the material intellect should be understood in accord with the nature of matter and that conjoining should be considered on analogy with the composition of matter and form insofar as matter has the nature of potency. But Alexander, he continues, thought of material intellect only as a disposition in the soul and a substance receiving the forms of existing things. For Averroes, however, this is severely problematic since it means that the material intellect will be composed with the forms it receives. If it is like what it receives, then it will be like sensible forms, with the result that the material intellect would be a composite plurality and not be able to know the sensible forms *as intelligibles.* What is more, the material intellect was in fact asserted by Aristotle in *De Anima* 3.4 to be a power which understands the essences of things—that is, the intelligible forms of things without their matter—in order to account for human knowing, which is so different from the sense perception of individuals. The intelligibles in the material intellect, then, have in them "nothing other than the quiddity of the intelligible. And if it were not so, then [the intellect] would not be able to know its own essence. Thus, a thing [which is not of this order] does not know its own essence."[86] Filling in the argument of Averroes, we may say that the material intellect as intellect is an immaterial entity and a unity which should be able to know its own essence. (Recall the discussion above of the material intellect's knowledge of privations within itself in the *Middle Commentary.*) Hence, given that the material intellect knows its own essence and given that the agent intellect is its perfection as its agent, formal, and final cause,[87] what the material intellect knows in knowing itself

86. Geoffroy and Steel (2001), 208.

87. Geoffroy and Steel (2001), 216: "The agent intellect is not cause of the material intellect in as much as it is agent only, but in such a way that it is also its final perfection in the way of formal and final cause, as is the case of sense in relation to the sensed."

and its own essence would be the agent intellect in its actuality in the material intellect.

That course of reasoning could—with additional premises—lead to the assertion that there is one material intellect for all human beings, but Averroes does not draw that consequence. He elects instead to expound the view that the actualization of the material intellect results in the theoretical intellect, which contains the intelligibles abstracted from the experience of things.[88] He writes that "it seems that this disposition by which a human being receives the separate intellects[89] is what is received by and comes to be in the theoretical intellect at the completion of its realization, so that the relation of this disposition to the realized acquired intellect is [similar to] the relation of the disposition that is called the material intellect to the soul."[90] This takes place in relation to individual souls, so Averroes goes on to consider the question of why the intellectual excellence of the material intellect does not take place in each person's soul. Teleological necessity in nature requires that the material intellect, which is in potency, be actualized at the level of the species.[91] That is, it is not necessary that each person manifest the presence of the material intellect and each person be conjoined with the agent intellect via the material intellect, though it is necessary that it be attained for the species by some individual. This is dictated by the nature of the material intellect and the nature of human community in the context of divine providence, which makes nothing in vain.[92]

These three considerations are relevant to the issue of the material intellect, but neither separately nor together are they sufficient to provide a substantive philosophical argument for a single shared separate material intellect, even though Averroes himself makes precisely that suggestion in *Epistle 1 On Conjunction*. Must we, then, take Averroes at his word when he says he must leave the issue because it requires a more profound study in its own right? As indi-

---

88. Geoffroy and Steel (2001), 218. Cf. pp. xxiii–xlii above for the account of generation of intelligibles in the *Middle Commentary*. As will be evident in what follows, the underlying problematic issue is that of the unity of intelligibles in act and the unity of human knowing. That is, are the intelligible essences of scientific discourse multiplied with the multiplication of individual material intellects, or are intelligibles in act a single set of unique intelligibles to which human discourse refers?

89. That is, the material and agent intellects.

90. Geoffroy and Steel (2001), 218.

91. Averroes provides the argument for the necessity of what is in potency to come to be in act. He concludes the discussion with these words: "Then the consequence necessarily is that the material intellect must become an intellect in act at some moment." Geoffroy and Steel (2001), 214.

92. Remarks by Averroes at Geoffroy and Steel (2001), 218 and 220, imply this.

cated above, Averroes does not assert the existence of a unique material intellect shared by all human beings in *Epistle 1 On Conjunction* but rather asks what would prevent one from asserting the existence of a material intellect, "one in number for all human beings in itself, but many by accident." The answer to the question can be found through a careful analysis of the issue of "separation" as raised in *Epistle 1 On Conjunction*.

As indicated above, the account of the human material intellect in the *Middle Commentary* had this human receptive disposition as a power not composed with or in the body as sight or imagination but rather as a separate power of an immaterial nature which, qua immaterial, cannot literally be in or composed with the body. Its nature as a power receptive of intelligibles in act abstracted from intentional images provided by imagination thanks to sense perception required that this power, the material intellect, be itself immaterial and separate for the reception of immaterial intelligibles in act. This is dictated by the very natures of the immaterial intelligibles in act by which human knowing comes to exist. Still, like the relationship of the celestial intellect to the celestial soul or the celestial soul to the celestial body, the relationship of the material intellect to the human soul must be one whereby a particular material intellect is "in" or necessarily associated with a particular human soul. This analogy breaks down insofar as the celestial body, the celestial soul, and the celestial intellect are separate substances in their own natures, while the material intellect—which is indeed separate from the human being insofar as the material intellect is neither a body nor a power in a body—is not separate from the human corporeal soul inasmuch as it is a particular power belonging to a particular human being.

In this context "separation" is an equivocal term with two very distinct senses which require clarification with precision. Separation$_1$ denotes a relation such that there is an essential connection of what is separate with a determinate subject. Separation$_1$ is found in the *Middle Commentary* in the essential relation of a separate particular material intellect to its particular subject, the human soul. On that account, the being of the separate particular material intellect was that of a disposition dependent on the subject to which it belongs or which it is equivocally "in." In *Epistle 1 On Conjunction*, Averroes appears to criticize this view when he explains that by "separation" Aristotle may have meant merely that it is not a power of the body nor divisible with the division of the body.[93] Separation$_2$ denotes a complete ontological separation such as that of the first separated power (the First Mover) of *Physics* 8, which is not

---

93. "Perhaps he meant to indicate by 'separation' that it is not a power [in the body], divisible according to its division, even if it displays necessarily a dependence in relation to the body by way of the soul." Geoffroy and Steel (2001), 210.

divisible in relation to what it affects, "not divisible according to body or mixed with matter."[94] Separation$_2$ properly characterizes the celestial body, the celestial soul, and the celestial intellect. The view that the material intellect is "one in number for all human beings in itself, but many by accident" requires this separation$_2$ and is precisely the mature teaching of the *Long Commentary*, in which one material intellect is shared by a plurality of individuals, as will be explained at length below. Yet what prevents precisely such an assertion?

The controlling issue present here is that of the nature of intelligibles in act and their required subject. In the *Middle Commentary* each human being has an immaterial, separate$_1$ individual material intellect into which intelligibles in act are received. These intelligibles in act constitute the content and activity of human knowing brought about by the presence of the agent intellect and its activity in each human material intellect. The content of those intelligibles in act comes from human experience of the world by way of intentions of the imagination abstracted by the agent intellect and brought about in the individual material intellect of the human being who provides those intentions. As such, the agent intellect does not provide the intentional content of intelligibles in act in the human material intellect. In this case, then, the intelligibles in act are multiplied in accord with the multiplication of individual human knowers. The intelligible in act or essence of "horse" will be multiplied and idiosyncratic to each individual human knower. However, on such a view the unity of scientific understanding and intelligible discourse would seem to be undermined since there would be no common referent for the intelligible understandings taking place in each distinct human being.

It is precisely this conception of intelligibles in act as multiplied in the material intellects of many human beings in the teaching of the *Middle Commentary* that prevents the assertion of a single transcendent material intellect, "one in number for all human beings in itself, but many by accident." As seen above, in the *Middle Commentary* Averroes scoffingly rejected this notion of a material intellect existing in separation$_2$.[95] In order to overcome the limitations of his earlier view, then, Averroes had to come to a new understanding of the nature of intelligibles in act such that there is a single set of intelligibles in act which are the common referents for scientific understanding and discourse. Such a view is found in the *Long Commentary* and is developed by Averroes in critical dialogue with the teachings of Themistius in his *Paraphase* of the *De Anima*.

---

94. Ibid. Geoffroy identifies the precise reference to the *Physics* of Aristotle as 266a 10–b6. Geoffroy and Steel (2001), 261.

95. *Middle Commentary* (2002), 111.

Averroes' Final Position on Intellect:
The Long Commentary on the De Anima

With its 325 sections of Text and Comment, the *Long Commentary* provides detailed critical reflections on all the parts of the *De Anima* in the order of the work set forth by Aristotle, from the First Book's opening considerations of methodology, through its mention of issues and the positions of the predecessors of Aristotle, through the Second Book's discussion of soul, body, and external and internal senses, and on through the Third Book's detailed discussions of intellect and concluding sections concerned with movement on the part of the soul. For his commentary, Averroes draws on works on soul and intellect by Alexander, Theophrastus (through Themistius), Themistius, al-Fârâbî, and Ibn Bâjjah, while making references to the thought of Plato, Galen, Avicenna, and others, as well as to other works of the Aristotelian corpus. While the *Middle Commentary* makes no reference to the *Short Commentary*, as noted above the later version of the *Short Commentary* contains a note referring the reader to Averroes' mature views in the *Long Commentary on the De Anima*. For its part, the *Long Commentary* does contain implicit reference to the teachings of the *Short Commentary* by way of its refutation of Ibn Bâjjah and the doctrine that the material intellect is the imagination insofar as the forms of the imagination are the subjects for the disposition called material intellect.[96] Nevertheless, the Arabic version of the *Long Commentary*, which survives only in Latin translation and in Arabic fragments, is a work which stands alone without any requisite argumentative reference in its teachings to Averroes' earlier commentaries on the *De Anima*.

With a structure different from the topical divisions of the *Short Commentary* and the traditional division of the work into three "discourses" or books (مقالات *maqâlât*) of the *Middle Commentary*, the *Long Commentary* also charts a distinctive course.[97] In this work Book 3 begins with the discussion of intellect traditionally placed in Book 3, chapter 4. That is, Averroes has chosen to extend the account of Book 2 up to the end of Aristotle's discussion of imagination and to begin Book 3 where Aristotle initiates discussion of the soul which **"knows and understands"** {379}.[98] Thus, the doctrine of the intellect, and es-

96. See above, pp. xxv–xxviii. It may also refer to Averroes' *Commentary on the De Intellectu of Alexander.*

97. On the divisions of the text of the *De Anima* in the Arabic tradition, see Elamrani-Jamal (2003), 351.

98. Averroes makes no comment on his procedure, so perhaps he took it to be self-evident that discussion of all bodily powers of soul should be placed with discussion of soul and sensation in Book 2 and the non-bodily powers of intellect should be seen to be the key concern of Book 3.

pecially that of the material intellect, in the *Long Commentary* can be considered a distinct study of intellect and its issues where Averroes sets forth his considered final position, with arguments for the most part located in Book 3, though important and relevant issues arise in the earlier books.

The Science of the Soul
and Metaphysics

That Averroes thought the most compelling issue addressed by his commentary on the *De Anima* was that of the nature and status of the material intellect is evident early on when he comments on Aristotle's remarks in Book 1 that the science of the soul has a special position of priority among the sciences because of its exactness and because of its objects. Its exactness is constituted in its use of the method of demonstration; its objects are living things in which the presence of soul is evident. But for Averroes the science of the soul has a function in reference to the science of metaphysics not mentioned in any explicit way by Aristotle: "The practitioner of divine science gets from it the substance of his subject. For here [in the science of the soul] it will be explained that the separate forms are intelligences and also many other things concerning the knowledge of states consequent upon intelligence considered as intelligence and intellect" {5}. It is in the science of the soul that the existences of the agent intellect and the material intellect as separate, immaterial entities are established. Thinking ahead to his understanding of Aristotle's account of these two intellects in *De Anima* 3.4 and 3.5, Averroes has in mind that the particular intentions grasped in the perceptions and activities of the external and internal senses require the involvement of transcendent intellectual powers. Intelligibles in potency found in the world and in the soul's powers give rise to the intelligibles in act constituting the intellectual understanding of things characteristic of human thought. This knowledge of intelligibles in act as universals is the essence of science applicable to many particulars and not bounded by reference only to a certain individual. Understanding this to be necessarily the activity of what is intellectual and immaterial, Averroes considers the science of the soul to be responsible for establishing the existence of immaterial entity as intellectual in nature. While physics had proven for him the existence of an ultimate separate mover, the proof of the nature of this mover was beyond the limits of the science of physics. Philosophical psychology's proof that intellect exists and is necessarily immaterial provides one instance of the evidence sought by Aristotle in *Metaphysics* 6, where he wrote, "If there is no substance other than those which are formed by nature, natural science will be the first science; but if there is an immovable substance, the science of this must be prior and must be first philosophy, and universal in this way, because it is first. And it will belong to this to consider being *qua* being—both what it is and the attributes which belong to it *qua* being."[99]

The full import of this for Averroes' philosophical methodology is evident when he cites the same issue in his *Long Commentary on the Metaphysics*, a work written after the final version of the *Long Commentary on the De Anima*:

> It is fully clear that these celestial bodies are alive and that among the powers of soul they have only intellect and the power of desire, i.e. [intellect] which causes motion in place. This is perhaps evident from what I say, for it has been explained in the eighth book of the *Physics* that what causes motion belonging to the celestial bodies is not in matter and is a separate form. And it was explained in the *De Anima* that the separate forms are intellect. So, consequently, this mover is an intellect and is a mover insofar as it is an agent of motion and insofar as it is the end of motion.[100]

Averroes does not elect here to exploit philosophical psychology's epistemological arguments for constructing a proof of the existence of immaterial being, but instead chooses only to draw on its identification of immaterial substance as intellect. Averroes does exploit the results of the study of psychology for another key metaphysical principle. Not only has philosophical psychology provided the establishment of the subject matter of the science of metaphysics by showing the existence of a substance immaterial, intellectual, and not formed by nature (and hence not included under the science of physics), but it has also given evidence of the existence of a form of potency existing in separate intellectual substances. By its proof of the nature and separate existence of the material intellect, psychology has proven that a kind of potency can exist in what is intellect, for the material intellect, as discussed in detail below, is essentially a receptive disposition for intelligibles of things of the world while itself being separate intellect. And by establishing that a kind of potency can exist in what is separate intellect, psychology, as Averroes understands it, provides metaphysics with the basis for a ranked hierarchy of intelligences or intellects distinguished from one another and from the pure actuality of the First Cause.[101] In Book 3 of his *Long Commentary on the De Anima*

99. Aristotle, *Metaphysics* (1984), 6.1, 1026a27–32.

100. *Long Commentary on the Metaphysics* (1952), Book Lâm (Lambda, XII), c. 36, 1593–1594. My translation. Cf. (1962), XII, c. 36, f. 318v G–H, and (1984), 149.

101. "One should hold that it [scil. the material intellect] is a fourth kind of being. For just as sensible being is divided into form and matter, so too intelligible being must be divided into things similar to these two, namely, into something similar to form and into something similar to matter. This is [something] necessarily present in every separate intelligence which understands something else. And if not, then there would

he writes with full awareness of the importance of this for the metaphysical issues: "If it were not for this genus of beings which we have come to know in the science of the soul, we could not understand multiplicity in separate things, to the extent that, unless we know here the nature of the intellect, we could not know that the separate moving powers ought to be intellects" {410}.[102]

Yet, not unlike Aristotle's own text of Book 1, Averroes marshals few detailed arguments regarding intellect in his Comments in the First Book. Instead, employing the results of his arguments yet to come in Book 3 to interpret Aristotle's statements in Book 1, Averroes explains his understanding of Aristotle's own hints on key characteristics of intellect: "This is his opinion concerning the material intellect: it is separate from the body and it is impossible that it understand anything without the imagination. He did not mean by this what appears superficially [to be the case] from this account, that if understanding comes to be only with imagination, then the material intellect will be generable and corruptible, as Alexander thought from [this account]" {18}. And it is only by this paradoxical separation from body while at the same time requiring involvement with imagination, which is a bodily power, that the material intellect can be what "discerns the intentions of all beings" {88}. Distinct from the imagination, which Averroes sometimes calls the imaginative intellect or passible intellect {88}, the material intellect, he asserts, "discerns universal intentions" {90}. The full meaning of these statements on the material intellect in Book 1 becomes evident only in the extended treatments of Book 3.

The Senses and Internal Powers
of Particular Human Beings

The distinction between the senses, internal and external, and the intellect is explained at greater length in Book 2, Comments 60ff., where Averroes stresses the differences between sense and intellect: "The reason for the difference between sense and intellect in the acquisition of complete actuality lies in the fact that the mover is external in the case of sense and it is internal in the case of intellect. For sense in act is moved only by a motion which is called apprehending and [is dependent] upon sensible particular things which are outside the soul. Intellect, however, is moved to complete actuality by universal things and those are in the soul" {220}. What come from the senses, he goes on to

---

be no multiplicity {410} in separate forms. It was already explained in First Philosophy that there is no form free of potency without qualification except the First Form which understands nothing outside itself. Its being is its quiddity. Other forms, however, are in some way different in quiddity and being."

102. This issue is treated at greater length in Taylor (1998a).

explain, are intentions which can be grasped by imagination, while what the intellect has in it are "universals in potency" or what he calls a "universal intention . . . different from an imagined intention." It is by means of these that human beings are able to form concepts when they wish, in contrast to sensation which "needs sensibles which are outside the soul." Sensibles move the soul not in accord with their manner of existence in matter outside the soul but as intentions received by the sense and caused by the external objects {220}. As a potency limited in its objects and range, sense is directed intentional potency and disposition for receiving intentions which are both sensible in potency and intelligible in potency {221}. These intentions apprehended by sense are intentions of individuals. And "that individual intention is what the cogitative power discerns from the imagined form and refines from the things which were conjoined with it from those common and proper sensibles {226}, and it deposits it in the memory. This same [individual intention] is what the imaginative [power] apprehends, but the imaginative [power] apprehends it as conjoined to those sensibles, although its apprehension is more spiritual."

Later Averroes explains that this cogitative power or cogitation, an internal bodily power located in the brain, is "an individual discerning power . . . which discerns the intention of a sensible thing from its imagined image"{415}. It is third in the order of spirituality, with common sense and imagination less spiritual and the power of memory more spiritual than cogitation. Yet while these powers are spiritual insofar as they discern or separate intentions from things of the world, they are not intellectual or rationally discerning since they still concern the intentions of individuals. "Although, therefore, a human being properly has a cogitative power, nevertheless this does not make it that this power is rational and discerning, for [the rational power] discerns universal intentions, not individual ones" {416}. What Averroes calls "the discerning rational power," intellect, cannot be a power in a body since it would require an organ. But such a thing is impossible since the intellect cannot be a power mixed with body and still be intellect which grasps intelligibles in act. In short, the function of the bodily yet spiritual cogitative power is to discern and refine sensible intentions presented by the internal power of imagination by denuding the intentions as much as possible of accretions extraneous to the intention itself. Nevertheless, what it deposits in memory is not an intelligible but rather a denuded individual intention still "material" insofar as it is the intention of an individual particular which is intelligible in potency, not intelligible in act. By the action of the cogitative power and memory, the individual intention, refined as much as possible, is prepared for the activity of a higher and completely immaterial power, the intellect, in what Averroes later describes as a process in which the refined imagined intention "is transferred in its being from one order into another" {439}—that is, from intelligible in potency to intelligible in act.

From the foregoing it is evident that the most important role among the internal sense powers is reserved for the cogitative power, which received little mention in the *Short Commentary* and the *Middle Commentary*. Regarding "the passible intellect," which "is necessary for conceptualization," in the *Long Commentary* Averroes writes that this term is used by Aristotle to mean "the forms of the imagination insofar as the cogitative power proper to human beings acts upon them. For that power is a kind of reason and its activity is nothing but the placing of the intention of the form imagined in its individuality in memory or the discerning of it from [the individual] in conceptualization and imagination.[103] And it is evident that the intellect which is called material receives the imagined intentions after this discernment" {449}. So important in the epistemological account are these internal powers in the particular human being that Averroes asserts, "without the imaginative power and the cogitative [power] the intellect which is called material understands nothing" {450}. But as these citations indicate, it is in Book 3 that Averroes, while still following Aristotle's text, fully sets forth his final position on the intellect. So the completion of this account of the role of the cogitative power must await a detailed exposition of his new teachings on the separate intellects.

The Material Intellect

In the 68 Comments on the Texts of Aristotle's Book 3, chs. 4–13 of the *De Anima*, Averroes mentions the material intellect some 182 or more times and spells out his teachings in several key sections. As indicated, however, the order of his account is not driven primarily by his own systematic doctrine but rather follows the order of Aristotle's Texts. Still, the doctrine he sets forth is itself a detailed and methodical account of the principles which yield the novel doctrine of intellect expounded in this work. In Comment 5 he sets forth his understanding of the nature of the material intellect in critical dialogue with the views of Alexander, Theophrastus, Themistius, and Ibn Bâjjah as Averroes understands them; in Book 3, Comments 18–20, he expounds his understanding of the grounds for asserting the existence of separate agent and material intellects; and in Comment 36 the natures of understanding and conjoining

103. Since conceptualization properly speaking can take place only at the level of intellect, here *formationem* is used to indicate image formation as an activity of imagination or cogitation working still at the level of particulars rather than a properly intellectual activity. The Arabic is surely تصوّر *taṣawwur*, which literally means "image forming." With the addition بالعقل *bi-l-ʿaql* it denotes intellectual conceptualization. Here, however, I translate *formatio* as it is translated elsewhere in the *Long Commentary*.

with separate intellect as such are the primary focus. Throughout Book 3 Averroes' new understanding of the function of cogitation in the process of conceiving and reconceiving knowledge emerges as a fundamental part of his mature teaching.

Following Aristotle, Averroes begins his Third Book with consideration of the nature of human understanding's conceptualizing (تصوّر *taṣawwur, formare per intellectum*) as both similar and dissimilar to sense perception. Each is an apprehensive power of the soul and so is receptive. But unlike sensation, which is "a power in a body," intellect's power of conceptualizing "does not undergo affection equivalent to the affection of the sense, namely, there does not come about for it a change similar to the change which comes about for the sense, but it is only likened to sense in regard to receptivity, because it is not a power in a body" {381}. The reason for this difference lies in the change which takes place in sensation, whereby what is a body or a power in a body is changed in its accidental being as a determinate particular {382}, whereas the intellect "is neither a body nor a power in a body" {383}.[104] Consequently, intellect is not changed by its reception of intelligibles because these are not determinate particulars which are intelligibles in potency but rather intelligibles in act under the very notion of knowledge. And as Anaxagoras held, "it is necessary that it be unmixed so that it may apprehend and receive all things. For if it is mixed, then it will be either a body or a power in a body, and if it is {384} either of these, it will have its own form and this form will impede its reception of another foreign form."

Thus, insofar as conceptualizing comes about in the intellect, the subject in which this takes place must be one which is immaterial and yet receptive. Since knowledge concerns things of the material world, the rational soul is receptive insofar as "the rational soul needs to consider the intentions which are in the imaginative power, just as sense needs to view sensibles" {384}. Yet it must also be active "since it seems that the forms of external things move this power in such a way that the mind (*mens*) abstracts them from matters and makes them first to be intelligibles {385} in act after they were intelligibles in potency." It is for this reason, writes Averroes, that Aristotle found it "necessary to assert that these two differences are in the rational soul, namely, the power of activity and the power of affection" {385}. Averroes is able to conclude that "this substance which is called the material intellect has none of those material forms in its nature" on the basis of two principles derived from these

---

104. "Determinate particular" reflects the Latin *aliquid hoc*, which corresponds to Aristotle's τόδε τι at *De Anima*, 402a24, and المشار إليه *al-mushâr ilaihi*, meaning "designated" or "determinate" in the *Middle Commentary* on the *De Anima*. See *Middle Commentary* (2002), 113.14 and 113.22. For a discussion, see Bauloye (1997), 74–76.

considerations. First, this intellect is receptive of the intentions of all worldly material forms without restriction; second, "everything receiving something else must be devoid of the nature of the thing received and its substance must not be the same in species as the substance of the thing received" {385}. In this way he has shown that "this substance which is called the material intellect {386} is neither a body nor a form in a body; it is, therefore, altogether unmixed with matter." It is then a being which is a receptive potency, separate, without a material form, and in itself simple and not changeable as are determinate particulars subject to substantial or accidental change {386}.

Averroes' solution to the key epistemological and metaphysical issues comes in a discussion of considerations central to the doctrine of the material intellect, which he finds prompted by study of the Greek commentators Theophrastus, Themistius, and Alexander, with Ibn Bâjjah's view critically evaluated as well. The three issues are these: (1) If the agent intellect is eternal and the material intellect is also eternal, what then must be the nature of the theoretical intellect in human beings? Must not the product of the agent intellect and the material intellect be eternal if these intellects are eternal? (2) How can the power called the material intellect be one and the same in all human beings at birth and yet individual for each in its final perfected state? (3) How is the material intellect an existing being of a nature essentially consisting in receptivity without being a material form or matter?[105] It is in this context that Averroes forms the set of two philosophical principles required to enable him to assert what he only raised as a question in his *Epistle 1 On Conjunction* as indicated above—namely, the existence of a single, shared material intellect for all human beings: "That part of the soul which is called the material intellect has no nature and being by which it is constituted inasmuch as it is material except the nature of possibility, since it is devoid of all material and intelligible forms. . . . The definition of the material intellect, therefore, is that which is in potency all the intentions of universal material forms and is not any of the beings in act before it understands any of them" {387}. The pure potentiality of the material intellect is distinct from that of prime matter, he continues, because the material intellect is a potency for the apprehensive reception of "all the intentions {388} of the universal material forms." Prime matter, in contrast, is a potency for the actual material reception of sensible forms without apprehension of any kind. Prime matter is receptive of "individual and particular forms," while the material intellect is receptive of universal forms which are intelligibles in act. Forms received into prime matter become determinate particular entities, with those forms existing as principles in substantial composition. The forms of things are then individual entities existing as intelligibles in potency—that is, intel-

---

105. This is the "question of Theophrastus." See below, pp. lxxx–lxxxi.

ligible only by reference to an external power which might apprehend them, discern their particular intentions, and abstract the intelligible intention to form an intelligible in act. The material intellect, however, which itself "is not a determinate particular nor a body nor a power in a body," is an entity which "must receive forms by a mode of reception other than that by which those matters receive the forms whose contraction by matter is the determination of prime matter in them." According to Aristotle, writes Averroes, the material intellect is a nature "which is other than the nature of matter, other than the nature of form, and other than the nature of the composite" {388}.

From this account Averroes is able to conclude that the material intellect is an entity unlike prime matter because of its apprehensive nature and unlike the apprehensive external and internal powers of the soul because all these are receptive of intentions of determinate particulars. As indicated above, even the more spiritual of the internal senses, cogitation and memory, work with determinate particular intentions and require the abstraction of an intellectual power to "transfer" the intention from the mode of being of a determinate particular to the mode of being of an intelligible in act. Yet since the intelligibles in act which come to exist in the material intellect cannot have the mode of being characteristic of a determinate particular, they cannot be received into a subject which is itself a determinate particular. Were that to happen, they would be contracted in their recipient subject from a mode of being an intelligible in act to that of what is an intelligible in potency only. Thus, the material intellect cannot itself be a determinate particular entity (*aliquid hoc,* المشار إليه *al-mushâr ilaihi*). As such, the material intellect then has a unique mode of existence since, on the one hand, it is required by each human being for conceptualization and intellectual understanding to take place, but, on the other hand, it is unique in its species and not a determinate particular belonging individually to any determinate particular human being. This account provides part of the argument for the assertion of the existence of one separate material intellect contemplated but not argued in *Epistle 1 On Conjunction.* It remains for Averroes to explain how there can be one material intellect for all and yet knowing somehow takes place differently in distinct human subjects such as Zayd and ʿAmr or Plato and Socrates.

That explanation comes toward the end of Comment 5, where he explains regarding the material intellect that "it is not necessary that the recipient be nothing at all in act but rather that it not be in act something of what it receives" {410}. That is, the material intellect has a nature of its own, consisting in receptivity and receptivity actualized by what is extrinsic to it. Likening the relation of the agent intellect and the material intellect to that of light and the transparent medium, Averroes extends the analogy to the forms of things of the world when he adds,

The relation of the material forms {411} to [the material intellect] is [the same as] the relation of color to the transparent [medium]. For just as light is the actuality of the transparent [medium], so the agent intellect is the actuality of the material [intellect]. Just as the transparent [medium] is not moved by color and does not receive it except when there is light, so too that intellect does not receive the intelligibles which are here except insofar as it is actualized through that [agent] intellect and illuminated by it. Just as light makes color in potency to be in act in such a way that it can move the transparent [medium], so the agent intellect makes the intentions in potency to be intelligible in act in such a way that the material intellect receives them. This, then, is how the material intellect and the agent [intellect] should be understood.

When the two intellects are joined in this fashion, abstraction of the intention intelligible in potency (the intention existing as a determinate particular in the internal senses subsequent to sense perception) takes place, with the result that the acquired intellect (العقل المستفاد, *al-ʿaql al-mustafâd, intellectus adeptus*) comes to be in the soul of the human agent who initiated the act of knowing by "our will."[106] This is the theoretical intellect (العقل النظري, *al-ʿaql al-naẓarî, intellectus speculativus*), whereby knowledge is, in a way, retained in the individual human being. In virtue of this human beings can be denominated knowers. This is so thanks to an understanding of knowing which Averroes borrows from his understanding of sense perception, his two-subject theory.

In his *Short Commentary* Averroes speaks of two subjects for intelligibles, a subject external to the soul in virtue of which the intelligible is true and another subject in virtue of which the intelligibles exist.[107] In the *Long Commentary* he expounds a slightly modified version of this notion, derived from consideration of sense perception, to account for the duality by which knowing can be said to belong to both the separate material intellect and the particular human knower.

Apprehending by sense is something which is actualized through two subjects, one the subject in virtue of which the sense is true (this is the

106. {390}. Also see {439}, {490}, and {495}. That this comes about by will or "whenever we wish" is also asserted by Themistius. See Themistius, *De Anima Paraphrase* (1899), 99; (1973), 179; (1996), 123; (1990), 90.

107. *Short Commentary on the De Anima* at (1985), 116–117, and 124–125 respectively; (1987), 203–204 and 210. Cf. Book 3, n. 59. Also see Blaustein (1984), 63ff. The inspiration for this two-subject analysis is probably Ibn Bâjjah's reflection on the status of intelligibles in perishable particular human beings as spiritual forms and in themselves as intelligible forms. See Ibn Bâjjah, *Treatise on the Conjoining of the Intellect with Man* (1942), 15–16; Spanish, 33–35; (1968), 163–164; (1981), 188.

thing sensed outside the soul) and the other the subject in virtue of which the sense is an existing form (this is the first actuality of the sense organ). Hence, the intelligibles in act must also have two subjects, one the subject in virtue of which they are true, namely the forms which are true images, and the other that in virtue of which the intelligibles are among the beings in the world, and this latter is the material intellect. For there is no difference regarding this between sense and intellect except that the subject of the sense in virtue of which it is true is outside the soul and the subject of the intellect in virtue of which it is true is inside the soul[108] {400}.

Thus, the subject by which they exist is the material intellect, which is the immaterial and separate subject for intelligibles in act following the agent intellect's "illumination," which both transforms intelligibles in potency into intelligibles in act and also makes possible the reception of these by the receptive material intellect, their subject of existence.[109] The subject by which they are true is the particular human being's more spiritual internal sense powers— namely, imagination, cogitation, and memory—which presented the refined image before the agent intellect. "For, just as the subject of vision moving [vision], which is color, moves it only when color is made to exist in act through the presence of light after it was in potency, so too the imagined intentions move the material intellect only when the intelligibles are made to exist in act after they were in potency" {401}.

This theory of two subjects then also has a role to play in the explanation of how it is possible for differences in knowledge between two particular human subjects while there is nevertheless one shared material intellect by which all human beings are knowers. "If the thing understood in me and in you were one in every way, it would happen that when I would know some intelligible you would also know it, and many other impossible things [would also follow]. If we assert it to be many, then it would happen that the thing understood in me and in you would be one in species and two in individual [number]. In this way the thing understood will have a thing understood and so it proceeds into infinity" {411}. What is understood—that is, the intelligible in act—cannot be shared such that when one person knows, any other human being also knows, an impossible consequence given human experience. Like-

---

108. See Book 3, n. 66.

109. "For to abstract is nothing other than to make imagined intentions intelligible in act after they were [intelligible] in potency. But to understand is nothing other than to receive these intentions. For when we found the same thing, namely, the imagined intentions, is transferred in its being from one order into another, we said that this must be from an agent cause and a recipient cause. The recipient, however, is the material [intellect] and the agent is [the intellect] which brings [this] about" {439}.

wise, what is understood cannot be many such that the intelligible in act is existing multiple times in multiple particular human beings, since the Third Man Argument would require the assertion of a third intelligible in act over those in particular human beings, and so forth into infinity. Knowing, then, is not something generated and created "in the student, in the way in which one fire generates another {412} fire similar to it in species." This impossibility together with the fact that "what is known is the same in the teacher and the student . . . caused Plato to believe that learning is recollection" {412}. Yet that cannot be the case simply because knowing is the grasp of things of the world intelligible in potency under the power of intellect whereby they come to exist as intelligible in act. On the basis of these considerations, Averroes concludes, "Since, then, we asserted that the intelligible thing which is in me and in you is many in subject insofar as it is true, namely, the forms of the imagination, and one in the subject in virtue of which it is an existing intellect (namely, the material [intellect]), those questions are completely resolved" {412}.

Hence, the intelligible can be said to belong to each individual human being only insofar as that human being is the subject of the truth of the intelligible—that is, only insofar as that human being had formed in imagination, cogitation, and memory the denuded intention which is that human being's contribution to the process of knowing taking place at the transcendent level of the separate material and agent intellects. Knowledge, then, belongs to individuals in virtue of their causal contribution to its formation in the separate intellects, where that intelligible in act comes to exist in a subject which is the material intellect itself. Without that causal link, the particular human being does not have knowledge and is not linked with the material intellect. In this way, for example, one person who in the past has seen and studied giraffes with individual effort is able to make his knowledge actual again by reconnecting with the material intellect when he encounters this remarkable animal in the jungle. But another person, who has no image in memory and has not linked with the material intellect to apprehend the intelligible in act of the giraffe, cannot identify this animal correctly.[110]

Thus, as indicated above, this intelligible in act is not literally and actually present with the individual human soul as its subject since that subject is a particularizing power in a body. Rather, it must exist in the material intellect, which, as unique and itself a distinct and complete species (as is each of the separate intellects), is not a determinate particular (*aliquid hoc*, المشار إليه *al-mushâr ilaihi*). Its nature in this way is such that it can receive and contain intelligibles

110. As indicated above at p. x, at *Middle Commentary* (2002), 123 (314), Averroes writes that "one who does not sense a genus of sensible objects cannot know it, nor can an intelligible [of the genus] ever reach him."

in act without particularizing them, while at the same time being itself a thesaurus of actualized intelligibles to which all human beings who have provided
images for their abstraction may refer. This then provides the second of the two
principles required for the doctrine of the separate material intellect.

With this doctrine, Averroes has provided the grounds for the assertion of
the material intellect as required by the metaphysics of the nature of intelligibles
and their subjects. With reasons and arguments not mentioned in *Epistle 1 On
Conjunction*, where he could only raise the question of the possibility of conceiving the material intellect to be unique, separate, and shared, here Averroes has
supplied the needed principles and accounts for setting forth his new understanding of the material intellect. And while he saw this to be in accord with
the relevant philosophical principles and also as the only sound account of
Aristotle, his teaching on the material intellect was fully understood by Averroes to be new in the tradition: "One should hold that it is a fourth kind of being"
{409}.[111] That is, it is neither matter nor form nor a composite of these, but rather
a unique entity which the philosophical principles and issues led Averroes to
assert. It is an intellect unique in its species with the nature of receptivity.[112]

Averroes did not take his understanding of the unique and shared material
intellect from Themistius, but in forming his thought on it, he did take several
principles from Themistius in his critical engagement with the *Paraphrase of
the De Anima* in the course of his third reading of that work while composing
the *Long Commentary*. The notion of the unity of science in a single set of intelligibles in act, key in enabling Averroes' move to the assertion of a unique
material intellect as explained above, was adopted in rejection of the doctrine
of the *Middle Commentary*, where a plurality of individual material intellects,
each with its own set of intelligibles in act, is set forth. The source of the new

111. The complexity of the issues at stake and the difficulty of their reconciliation
were daunting to Averroes, but he was intent on working toward their resolution to the
extent of his ability. "Since there are all those things [which can be raised regarding
the material intellect], for this reason it seemed [best] to me to write what seemed to
me to be the case on this topic. If what appears to me is not complete, it will be a start
for a complete account. So I ask my brothers seeing this exposition to write down their
doubts and perhaps in that way what is true regarding this will be found out, if I have
not yet found [it]. If I have found [it], as I suppose, then it will be clarified through those
questions. For truth, as Aristotle says, is fitting and gives testimony to itself in every
way"{399}.

112. See pp. lviii–lix. In his late *Commentary on the De Intellectu of Alexander*, Averroes
asserts that "the material intellect is one power shared by individual souls" and that
the theoretical intelligibles are "in essence ungenerable and incorruptible." *Commentary
on the De Intellectu of Alexander* (2001), 29. See Book 3 {406–408} and the notes there.

teaching is Themistius. This Greek thinker is also a foundational source for Averroes' difficult doctrine that the agent intellect is not only agent or efficient cause in the generation of intelligibles, but also "in" the soul as "form for us." However, while Themistius is a source for Averroes, his teachings are not taken uncritically but rather serve as points of philosophical inspiration which Averroes crafts to fit coherently with other principles of his own Aristotelian account.

Quite different from the teachings of the *Long Commentary*, Themistius' *Paraphrase of the De Anima* sets forth the view that a potential intellect and an actual intellect are found in each individual human soul. According to Themistius, the actuality of these is founded in a relationship to the unique productive intellect: "There is no need to be puzzled if we who are combined from the potential and the actual [intellects] are referred back to one productive intellect, and that what it is to be each of us is derived from that single [intellect]. Where otherwise do the notions that are shared (*koinai ennoiai*) come from? Where is the untaught and identical understanding of the primary definitions and primary axioms derived from? For we would not understand one another unless there were a single intellect that we all shared."[113] The productive intellect "has all the forms all together and presents all of them to itself at the same time,"[114] while individual intellects are characterized as "combined from the potential intellect and actual [intellects]."[115] Identifying the individual human intellect more with the actual intellect insofar as this is the source of actuality, Themistius asserts that the actual intellect itself has as its source the transcendent productive intellect, which "alone is form in a precise sense, and indeed this is 'form of forms,'" such that "we are the productive intellect" properly speak-

113. Themistius, *De Anima Paraphrase* (1899), 103.36–104.3; (1973), 188–189; (1990), 105; (1996), 129. Note that for Themistius this "productive intellect" is not the most transcendent entity or God, but rather an intellect at a lower level of reality and involved with human understanding. The corresponding Arabic of the *Paraphrase* has, "There need be no wonder that we all are as a group composites of what is in potency and of what is in act. All of us whose existence is by virtue of this one are referred back to a one which is the agent intellect (العقل الفعال *al-ʿaql al-faʿʿāl*). For if not this, then whence is it that we possess known sciences in a shared way? And whence is it that the understanding of the primary definitions and primary propositions is alike [for us all] without learning? For it is right that, if we do not have one intellect in which we all share, then we also do not have understanding of one another."

114. Themistius, *De Anima Paraphrase* (1899), 100.9–10; (1973), 181; (1990), 93; (1996), 124.

115. Themistius, *De Anima Paraphrase* (1899), 100.16–20; (1973), 182; (1990), 93–94; (1996), 124–125.

ing since it is the source of our actuality.[116] In this account each human being has a potential intellect, and an illuminating and abstracting actual intellect which is responsible for the formation of intelligibles from a storehouse of experience in the potential intellect, which contains "the imprints from perception and imagination through the agency of memory."[117] However, this abstracting takes place only thanks to the individual actual intellect's sharing of the power of the transcendent productive intellect: "The intellect that illuminates (*ellampôn*) in a primary sense is one, while those that are illuminated (*ellampomenoi*) and that illuminate (*ellampontes*) are, just like light, more than one."[118] When this abstraction on the part of the actual intellect takes place, the productive intellect "encounters it and takes over" it,[119] such that the productive intellect is "not outside" but "settles into the whole of the potential intellect," as if "to pervade it totally," and "becomes one with it."[120] In this way, as "'form of forms,'" the productive intellect comes to act as an intrinsic formal cause of the potential intellect through the individual's actual intellect, although the productive intellect retains its transcendent existence. Only by this sort of participation of the power of the productive intellect, which comes to be intrinsic to the human intellect, does abstraction of intelligibles in act from the storehouse of images in the potential intellect take place for Themistius.

The productive intellect, then, contains and thinks all the transcendent forms, something Themistius confirms with the rhetorical question, "From what source will the potential intellect also come to think all objects, if the intellect that advances it to activity does not think all objects prior to it?"[121]

---

116. Themistius, *De Anima Paraphrase* (1899), 100.31–32 and 100.35–101.1; (1973), 182–183; (1990), 95; (1996), 125.

117. Themistius, *De Anima Paraphrase* (1899), 99.6–8; (1973), 179.5–6; (1990), 89; (1996), 12 3. For the Arabic Lyons suggests ذخيرة *dhakhîrah* (storehouse) in place of كثرة *kathrah* (multitude), found in the sole extant Arabic manuscript.

118. Themistius, *De Anima Paraphrase* (1899), 103.33–34; (1973), 188.13–14; (1990), 104; (1996), 128–129.

119. Themistius, *De Anima Paraphrase* (1899), 99.8–10; (1973), 179.6–7; (1990), 89–90; (1996), 123.

120. Themistius, *De Anima Paraphrase* (1899), 99.13–18; (1973), 179.6–7; (1990), 90; (1996), 123.

121. Themistius, *De Anima Paraphrase* (1899), 103.30–32; (1973), 188.11–13; (1990), 104; (1996), 128. The extant Arabic text has: "Whence does the intellect in potency come to know all things if what brings it to act is *first* knowing all things?" Lyons (1973) reads أولا *awwalan* (first), while the original translation likely had لا *lâ* (not)—that is, "Whence does the intellect in potency come to know all things if what brings it to act is *not* knowing all things?"

Abstraction by the individual human being's actual intellect takes place only under the intrinsic presence of the productive intellect, which already itself contains the intelligible forms. This is something which may function as guaranteeing that abstraction of intelligibles by the individual actual intellect matches with the real transcendent intelligible forms.[122]

In the account of Themistius, then, Averroes finds the needed principle asserting that there must be but one thesaurus of intelligibles in act for the unity of intellectual understanding and scientific discourse. Where Themistius wrote, "For we would not understand one another unless there were a single intellect that we all shared," Averroes found in the Arabic, "For it is right that, if we do not have one intellect in which we all share, then we also do not have understanding of one another." In adopting this conception of intelligibles in act, Averroes responded to the question raised in *Epistle 1 On Conjunction* which had to be resolved before the material intellect could be asserted as unique and shared by all human beings.

In the *Long Commentary*, however, Averroes does not follow Themistius in holding that the agent intellect (corresponding to productive intellect in Themistius) precontains the intelligibles in act. Rather, Averroes insists that the human attainment of intelligibles in act comes about only through external and internal powers of individual human souls existing in bodies. As indicated above, if images and intentions from personal worldly experience are not present in the soul's powers, an individual human being has no means of attaining intelligibles in act of things of the world. For human beings all intellectual understanding of the world necessarily comes through or with sense perception. Nevertheless, while rejecting the conception of the agent intellect as containing exemplar intelligibles in act, Averroes embraces and makes his own the Themistian notion that the agent intellect must necessarily be understood to penetrate the human soul so profoundly in the activity of intellectual understanding as to be "in" the soul as "form for us"—that is, as its formal cause in a fashion discussed at length below.[123]

Thus, Averroes answers the three key questions motivating this portion of his detailed study as follows. (1) The agent intellect and the material intellect are eternal substances and are related to the perishable theoretical intellect as first and final actualities, functioning intrinsic to the human intellective soul yet existing separately. The intelligibles in act shared in the perishable theoretical intellect are themselves eternal when in the material intellect as their subject; as shared by the individual human being, they are perishable with the perishable nature of their human subject. (2) This material intellect can be

---

122. Cf. the remarks of Todd at Themistius, *De Anima Paraphrase* (1990), 104, n. 119.
123. See below pp. lxvii–lxxv.

shared by all human beings insofar as the disposition for understanding as first actuality is common to the human species. Nevertheless, intellectual understanding is individual for each human being since it is linked to an individual's personal will and effort, as evidenced in the formation of denuded particular intentions by the individual's cogitative power or imaginative power generally so called. These are presented to the separate intellects in the process of abstraction, a process which remains rooted in the experiences and efforts of the individual for its content. The final perfected state of knowing is in this way achieved individually when the knower is the subject on which the truth of the intelligible rests and that individual is linked to the material intellect, which is the subject for the intelligible's existence in act. (3) The coherence of this doctrine requires that the material intellect be an immaterial receptive substance and an intellect insofar as it is receptive of intelligibles in act and functions as a thesaurus of intelligibles in act, which is the single, distinct set of referents or scientific universals in thought and speech. As such, it is a unique "fourth kind of being" {409}, something which is both receptive and at the same time an immaterial intellect and, in a way, eternally in act.

Two Separate and Distinct Intellectual Substances: Material Intellect and Agent Intellect

The relationship of this material intellect and the agent intellect is taken up in some detail in Book 3, Comments 18–20. Working from a faulty Text of *De Anima*, 430a14–17, where Aristotle speaks of two intellects while Averroes' Arabic Text of the *De Anima* mentions three, Averroes skillfully makes sense of the passage by reading it as a discussion of the material intellect, agent intellect, and the intellect in a positive disposition (العقل بالملكة *al'aql bi-l-malakah*, *intellectus in habitu*). This last is the intellect insofar as it is in a particular human being subsequent to the formation of an intelligible in act in the material intellect since it concerns "the generated intelligible." All three of these are distinct in substance for Averroes, who holds the agent intellect and material intellect to be two intellectual substances and the intellect in a positive disposition to be a power of the particular human being.[124] The reasoning, he writes, "which forced us to suppose the agent intellect" involves the analogy with sight and light. "For just as sight is not moved by colors except when they are in act, which is not realized unless light is present since it is what draws them

---

124. "Two of these three are eternal, namely, the agent and the recipient; the third is generable and corruptible in one way, eternal in another way" {406}. "And because the intellect which is in a positive disposition is one of the generable beings, it is necessary that, when it will have come to the end in generation, it come to the end in its activity" {489}.

from potency into act, so too the imagined intentions do not move the material intellect except when the intelligibles are in act, because it is not actualized by these unless something else is present, namely, the intellect in act" {439}. In this way the contribution of the higher internal human powers of imagination, cogitation, and memory, based on sense perception, provides the content of knowing originally as intelligibles in potency to be made into intelligibles in act by the agent intellect and received by the material intellect. Expressly rejecting the notion that "the intelligibles" are able to "enter into the material intellect from the agent intellect, without the material intellect needing to behold sensible forms" {438}, he concludes, "Hence, in view of our having asserted that the relation of the imagined intentions {439} to the material intellect is just as the relation of the sensibles to the senses (as Aristotle will say later), it is necessary to suppose that there is another mover which makes [the intentions] move the material intellect in act (and this is nothing but to make [the intentions] intelligible in act by separating them from matter)." This, he writes, "forces the assertion of an agent intellect different from the material intellect and different from the forms of things which the material intellect apprehends" {439}. "It was necessary to ascribe these two activities to the soul in us, namely, to receive the intelligible and to make it, although the agent and the recipient are eternal substances, on account of the fact that these two activities are reduced to our will, namely, to abstract intelligibles and to understand them" {439}.

The nature of the agent intellect in itself has no receptivity of the sort found in the material intellect and does not have understanding of worldly forms: "the agent intelligence understands nothing of the things which are here" {441}. Still, like all entities other than the First Cause, it has a different sort of receptivity insofar as its being has within it a reference to something outside itself, scil. the First Cause, which is the final cause of all and equivocally also the formal and efficient cause of all.[125] While it is an eternal entity posited to

125. See n. 101 above and also see Taylor (1998a), nn. 30, 31, and 48. The First Cause is also "the First Knower, who understands nothing outside Himself" {420}. In his *Incoherence of the Incoherence*, Averroes writes: "The difference between the First's understanding of Itself and the understanding of themselves which the rest of the intellects have is that the First Intellect understands Itself as existing through Itself, not as what is related to a cause, while the rest of the intellects understand themselves as being related to their cause so that plurality enters into these in this way. For it is not necessary that they all be in one grade of simplicity since they are not in a single grade in relation to the First Principle and none of them exists simply in the sense in which the First is simple, because the First is considered to exist by Itself, while they are in related existence (في الوجود المضاف *fî-l-wujûd al-muḍâf*)." *Incoherence of the Incoherence* (1930), 204. My translation. Cf. *Incoherence of the Incoherence* (1969), 122. Also see *Long Commentary on the Metaphysics* (1952), 1697, ll. 6–9; (1962), c. 51, 335vI, where he explains, "The

account for human intellectual abstraction and its operation is an intellectual one which thereby might be called understanding, properly speaking the agent intellect functions as what "transfers" intelligibles in potency to the realm of the intellect, where they are intelligibles in act in the material intellect. "After he had recounted these things which it has in common with the material intellect, he gave the disposition proper to the agent intellect. He said: **and in its substance it is activity**, that is, there is in it no potency {441} for something, as there is in the recipient intellect potency for receiving forms. For the agent intelligence understands nothing of the things which are here. It was necessary that the agent intelligence be separate, unmixed and impassible, insofar as it is what makes all forms intelligible."[126] However, Averroes' description of these two intellects in Book 3, Comment 20, has led some to consider that these are in themselves just one intellectual substance.[127] There he writes, "Generally, when someone will consider the material intellect with the agent intellect, {451} they will appear to be two in a way and one in another way. For they are two in virtue of the diversity of their activity, for the activity of the agent intellect is to generate while that of the former is to be informed. They are one, however, because the material intellect is actualized through the agent [intellect] and understands it. In this way we say that two powers appear in the intellect conjoined with us, of which one is active and the other of the genus of passive powers." His meaning here is that these distinct substances can be regarded

---

intellect of that which thinks any thing whatever follows that thing which it thinks, that is, it is always below it in rank; it is a primary notion of ours that the divine intellect must be in the highest degree of excellence and perfection." Ibid. (1984), 193. In the *Incoherence of the Incoherence* he explains as follows: "It is not necessary that the existence of the intellect and the intelligible in separate intellects as one and the same be such that they are all equal in simplicity. For [the philosophers] hold that in this notion the intellects surpass [one another] to greater or lesser degrees and that this [simplicity] exists in reality only in the First Intellect. The reason for this is that the essence of the First Intellect is subsistent per se, while the rest of the intellects understand by their essences that they subsist through [the First Intellect]." *Incoherence of the Incoherence* (1930), 204. My translation. Cf. ibid. (1969), 123.

126. Cf. "This is one of these things by which this intellect is distinguished from the agent intellect, namely, that in this intellect each is found, while in the agent [intellect] only act [is found], not potency. For this reason Aristotle rightly called that intellect *material*, not because it is mixed and has matter, as Alexander held" {463}.

127. For example, this was the view of Alfred L. Ivry in Ivry (1991), 693. However, in Ivry (1999), 210–211, Ivry has come to understand the two intellects to be distinct substances in the *Long Commentary*. My understanding of Averroes is that these are two distinct intellectual substances existing in separation from matter, in accord with the view of Davidson (1992), 292–293, 332–333.

as one insofar as the actuality of the agent intellect takes place in the recipient material intellect, following the Aristotelian notion that the actuality of the agent and that of the patient are one but under two descriptions.[128] In this context, however, this does not entail that they are literally one substance. Rather, in light of the foregoing, it is evident that the argument of Averroes required two distinct substances and that he held to this view.

The Cogitative Power and Conjoining with Separate Intellect

With the establishment of the natures of the material intellect and the agent intellect, it remains to return to a consideration of the cogitative power and to recount the more robust explanation of individual human thinking and the nature and role of the higher internal senses in Averroes' new doctrine of intellectual understanding in the *Long Commentary*. The initial account of the cogitative power, "a particular material power" {476}, given above, stresses its role in the distillation of denuded particular intentions from imagination {415} and the placement of purified intentions of particulars in memory. In this way the particular human soul's cogitative power is responsible for the processing of the particular intentions then presented to the rational power properly so called—namely, the material intellect and the agent intellect in their combined activity, which "discerns universal intentions" {416} or intelligibles in act. When that activity takes place, a human being is in the state called "acquired intellect" since it is involved in the immediate activity of knowing. This acquisition of intelligibles results in the actualization of the human soul as "intellect in a positive disposition" of knowing. In reference to the content of knowledge realized in the material intellect thanks to the contribution of the cogitative power and the intellectual actualizing of the intelligibles in potency by the agent intellect, the term "theoretical intellect" is used to denote the content of knowing now present to the particular human knower.

This activity belonging to particular human beings and called knowing can also be considered as a form of joining, conjoining, or uniting with the agent intellect: "when the theoretical intelligibles are united with us through forms of the imagination and the agent intellect is united with the theoretical intelligibles (for that which apprehends [theoretical intelligibles] is the same, namely, the material intellect), it is necessary that the agent intellect be united with us through the conjoining of the theoretical intelligibles" {500}. However, this conjoining is not merely the generation of intelligibles by the

---

128. "There is nothing to prevent two things from having one and the same actualization (not the same in being, but related as the potential to the actual)." Aristotle, *Physics* (1984), 3.3, 202b9–10.

agent intellect in some particular human subject as "a cause acting upon us only," as al-Fârâbî is alleged to have taught in his lost *Commentary on the Nicomachean Ethics* {485}. Rather, it must involve a relation of the human subject to the agent intellect, described analogically as that of matter to form.

> It is also evident that, when we assert that the material intellect is generable and corruptible, we will then find no way in which the agent intellect will be united with the intellect which is in a positive disposition by a uniting proper to it, namely, with a uniting similar to the conjoining of forms with matters.
>
> When that conjoining has not been asserted, there will be no difference between relating it to a human being and relating it to all beings except in virtue of the diversity of its activity in them. In this way its relation to a human being will be only the relation of the agent to the human being, not a relation of form, and the question of al-Fârâbî which he voiced in his *Commentary on the Nicomachean Ethics* arises. For assurance of the possibility of the conjoining of the intellect with us lies in explaining that its relation to a human being is a relation of form and agent, not a relation of agent alone. {502}

The appropriate sort of conjoining must be such that the agent intellect is not merely an extrinsic generating cause bringing about intelligibles in act in the human subject for the reason cited above—namely, because the metaphysics of the issues as analyzed by Averroes precludes the particular human subject from receiving the intelligibles in act as such without particularizing them. Further, were the agent intellect only extrinsic, the intellectual or rational nature would not be intrinsic or per se but rather seemingly *per aliud* and *per accidens*. Averroes does not explicitly cite these reasons, but they follow from principles adopted earlier in this work. For Averroes, to describe the conjoining suitably requires that we be conjoined to the agent intellect in an intrinsic way, having it as "form for us" and "our final form."[129]

In a composite material entity, the conjoining of matter to form is such that the potentiality intrinsic to the matter is brought to actuality by the form in a genuine hylemorphism of a single actual being, not such that matter and form remain two distinct things in the material entity. Rather, these two are principles of the being of one thing, one entity. Similarly, the relation of the material intellect to the agent intellect is such that the agent intellect is form or formal cause for the material intellect, although the two remain distinct sub-

---

129. {445}, {486}, {490}. This notion is derived from Alexander of Aphrodisias as Averroes understood him. See below, pp. lxxxii–lxxxiii and lxxxvi. For a detailed discussion, see Taylor (2005).

stances even though the agent intellect is "in" the material intellect. "When he said: **And when it is separate, it is only what it is**, not mortal, he means the agent intellect insofar as it is form for the material intellect, and this is the theoretical intellect according to him. That question will concern the agent intellect insofar as it is in contact with the material intellect (this is the theoretical intellect)" {445}. The result of this "composition" or presence of the agent intellect "in" the material intellect is manifold: it brings about the actualization of intelligibles in potency in the material intellect as intelligibles in act through the actuality of the agent intellect, and it brings about the acquired intellect and the consequent theoretical intellect in the intellect in a positive disposition in the human subject, as explained above.

> When the theoretical intelligibles are united with us through forms of the imagination and the agent intellect is united with the theoretical intelligibles (for that which apprehends [theoretical intelligibles] is the same, namely, the material intellect), it is necessary that the agent intellect be united with us through the conjoining of the theoretical intelligibles. It is evident [then] that, when all the theoretical intelligibles exist in us in potency, it will be united with us in potency. When all the theoretical intelligibles exist in us in act, it will then be united with us in act. And when certain [theoretical intelligibles] exist in potency and certain in act, then it will be united in one part and not in another. Then we are said to be moved to conjoining. {500}

What is more, it is also "form for us" because we are "able to generate intelligibles when we wish" {499}. And this follows, "For, because that in virtue of which something carries out its proper activity is the form, while we carry out {500} our proper activity in virtue of the agent intellect, it is necessary that the agent intellect be form in us."

The analogy of matter and form, however, has its limit, which must be noted. The agent intellect supplies the "light" by which the intelligibles in potency are affected so as to give rise to the intelligibles in act which are received into the material intellect. However, as already stated, unlike form in the material composite, the agent intellect does not provide from itself the quidditative content of the understood intelligible.[130] Rather, that content comes from the world by way of the senses and internal powers of the particular person.

> Now he gives the way on the basis of which it was necessary to assert the agent intelligence to be in the soul. For we cannot say that the relation of

---

130. What the agent intellect brings about must be sound abstractions of natural intelligibles because "It is impossible for false intelligibles to have conjoining, since they are not something occurring naturally" {502}. Cf. Black (1997).

the agent intellect in the soul to the generated intelligible is just as the relation of the artistry to the art's product in every way. For art imposes the form on the whole matter without it being the case that there was something of the intention of the form existing in the matter before the artistry has made it. It is not so in the case of the intellect, for if it were so in the case of the intellect, then a human being would not need sense or imagination for apprehending intelligibles. Rather, the intelligibles would enter into the material intellect from the agent intellect, without the material intellect needing to behold sensible forms. And neither can we even say that the imagined intentions are solely what move the material intellect and draw it out from potency into act. {438}

Sensation and consequent intentions in the imagination alone do not give rise to intelligibles in act. Agent intellect alone does not generate the content of intelligibles in act since in that case the apprehensive powers of sensation and imagination would be superfluous. The relationship of the material intellect, and thereby the theoretical intellect in a particular human knower, to the agent intellect, then, is appropriately described as a relationship in which the agent intellect is "form for us" as shared by us in the very act of intellectual abstraction. "When he said: **And when it is** separate, **it is what it is alone**, not mortal, he means when that intellect has been united to us and in virtue of it we understand other beings insofar as it is form for us, then this alone of the intellect's parts is not mortal. Next he said: **We do not remember**, etc. This is a question concerning the agent intellect insofar as it is united to us and in virtue of it we understand" {444}. And this conjoining comes about consequent to the voluntary efforts of particular human beings seeking intellectual understanding. Nevertheless, the cause of understanding is conjoining, not the reverse {501}. This conjoining is a means to intellectual understanding of the world for Averroes; intellectual understanding of the world is not a means to some sort of higher state of conjoining, as is the case for Ibn Bâjjah.[131]

This well-developed notion of agent intellect as an intrinsic formal cause that comes to be active in the soul of human beings in the course of intellectual understanding by conjoining is remarkably similar to the account of the agent intellect Averroes read in the *Paraphrase of the De Anima* by Themistius. Though different in ways mentioned above, the teachings of Themistius and Averroes coincide in the very special way that the productive intellect/agent intellect comes to be present formally and actively in the human process of forming intelligibles in act out of the imagination's intentions constituted from sense perception. For Themistius that abstraction could not take place without the participation of the productive intellect in the very activity of the indi-

131. See above, p. xxvi, and below, p. xci.

vidual actual intellect. Similarly, for Averroes the transference of intentions from the level of images potentially intelligible to the level of intelligibles in act can take place only insofar as the agent intellect comes to be "in" the soul and "form for us"—that is, only insofar as it is formally intrinsic to the individual human soul, providing the intellectual power for abstraction and the formation of intelligibles in act in the material intellect. For both Themistius and Averroes it is we who act when we wish or by will in the apprehension of intelligibles in act but only insofar as the power of the productive intellect/ agent intellect is formally present and active in us, drawing from forms in the imagination the content of the intelligibles in act.[132] This sort of participation or sharing in the power of the agent intellect is an essential part of Averroes' noetic doctrine which has gone unrecognized, perhaps due to the attention drawn to his novel doctrine of the material intellect.

The agent intellect, according to Averroes, is "form for us" also as "our final form" {490} "in the end" {499}. "In the beginning it is not conjoined with us" {450} since human beings are at that stage in "the first actuality of the intellect," which "is not a power in a body" {381}. That first actuality for knowing is "the disposition for intelligibles which is in the imaginative power" {405} together with "the material intellect in its first conjoining with us, namely, [in] the conjoining which is through nature" {450} at birth. The second or final actuality is the perfection of the potentiality for intellectual understanding in particular human beings, and its realization in us is the culmination of our fulfillment as rational beings. As intrinsic formal cause coming to the soul from outside by a sort of participation, the agent intellect is not separate from us when we are in the activity of knowing for "it is necessary that a human being understand all the intelligibles through the intellect proper to him and that he carry out the activity proper to him in regard to all beings, just as he understands by his proper intellection all the beings through the intellect which is in a positive disposition, when it has been conjoined with forms of the imagination" {500}. This development of intellect in human beings is natural but only realized in act if the innate potentiality for its actualization by way of the separate intellects in intellectual understanding is pursued by the particular human being. This is because "the material intellect is not united with us per se and initially but is united with us only in virtue of its uniting with the forms of the imagination" {486}. Thus, this "intellect proper to" a human being {500} is constituted in understanding by way of the internal powers of imagination, cogitation, and memory {476}, known collectively as "the passible intellect."

132. See Themistius, *De Anima Paraphrase* (1899), 91.20–21; (1996), 115; and (1899), 99.22–23; (1973), 180.5; (1990), 91; (1996), 123. For Averroes, see {439}.

This is confirmed by consideration of the use of intellect in the context of identifying and classifying particulars of experience. When a soldier sees a distant fire as a signal, he "puts the starting point of his consideration of possible things in present things which he sees" {474–475}. That is, we begin with consideration of experience and are able to understand present things and experiences in terms of prior intellectual understanding. In this way a human being manifests the presence of knowledge—that is, manifests the ability of the intellect in a positive disposition to reestablish its contact with the material intellect and thereby to understand a present particular in terms of the intelligible in act. This is simply understanding it *qua* instance of a universal notion. One power at work in this action is the cogitative power, which "draws aid for itself from the informative and the memorative [powers]." It forms "on the basis of the images of things something which it never sensed, in the same disposition according to which it would exist if it had sensed it, by means of assent and conceptualization. Then the intellect will judge those images with a universal judgment" {476}. In this mixed action involving particulars and universals, it is the particular human being who voluntarily initiates by will the action of intellect used in judgment involving reference to intelligibles in act as universals. And it is the cogitative power which moves the will insofar as desire prompted by cogitation is properly speaking will (اراده *irâdah voluntas*), while desire initiated in the absence of cogitation is appetite {519}. In this sense, then, human agency in the original attainment of knowledge and also in the use of already attained knowledge for understanding particulars of experience belongs primarily to the cogitative power or to the ensemble of the imagination, cogitation, and memory, which together can be generally called the imaginative power.[133] To this extent, then, will has to be conceived as being a particular bodily power, as is the cogitative power, and not a power of intellect per se, since the cogitative power is not a power of intellect per se. As a consequence, Averroes' account of the soul in the *Long Commentary* has no provision for the continued existence after death of the individual human agent responsible for moral activity.[134]

The foregoing explains, regarding the material intellect (together with our own particular intellects), "how it understands what has long existed with a

133. "The intellect existing in us has two activities insofar as it is ascribed to us, one of the genus of affection, namely, understanding, and the other of the genus of activity, namely, to extract forms and denude them of matters, which is nothing but making them intelligible in act after they were such in potency. [Hence] it is evident that, after we have possessed the intellect which is in a positive disposition, it is in our will to understand any intelligible we wish and to extract any form we wish" {495}.

134. See Taylor (1998b). Regarding this issue and the attack upon Averroes by Aquinas over the will, see Taylor (2000a) and (1999b).

new intellection" and "why we are not conjoined with this intellect in the beginning but rather in the end" {501}. In order for a particular person to come to have knowledge, it is required for that person to supply intentions intelligible in potency to the separate rational power (agent intellect and material intellect) with personal effort by the directing cogitative power. This is nothing more than to undertake voluntarily the pursuit of knowledge and understanding. Such a thing is possible for human beings because of a natural affiliation of the human soul with the separate material intellect and agent intellect which makes possible the fulfillment of the end of human beings consequent upon their natures as rational beings. This is affirmed by Averroes in his *Commentary on Plato's Republic* (perhaps written around 1195), where he writes, "The purpose of man, inasmuch as he is a natural being, is that he ascend to . . . the intelligibles of the theoretical sciences."[135] There he also writes, "This [intellectual understanding of the theoretical sciences] is man's ultimate perfection and ultimate happiness."[136] The end of human beings is just this realization of knowledge, with the agent intellect as the final perfective form, something toward which the human species is naturally directed but something which is attained individually, not collectively.[137]

This attainment of the end of human beings is for Averroes an epistemological account of human intellectual perfection and not a religiously based experience of the divine. Conjoining (اتصال *ittiṣâl continuatio*) with separate intellect is neither some mystical moment nor a non-intellectual experiential stage in human fulfillment. Rather, it is the grasping of intelligibles in act, knowing, and the philosophical understanding consequent upon that which is the end of human beings, not conjoining as such. As indicated above, conjoining with separate intellect is better characterized as the means to the attainment of the true end of human beings—namely, the fulfillment of knowledge. The pursuit of this goal, particularly in its metaphysical investigation of the nature of being, constitutes the Sharî'ah, religious law or set of religious duties, incumbent on philosophers:

> The *Sharî'ah* specific to the philosophers (الحكماء *al-hukamâ'*) is the investigation of all beings, since the Creator is not worshipped by a worship more noble than the knowledge of those things that He produced which

135. *On Plato's Republic* (1974), 88.

136. *On Plato's Republic* (1974), 86. My addition.

137. In *Epistle 1 On Conjunction* Averroes mentions that the fact that some human beings are unable to have higher contemplation of intelligibles does not mean that it is not something possible for others. Geoffroy and Steel (2001), 218. That is, it is a perfection characteristic of the human species as its end but not shared by all human beings in its ultimate perfection or actuality. Cf. Taylor (2007), 50.

lead to the knowledge in truth of His essence—may He be exalted! That [investigation philosophers undertake] is the most noble of the works belonging to Him and the most favored of them that we do in God's presence. How great is it that one perform this service which is the most noble of services and one take it on with this compliant obedience which is the most sublime of obediences![138]

Averroes' Major Philosophical Resources for the *Long Commentary*

Aristotle's *De Anima*

Averroes' *Long Commentary on the De Anima* is a continuation of the Greek commentary tradition and makes extensive use of the work of Alexander and Themistius, as well as that of his Andalusian predecessor, Ibn Bâjjah. Al-Fârâbî's work on intellect also plays an important role in Averroes' reflections even if, as with his other sources just mentioned, he rejects its apparent conclusions. And while there is little mention of Avicenna, Averroes was well aware of the approach to intellect and soul taken by his important predecessor. Still, first and foremost, Averroes was engaged with the text of Aristotle's *De Anima*.

In composing his *Long Commentary*, Averroes made use of two different translations of the *De Anima*. He quotes his alternate or secondary translation some ten times and at various other times seems to consult it without citation.[139] This translation, which is the sole complete medieval Arabic translation extant today, has been edited by 'Abdurrahman Badawi, who, following the manuscript attribution, incorrectly identified this as the reported second, improved and complete, translation by Isḥâq Ibn Ḥunayn.[140] This anonymous Arabic translation, less accurate and precise, is likely of an era earlier than the Text quoted in its entirety in the *Long Commentary*.[141] In the notes to the present English translation the corresponding Arabic text from the edition by Badawi is quoted with English translation where substantive difference between the Latin and Arabic is noted.

The primary translation found complete in the Latin Text of the *Long Com-*

---

138. *Long Commentary on the Metaphysics* (1952), 10.11–16. This text was not available in the Latin translation.

139. See {46}, {86}, {218}, {284–285}, {452}, {469}, {480}, {514–515}, {519}, and {526}.

140. Aristotle, *De Anima* (1954), (16). Also see Arnzen (1998), 690–707. For the *status questionis* regarding the translations of the *De Anima* into Syriac and Arabic, see Elamrani-Jamal (2003).

141. Frank (1958–1959) established that this was not the work of Isḥâq Ibn Ḥunayn. Also see Gätje (1971), 20–44, esp. 42–44, where he suggests the translator may be the Christian Ibn Nâ'ima.

mentary is not extant in Arabic, though it does bear some relation to quotations by Avicenna in his surviving marginal notes on the *De Anima* published by Badawi.[142] However, in addition to the Latin, this text of the *De Anima* has also survived in Hebrew translation attributed to Zeraḥyah ben Isaac ben Shealtiet Ḥen (fl. late thirteenth century), recently edited by Gerrit Bos, who established the Hebrew and Latin to be ultimately from the same Arabic translation. The precise provenance of this lost Arabic translation of the *De Anima* is a matter of considerable scholarly dispute and has yet to be fully determined. Bos prefers to follow Helmut Gätje in part and Moritz Steinschneider in holding that this version of the *De Anima* was partially translated into Syriac by Ḥunayn Ibn Isḥâq, completed by his son Isḥâq, and finally rendered into Arabic by Ibn Zur'a.[143] In a study published in 2001 Alfred Ivry confirmed that these Latin and Hebrew texts come for the most part from a single Arabic translation, though he argues "for Isḥâq ibn Ḥunayn as the common source for most of the *De anima* quotations and paraphrases brought by Avicenna, Averroes and Zeraḥyah."[144] Ivry observes that for the *Middle Commentary* "Averroes frequently utilized Themistius' undeclared quotations and paraphrases of Aristotle (often practically identical with their sources)" and also a text of the *De Anima* from the same translator as that of the *Long Commentary*.[145] After establishing to his satisfaction by way of detailed consideration of seven significant textual examples that Isḥâq is the translator of the lost Arabic *De Anima* and also the translator of the *Paraphrase* of Themistius, Ivry concludes with an important qualification: "The above illustrations are not meant to claim that Averroes, Zeraḥyah and the Latin translator always had the exactly identical text before them, given the inevitable corruptions in the transmission of texts, and the likelihood of different recensions of Isḥâq's translation. But the Aristotle who emerges from all this is nevertheless predominantly the one Isḥâq ibn Ḥunayn presented to the Muslim philosophers, giving them thereby a common basis for their deliberations."[146]

The importance of that qualification becomes evident from the careful con-

142. See Ibn Sînâ, *Notes on the De Anima* (1947). The *Long Commentary*'s Text begins its third book at *De Anima* 3.4, 429a10–13, as did the version used by Avicenna. See Gutas (1988), 61, n. 3. Also see Elamrani-Jamal (2003), 351.

143. Aristotle, *De Anima* (1994), 9–12, particularly 10, n. 3. Steinschneider (1893), (1956), 146. See Elamrani-Jamal (2003), 350, regarding an unfortunate misstatement of his own position by Bos at Aristotle, *De Anima* (1994), 12.

144. Ivry (2001), 64.

145. Ivry (2001), 65. As noted above, Ivry's view is that the *Long Commentary* preceded the *Middle*. He holds that Averroes used Aristotelian lemmata from the *Long Commentary* and his copy of the *De Anima* while writing the *Middle Commentary*.

146. Ivry (2001), 77. The literature and issues concerning the medieval Arabic texts of the *De Anima* are also reviewed by Elamrani-Jamal, who concludes that there were

sideration of the use of the vocabulary of cogitation (*cogitatio, cogitare, virtus cogitativa, cogitabile*) in the Text of the *De Anima* in the *Long Commentary*. As indicated above, the cogitative power is a particular discursive power of the brain for sorting through and denuding images in its role in the process of the formation of intelligibles in act. And it likewise plays an important role in the calling back to mind intelligibles in act previously attained. Moreover, Averroes regards this bodily power as bearing most of the responsibility for activities of will and effort on the part of individual human beings dealing with particular matters and concerns. What is remarkable in the case of the *Long Commentary* is to find just this sort of doctrine in the very Text of the Latin *De Anima* though it is not found in the original Greek. As I have argued elsewhere,[147] while the Text of the *Long Commentary* is from the same Arabic translation as the Hebrew translation by Zeraḥyah, they are from different recensions of that translation. This is evident because the Latin Text often renders a wide array of Greek terms (λογιστικός, λογισμός, λογίζομαι, διανοέομαι, διάνοια, perhaps ὑπολαμβάνω, βουλεύω, βουλευτικός, and δόξα) by *cogitare, cogitatio* and other forms of the same root, although the Hebrew generally reflects the Greek more precisely in preserving distinctions between these terms. Careful consideration of the Latin translation gives no support to the view that

---

three Arabic versions: a first incomplete translation by Isḥâq Ibn Ḥunayn; an anonymous complete translation edited by Badawi; and a second complete translation, possibly the purported second version by Isḥâq Ibn Ḥunayn, preserved today in the Latin of the *Long Commentary* and in the Hebrew of Zeraḥyah ben Isaac ben Shealtiet Ḥen. Elamrani-Jamal also notes that the *Middle Commentary* follows the traditional Greek divisions of the text in contrast to the non-traditional divisions found in Avicenna and in Averroes' *Long Commentary*. Elamrani-Jamal (2003), 351. However, the traditional divisions of the *Middle Commentary* may well be a consequence of Averroes' heavy dependence on the *Paraphrase* of Themistius rather that an indication of his possession of a text of the *De Anima* with the traditional divisions of the books different from the text used for the *Long Commentary*. In a forthcoming entry on Ibn Bâjjah in the online *Stanford Encyclopedia of Philosophy*, Josep Puig Montada includes a supplement on the Arabic translations of the *De Anima*. He holds that the first was the extant anonymous translation edited by Badawi (Aristotle, *De Anima* [1954]), a later second translation was done by Isḥâq Ibn Ḥunayn, and, completing the second, a third translation was perhaps by Ibn Zurʿa, which begins at 431a14. As indicated above, Averroes cited the first, older translation just ten times and included all of the Isḥâq translation with his commentary without indicating any awareness that it may have been completed by a text from another translator. In a reading of the Isḥâq translation through the extant Latin Text, it is far from evident that its Arabic source after 431a14 is by a different translator. Further research on these matters is necessary before definitive determinations may be made.

147. Taylor (1999a), 243ff.

this is the result of changes by the Latin translator. Moreover, Averroes' Comments reflect precisely these Texts, indicating the changed Text was before his eyes. Nor can it be argued that the translator rendering the text into Arabic was responsible for this since the Hebrew retains distinctions of the Greek. To that extent, at least on the issue of the rendering of these distinct terms, the Hebrew bears witness to a superior Arabic rendering of the Greek.[148] For example, Text (18) of the *Long Commentary*, at 430a14–17 {437}, incorrectly refers to three intellects, though the Greek mentions only two. In this case the Hebrew is in accord with the Greek. And in this case one can see that the *Middle Commentary on the De Anima*, for which Averroes appears to have used just one translation, seems to access a redaction different from that of the *Long Commentary* since the corresponding passage of the *Middle Commentary* is in accord with the Greek, not the Text of the *Long Commentary*.[149] How it came to pass that Averroes used different redactions of the Isḥāq translation in the *Middle Commentary* and in the *Long Commentary* and how it happened that the *Long Commentary* came to have a faulty Text more congruous with Averroes' new teachings on the cogitative power than the original Arabic *De Anima* are unclear at present and must remain issues for future research.

Theophrastus

Averroes' knowledge of the doctrines of Theophrastus (371–287 B.C.) on the intellect as discussed in the *Long Commentary* comes solely from the citations of Theophrastus in the *Paraphrase* of Themistius.[150] For the most part the name of Theophrastus occurs in the company of that of Themistius though once with that of Nicolaus of Damascus (ca. 64–4 B.C.) {432}. Consideration of the notion that the material intellect cannot be of the genus of the receptivity found in composite substances or in prime matter is said by Averroes to have "brought Theophrastus, Themistius, and several commentators to hold the opinion that the material intellect is a substance which is neither generable nor corruptible" {389}. "Theophrastus, Themistius, and others" are also said to hold that the theoretical intellect (the intellect in a positive disposition) is affected by its mixture with the powers of particular individuals, sometimes weakening it and at other times strengthening it {390–391}. On another occasion Averroes

148. "The Hebrew, however, clearly uses different terms in at least seven cases in which forms of *cogitatio* in the Latin are used to render forms of διανοέομαι (two times), διάνοια (two times), and βουλευτικός (three times)." Taylor (1999a), 246.

149. See {437} and the note to that Text with references to the *Middle Commentary* and the Hebrew *De Anima*.

150. This is clearly established by Gutas (1999b). The text is at Themistius, *De Anima Paraphrase* (1899), 107.30–109.3; (1973), 195–198; (1990), 113–117; (1996), 133–134.

remarks that he shares with these thinkers the view "that the material intellect is a power which has not come into being" {392}.

Of greatest philosophical significance for present concerns are Averroes' comments on the so-called

> question of Theophrastus, namely, that it is necessary to assert that this intellect has no form and it is necessary to assert also that it is a being; and if not, there would be neither a reception nor a disposition. For the disposition and reception result from the fact that they are not found in a subject. Since it is a being and does not have the nature of a form, then it remains that it has the nature of prime matter, which is altogether unthinkable, for prime matter is neither apprehensive nor discerning. How can this be said regarding something the being of which is such that it is separate?[151] {399}

It is in part this issue which prompts Averroes to take the radical step of asserting his doctrine of the separate and unique material intellect shared by all human knowers. To accommodate the requirements of his analysis of the problems of Aristotle, and in particular that of the necessity that the material intellect be a power in the soul, Averroes takes what for loyal disciples of Aristotle is the ironic step of setting forth a novel interpretation on the nature of the material intellect. As already noted above, he writes that "one should hold that it is a fourth kind of being. For just as sensible being is divided into form and matter, so too intelligible being must be divided into things similar to these two, namely, into something similar to form and into something similar to matter" {409}. That is, the material intellect is both intellect and also receptivity so that the intelligibles may be understood as received into an immaterial intellect. The novelty lies in the contradiction of the common notion of the Greek and Arabic tradition that immaterial intellect—that is, separate existing form—must be actuality without potency. Yet the solution of the problem of the understanding of intelligibles in act requires that these be in an immaterial intellect, indeed, in an immaterial intellect which is not a determinate particular of a species. For the intelligibles understood by human beings to exist as the unique intelligibles in act which make possible the unity of human thought and its referents (and not merely spiritual forms derivative upon the true intelligibles in act, after the fashion of Ibn Bâjjah),[152] they must be unique, immaterial, and present in one shared intellect.[153]

As indicated above, this new doctrine prompted by the "question of Theo-

---

151. See Themistius, *De Anima Paraphrase* (1899), 107.30–108.8; (1973), 195–196; (1996), 133. The Arabic of the account of Theophrastus is translated by Gutas in Huby (1999), 120.

152. See below, p. xci.

153. The "question of Theophrastus" presented Averroes with an account of the material intellect quite different from that of Themistius, in whose *Paraphrase* the cita-

phrastus" proved for Averroes that receptivity exists in separate intellect—
namely, the material intellect. By extending this receptivity to all separate
intellects with the sole exception of God, Averroes provided grounds on the
basis of which he was able to assert a hierarchy of separate intellects distinguished not only *per accidens* by the various motions they cause in the heavens,
but also *per se* by their very natures.[154]

Alexander of Aphrodisias

The *De Anima* and the *De Intellectu* of Alexander of Aphrodisias (fl. ca. 200 CE)
in Arabic were studied carefully, used, and quoted by Averroes in the *Long Commentary*.[155] On the challenging issue of the material intellect, Averroes read Al-

---

tion of Theophrastus on intellect was contained. While for Themistius what Averroes
calls the agent intellect was shared and the ground for intersubjective discourse and
knowing, Averroes saw Theophrastus as giving reasons for that grounding in a single
shared material intellect. This provides the response to the issue raised by Dimitri
Gutas when he writes, "The conclusions reached here raise the question why *Averroes*
bothered to mention Theophrastus if he had no access to an independent work by him
and if Theophrastus' views were shared by Themistius, and what this indicates about
Averroes' conception of the praxis of philosophy. This very significant question deserves
separate study." Gutas (1999b), 144. Theophrastus pointed out the need for the receptive
(material) intellect to be intellect yet also receptive, to have at once the nature of form
and the nature of receptivity, two normally incompatible characteristics in immaterial
entities insofar as form without matter is per se actual and determinate.

154. See Taylor (forthcoming a) and Harry A. Wolfson's (1958) discussion of the issue
of the plurality and distinction of separate substances: "According to the mediaeval explanations there is some kind of distinction of prior and posterior in the immaterial
movers themselves, whereas according to our explanation [of Aristotle] there is no distinction at all in the immaterial movers themselves; the distinction between them is only
a distinction in their relation to things outside themselves—a distinction of external relation which, as we have shown, does not affect their nature. Now the assumption on the
part of the mediaevals of a distinction of prior and posterior, whether that of cause or
that of nobility, in the immaterial movers themselves has led to those endless questions
as to whether that distinction does not after all imply a relationship of matter and form
and also as to whether that relationship of matter and form is compatible with the initial
assumption that these immovable movers are immaterial. But to assume, as we do, that
the distinction between the immaterial immovable movers is only a distinction in their
relation to things outside themselves does not lead to any of those questions" (248–249).

155. The *De Anima* of Alexander is not extant in Arabic (see Alexander, *De Anima*
[1887], [1979]), but the *De Intellectu* is. See Alexander, *De Intellectu* (1887), (2004), (1990),
(1971), (1956). Regarding the *De Intellectu* in Arabic, see Geoffroy (2002). The work of
Alexander is also discussed in the *Short* and *Middle Commentaries*. For precise passages,

exander as wrongly holding that the material intellect was nothing but the disposition (ἐπιτηδειότης اسـتعداد, *isti'dâd*) itself for the reception of intelligibles, not itself in a subject {395, 430–433, 443–444}. Averroes understood Alexander to believe that this disposition was something which arose from a mixture of physical causes {118, 397–398}. He expounded this as set forth in the *De Anima* of Alexander and then went on to quote the *De Intellectu*: "It is a power made from a mixture which occurred in bodies, [a power] disposed to receive the intellect which is in act" {394}. Both of these views are vehemently attacked by Averroes in the *Long Commentary*. Aristotle writes of the material intellect as a substance which is a disposition and *subject* for the reception of immaterial intelligibles, argues Averroes, not the mere disposition itself {395}. In this Alexander was confused by equivocation regarding the notion of first actuality, writes Averroes. Following Aristotle on the notion that the soul was the first actuality of the body, Alexander thought the first actuality of intellect—that is, the material intellect—must itself also be an actuality of body. Yet "to say *form* and *first actuality* is to speak equivocally about the rational soul and about the other parts of the soul" {397} simply because the activity of the rational part is immaterial while those of other parts of the soul take place in the body or are powers of a body. "It has therefore been explained that the first actuality of the intellect differs from the first actualities of the other powers of the soul and that this word 'actuality' is said of these in an equivocal way, contrary to what Alexander thought" {405}. Although soul and receptive material intellect are both first actualities, they are first actualities of completely different sorts: soul is the first actuality of body and material intellect is the first actuality of incorporeal intellect.

Averroes also railed against what he saw to be Alexander's contradictory accounts of the material intellect and its ability to know the agent intellect and separate forms in these two works. In the *De Anima* of Alexander, writes Averroes, the material intellect and the intellect in a positive disposition are both corruptible with their particular corporeal human subject, yet the intellect which is in us for understanding separate forms must be ungenerated and incorruptible for intellect's understanding to be possible. If understanding involves a noetic identity of knower and known, then a generated and corruptible material intellect will have to come to be eternal and incorruptible if it is to know the eternal intelligibles {481ff.}. Thus the intellect which understands intelligibles and the separate agent intellect can only be the acquired intellect which has come from outside, not the human material intellect {483}. Yet in his *De Intellectu* Alexander said that the intellect in potency (the material intellect), when "complete and fulfilled . . . will understand the agent intellect"

---

see the indices of the *Short Commentary on the De Anima* (1985) and the *Middle Commentary* (2002).

{483}. Reflecting on these accounts, Averroes concludes that Alexander's true meaning is that the actualization and fulfillment of the material intellect comes in conjoining with the agent intellect so that it is "the form effected in us" {484}. That is, the agent intellect comes to be *form for us* and, by its being our form, it is we who are able to understand the agent intellect and also the intelligibles which come to be in act from sensibles where they were in potency. Hence, the end is understanding, and the means to this is conjoining with the agent intellect.

For the development of Averroes' own thought on the nature of the material intellect and human knowing, Alexander's writings provide three crucial notions, though Averroes makes it clear he is no "Alexandrian" {433}. First, Averroes adopted the notion that the agent intellect is "form for us" as "our final form," as explicated above. This made it possible for him to argue that the activity of knowing is an activity intrinsic to individual human knowers thanks to this natural presence of the power of agent intellect "in" and at the disposal of our will {439–440}. Here also Averroes follows Alexander in understanding the human intellect in a positive disposition as the theoretical intellect to be an entity not fully identical with the agent intellect {448}. Second, he adopted the rationalist philosophical view that the human end is intellectual understanding via conjoining with the agent intellect. That conjoining is the means to the human end. There is no role here for mystical ascent or postmortem higher enlightenment. Intellectual understanding on the part of individual perishable human beings is the end for human beings, not a stage to something more. Third, he adopted Alexander's notion of the perishable nature of individual human knowers—that is, the perishable nature of what Averroes calls the theoretical intellect in individuals and the intellect in a positive disposition. Human beings, their corporeal powers of imagination, cogitation, and memory, and their sharing of knowledge in the theoretical intelligibles are all perishable with the natural perishability of their ultimate subject, the body.

Themistius

Averroes made use of the *Paraphrase of the De Anima* by Themistius (ca. 317–388 CE) for all three of his *Commentaries* on the *De Anima*, but it was particularly important for his *Middle Commentary* and his *Long Commentary*. For these works he appears to have made distinct readings of the *Paraphrase*.[156] As the notes to the present translation show, for all three books of his *Long Commentary* Aver-

156. Regarding the Arabic translation, see Lyons' introduction in Themistius, *De Anima Paraphrase* (1973) and Elamrani-Jamal (2003), 352–353. Also see Lyons (1955) and Browne (1986). Themistius' teachings on the soul are also mentioned by Averroes in his *Short Commentary*. For precise passages, see the indices of *Short Commentary on the De Anima* (1985). Lyons, in Themistius, *De Anima Paraphrase* (1973), 169–178, provides a

roes frequently consulted and employed this work by Themistius, often without explicit citation of his source. While there is some ambiguity in the *Paraphrase* itself concerning the nature of the intellect, Averroes understands Themistius to discuss four intellects. For Themistius these are the common intellect, the actual intellect, the potential intellect, and the productive intellect. In Averroes' terminology these correspond respectively to the passible intellect (the corporeal internal senses of the human soul—that is, common sense, imagination, cogitation, and memory); the trio acquired intellect—theoretical intellect—intellect in a positive disposition (in the human soul as formed by the action of the next two); the material intellect; and the agent intellect. They differ, however, regarding the natures of these. For Themistius the productive intellect is both transcendent and immanent, with each individual human being possessing, together with a particular potential intellect, a particular actual intellect which is also itself illuminated by the light of the single separate productive intellect. The intersubjective nature of human understanding comes about thanks to this connection of all particular actual intellects illuminated in their actuality by the one separate productive intellect, which contains the forms in act.[157] For Averroes in all his works there is a unity of the agent intellect as the cause of intellectual abstraction and as a cause of primary intellectual principles. However, for the *Long Commentary*, since the agent intellect is only one and in the individual it is the intrinsic formal cause of the activity of abstraction from sensed intentions in the imagination, the unity of human understanding is due to the unity of the material intellect.[158]

With Themistius, Averroes rejects Alexander's account of the material intel-

<hr/>

list of some citations of Themistius by Averroes in various works dealing with the issue of the intellect.

157. Themistius, *De Anima Paraphrase* (1899), 103.20ff; (1973), 187ff.; (1990), 103ff.; (1996), 128ff. "There is no need to be puzzled if we who are combined from the potential and the actual [intellects] are referred back to one productive intellect, and that what it is to be each of us is derived from that single [intellect]. Where otherwise do the notions that are shared (*koinai ennoiai*) come from? Where is the untaught and identical understanding of primary definitions and primary axioms derived from? For we would not understand one another unless there were a single intellect that we all shared." Ibid. (1996), 129. Ibid. (1899), 103.36–104.3; (1973), 188.17–189.4; (1990), 105. I understand Themistius to hold for a form of participation whereby the transcendent productive intellect comes to be present and acting in individual actual intellects. That the views of Themistius are decidedly influenced by Neoplatonism is held by a number of scholars. See Verbeke in Themistius, *De Anima Paraphrase* (1957), introduction, xl ff.; Ballériaux (1989); and Falcon (2005). Blumenthal (1979) understands the account to be more genuinely Aristotelian.

158. The *Paraphrase* of Themistius, its Arabic translation, and Averroes' understanding and use of that text require more study and discussion than permitted here. The

lect as solely a disposition associated with the perishable human body and instead holds it to be an eternal substance in its own right and ungenerated {392, 432–433}. The material intellect or "the intellect which is in potency is conjoined with us before the agent intellect" {447}, and it is this which "has the power to separate forms from matters and to understand them" {487}. For Averroes, Aristotle saw that the material intellect was not form or matter or composite and was followed in this by "Theophrastus, Themistius and several commentators" who "hold the opinion that the material intellect is a substance which is neither generable nor corruptible. For everything which is generable and corruptible is a determinate particular; but it has already been demonstrated that [the material intellect] is not a determinate particular nor a body nor a form in a body" {389}. According to Themistius and himself, Averroes writes, the material intellect and the agent intellect have something in common—namely, the theoretical intellect manifested in the individual human being {447}. For Themistius this theoretical intellect is nothing more than the very contact and conjoining of the agent intellect with the material intellect {444–446, 448, 406}. And the understanding which comes about for us thanks to a "conjoining with the intentions of the imagination" {452} is in fact learning as recollection. It is by our will and effort that the intelligibles of the theoretical intellect come to exist for us as we use intentions of the imagination (intelligibles in potency) to prompt the actualization of the material intellect with intelligibles in act by "the agent intellect insofar as it is form for the material intellect, and this is the theoretical intellect according to him" {445}. On this account of the thought of Themistius, the intelligibles in act are understood to exist first in the agent intellect and then in the material intellect, with recollection and learning being their realization in the material intellect through abstraction founded on sensory experience. This is why it can be said that they "are in [the material intellect] in a disposition diverse from their be-

---

Arabic text of the *Paraphrase* was far from clear, and in some passages it was up to Averroes to determine both what Themistius meant and what value it had for the issue at stake. In the important case of the nature of the agent intellect and its relation to the material intellect, the views of Themistius himself are complex, and the Arabic text required thoughtful interpretation by Averroes. The Arabic *Paraphrase* is extant in only one faulty manuscript, which has significant omissions and also displays some confusion in the understanding of the text. While it is clear that Averroes had more of the text than is now extant, it is not clear precisely how well the doctrines of Themistius were conveyed throughout. Note that in the *Middle Commentary*, as discussed above, Averroes embraced the view of Themistius that there are a plurality of individual material intellects deriving from the single separate agent intellect, though Averroes did not accept the plurality of agent intellects or actual intellects in individual human beings.

ing in the agent intellect" {452}. Averroes, however, rejects this particular sort of Platonic approach to the issue and holds instead for a genuine abstraction of the intelligible content of human understanding from experience of the world thanks to the enabling activity of the unique agent intellect and the receptive nature of the unique material intellect. For Averroes intelligibles in act do not preexist in the agent intellect.

The Themistian assertion of the separate material intellect was an important source of philosophical inspiration for Averroes, even if Themistius had asserted it to be many. For Averroes it contributed valuably to his reflections on the nature of theoretical intelligibles. He agreed with Alexander that the agent intellect was form for the generation of theoretical intelligibles in the material intellect but disagreed on the perishable nature of the material intellect. He agreed with Themistius on the separate nature of the material intellect but disagreed with him on the intellect in a positive disposition (the theoretical intellect) as constituted by recollection. Rather, as indicated above, for Averroes intelligibles in act are truly generated from intentions of the imagination derived from the world. The intellect in act is generated by the agent intellect's abstractive "light"; the intelligible is "transferred in its being from one order into another" {439} by the power of the agent intellect without the agent intellect itself giving forms as the content of understanding from its own nature. The only forms from the agent intellect are the first principles of reason, the primary natural intelligibles, which yield voluntary intelligibles—that is, intelligibles brought about by our will—when used with the abstractive power of the agent intellect and intentions of the imagination {496–497}. These theoretical intelligibles for Averroes have two subjects, the material intellect as their subject for existence and the human general imaginative power as their subject of truth. They are in the individual human theoretical intellect, where they are perishable, as is their subject, and they are in the material intellect, where they are eternal and imperishable, as is their subject, as explained above. Yet in spite of differences, Averroes does find in Themistius support for the Alexandrian notion that the agent intellect is form for the material intellect and in virtue of that it is "form for us" {445}.

al-Fârâbî

The work of al-Fârâbî (870–950 CE) on the intellect is foundational for later discussions of soul and intellect in Arabic philosophy, and Averroes drew on it for terminology and philosophical issues.[159] In the *Long Commentary* Averroes cites al-Fârâbî's lost *Commentary on Aristotle's On Generation and Corruption* {493} and

---

159. Regarding terminology, see Book 3, nn. 32 and 90. The language of "intelligibles in potency" and "intelligibles in act" found throughout the *Long Commentary* is also

his lost *Sophistic Refutations* {444},[160] makes extensive use of al-Fârâbî's *On Intellect and the Intelligible*—that is, *Letter on the Intellect* {420, 483, 486, 491, 493}—and contends strongly against the reported doctrine of the lost *Commentary on the Nicomachean Ethics* {433, 481, 485, 502}. The chief philosophical concern of Averroes regarding al-Fârâbî's account of intellect has to do with a notion central to Averroes' reading of Alexander and Themistius: the relation of the agent intellect to the intellect in us and the characterization of the agent intellect as "form for us."

Averroes understands al-Fârâbî to follow Alexander in holding the receptive material intellect to be a power of the perishable human soul which "abstracts the intentions of things which are outside the soul" {420}. This abstraction of intelligibles in potency brings about distinctly existing intelligibles in act in what al-Fârâbî called the acquired intellect only thanks to the assisting activity of the separate agent intellect which "is nothing but a cause acting upon us only" {485}. Through this a human being by the perfection of the acquired intellect approaches nearer to the agent intellect, no longer needing the body, and in this intellectual fulfillment attains its ultimate happiness.[161] Yet this is problematic in multiple ways, according to Averroes.

First, on this account of understanding, something generated and perishable

---

derived from al-Fârâbî. See, for example, al-Fârâbî, *Letter on the Intellect* (1983), 15–17; (1973), 215–216; (1974), 97–98. Al-Fârâbî found this language in the *De Intellectu* of Alexander of Aphrodisias: νοητὰ γίνεται ὄντα δυνάμει ὀητά; Alexander, *De Intellectu* (1887), 108.3–4; "potentially objects of thought become such [i.e., in actuality]"; ibid. (1990); تصير معقولة بالفعل إذ كانت بالقوة معقولة; ibid. (1971), 34.5; (1956), 185.1–2. On al-Fârâbî's doctrine of intellect, see Davidson (1992), 44–73; Lucchetta in al-Fârâbî, *Letter on the Intellect* (1974), 18ff.; and Geoffroy (2002). Geoffroy argues that the teachings of al-Fârâbî are based on Alexander rather than a direct study of Aristotle's *De Anima*.

160. Al-Fârâbî, *Book of Sophistic Refutations* (1983), is not the work to which Averroes refers here.

161. Al-Fârâbî, *Letter on the Intellect* (1983), 31; (1973), 219–220; (1974), 104–105. Al-Fârâbî's teaching in this work is that the extrinsic agent intellect by efficient causality provides to the human soul the power required for the abstraction of intelligibles, thereby actualizing potential intellect into actual intellect: "The agent intellect which Aristotle mentioned in the third treatise of the *De Anima* is a separate form which never existed in matter nor ever will exist in it, and it is in a certain manner an intellect in actuality close in likeness to the acquired intellect. The agent intellect is that principle which makes (جعل *ja'ala*) that essence which was an intellect in potentiality, an intellect in actuality and which makes (جعل *ja'ala*) the intelligibles which are intelligibles in potentiality, intelligibles in actuality." Al-Fârâbî, *Letter on the Intellect* (1983), 24–25; (1973), 218; (1974), 102. Translation slightly modified. In *The Political Regime* al-Fârâbî writes that the agent intellect "makes (يجعل *yaj'alu*) the things which are not in their essences intelligible to be intelligible." It raises (يرفعها *yarfa'u-hâ*) things which are not per se

(the human material intellect) will come to be something eternal, if knowing is a noetic identity. That is, "it will happen that something generated receives something eternal and is made like it, and in this way what is generated will become eternal, which is impossible" {485}. Second, the nature of the intelligibles in the acquired intellect is problematic since they are not the very intelligibles in act but rather are distinct from the intelligibles in act in the agent intellect. Another intellect will be needed to abstract from the intelligibles in the acquired intellect more intelligibles, and so forth to infinity, unless somehow the intelligibles in the acquired intellect are the very intelligibles in act in the agent intellect {493}. Third, if the human perfection or end is merely the perfection involved in the reception of theoretical intelligibles in a perishable substance and not a true conjoining with the separate agent intellect as intrinsic to the soul, then the agent intellect's "relation to a human being will be only the relation of the agent to the human being, not a relation of form" {502}. According to Averroes the result of this will be that the abstractive process of understanding intelligibles in act will belong not to human beings but to the separate agent intellect alone, and humans will only be recipients of its agent causality. That is, the agent intellect will be what provides forms through its own abstractive power to human beings, and "there will be no difference between relating it to a human being and relating it to all beings except in virtue of the diversity of its activity in them" {502}. Such a relationship of an extrinsic efficient cause (the agent intellect) giving forms intelligible in act to distinct human material intellects (resulting in acquired intellects) may by implication raise the question of whether human beings are per se rational or are denominated so only thanks to what they receive from the agent intellect.

As Averroes sees it, these issues arise if the relationship of the agent intellect is that of external efficient cause and not that of formal cause—precisely what Averroes reports regarding al-Fârâbî's teachings in his lost *Commentary on the Nicomachean Ethics*. "For in his *Commentary on the Nicomachean Ethics* he seems to deny that there is conjoining with the separate intelligences.[162] He says that this is the opinion of Alexander and that it should not be held that the human end is anything but theoretical perfection" {433}. If the fulfillment

---

intelligibles to a rank of existence higher than they possessed naturally so that they are intelligibles for the human intellect in act. In this way the agent intellect causes them to become intelligibles in act for the human rational power, assisting it to reach the rank of the agent intellect, which is the end of human beings in their perfection and happiness. al-Fârâbî, *Political Regime* (1964), 34–35.

162. See Pines (1978), (1979), and (1990), and Davidson (1992), 70–73. For the source of this in Ibn Bâjjah, see Harvey (1992a) 225, n. 56. My thanks to Joshua Parens for assistance with references.

of the perishable theoretical intellect is the only perfection possible, this is because conjoining is not possible. And that conjoining in noetic identity of the acquired intellect with the agent intellect is not possible because it makes no sense to think that what is generated and corruptible can become eternal and incorruptible. But the problem lies in al-Fârâbî's failing to conceive of the agent intellect as formal cause. "In this way its relation to a human being will be only the relation of the agent to the human being, not a relation of form, and the question of al-Fârâbî which he voiced in his *Commentary on the Nicomachean Ethics* arises. For assurance of the possibility of the conjoining of the intellect with us lies in explaining that its relation to a human being is a relation of form and agent, not a relation of agent alone" {502}. That is, al-Fârâbî did not understand that the agent intellect must have its activity as genuinely *in* our souls as formal cause in the abstractive process of understanding {438}. What is more, for Averroes the material intellect too must be *in* our souls {406}, such that there are not two sets of intelligibles and a consequent generation of an infinite regress of abstractions. Rather, there must be one set of unique intelligibles in act realized in the separate material intellect, which is also somehow present *in* our souls as the theoretical intelligibles in us.

Ibn Bâjjah

The works of Ibn Bâjjah[163] (ca. 1085/90–1138 CE) cited by Averroes in the *Long Commentary* are his *Book on the Soul*,[164] *Treatise on Conjoining with the Intellect*, and *Letter of Farewell*. In these works Ibn Bâjjah was intensely concerned with the issue of the nature of the receptive human intellectual power, the material intellect, so much so that Averroes writes, "This question did not leave his mind nor over time did he take his eye off it. . . . For this topic is extremely difficult, and since such was the case for Ibn Bâjjah in regard to this question, how much more [can be expected] of any one else?!" {487}.

As indicated above concerning Averroes' *Short Commentary on the De Anima*, Ibn Bâjjah's teaching on the material intellect as a disposition having the forms of the imagination as its subject was adopted by Averroes in that work. The *Middle Commentary* rejected that approach in part because it entailed that the material intellect be body or a power in a body, an objection the *Long Commentary* repeats. There Averroes explains that Ibn Bâjjah had thought locating

163. Ibn Bâjjah is referred to as Avempace in Books 2 and 3 except for two references to him as Abubacher (that is, Abû Bakr) at {397}. Interestingly enough, Albertus Magnus thought Abû Bakr referred to the physician Abû Bakr Muḥammad Ibn Zakarîyah al-Râzî (d. 925), known in Latin as Rhazes. See Bach (1881), 122–129.

164. Ibn Bâjjah, *Book on the Soul* (1960), (1961). This work is incomplete in manuscript, ending abruptly shortly after the beginning of the section on the rational power.

the material intellect as a power in the imagination would enable him "to avoid the impossible results [reached] by Alexander, namely, that the subject receiving the intelligible forms is a body made from the elements or a power in a body" {397}. Averroes also objects that Ibn Bâjjah considers that "the disposition for intelligibles which is in the imaginative power is similar to the dispositions which are in the other powers of the soul" {405} because common to both these dispositions is that they are generable and corruptible. That is, for each the disposition is "generated through the generation of an individual, corrupted through its corruption, and generally numbered through its numbering. They differ in this: one is a disposition in a mover insofar as it is a mover, namely, the disposition which is in the intentions {406} imagined;[165] the other is a disposition in the recipient and is a disposition which is in the first actualities of the other parts of the soul." The disposition in the imagination is one which actively provides intelligibles in potency for abstraction, while the disposition which is the material intellect is receptive in nature. Yet, as Averroes says, "these two dispositions differ as [much as] the earth from the heavens. For one is the disposition in the mover insofar as it is a mover and the other is a disposition in the moved insofar as it is moved and receptive" {406}. That is, there is an equivocation on the term "disposition" here: the material intellect is posited as a disposition receptive of immaterial non-particular intelligibles in act that is completely different from the disposition of the imagination, which provides only particular, individual intentions intelligible in potency. This criticism of Ibn Bâjjah corresponds with the stage which the *Middle Commentary* represents in its argument that receptive material intellect is a remote disposition caused by the agent intellect and belonging individually to each human being as a power associated with that human being's soul but not present in the human soul as in a subject. This immaterial power, provided at birth by the agent intellect, is capable of being fully actualized when mature, again by the power of the agent intellect. That approach took into account the difference between the disposition of imagination and that of material intellect.

Ibn Bâjjah's assertion of a plurality of individual human receptive material intellects actualized as theoretical intellects posed a serious challenge to Averroes' doctrine of a single, shared, immaterial intellect for all human beings. Ibn Bâjjah had already spelled out objections to it.[166] If it is the case that all intelligibles are one in number for each human being, individual talent or ef-

165. "The imaginative form is the first mover in man." Ibn Bâjjah, *Treatise on the Conjoining of the Intellect with Man* (1942), 12; Spanish, 29; (1968), 159; (1981), 185.

166. "Generally it is thought that the impossible things which result for this position result for our position because the intellect which is in a positive disposition is one in number. Ibn Bâjjah already listed most of these in his short work which he called *The Conjoining of the Intellect with Human Beings*" {404}.

fort would be in vain since each human being would have those intelligibles insofar as that human is a member of the species. And if those intelligibles are not one in number for all, the distinct intelligibles in two different persons would require a third intelligible in act as what is common to those two, with a resultant infinite regress, which cannot be the case if there is actual understanding of intelligibles in act. Furthermore, if intelligibles are apprehended by individuals in their own material intellects, since an individual's intelligibles arise from sensory experience of particulars, then those intelligibles are tied to the experience of particulars or a set of particulars which gave rise to them. Anyone who has not, for example, had the sensory experience of a giraffe cannot possess the intelligible form of a giraffe. And if the intelligibles are related in this way to the individual, when the individual perishes, so too would the intelligibles. The solution for Ibn Bâjjah is that the forms existing in individual human material intellects are spiritual forms or intentions, and it is by way of these that human beings are conjoined to the intelligible forms.[167] And for Ibn Bâjjah the proximate end is the unity of all human intellects in the agent intellect, and the ultimate end is unity of all intellects in complete conjoining, described as the attainment of divinity, as indicated above.

Averroes saw another challenge from the accounts of Ibn Bâjjah to his teaching on the unity of the material intellect concerning the model for the material intellect and its relation to individual human beings in the *Middle Commentary*—namely, the relationship of the celestial bodies and their associated intellectual souls. In that work the material intellect was understood to be related to the human soul as the celestial intellectual soul is related to the celestial body—that is, as associated with but not present in the soul or celestial body as in a subject. There it was argued that each human soul has its own associated material intellect. In light of that, how could Averroes' final teaching on the unique and shared separate material intellect hold that there was one intellect for many human souls? In the case of the separate celestial bodies, which are unique in species, there is also only one intellect for each, and it would be superfluous to have more than one intellectual mover, since the celestial body is moved by one intention, for which one intellect suffices. Similarly, one sailor does not pilot more than one ship at a time, nor does one artisan need and employ more than one tool of a kind at a time. Hence, it seems each soul should have its own intellect and that one intellect with the same intention shared by all would be useless. Indeed, if the latter were the case, there should be only one theoretical intellect, not many {403–404}. But there is a plurality of theoretical intellects, so why should there not be a plurality of material intellects?

---

167. Ibn Bâjjah, *Treatise on the Conjoining of the Intellect with Man* (1942), 14–16; Spanish, 32–35; (1968), 162–164; (1981), 187–188.

These challenges from his analysis of the thought of Ibn Bâjjah were dealt with directly and at length by Averroes. One task was to explain how there could be a plurality of individual theoretical intellects without the generation of an infinite regress of intelligibles. Another was to explain how there could be a unity of intelligibles such that what was in one theoretical intellect as an intelligible in act was also in another theoretical intellect as the same intelligible in act. As explained above, Averroes' ultimate solution was the assertion of the unique material intellect as existing *in* human souls as shared by all human beings. It was to locate both the material intellect and the agent intellect as powers *in* the soul, thanks to his positing of the unique shared material intellect and of the special nature of the agent intellect as intrinsic form for us. Averroes' response to Ibn Bâjjah is twofold. First, he accuses Ibn Bâjjah of equivocation on the term "intellect" when used in reference to the agent intellect and the theoretical intellect. "This name, however, namely, 'intellect,' is said equivocally of the theoretical and the agent [intellects]" {412}. If the theoretical intellect is truly to be intellect and its theoretical intelligibles truly to be intelligibles in act, then it must be intellect in the same sense as the agent intellect, which contains the intelligibles in act. But this is not so, since it is only the agent intellect, which contains the ultimate intelligibles in act for Ibn Bâjjah. The theoretical intellects in individuals do not contain the intelligibles in act for Ibn Bâjjah but rather only spiritual forms or intentions related to and representative of the true intelligibles in act properly located in the agent intellect. In this sense, then, intellect is not predicated in the same way of the agent intellect and the theoretical intellect {412–413}. For Averroes this challenge can be fully met only if the theoretical intelligibles are both present in the separate material intellect as eternal in accord with their subject and at the same time present in the theoretical intellects of the perishable subjects that human beings are. Again, this is to locate the material intellect and its actualization by the agent intellect as *in* the soul.

Second, on Averroes' view, Ibn Bâjjah's difficulties resulted from a failure to understand that both the material intellect and the agent intellect must somehow be located *in* the soul for it to be the case that human beings have intellectual understanding of things of the world. Ibn Bâjjah's argument for the theoretical intellect as coming to have the intelligibles in act—if there is no equivocation on the term "intellect"—necessarily entailed that the agent intellect must be the form of the theoretical intellect. To say otherwise is to say either that (a) the intelligibles in the theoretical intellect are not the same intelligibles in the agent intellect and so are not intelligibles in act, or (b) the theoretical intellect is not intellect. With the agent intellect as form of the theoretical intellect, the activity of abstraction of intelligibles is our activity by our will. Moreover, when the agent intellect by its power of abstraction transfers what is intelligible in potency into a new mode of being as intelligible in act {439}, it has two activities, abstraction or separation of the intention from its material conditions and the enabling of the realization of the intelligible in act in the material intellect. Since it is the individual person who goes from not understanding the intelligible to understanding the intelligible, these activities take place in us. Such a thing can only happen by our will if the power of such abstraction and reception is truly ours—that is, only if the agent intellect is in us as form for us and the theoretical intelligibles of the material intellect are also in us. Simply put, the potentiality for the presence of the material intellect and the agent intellect intimately involved in human understanding must be part of the definition of human beings as rational animals, even if their presence does not manifest itself equally in every member of the species.[168]

Other Sources for Averroes:
Plato, Galen, Avicenna, Nicolaus of Damascus, the De Aspectibus, and Abû al-Faraj Ibn al-Ṭayyib

Averroes' understanding of Plato (427–347 BC) in the *Long Commentary* is for the most part dependent on the works of Aristotle, Galen's *Compendium of the Timaeus*, and the *Paraphrase of the De Anima* by Themistius, though Averroes did himself know the *Republic*, on which he wrote a paraphrasing commentary toward the end of his life.[169] Attributing to Plato the use of the method of division in the study of the soul {9}, Averroes recounts Aristotle's criticism that Plato's views concerned every soul, not just the human soul {12}. According to Averroes, on Plato's account in the *Timaeus* the powers of the soul correspond to distinct parts of the body {120–121}, understanding to the brain, the concupiscible to the heart, and the nutritive to the liver {10}, such that the bodily subject for knowing and understanding is not the same as for other powers {380}. Averroes portrays the Platonic doctrine of forms as intelligibles existing in themselves outside the soul {12, 409} as eternal {452} "universal things" {12} which are not apprehended by way of sensibles {425}. Rather, knowing and learning consist in the recollection of those universals {218, 412, 452}. Averroes also mentions Plato's understanding of flavors, relying on the account of the *Timaeus* in Galen {322} that the soul has three parts: the rational, the emotional, and the desiderative {509}.

Averroes makes critical reference to Galen (129–ca. 210 CE) in regard to three distinct issues: respiration, flavor, and the bodily nature of the rational power.[170] Averroes mentions that he does not have access to the discussion of respiration in Aristotle's *On Youth, Old Age, Life and Death, and Respiration* and that what

---

168. See above, p. xlvii.

169. See *On Plato's Republic* (1974).

170. Averroes was well acquainted with the thought of Galen and commented on a number of his treatises. See *Commentaria Averrois in Galenum* (1984), (1998), and *Medical*

Galen had said on respiration is not adequate.[171] He goes on to say that for Aristotle breathing takes place for the sake of cooling the heart by inhaling cool air into the lungs and exhaling for the sake of the lungs, which are cooled by this exhalation of warm air {266–267}. Apparently Averroes understood Galen, who rejected Aristotle's explanation that respiration was primarily for cooling the heart,[172] to attribute the movement only to the chest, while Averroes thought the accumulated warmed air in the lungs also to be a cause. Galen is also incorrect in holding the association of flavors and temperature, believing that the acrid is cold and the pungent warm, says Averroes, since bitterness is found in warm and cold things {291–293}. Galen was correct in following Plato in asserting a role for texture in flavor, remarks Averroes {322}. Yet Galen was incorrect in asserting that the rational power was a bodily power identical to the cogitatîve power. In this, says Averroes, Galen made a logical mistake with the second figure of the syllogism. From the facts that human beings have a rational power and that they have a cogitative power located in the brain, it does not follow with necessity that the rational power is the same as the cogitative power {415–417}.

Averroes gives scant explicit attention to the teachings of Avicenna (980–1037 CE) in the *Long Commentary*, though he is aware of important Avicennian teachings. In explaining that universal propositions in judgments concern things potentially infinite in number, Averroes asserts that the particular powers of the soul can judge only finite or particular intentions. Hence, what judges regarding universal or infinite propositions should itself not be a power of the soul mixed with the body and finite in nature. That is, it should be a power unmixed with the body. From this Averroes concludes that "judgment and discernment in us are ascribed only to the material intellect" and asserts that this is a proposition Avicenna held {442}.[173] Certainly this is correct since Avi-

Manuscripts of Averroes (1986). On Galen in Arabic, see the account of Anawati and Ghalioungui in *Medical Manuscripts of Averroes* (1986), 16–36; Bürgel (1967); Sezgin (2000); and Walzer (1965).

171. In his well-known medical compendium, *Kitâb al-Kullîyât*, he also makes the remark that this is an issue which requires more study. See *Kitâb al-Kullîyât* (2000), 88.

172. See Siegel (1968), 162.

173. Gutas (1988), 61, calls attention to Avicenna's *Letter to Kiyâ*, where Avicenna asserts that a key principle for Aristotle is found in the latter's discussion of Democritus, which presupposes that intelligibles can exist only in immaterial subjects. In his own context Averroes is asserting that universal judgments concerning intelligibles can take place only in immaterial subjects. Hence, the cogitative power located in the brain cannot be the rational power by which human beings make universal judgments. Regarding the issue of the material intellect with which Averroes was much obsessed, Davidson (1992), 258, remarks: "Avicenna took up the nature of the human material intellect

cenna understood the human soul, insofar as it was rational, to be separable and distinct in its own right from the body {441–442}. Yet Avicenna, writes Averroes, "followed Aristotle only in dialectics, but in other things he erred, and chiefly in the case of metaphysics . . . because he began, as it were, from his own perspective"{470}. Although these are the only remarks on Avicenna in the *Long Commentary*, Averroes was well aware of the teachings of Avicenna on the soul. For example, Averroes' remarks in his *Long Commentary on the Metaphysics* and elsewhere make it clear that he was familiar with Avicenna's doctrine of the separate agent intellect. There he refers to Avicenna's doctrine of substantial change taking place only by way of the agent intellect as Giver of Forms (واهب الصور *wâhib al-ṣuwar, dator formarum*).[174] He was also aware of Avicenna's teachings on the internal sense powers and rejected Avicenna's account of *wahm*, the estimative faculty which apprehends and judges non-sensible intentions. What is more, Averroes declines to follow Avicenna's distinction of the retentive imagination and the compositive imagination, instead absorbing the functions of the latter into the cogitative power. Still, Avicenna's teachings on the inner senses and the powers of the brain were an important influence on the development of Averroes' thought, even if he revised it in accord with his own interpretation of the texts of Aristotle.

Averroes makes brief references to a summary of Aristotle's *Movement of Animals* by Nicolaus of Damascus (ca. 64–4 BC) in the context of a discussion of appetite as the form of the body of an animal in motion {524} and remarks that Nicolaus is among the reliable interpreters of Aristotle {432}. He also makes two references to a work called *De Aspectibus* (*On Perspectives*) for the notions that light travels in a straight line and that a bright sphere is so owing to its being a "body . . . luminous from all its parts" {253–254}. These are likely references to the *Optics* of Ibn al-Haytham (ca. 965–1039 CE), which was widely known, though in context the issue concerns the geometry of light, something taken up by al-Kindî (ca. 801–873 CE) in *On the Causes of Differences of Perspective and On the Geometrical Demonstrations for Them*, which was also known in Latin as *De As-*

---

only indirectly, in the course of treating a different issue that preempted the question of the material intellect's nature. He maintained that the human soul, and not merely the intellect, is 'an incorporeal substance,' which is brought into existence together with the generation of each human body."

174. See *Long Commentary on the Metaphysics* (1952), 882, 1496, 1498; (1962), 181rA, 304rA–vG; (1984), 107–109; and Davidson (1992), 245. Hasse (2000), 188, remarks regarding Avicenna's use of the description "giver of forms" (*wâhib al-ṣuwar, dator formarum*) that "Avicenna himself never seems to explicitly identify the giver of forms and the active intellect." He adds that "Averroes writes that Avicenna identifies the active intellect and the giver of forms, but he clearly refers to substantial and not to intelligible forms."

pectibus. One reference is also made to a contemporary rival of Avicenna, the Nestorian physician, theologian, and philosopher Abû al-Faraj Ibn al-Ṭayyib, whom Averroes criticizes for holding that the cogitative power is the rational power in Ibn al-Ṭayyib's lost *Commentary on Sense and Sensibilia* {416}.[175]

The Influence of the *Long Commentary on the De Anima*

In the Arabic tradition the *Long Commentary* is not known to have had any substantive influence. Puig (1992) has found references to some ten disciples of Averroes in Arabic sources, but few are philosophers and none is known to have pursued issues concerning the nature of the intellect with the exception of his son, Abû Muḥammad ʿAbdallâh Ibn Rushd. A physician and scholar who wrote on medical matters, he is also the author of a treatise apparently written during the lifetime of Averroes, *On Whether the Active Intellect Unites with the Material Intellect Whilst It Is Clothed with the Body*, which has been edited in its Arabic, Hebrew, and Latin versions and translated into English by Charles Burnett and Mauro Zonta.[176] The historical evidence indicates that the suppression of philosophy in Andalusia which took place toward the end of Averroes' life sorely affected the study and transmission of his thought in the Arabic tradition.[177] Present knowledge for the most part supports the view that while many works survived in Arabic, his philosophical writings played no detectable part in the development of philosophical tradition in Arabic until a revival of interest came about following the appearance of Renan's *Averroès et l'averroïsme* in 1852.[178] As von Kügelgen has explained, there was a rediscovery of Averroes in the nineteenth century, followed by much use of his work and name for the furthering of various political causes espoused by nineteenth- and twentieth-century thinkers of Egypt and elsewhere.[179] Yet there is little evi-

175. This commentary is not extant, but Peters (1968), 46, remarks that it is mentioned by the biographer Hajji Khalifah and cited by a disciple of Avicenna. On Ibn al-Ṭayyib, see Vernet (1971), 955a; Yousif (1997), 137–142, and (2003), 227–234; and Gyekye (1979), 20.

176. Burnett and Zonta (2000). Note that this treatise is precisely concerned with the issue of *De Anima* 3.7, 431b17–19, that of whether it is possible to have knowledge while in the body.

177. See Puig (1992), 251–255.

178. Renan (1852). Burnett (1999) provides references to a few studies indicating some knowledge of Averroes' work among Western Muslims and also argues that some credence might be given to the traditional story of the sons of Averroes at the court of Emperor Frederick.

179. Von Kügelgen (1994), (1996).

dence of the Arabic *Long Commentary* being studied or even surviving among Arab thinkers, aside from the extant Arabic fragments.[180]

In the Jewish tradition the translated works of Averroes were powerfully influential up to the middle of the sixteenth century, but his works translated into Hebrew were mostly different from those translated into Latin.[181] While the thirteenth-century Latin West had Averroes' mature *Long Commentaries* on the *De Anima, Physics, De Caelo,* and *Metaphysics,* it had few of his *Middle Commentaries* and nothing of his dialectical and religious writings.[182] In contrast, the *Decisive Treatise;* the *Incoherence of the Incoherence;* many *Short Commentaries;* the *Middle Commentaries* on the *Physics, De Caelo, De Anima,* and *Metaphysics;* and the *Long Commentaries* on the *Posterior Analytics* and *Physics* came to be available in Hebrew and were extensively used, even more than the works of Aristotle. As Steven Harvey puts it, "At the heart of this translation movement was not, as one might have expected, the works of Aristotle, *the* philosopher, but rather the many commentaries of Averroes on the Aristotelian corpus."[183] However, the mature *Long Commentary on the De Anima* is not known to have been translated from Arabic into Hebrew, and its influence on Jewish thinkers came via Latin thinkers such as Thomas Aquinas. At least portions of an early version of the *Long Commentary* were available in Jewish schools, as evidenced in the extant fragments, some of which have been studied in depth by Geoffroy and Sirat in research preliminary to the future publication of fragments only in part published by Ben Chehida.[184] The *Long Commentary* was translated into Hebrew by Ibn Ya'ish (Abraham di Benevento) in the late fifteenth century from the Latin. The alternate versions of Book 3, Comments 5 and 36, by Jacob Mantino, found in the Giunta editions may be from this Hebrew-from-Latin translation.[185]

In contrast with the Arabic tradition, the works of Averroes translated into

180. *Long Commentary* Fragments (1985), (2005). These are found as marginal notes to the *Middle Commentary on the De Anima* in the Arabic in Hebrew script manuscript, Modena, a.j.6.23, one of the two primary manuscripts used in *Middle Commentary* (2002). For more information, see Geoffroy and Sirat in *Long Commentary* Fragments (2005).

181. See Ivry (1983) and Harvey (2005).

182. See n. 1 for bibliographies of his works, particularly Anawati (1978), which has a foldout chart of works and translations, and Wirmer, Thomas Institut (2006).

183. Harvey (2003), 268. On the role of Maimonides in the determination of the importance of Averroes in the Jewish tradition, see Harvey (1992b) and (2003).

184. See *Long Commentary* Fragments (2005) and (1985) respectively.

185. See Davidson (1992), 263, n. 24, on the various possible sources for these Latin texts. Also see Wolfson (1963), appendices I and II, 445–454 in the 1973 reprint. Zonta (1994) provides a list of extant Hebrew manuscripts of the *Long Commentary* and a discussion of Mantino's translations of Book 3, Comments 5 and 36. Tamani and Zonta (1997) contains lists of Hebrew manuscripts in Italian libraries and two important essays

Latin from Arabic mostly in the thirteenth century (and from Hebrew in Renaissance times) were ubiquitously present wherever the study of Aristotle and the interpretation of his philosophical doctrines took place through the time of the Renaissance and beyond.[186] The term "Averroism" (sometimes relabeled "heterodox Aristotelianism") is generally applied to selected writings of philosophers supportive of one or more of three characteristic notions: the world had no beginning, happiness can be attained naturally in the present life, and the single unitary material intellect is shared by all human knowers—all genuine doctrines of the mature Averroes.[187] Siger of Brabant (ca.1240–after 1282) of the Arts Faculty at Paris, the most well-known proponent of a philosophical psychology conceived under the influence of Averroes' *Long Commentary* in the mid-thirteenth century,[188] was in all likelihood the unnamed target of the vehement attack on Averroism and the doctrine of the material intellect in Averroes by Thomas Aquinas in his *On the Unity of the Intellect against the Averroists*.[189] The Condemnation of 1270 and, most important, the Condemnation of 1277 had a substantial effect on the study and use of the thought of Averroes in the Latin West, but the study of Averroes on intellect by no means ceased.[190] Siger was later followed by John of Jandun (ca. 1285–1328), who, like Siger, died while in some form of exile and condemnation.[191] For the Latin tradition, the *Long Commentary on the De*

in Italian, one on "Aristotle and Aristotelianism in Medieval Judaism," by Zonta, and "Diffusion, Conservation and Study of 'Aristotelian' Manuscripts," by Tamani. For brief accounts of Jewish Averroism, see Harvey (2003) and (2005) and Leaman (1996) and (1998b). Also see Zonta (1996) and the classic Steinschneider (1956).

186. See Wolfson (1961) and Schmitt (1979) and (1983).

187. For a brief account of Averroism, see Ebbesen (1998).

188. See Bazán (2003) for a brief account of Siger's work and the progressive development of his views on the nature of the intellect from his early embrace of Averroes' view of the unity of the separate, shared material intellect to "the traditional anthropological dualism that was pervasive during the first half of the thirteenth century" (638). For a list of important recent primary and secondary sources for the study of the thought of Siger, see Bazán (2003), 639–640. Fernand Van Steenberghen (1977) provides a comprehensive account of the scholarship up to 1977 in his *Maître Siger de Brabant*. Also see Wippel (1998). The famous work of Pierre Mandonnet (1899) prompted modern interest in Siger.

189. See Thomas Aquinas, *De unitate* (1976). For an analysis of Aquinas' various critiques of Averroes, see Mahoney (1994). For a different approach to the issue, see Taylor (1999b). For an account of positive contributions of Averroes' thought to that of Aquinas, see Wéber (1978). Albert the Great also wrote a *De unitate intellectus contra Averroistas*. See Albertus Magnus *De unitate* (1975). Also see Wéber (1994).

190. See Wippel (1977), (1998), and (2003).

191. For a brief account of John of Jandun and his thought, see South (2003). For a comprehensive study of his Averroist noetics, see Brenet (2003).

Anima was deeply important and widely studied by so many of the important philosophical and theological figures of the later Middle Ages and Renaissance after its translation around 1220 that it is far beyond the parameters of this introduction to recount the issues and developments.[192] Nevertheless, some important clarifications must be made regarding the present-day understanding of the reception of the *Long Commentary* and its teachings in the thirteenth century.

Averroes' teachings on the nature of the soul in the *Long Commentary* were initially welcomed in the Latin West, in part as a corrective of the views on the soul set forth in the *De Anima* treatise by Avicenna, which was available in Latin well prior to the *Long Commentary*. In his *De Anima* Avicenna taught that the agent intellect was a distinct immaterial and separate substance functioning as a giver of forms both to the physical world and to the individual receptive rational souls of human knowers. According to Avicenna in this work, sense perception and imagination prepared the immaterial rational soul for the reception of intelligibles from the agent intellect.[193] While this account may have some affinity to Augustinian illuminationist views, it still has the untoward consequence that it separates the abstractive power of intellect from the individual human being in whom the powers of knowing, willing, and acting were held naturally to reside. Hence, when Averroes writes that the agent intellect is "in the soul,"[194] that the agent intellect, the material intellect, and the theoretical intellect are "in the soul,"[195] and that universals are "in the soul,"[196] he provides what appears to be a welcome correction based on a proper reading of Aristotle's own text of the *De Anima*.[197]

In 1937 Dominique Salman introduced the notion that the influence of Aver-

192. See Nardi (1945) and (1958), Van Steenberghen (1966), Kuksewicz (1968), Schmitt (1979), Kessler (1988), and Poppi (1991), as well as the more recent studies listed in Bazán (2003).

193. *Sed causa dandi formam intelligibilem non est nisi intelligentia in effectu, penes quam sunt principia formarum intelligibilium abstractarum.* Ibn Sînâ, *Kitâb al-Nafs* (1968), 126–127; (1959) 234. *Restat ergo ut ultima pars sit vera, et ut discere non sit nisi inquirere perfectam aptitudinem coniungendi se intelligentiae agenti, quousque fiat ex ea intellectus qui est simplex, a quo emanent formae ordinatae in anima mediante cogitatione.* Ibid. (1968), 148–149; (1959), 246–247. This traditional understanding of Avicenna has recently been challenged. See Gutas (2001) and Hasse (2001).

194. See {390}, {438}.

195. See {406}, {437}.

196. See {220–221}.

197. The importance to the theological and philosophical tradition in the Latin West that the agent intellect be an individual power of each human soul is stressed by Bazán (2001), 179, when he writes in reference to the Condemnation of 1277, "It is of great philosophical interest to see this doctrine receive official sanction by the ecclesiastical

roes in the Latin West, particularly with respect to his teachings on the soul, took place in two distinct steps.[198] The first encounter with Averroes was a positive one in which the perceived teachings of Averroes on the presence of the powers of the agent and material intellects in the soul were much welcomed, while the teaching on the separately existing material intellect went undetected.[199] Later, when the full import of Averroes' doctrines on the intellects came to be understood, a very different and adversarial approach was taken by the likes of Albert the Great and Thomas Aquinas.

René Antoine Gauthier further refines this thesis in a series of articles and in the introduction to the critical edition of the *Commentary on the De Anima* by Thomas Aquinas.[200] According to Gauthier, the psychological doctrines of First Averroism correspond precisely to the genuine teaching of Averroes, while the later Second Averroism, which gave rise to the famous conflict on the unity of the intellect in the thirteenth century and beyond, was in fact an invention on the part of Christian theologians. He notes that the doctrine that came to be considered most characteristic of the philosophical psychology of Averroes and of thirteenth-century Latin Averroism, the unity of the possible or receptive human intellect (which Averroes called the material intellect), was first distinctly condemned by Robert Kilwardby and Bonaventure around 1252.[201] Gauthier then goes on to state that "One admits actually more and more today that Averroes was not an averroist," citing the work of Salvador Gómez Nogales.[202]

---

authorities of Paris because of its direct impact on the nature, object and scope of human knowledge. In the final analysis, it is the agent intellect, as an active faculty of the intellective soul, that determines what we, as human beings, can or cannot understand scientifically, including Metaphysics."

198. Salman (1937).

199. "Breaking from the tradition of 'all the philosophers' (Alfarabi, Avicenna, Algazel, Isaac [Israeli]) and of the 'theologians,' this averroism according to the first way makes acceptable to the young Albert the Great a conception of the agent intellect to which he will always remain faithful, and which he will transmit to his disciple Thomas Aquinas. Later undoubtedly, Albert will correct his historical interpretation of Averroes and then will rely only on the sole authority of Aristotle." Salman (1937), 211–212. Bazán (1989), 10, points out that Salman's notion "that the first Latins who used Averroes attributed to the Arab master the theory of the multiplicity of agent and possible intellects, and opposed this doctrine to Avicenna's separate Agent Intellect . . . was repeated by G. de Mattos in 1940, Miller in 1954 and by F. Van Steenberghen in 1966."

200. See Gauthier (1982b) and his preface in Thomas Aquinas, *Sententia libri De anima* (1984), 221*–222*. Also see Gauthier (1982a), (1983), and (1984).

201. Thomas Aquinas, *Sententia libri De anima* (1984), 221*–222*.

202. Ibid. Cf. Leaman (1994) for a quite different approach to the issue of Averroes and Averroism.

In 1976 Gómez Nogales published a short article entitled "Saint Thomas, Averroès et l'averroïsme," in which he argued that Averroes did not profess the unity of the human intellect but rather held for individual immortality of the soul, as well as the individual material intellect.[203] This Gómez Nogales sees supported by the fact that Averroes writes of individual personal moral responsibility and reward and punishment in the next life in his theological writings. In point of fact, however, what has happened in this case is that Gómez Nogales, editor of one of the two editions of the *Short Commentary on the De Anima*, has imposed upon the teachings of the *Long Commentary* something of the doctrine of the *Short Commentary*, together with a partial understanding of the religious writings of Averroes.[204] On his view the *Long Commentary* is replete with aporiai on the issue of the material intellect, and the proper understanding of Averroes requires that he be read as teaching a doctrine of intellect distinct from that of the Latin averroists: "Averroes is not an averroist. If it is true that there were some averroists who admitted the unity of the human intellect, this is not the case for Averroes, who admits the individual immortality of the human soul, even in the material intellect."[205]

It is Gauthier's reliance on this incorrect interpretation of the doctrine of intellect in Averroes' *Long Commentary* that led him to assert that the genuine understanding of Averroes in the *Long Commentary* is that of the pre-1250 "First Averroism" account, according to which the agent and material intellects are multiplied and exist solely "in the soul."[206] Hence, contrary to the view of

203. Gómez Nogales (1976). Much of his account presumes what he argued in Gómez Nogales (1967).

204. "As a good Muslim, Averroes accepts in his theological writings the dogmas proper to human responsibility. He is Sunni in what concerns otherworldly sanctions, which supposes additionally the individual immortality of each human being, and even with a material aspect, because he supposed that all human beings after death take on bodies adapted to the degree of spirituality to which they will have arrived during earthly life." Gómez Nogales (1976), 177. I have argued against this sort of understanding of certain of Averroes' statements in the *Incoherence of the Incoherence* in Taylor (1998c). Regarding the meaning of religious statements in Averroes, see Taylor (1998b), (2000b), (2003), and (2007).

205. Gómez Nogales (1976), 177. Also see Gómez Nogales (1978a), where this view is repeated.

206. Another curious example of misunderstanding Averroes is found in Roger Arnaldez's *Averroès. Un rationaliste en Islam*. Arnaldez devotes only a few pages to Averroes' doctrine of the intellect, seemingly ignoring the account of the *Long Commentary on the De Anima*. At the end of his chapter on Averroes as philosopher and theologian, he cites Mahmoud Kassem's reported discovery of a text of Averroes in which the agent and receptive intellect are said to be in one and the same entity. Arnaldez (1998), 173; (2000), 117–118. This text was reported by Kassem in his *thèse de lettres* at the Sorbonne

Gauthier, so-called First Averroism does not in fact well represent the views of Averroes on the intellect. Ironically, it is Second Averroism, as described by Bonaventure, Kilwardby, Aquinas, and others, which rightly represents the actual views of Averroes on the intellect.

Gauthier's thesis that the doctrine of the unicity of the material intellect in Averroes was a product of a misreading of the text of Averroes by the theologians was refuted on the basis of study of the Latin text of the *Long Commentary* by Bernardo C. Bazán, who nevertheless accepted the view of two stages in the understanding of Averroes.[207] In accord with the account of the material intellect I have given above, Bazán argues that the post-1250 view of the theologians is in fact well founded in the philosophical principles and text of Averroes. He rightly holds that First Averroism "might be the fruit of a naive approach and . . . insufficient comprehension" on the part of Latin thinkers of that era.[208] That the earliest Latin readers of Averroes' *Long Commentary* would find it difficult to understand his teaching on the unitary, separate, and shared nature of the material intellect is hardly surprising since, as Averroes himself well knew, this was a novel proposal in solution of very difficult issues of Aristotelian noetics.[209]

(Paris, 1945), later published in Arabic in 1964 (two of its three sections) and in French (complete) in 1978. See Qasim (1964) and Kassem (1978). In fact, this text is nothing but the *Middle Commentary on the De Anima* in Paris, *hébreu* 1009, Bibliothèque Nationale, one of the manuscripts used by Ivry for his edition.

207. See Bazán (1985) and (1989). Also see Bazán (1972) for his account of the views of Averroes on intellect. There he writes, "Averroes has sought to be strictly faithful to the principles that Aristotle had held with respect to the immaterial separate substances. It led him to a consequence of unexpected scope: the affirmation of the separate and unique character of the two intellective principles." Bazán (1972), 48.

208. Bazán (1985), 530.

209. See above pp. lxxx–lxxxi. At {409–410} he calls the material intellect "a fourth kind of being" insofar as it is immaterial separate intellect and yet has a sort of potency. This is essential for his solution of epistemological issues and also for his metaphysical account of separate intellects and God, though it is novel in the tradition. At {399} Averroes writes, "Since there are all those things [which can be raised regarding the material intellect], for this reason it seemed [best] to me to write what seemed to me to be the case on this topic. If what appears to me is not complete, it will be a start for a complete account. So I ask my brothers seeing this exposition to write down their doubts and perhaps in that way what is true regarding this will be found out, if I have not yet found [it]. If I have found [it], as I suppose, then it will be clarified through those questions. For truth, as Aristotle says, is fitting and gives testimony to itself in every way." Another interesting issue is that of just how the agent and material intellects were understood by the Latin translator. On his different choices of *intelligentia agens* and *intellectus agens* to translate العقل الفعال *al-ʿaql al-faʿâl*, see Book 2, n. 138, and Book 3, n. 43.

According to Bazán, however, what led to the First Averroism account was the preconceived understanding of human nature on the part of early Latin readers of the *Long Commentary*. He writes, "A dualistic conception of human beings explains, in my opinion, why the readers of Averroes were so receptive to his writings and why it took them so long to discover that there was more than what met the eye in the *Long Commentary*."[210]

In an article published in 2002 Bazán persuasively argues for the complete rejection of the conception of the existence of a First Averroism. On the basis of his analyses of early works on philosophical psychology, he concludes that Latin thinkers of what he calls "the eclectic period" often approached the consideration of the soul and its powers with the conviction that the soul was itself an individual substance in its own right, a *hoc aliquid*,[211] and also related to the body as its form. As he sees it, this led to the employment of words and arguments from Averroes in a supplementary way to form a novel understanding of the agent intellect as "a faculty of the soul that is the form of the body." In another article Bazán points out the basis for this as follows:

> The theoretical foundation of this thesis is the double consideration of the soul as *forma et hoc aliquid*. Being a substance, the soul must be composed of potential and actual co-principles, to which the Latins linked the receptive and agent intellects. The textual foundation of this doctrine was *De anima* 430a10–14, although some Latin Masters, for dialectical reasons, also appealed to Averroes in its support, quoting him out of context, even if they were aware of the true meaning of his own views. The doctrine is basically an eclectic neoplatonic Aristotelianism. To call it "First Averroism" obscures not only its historical originality, but also its doctrinal meaning.[212]

In his analysis of thirteenth-century commentaries on the *De Anima*, Bazán finds three major categories of classification: the eclectic period; the period of the genuine Averroistic reading, to some degree found in the work of Siger of Brabant; and the period of the post-1250 theologians and the synthesis of Thomas Aquinas. The middle of these periods he characterizes as one in which a genuine attempt was made to provide a consistent account of Aristotle's philosophical psychology of intellect using the work of Aver-

210. Bazán (1989), 20.

211. Bazán (2002), 125ff. Surely this was founded in part if not wholly on religious presuppositions about the nature of human beings as morally responsible agents and as possessing immortal souls. Note that this usage of *hoc aliquid* or *aliquid hoc* as substance in its own right is different from what Averroes appeals to. For Averroes the material intellect is a unique immaterial substance and not a determinate particular as a member of a species. As immaterial, it cannot be multiplied in number.

212. Bazán (2000), 53.

roes.[213] The final period was one of critique of the genuine Averroes and the analyses the *Long Commentary* inspired, culminating in what Bazán calls

> the personal synthesis of Thomas Aquinas, who tried to avoid the dangers of anthropological and metaphysical dualism by providing an interpretation that could satisfy at the same time the concerns of the "Eclectic" commentators regarding the incorruptibility of the human soul, and the concerns of the "Averroists" regarding consistency with the principles of hylemorphism. Thomas' interpretation is based on the conception of the human soul as a subsistent-substantial-form, a notion that secures both the unity of the human composite and the incorruptibility of the intellectual soul, and that evolves from the Aristotelian notion of form as actuality, brought to the limits of its ontological possibilities.[214]

As the foregoing makes clear, the historical account of the reception of Averroes' doctrine of the intellect in the thirteenth century is still in the process of being written and rewritten in spite of the many valuable works by scholars of the twentieth century.[215] The same is true for the importance of Averroes

213. Bazán (2002), 122.

214. Ibid. For a broader account of the role of Averroist thought in the thirteenth century, see Van Steenberghen (1966), 357ff., and (1970), 198ff. Bazán's recent essay, "Radical Aristotelianism in the Faculties of Arts. The Case of Siger of Brabant" (2005), and some of his articles cited above are prompting a rethinking among present-day scholars of the part played by the thought of Averroes in the development of philosophy in the thirteenth-century Latin West. Whether there was such a thing as Latin Averroism and just what that term might be meant to denominate is a matter of considerable discussion among some experts in the field. These and related issues are likely to appear as topics in periodicals, conference proceedings, and books in coming years.

215. For example, in 1994 Kuksewicz, a leading scholar in Latin Averroist studies, reasoned that he must revise his view that some authors of late thirteenth-century commentaries should be considered "undercover Averroists." (Cf. Kuksewicz [1968], 98.) He writes, "It seems to me that the interest in Averroes' philosophy, testified in different degrees by several commentaries at the end of the thirteenth century allows me to speak about an *initial phase* of the Averroistic reborn in Paris. This initial phase gave way to different manifestations: Not-Averroistic texts with some positive interest in Averroes' heterodox solutions and nearly clear Averroistic works were among these manifestations as well. Texts of this category were, however, the representation of only two extreme limits of the new current: its main body consists of works of ambivalent character, and I think these texts present no clear solutions, remaining hesitant between orthodox and heterodox theses. This interpretation, which seems historically acceptable, lets me explain and understand the contradictions and the doctrinal inconsistency proper to these works." Kuksewicz (1994) 109. The starting point for understanding the Latin Averroists and their various "Averroisms," however, has to be a sound under-

and his doctrine of the intellect among Renaissance thinkers. Katherine Park writes, "Many of the most important disputed questions in Latin psychology in fact had their roots in the parts of Averroes' *Commentarium magnum in Aristotelis De anima libros* where he pointed out issues on which he thought Aristotle had been incomplete or unclear."[216] This was certainly the case for the doctrine on the intellect in Aristotle, which Averroes in the *Long Commentary* set forth as a philosophical account devoid of explicit religious presuppositions.[217] Renaissance philosophical psychology has been held to take its start at the end of the fourteenth century in Italy, following Pietro d'Abano's move to Padua. According to Eckhard Kessler, "The period's main characteristic was the attempt to synthesize 'radical' naturalistic Aristotelianism, based on Averroes and imported from Paris to Padua by Pietro d'Abano, with the Oxford tradition of logical and mathematical analysis developed by Ockham and his followers. This attempt was accompanied by the humanist polemic against both the 'Averroist dogs' and the *barbari Britanni*, and, as time went on, was more and more censured, until finally suppressed by the church."[218]

This was a renewal of life for Averroist philosophical psychology, though Averroes' *Long Commentary* was continuously discussed and consulted through the entire later medieval period.[219] All the major figures of Renaissance philosophical psychology found in Averroes an approach worthy of consideration and, for many, adoption in one or another form or part. In many cases, the questions and issues as framed by Averroes provided the context for discussion. Paul of Venice (1369/72–1429), Cajetan (1480–1547), and Nicoletto Vernia (d. 1499) drew deeply upon Averroes' doctrine of intellect, adopting parts and rejecting others, while Alessandro Achillini (1463–1512) accepted much of Averroes on intellect. Agostino Nifo (ca. 1470–1538) initially drew upon the work of Siger of Brabant and John of Jandun in the Averroist account he was later to abandon. Pietro Pomponazzi (1462–1525), who was trained in the Averroist tradition, determined that both Aristotle and Averroes had to be rejected as Aquinas had rejected Averroes, since their positions did not allow suffi-

---

standing of Averroes' thought in relation to that of Aristotle, as de Libera (1994), 76, remarks: "To take a more exact measure of the true philosophical significance of the averroïst noetic, it would be opportune to start by reinstalling Ibn Rushd in the long duration of Aristotelianism. It is a task which largely remains to be achieved."

216. Park (1988), 474.

217. "Averroes' theory of the unicity of the intellect, or, more precisely, the unicity of the material intellect, was the most controversial thesis of Arabic philosophy in the Renaissance." Hasse (2004), 131.

218. Kessler (1988), 486.

219. See Wolfson (1961).

ciently for the rational nature of human beings.[220] Pomponazzi also rejected the account of Aquinas that the soul could be shown to be immortal on philosophical grounds insofar as that required the soul be created by God. His own view was close to that of Alexander. "Pomponazzi—referring to the principle that the intellectual soul cannot operate without imagination and is therefore dependent on matter *ut obiecto* (as its object) even if it is independent from it *ut subiecto* (as its subject) in terms of natural philosophy—chose the material solution and maintained that the human soul was the highest material form, attaining in its most elevated operations something beyond materiality."[221] In the end, however, he determined that the issue of the immortality of the human soul was not one which could be settled by analysis on the part of human natural reasoning.

The philosophy of Averroes continued to be read in the Renaissance volumes of the works of Aristotle in which the commentaries of Averroes were also printed.[222] And the *Long Commentary* continued to be consulted, studied, commended, and condemned for its teachings on the intellect by famous scholars such as Elijah Delmedigo (ca. 1460–1493), Jacopo Zabarella (1533–1589), Francisco Suarez (1548–1617), and many more too numerous to mention here. In light of the diverse uses of Averroes by these many thinkers, it perhaps becomes questionable whether the label "Averroism" continues to have descriptive value sufficiently specific to allow for the diverse ways the thought of Averroes was employed in the Renaissance period. When we speak of Renaissance philosophy, just as it is helpful to speak of "Aristotelianisms" rather than to assume a single shared reading of Aristotle,[223] so too the same can be said of the thought of Averroes and the "Averroisms" of varying degrees and sorts it generated.[224]

The Present Translation

This first complete translation of the *Long Commentary on the De Anima* into a modern Western language is preceded by two incomplete French translations of Book 3[225] and a modern Arabic translation of the entire work.[226] All these

220. Kessler (1988).

221. Kessler (1988), 503.

222. See Cranz (1976) and Schmitt (1979).

223. Mahoney and South (1998).

224. My thanks to James South for suggesting the term "Averroisms."

225. See *Long Commentary. Book 3* (1980–1981, 1982–1983) and *Long Commentary. Book 3* (1998).

226. *Long Commentary Modern Arabic Trans.* (1997). Selections from the *Long Commentary* are also translated into Spanish in Martínez Lorca (2004) and in Puig (2005).

are based on the 1953 edition of Crawford, who provided an austere edition based solely on the evidence of the Latin manuscripts.[227] While Crawford identifies the Text sections of Aristotle with the corresponding Bekker numbers, the edition contains no notes on any of the sources mentioned by Averroes; no indications of any corresponding teachings in related works extant in Arabic, Latin, or Hebrew; no explanations of complicated phraseology or technical terms; no explanations of doctrines; no consideration of differences between the Text of Aristotle embedded in the *Long Commentary* in relation to the Greek of Aristotle as known today; and no consideration of modern literature on Averroes and his philosophical psychology. The present translation in its notes and introduction provides much of what is missing in Crawford. The notes contain the following: (1) identification of Averroes' source references; (2) the extant Arabic fragments as currently available corresponding to the Latin, with English translations where the texts differ substantially; (3) the Arabic of Averroes' citations of his alternate text of the *De Anima*, again with English translations where the texts differ substantially; (4) remarks on significant variations of Averroes' Text of the *De Anima* from the Greek; (5) identification of the passages of the Arabic *Middle Commentary* which are identical to what is found in the *Long Commentary*; and (6) brief explanations of phraseology, technical terms, and complex argumentation. Since I have not undertaken a comprehensive study of the Latin manuscripts, I have seldom strayed from the text of Crawford, though where I have felt compelled to read the text differently, I have done so with indication in the notes. Consideration of the extraordinary influence of the *Long Commentary* in the Latin tradition, as indicated above in this introduction, is beyond the constraints of this book.[228]

This is a translation of Crawford's edition of the medieval Latin text presumed to have been rendered from Arabic into Latin by Michael Scot perhaps around 1220.[229] First evidence of Michael's activity as a translator is with his rendering of al-Biṭrûjî's *De motibus caelorum*, dated 1217 at Toledo, where Michael was likely in the company of Archbishop Rodrigo, whom he had

227. *Long Commentary* (1953). I leave out of consideration various very brief extracts of the *Long Commentary* that have been published in English and other languages.

228. Alain de Libera provides impressive analyses and insightful discussions of the arguments of the *Long Commentary* and their influence in his introduction and the substantial notes to his translation of Book 3, Texts and Comments 1–39, in *Long Commentary. Book 3* (1998). In *Long Commentary Modern Arabic Trans.* (1997) Gharbi provides only a short introduction and a table of terms, no notes. In *Long Commentary. Book 3* (1980–1981, 1982–1983) Griffaton provides only notes, with corresponding modern French translations of some of the texts of Aristotle.

229. See the remarks of Gauthier in Thomas Aquinas *Sententia libri De anima* (1984), at *221a, on the evidence that the *Long Commentary* was in Paris in 1225.

accompanied to the Fourth Lateran Council at Rome in 1215.[230] At Toledo Michael was part of a school of *verbum de verbo* translators partronized by the archbishops of Toledo for well over fifty years.[231] Michael was in Bologna in 1220, and in the following years enjoyed the support of Popes Honorius III and Gregory IX regarding various benefices in England and elsewhere, though he declined elevation to archbishop at Cashel.[232] This favor apparently continued until 1227, when Michael seems to have taken a place at the court of Frederick II, who would remain his patron until Michael's death sometime shortly before 1236.[233] It may be that Michael is the translator of a number of the *Long Commentaries* of Averroes on Aristotle, though only the *Long Commentary on the De Caelo* is thought with some certainty to be his.[234] While no sufficiently comprehensive study of the translation work of Michael has been completed to enable researchers to identify his work by internal criteria,[235] similarities among the Latin versions of the *Long Commentaries* on the *De Caelo, De Anima, Metaphysics,* and *Physics* may generally support the view that they may have been translated by the same person or group. The *Long Commentary on the De Anima* has but one unequivocal attribution to Michael from among the fifty-seven manuscripts used by Crawford.[236]

Since this is a modern translation of a medieval translation and not a direct rendering from the Arabic, I have chosen a somewhat literal style of translation, reflecting more closely what is supposed to have been written by the Latin translator or team of translators. The *Long Commentary* is a dense, complicated, and highly technical work not meant by Averroes for common consumption by the public but rather one focused on all the technical details of Aristotle's *De Anima* in their deepest meaning and importance. As such, it is far from easy to read and understand in the extant fragments in Arabic and all the more challenging in its Latin translation. Yet its translator or translators and many thinkers of the Latin West did extraordinarily well in grasping the meaning of Averroes' text and in grasping his complex and subtle arguments

230. Burnett (1994), 102. On Michael and Archbishop Rodrigo, see Pick (1998) and (2004). For a brief account of Michael Scot, see Minio-Paluello (1974).

231. Burnett (1997), 66; (1994), 103.

232. Haskins (1927), 274–275.

233. Haskins (1927), 275–276; Thorndike (1965), 32–39.

234. "We infer from the similarity of style and the time of appearance of several of Averroes's commentaries on Aristotle's natural science that they were all translated by one person and that person was Michael Scot. But only one commentary—that on the *De caelo*—has Michael's name as translator firmly attached to it." Burnett (1997), 67. For a list of Latin translations and their possible translators, see Burnett (2005).

235. But see van Oppenraay (1990), Burnett (1997), and Schmieja (1999).

236. See Crawford's remarks in *Long Commentary* (1953), Prolegomena, xi.

only by intensively poring over the precise language of his *Long Commentary*. The present translation seeks to preserve his arguments as found in the Latin text in their precision and their complexity of phraseology and meaning, though explanatory notes are provided to assist readers. For example, I have frequently chosen to render the Latin *intentio* (for the most part corresponding to Arabic معنى *ma'nâ*) as "intention" rather than "notion," "idea," "form," "meaning," and other possible renderings because of its technical usage in Arabic and Latin philosophy. This is appropriate since the very text of the *Long Commentary* communicated in an important way to the Latin West the multiple meanings of the Arabic as involving at once the senses of form, notion, idea, purpose, and end by the use of *intentio*. This is a technical term whose meaning in English has been split into the usage of two words, "intention" and "intension," both of which derive from the same Latin. The use of "intention" in the present translation, which may appear awkward to the untrained modern ear, even if historically appropriate in English, has the advantage of highlighting what Latin readers and also Averroes understood as a sophisticated and complex philosophical usage.

Book 1

1. Since knowing something about things differing from one another is considered honorable either in virtue of exactness or because those are known through things more splendid and more noble,[1] **it is right for these two reasons to give the discourse on the soul a position of priority.** (1.1, 402a1–4)

By **exactness** he means the confirmation associated with demonstration. By what he said: **or because they are** known **through things more noble**, he means the nobility of the subject. For the arts differ from one another in just one of these two ways, either in the confirmation associated with demonstration or in nobility of subject, or in both ways. For example, Geometry surpasses Astronomy in the confirmation associated with demonstration, but Astronomy surpasses it in the nobility of its subject. He also said: **it is** necessary **for these two reasons**, etc. That is, because these two features are found in the science of the soul, it is necessary that an account of it take precedence over other sciences. This is obvious to those who give it consideration since the subject of this science is nobler than [those of] others and its demonstration is likewise more certain.[2] He began to give [his] account in this way to lead people to {4} a love of [this] science. His account is in the form of a categorical syllogism. It is as if he says: Because we hold that knowledge concerns things which are honorable and desirable and that such things surpass one another on account of the confirmation associated with demonstration, on account of the nobility of the subject, or on account of both, as we find in the science of the soul, because in these two features it surpasses other sciences, except for divine science,[3] we must hold that the science of the soul comes before the other sciences;

1. The Greek has a slightly different sense. "Holding as we do that, while knowledge of any kind is a thing to be honoured and prized, one kind of it may, either by reason of its greater exactness or of a higher dignity and greater wonderfulness in its objects, . . ." Aristotle, *De Anima* (1984).

2. Cf. Themistius, *De Anima Paraphrase* (1899), 1.11–14; (1996), 15; (1973), 1.10–2.9. Regarding the position of Themistius on the soul and Averroes' use of his commentary, see the introduction, pp. lxxxiii–lxxxvi.

3. *Scientiam divinam* was probably العلم الالهي in the Latin translator's Arabic manuscript. Cf. n. 9 below. In the Arabic context it is clear that this is metaphysics, not *kalâm* (philosophical and dialectical theology). Arabic fragments correspond to Book 1, (*Long Commentary* هو أشرف من جميع موضوعات سائر العلوم ما خلا العلم الالهي:1.32–33) Fragments [1985], 29).

1

and for this reason we placed it in a position of priority among all subjects of inquiry.

2. We also see that knowing it helps a great deal in regard to all truth, and especially in regard to nature. For [the soul] is, so to speak, the principle of living things.[4] (402a4–6)

After he had shown the reason why this science must be more honorable and take precedence over the other sciences in nobility, he also began to show the usefulness of this science, when he said, **We also see that** knowledge, etc. By **all truth** he means the theoretical sciences.[5] And by saying **and especially in regard to nature**, he means especially in regard to natural science. Next he gave the reason why it is more helpful to natural science than to any other, when he said, **For it is, so to speak, the principle of living things.** That is, the reason for this is that knowing about living things is the greatest knowledge [that can be had] of the divisions of natural things and the soul is the principle of living things. That is why it is necessary that knowing about the soul be not just useful but rather necessary for knowledge of living things.

You should be aware that the science of the soul {5} is found to be helpful to the other sciences in three ways. First, inasmuch as it is part of that science,[6] indeed the noblest of its parts—and this is the relationship it has to natural science. For living things are the noblest of generable and corruptible bodies, but the soul is nobler than all [others] among living things.[7] Second, because it supplies more principles for more sciences, for example, for moral science— that is, [the science] of governing states—and for divine science. For from this science moral science gets the final end of human beings considered as human beings and the knowledge of what their substance is.[8] The practitioner of divine science[9] gets from it the substance of his subject. For here [in the science of the

---

4. Cf. {132}.

5. *Scientias speculativas.*

6. That is, natural science.

7. Arabic fragments correspond to Book 1, 2.22–24: وهذا بين بنفسه اذ هو أشرف ما في الأشـــياء . . . لأن النفس أشـــرف ما في الحيوان والحيوان هو أشرف من جميع الموجودات الكائنة الفاسدة. (*Long Commentary* Fragments [1985], 29); "This is self-evident since it is the most noble of what is in things . . . because the soul is the noblest among living things and living things are more noble than all generable and corruptible beings."

8. Note that no mention of moral or political science is made at the corresponding parts of the *Middle Commentary* (2002), 1. Averroes is following Themistius, *De Anima Paraphrase* (1899), 1.28–2.5; (1973), 2.12–3.3; (1996), 15–16.

9. *Divinus*, the masculine of the adjective, likely reflects the Arabic العلم الالاهي for [العلم] الالاهي , "divine [science]," or is a corruption of an original Latin translation such as *Divina (scientia)*. The original Arabic was probably, "Metaphysics receives from it the

soul] it will be explained that the separate forms are intelligences and also many other things concerning the knowledge of states consequent upon intelligence considered as intelligence and intellect.[10] And third, it is generally helpful and enables the acquisition of confirmation regarding first principles, since from [this science] we acquire knowledge of the first causes of propositions, and knowledge of anything through its cause is more certain than [knowledge] only of its own being.[11]

3. And what is sought is knowledge of its nature and substance, and then all the things that accrue to it. It is thought that some of these attributes are affections proper to the soul and some accrue to the body because of the soul. (402a7–10)

After he had shown the usefulness of this science, he began to show his intention,[12] when he said, **And what is sought is,** {6} etc. That is, what is to be sought and thoroughly investigated in this science is knowledge of the nature

---

substance of its subject." Here *divinus* in the Latin has to be understood as referring to the metaphysician or, as I have phrased it, "the practitioner of divine science." Cf. n. 3 above.

10. Cf. {410}: "This was unknown to many modern [thinkers] to the extent that they denied what Aristotle says in the Eleventh Book of First Philosophy, that the separate forms moving the bodies must be in accord with the number of celestial bodies. To this extent knowledge of the soul is necessary for knowledge of First Philosophy."

11. On how the science of psychology provides principles for the science of metaphysics, see Taylor (1998a). This notion was already expressed by Averroes in his *Short Commentary on the De Anima* (1950), 93; (1985), omitted; (1987), 218, in his summary of Ibn Bâjjah's *Treatise on the Conjoining of the Intellect with Man* (1942), (1968), (1981).

12. *Intentionem suam.* Forms of the word *intentio* seem often to be translations of forms of معنى or قصد, although likely not in all cases. The Arabic term معنى *ma'nâ* has a long history in Arabic *kalâm* and philosophy, with a wide range of meanings in philosophical contexts, including intention, intension, form, meaning, and thing. See Frank (1967). Black (2005), 314–317, discusses معنى briefly and cites Avicenna's explanation of the term in his *Interpretation* from his *Shifâ'*. See Ibn Sînâ, *Interpretation* (1970), 2. There Avicenna identifies معنى with قصد (intention, design, purpose, object, goal, aim, sense, meaning), explaining that "What in the soul are indicative of things are what are called معانى, i.e., مقاصد." In the present translation, oftentimes I consider *intentio* a technical term and render it "intention," although at other times it has a less technical sense ("meaning," "notion"). This English word has in its history carried the meanings of both "intention" and "intension," which derive from the same Latin word, with the latter sense deriving at least in part from texts translated from Arabic. Cf. Book 1, Text 14, and n. 62, where *intentiones* corresponds to the Greek λόγοι and Averroes comments, "That is, it is therefore obvious that the forms coming to exist in that soul by affection and motion are forms in matter" {21}. Also see Book 1, Text 16 and n. 72.

of the soul, i.e., its substance, then knowledge of all the characteristics which accrue to it, just as with other things to be considered in natural science. For knowledge of any genus and its species will be realized only through knowledge of the substance of that species and knowledge of the characteristics which accrue to it, as was said in the *Posterior Analytics*.[13]

Next he said: **It is thought**, etc. That is, of the attributes accruing to the soul, it is thought that some are affections which belong to the soul alone, since the soul does not need the body to have these affections, for example, as in the case of representation by intellect.[14] Others, however, are thought to need the body, and [it is thought] that they will not be realized except through both, namely, the soul and the body.[15] That is what he meant when he said: **and some** accrue **to the body because of the soul.** These are the affections attributed to

13. This seems to be a general reference to the notion that complete knowledge of the genus and the species is dependent on a grasp of substance and its essential attributes. The particular text Averroes has in mind may be *Posterior Analytics* 2.13, 96b12–14: "We make the further assumption that the substance of each subject is the predication of elements in its essential nature down to the last differentia characterizing the individuals. It follows that any other synthesis thus exhibited will likewise be identical with the being of the subject." Aristotle, *Posterior Analytics* (1941).

In Comment 71 of Book 2 of his *Long Commentary on the Posterior Analytics* (1962), Averroes says, "We concede that the essence of singular material beings is the ultimate definition which is said of all the individuals" (508A, Abram.) and "[Aristotle] shows in the science of metaphysics that the definition truly is of individuals which are in act" (508B). My translations. Cf. *Metaphysics* 7.11, 1037a17–32, and the remarks of Averroes in C. 40 of the corresponding book of his *Long Commentary on the Metaphysics* (1952), 937–939; (1962), 192v–193r.

14. *Ut in ymaginatione per intellectum.* This is التصوّر بالعقل, literally "representation (or image forming) by intellect" but with the meaning of "conceptualizing" or "conceptualization," which is found in the corresponding passage of the *Middle Commentary* (2002), 2.5. This is the sole occurrence of the infelicitous translation *ymaginatio per intellectum* in this work, a term used frequently to render the Arabic التصوّر بالعقل in the *Long Commentary on the Metaphysics*, Book Lâm. See, for example, *Long Commentary on the Metaphysics* (1952), 1599–1600; (1962), 319H–I; (1984), 151. Here I render it literally to reflect what appears to be the understanding of the Latin translator at this moment in his work. Later, in Book 3 of the present work, *formare per intellectum* and *formare* are both rendered by forms of "to conceptualize." Cf. Book 3, n. 5. Also see {379–382}, {384}, {391}, {400}, {408–409}, {434}, and {446}. At {417} the phrase *in formatione per intellectum*, "in conceptualizing," corresponds to the Greek τοῦ νοητικοῦ. For further discussion, see the introduction, pp. lv–lviiiff.

15. Arabic fragments correspond to Book 1, 3.20–21: وان النفس لا يتم لها ذلك الفعل الا بالبدن (*Long Commentary* Fragments [1985], 29); "and that this activity is not realized by the soul except through the body."

the concupiscible power, namely, to the [part of the] soul which desires and avoids [things]. He introduced this division among the attributes of the soul because we want very much to find out concerning the affections of the soul whether or not among them there can be something separate, and this is impossible unless at least one of them is proper to the soul without the body. By **affections proper to the soul** he may also mean those which exist primarily in the soul and secondarily in the body, such as sense and imagination. By the others he means those which exist in the soul on account of the body, such as sleep and wakefulness. In this way he includes in this account all the things which accrue to soul and are attributed to it.[16]

4. It is very difficult and burdensome to find out anything certain regarding its being. For, since this investigation is common {7} to many other things—namely, the investigation concerning its substance and what that substance is—we have to think that the method is the same for all things whose substance we wish to know, just as the method of demonstration is the same for the affections accruing to a substance. And so this method must be explained. (402a10–16)

When he had shown that the things sought in this science are primarily of two sorts, one knowing the substance of the soul and the other knowing the things which accrue to the substance, he began first to show the reasons why it is difficult to know its substance. This is the difficulty of knowing the method and rule on the basis of which someone can find out the soul's definition. He said: **It is very difficult**, etc. That is, it is very difficult to have a rule and a method for learning the definition of the soul on the basis of which we can know its true definition, a method leading us perfectly to its definition. For, if we have such a rule, it will be easy to learn the definition of the soul.[17] Then he began to show why it is difficult to find such a method and to indicate the questions which arise because of this difficulty. He said: **For, since this investigation is common**, etc. That is, the reason for this difficulty is that,

16. Arabic fragments correspond to Book 1, 3.25–33: ان تشوق أكثر ذلك من معرفة انفعالات النفس وأفعالها * انما هو هل فيها ما هو يفارق أم لا وذلك شىء لا يمكن ان يكون فيها ما يخص النفس دون البدن. ويحتمل ان يريد ‹بـ› » الانفعالات التي تخص النفس« أي التي توجد للنفس وجودا أوليا وللبدن ثانية مثل الحس والتخيل ، ويعني » بالآخر« التي للنفس من أجل البدن ‹من› نوم ويقظة ، ويكون غرضه في هذا القول حصر جميع ما يلحق النفس (*Long Commentary* Fragments [1985], 29); *Where the Latin has "concerning the affections of the soul," the Arabic has "the affections and activities of the soul."

17. Arabic fragments correspond to Book 1, 4.17–22: ان أصعب الأمور في معرفة حد النفس ان يكون عندنا قانون وطريق يقينى نستنبط به حدّها الحقيقي التام ، فانه لو كان عندنا هذا القانون لكان يسهل معرفة حدّها علينا (*Long Commentary* Fragments [1985], 30); " . . . a rule and a *sure* method."

since this investigation of the soul, which consists in seeking knowledge of its substance, is common to [the soul] and to all things whose substance is sought, someone may say that the method by which we generally arrive at the knowledge of the definitions of things is the same when we seek knowledge of the substance [of the soul] and [knowledge] of the other substances of all things being sought after. He gives the reason {8} for this when he says that just as the method by which one produces a demonstration regarding the affections which accrue to things is the same for the soul and for other things, so is the method for knowing the substance. Thus it is necessary to know what that method is, and this is very difficult. After he described the difficulty that arises for one who says that the method is the same [for the soul and for other things], since one should seek to know from him what that method is, he began to show the difficulty arising for one who says that the method is not the same.

5. **If, however, that method is not the same and common,[18] then what is sought will be more difficult. For it will be necessary to find a method for each and every thing and to know what that method is. Even if it has been explained whether it is demonstration or division or some other method, afterwards many questions will remain regarding those [principles] from which we ought [to begin] to inquire. For there are different principles for different things, for example, the principles of numbers and of surfaces.** (402a16–22)

He means that, if this method by which we proceed in finding out the definitions of things and in learning their substances were not the same and common to all the things whose definitions are to be sought, but [were] more than one, then what is sought regarding the knowledge of the substance of the soul will be more difficult. For in that case for each and every thing whose definition is to be learned one must first learn some method proper to the things whose substances are to be known.

When we have explained that there is a method and that it is one, then we have to know first what that method is: {9} whether it is demonstration, as Hippocrates said,[19] or division, as Plato said,[20] or another method, for instance, the method of composition, which Aristotle presented in the *Posterior Analyt-*

18. The Greek περὶ τὸ τί ἐστιν, "for solving the question of the essence" (Aristotle, *De Anima* [1984]), is dropped here. The phrase is preserved in the other Arabic translation as في معرفة آنية الشيء (ibid. [1954]); "in knowing the being of the thing."

19. Themistius, *De Anima Paraphrase* (1899), 2.15–25; (1996), 16. Themistius is the source of this comment, including the mention of demonstration as a method for attaining definitions, although he makes no mention of the name of Hippocrates.

20. Cf. *Phaedrus*, 265D; *Sophist*, 218D–221C; and *Statesman*, 262A–B.

ics.[21] When this has been explained, many questions and occasions for error will remain **regarding** the things **from which** we ought **[to begin] to inquire** into the knowledge of the definitions of things. For, along with the knowledge of that method, we have to know the principles proper to every single genus to be examined.[22] For the principles of things differing in genus are themselves different.[23] That is why knowledge of that method is not enough for knowing the definitions of things, unless the principles proper to those things are known. For definitions can only be compiled from the proper principles which are in the thing.[24]

6. It is fitting and right that we first determine in which genus it exists and what it is, that is, whether it is a determinate particular[25] and a substance,

21. Cf. *Posterior Analytics* 2.13. Arabic fragments correspond to Book 1, 5.19–23: وان كانت هذه السبيل واحدة فقد يجب قبل ان نفحص أي سبيل هي : هل هي برهان ⟨كما يرى ذلك بقراط⟩ أو قسمة ⟨حسب قول أفلاطون⟩ أو سبيل أخرى مثل سبيل ألتركيب كما بينه أرسطو فى كتاب البرهان (*Long Commentary* Fragments [1985], 30). Part of this is identical to the *Middle Commentary*: وان كانت هذه السبيل واحدة فقد يجب قبل ان نفحص ;أي سبيل هي : هل هي برهان أو قسمة أو تركيب "If, then, this procedure is one, we ought first to investigate which it is, whether demonstration, division, composition." *Middle Commentary* (2002), 2.15–16. Since both the Arabic fragments and the *Middle Commentary* testify to the presence of قبل, "first" or "beforehand," I read *primo* at {8}, 5.20, with manuscript A in lieu of *post*.

22. Arabic fragments correspond to Book 1, 5.26–28: لا بد له أن يحتاج مع معرفة هذه الطريق ان يعرف المبادئ الخاصة بجنس جنس من الأجناس التي ينظر فيها. (*Long Commentary* Fragments [1985], 30).

23. Arabic fragments correspond to Book 1, 5.28–9: مختلفة هي مختلفة (*Long Commentary* Fragments [1985], 30).

24. Arabic fragments correspond to Book 1, 5.31–32: فان الحدود انما تتألف من المبادئ الخاصة الموجودة في الأشياء. (*Long Commentary* Fragments [1985], 30); "For the definitions are only compiled from the specific principles existing in the things." The Arabic has the plural (في الأشياء) while the Latin has the singular (*in re*).

25. *Hoc*: τόδε τι This term is used to refer to a particular, be that a particular form or a particular substance. At 403b1 Aristotle explains that the λόγος of a thing must be a "this" in matter of such a sort—that is, it must be a determinate particular existing in a suitable particular matter. See Averroes' remarks at {23–24}. In Book 3, at 429b14, *aliquid hoc in aliquo hoc* corresponds to τόδε ἐν τῷδε. Throughout I normally translate both the technical terms *hoc* and *aliquid hoc* as "a determinate particular" without distinction. *Aliquid hoc* occurs only in Book 3. Regarding Averroes' understanding of what is الشخص المشار إليه, *aliquid hoc*, and its correspondence with τόδε τι, see Bauloye (1997), 74–76. The phrase المشار إليه means "determinate" or "designated" in this context. It occurs in the *Middle Commentary* with some frequency. See, for example, *Middle Commentary* (2002), 113.14: الشخص المشار إليه, "a particular individual," and 113.22: تلك الماهية هى في ذلك الشخص المشار إليه, "a particular essence is in a given individual."

or a quality or a quantity or another of the categories which we have determined. And, furthermore, whether it is a being in potentiality or is nobler
as an entelechy,[26] since these two differ in no small way. (402a23–b1)

After he had shown the difficulty that arises for anyone who wants to define
the soul, he began to show the things which must first be investigated by anyone who wants to know its complete and true definition. He said: **It is fitting**,
etc. That is, anyone who wants to know its definition must first know in which
of the ten genera it is contained: whether in substance, in quality, in quantity,
or [in] the others.[27] Then, when he knows the genus in which {10} it is located,
he must know whether it is in that genus potentially or as an entelechy, that
is, in actuality[28] (for the difference between these two is great)—that is, he must
suppose that it is in one of the categories, but [its being in that category potentially or actually] will not be determined by that determination; for potentiality and actuality are differences which occur in all the categories, and they are
complete opposites.[29]

7. **Further, though, one must consider whether every soul is divisible or
not; and whether all souls are univocal in species or not; and, if they are not
the same, whether they differ in species or in genus. We find, however, that
everyone who discusses and investigates the soul seems to consider only
the human soul alone.** (402b1–5)

When he began to list questions that require investigation by anyone who
wants to consider the soul and showed first that he should seek out its substance,

---

For discussion of this notion and its importance in the thought of Aquinas, see Bazán
(1997). Cf. below Book 3, n. 137. See the discussion of this notion and its importance to
the formulation of Averroes' doctrine of the separate material intellect in the introduction, pp. lvi–lviii.

26. *Endelechia*: actuality. The Greek ἐντελέχεια, sometimes found as أنطلاشيا *anta-
lâshiyâ* or التمام *at-tamâm* in Arabic translations, was understood as actuality, perfection,
or completion, like the Greek. Cf. Walzer (1962), 90, 95–96. *Endelechia* is rendered "actuality" throughout, with the exception of the present Text and Comment.

27. Arabic fragments correspond to Book 1, 6.12–15: ⟨يعني لا بد لمن أراد معرفة حدّها
أن يعرّف أولاً⟩ تحت أي جنس من الأجناس هي داخلة: أعني هل هي داخلة في جنس الجوهر
أو في جنس الكمّ أو الكيف أو في غير ذلك من الأجناس ⟨العشرة⟩ (*Long Commentary* Fragments [1985], 30).

28. Arabic fragments correspond to Book 1, 6.16–17: وأيضا . . . ينبغي ان نعرف هل
هي داخلة تحت جنس ما هو بالقوة أو هي داخلة تحت ما هو ⟨انطلاخيا⟩ أي ما هو بالفعل
(*Long Commentary* Fragments [1985], 30).

29. Arabic fragments correspond to Book 1, 6.18 and 20–21: والفرق بين هذين النحوين:
⟨Long⟩ فرق ⟨كبير⟩ وذلك واجب فان القوة والفعل يلحقان جميع المقولات وهي ظاهرة التضاد
Commentary Fragments [1985], 30).

he also began to say what one should seek out after that. He said: **one must** also **consider whether it is divisible** [30]—that is, as regards its subject—**or not** divisible by means of a division [of its subject]. For Plato said that the intelligible power is in the brain and the concupiscible in the heart and the natural, i.e., the nutritive, in the liver.[31] Aristotle, on the other hand, holds that these powers are one as regards their subject and more than one considered as powers.

Next he said: **and whether all souls**, etc. That is, one should consider next whether the soul is the same in species in all animate things, e.g., the soul of a human being and a horse, or [whether] they are different.[32]

Next he said: **and if they are not the same**, etc. That is, if it has become apparent that they differ in species, it should also be considered whether the difference is only in species and they are still the same in genus, or the difference is in both [species and genus].[33] For their dismissal of this {11} investigation is the reason why the ancients did not consider any but the human soul alone, thinking that a consideration of [human beings] would be a consideration of soul as such.[34] This would be true if souls were the same in species; but, as it is, because they are different, it is necessary to consider whether they are the same in genus. Because

---

30. Arabic fragments correspond to Book 1, 7.11–12: قال : « وينبغي ان ننظر أيضا من
أمرها هل هي متجزئة» (*Long Commentary* Fragments [1985], 30).

31. *Timaeus*, 69B–73C, as known in Arabic through Galen, *Galen's Compendium of Plato's Timaeus* (1951), Arabic, 22–24; Latin, 72–76.

32. Cf. Themistius, *De Anima Paraphrase* (1899), 3.14–18; (1996), 17.

33. Arabic fragments correspond to Book 1, 7.21–23: ان كانت مختلفة بالنوع فهل هي
مختلفة بالنوع فقط – وهي في الجنس واحدة – أم هي بالنوع والجنس مختلفة؟ (*Long Commentary* Fragments [1985], 30). In his note to the corresponding passage of the *Middle Commentary*, Ivry remarks that the Latin of the *Long Commentary* has the same statement. However, this direct consideration of the Arabic fragments of the *Long Commentary* reveals that the Arabic texts of the *Long Commentary* and the *Middle Commentary* here are identical. ... ان كانت مختلفة بالنوع فهل هي مختلفة بالنوع فقط – وهي في الجنس
واحدة – أم هي بالنوع والجنس مختلفة; "If they differ in species, do they differ in species only but belong to the same genus, or do they differ in species and in genus?" *Middle Commentary* (2002), 4.3–5 and 152, n. 13.

34. Arabic fragments correspond to Book 1, 7.23–27: قال : فان هذا الفحص من أمر
النفس هو أحد ما أغفله البعض من القدماء لذلك كان بحثهم في نفس الانسان فقط
لاعتقادهم ان كل نفس هي واحدة باعتبار ﴿أنهم﴾ اذا نظروا في نفس الانسان نظروا في النفس
﴿على ٱلاطلاق﴾ وإن الفحص في نفس الانسان هو الفحص في كل نفس (*Long Commentary* Fragments [1985], 30). The Arabic has the additional text, "if the investigation of the soul of human beings is [an investigation] of every soul." Ivry also notes that this sentence is paraphrased in the *Middle Commentary*. *Middle Commentary* (2002), 152, n. 13. Again, detailed comparison with the extant fragments shows the texts to be nearly identical. The *Middle Commentary* has قال : فان هذا الفحص من أمر النفس هو أحد ما أغفله القدماء
ولذلك لم يتكلموا إلا في نفس الانسان فقط; "He said: This investigation of the [differ-

this is so we must concern ourselves first about the definition of that genus then afterward about the things that are proper to each soul, as Aristotle did.[35] It makes no difference whether that genus was predicated univocally or primarily and secondarily, as it is in the definition of the soul which he introduces later.[36]

8. **We must take care so that we do not ignore the question of whether its definition is the same as the definition of a living thing or is different for each [living] thing, e.g., the definition of a horse, a dog, a human being, and a god.**[37] **The universal living thing is either nothing or it is something derivative, as is the case if there is something else here of which the universal is predicated.** (402b5–9)

When he expressed his view that the master of this art must consider soul in general, he began to show that when he seeks the definition of soul in general, he must not disregard—as the ancients did—the question of whether that definition is like definitions of genera or like definitions of species. He said: **We** must **take care** when we seek one and the same general definition for [the soul] not to disregard the question of whether the generality of the definition for all animals is like the generality of animal in all its species or like the generality of the definition of a human being and the definition of horse in all their individuals. For, once that has been considered, we will not fall into thinking, {12} as Plato did, that we have spoken of every soul when we have spoken of the soul of a human being.

Next he said: **The universal living thing,** etc. This shows that he does not hold that the definitions of genera and species are definitions of universal things existing outside the soul. Rather, they are definitions of particular things outside the intellect, but it is the intellect that brings about the universality in them. It is as if he were to say that the being associated with the definitions is not attributed to species and genera in such a way that those universal things are existent outside the intellect. For the universal living thing either is nothing at all or its being is posterior to the being of sensible things, if there is any universal being per se. He said this because it appears here that definitions are of sensible things that exist outside the intellect. In that case either there are no universal

---

ent kinds of] soul is one of the things which the Ancients neglected, speaking, therefore, only of man's soul." *Middle Commentary* (2002), 4.6–7.

35. *De Anima* 1.1ff.

36. *De Anima* 2.3, 414b20ff. Cf. Book 2, Texts 30–31 {173–177}, esp. {176}.

37. Ivry notes that "dog" and "god" are not mentioned in the corresponding passage of the *Middle Commentary* probably because of the negative connotations of the former and because of the religious sensibilities concerning the latter. See *Middle Commentary* (2002), 152, n. 14. These are not discussed in the following Comment.

things existing per se, as Plato used to say, or, if there are, their being is not necessary for understanding the substances of sensible things. It is as if he were to say that in this passage he does not care how that may be, since it appears that those definitions are only in particular things existing outside the soul. But what is apparent here is that either they do not exist at all or, if they do exist, they are something posterior, that is, they are things posterior to sensible things. For, if they were to precede them in such a way as to be their causes, we would not be able to know the substances of sensible things until we had attained assent regarding the being of [the universals], as is the case for the other causes of things which [causes] exist in [sensible things], namely, form and matter.[38]

9. **Furthermore, if souls should turn out not to be many, but [each to have many] parts, should one first inquire about the soul as a whole or about its parts? What is very difficult to discern is which of those [parts] differ from one another in nature.** (402b9–11) {13}

Furthermore, once it has been explained that souls are many not in subject but in parts, while still one and the same in subject, we have to investigate whether we ought to begin first with consideration of the whole soul and then later [consider] its parts, or whether we ought to consider the parts first before [we consider] the soul as a whole insofar as it is soul.

Next he said: **What is very difficult** , etc. That is, even when we have supposed that it is more than one in parts, it is difficult for us to discern these parts and to indicate the differences by which they differ from one another. For in certain cases [those differences] are obvious and in certain cases they are obscure, for example, [the differences] between intellect and imagination and between imagination and sense.[39]

10. **And whether one should first investigate the parts or their activities, e.g., whether understanding before intellect, or sensing before the senses, and so forth. If we should investigate the activities first, one can raise questions as to whether one should investigate what is sensed before [investigating] sense, and what is understood before intellect.** (402b11–16)

Earlier he began to list the questions which arise about the ordering of the investigation of the soul and raised first the question of whether one should

---

38. Arabic fragments correspond to Book 1, 8.40–43: ولو كانت أسبابها لكان لم يتسنّ لنا أن نقف على الأشياء المحسوسة الا أن نعقل قبل جواهر الأشياء المحسوسة كما هو الحال في سائر الأسباب الموجودة فيه . أعني الصورة والهيولي (*Long Commentary* Fragments [1985], 31).

39. Cf. Themistius, *De Anima Paraphrase* (1899), 4.19ff.; (1996), 18. Arabic fragments correspond to Book 1, 9.15–17: لأن في بعضه الأمر ظاهر وفي بعضه خفي ، وخاصة الفرق الذي بين العقل والتخيل والتخيل وبين التخيل والحس (*Long Commentary* Fragments [1985], 31).

consider soul in general or in particular. He now begins to seek out whether, when we give consideration to the parts, one should begin with the parts and afterwards [consider] their activities, or vice versa.[40]

He said: **and whether one should first investigate**, etc. What he said [here] is understandable on its own.

Next he said: **If we should investigate the activities first, one can raise questions**, etc. That is, even if it has been explained that we must first inquire about their activities, {14} someone will raise questions about whether one should begin from what is sensed before [investigating] the sense, and from what is understood before the intellect, or vice versa.[41] He will raise questions about such things because one must go from things which are more known to us to things which are more hidden from us. The sciences differ in this respect,[42] for in some sciences things which are more known to us have precedence, as in mathematics, and in others it is the other way around, e.g., in some [of the sciences] contained in natural science.[43]

11. **Knowing what something is seems useful not only for knowing the causes of the attributes of substances (e.g., in Mathematics, since knowing what straight is and [what] curved [is], what a line is, and what a plane is, is useful for learning how many right angles equal the angles of a triangle); but conversely [it seems] also that the attributes provide a great deal of help for knowing what something is. For when we have given [an account of] something in [terms of] all or most of its attributes as they are presented to us by the imagination,[44] we will then also give a better account of the sub-**

40. Arabic fragments correspond to Book 1, 10.10–13: من أين ينبغي أن نجعل الفحص عن ذلك؟ هل نبتدئ فنفحص عن الأجزاء ثم بعد عن أفعال تلك الأجزاء أم الأمر ينبغي أن يكون بالعكس. (*Long Commentary* Fragments [1985], 31). This entire fragment is identical to the corresponding Arabic text of the *Middle Commentary*: "where to begin: with the parts first and then the functions of these parts, or the reverse?" *Middle Commentary* (2002), 4.17–19.

41. Arabic fragments correspond to Book 1, 10.18–19: هل ينبغي ان نبحث عن المحسوس قبل الحس وعن المعقول قبل العقل أم الأمر بخلاف ذلك؟ (*Long Commentary* Fragments [1985], 31). With the exception of three words, this is identical to what is found in the *Middle Commentary*: هل ينبغي ان نبحث عن المحسوس قبل الحس وعن المعقول قبل العقل الذى هو الفعل أم الأمر بخلاف ذلك; "ought we to inquire into the sensible object before the [faculty of] sense, and into the intelligible object before the intellect—which is the function—or is the matter otherwise?" *Middle Commentary* (2002), 5.3–4.

42. Arabic fragments correspond to Book 1, 10.20–22: هل ينبغي ان نصير من الأعرف 〈الأخفى〉 عندنا الى عندنا وهذا مخالف 〈للعلوم〉 (*Long Commentary* Fragments [1985], 31).

43. Cf. Themistius, *De Anima Paraphrase* (1899), 4.25–29; (1996), 18–19.

44. *Secundum viam ymaginationis*, "according to the way of imagination," is apparently a literal rendering in the Arabic of the Greek κατὰ τὴν φαντασίαν, "according

stance. For the starting point of every demonstration is [the account of] what something is. Therefore definitions which do not provide a knowledge of the attributes and do not make anything about them easily understood are patently nothing but empty words.[45](402b16–403a2)

After he had raised questions about whether the master of this art ought to begin from the posterior and proceed toward the prior, or conversely, he began to explain that each way is common in the sciences {15} and used by them. For, although it is more customary to go from the prior to the posterior,[46] still sometimes one will go from the posterior to the prior. He said: [Knowing what something is] seems, etc. That is, the knowledge of a thing's substance seems not to be the sole starting point of the acquisition of knowledge of its attributes, as happens in Mathematics. For in Geometry to know what a line is, what straight is, what concave is, and what a plane is, is the starting point of knowledge of the angles of a triangle, namely, how many right angles they equal. But also conversely[47] to know many posterior things is the starting point for knowing antecedent things. His account concerning this is understandable in its own right. After he had shown that knowing the posterior is sometimes the starting point for knowing the antecedent, he began to explain that this does not happen for all the attributes belonging to a thing, that they are the starting point of the knowledge of antecedent things, namely, of the substance. He said: **For when we have given [an account of] something as**, etc. That is, it is not possible for such a thing to happen, namely, to go from the knowledge of the attributes to the knowledge of the substance, except when we have acquired knowledge of a thing's attributes as presented to us by imagination, i.e., the attributes which are evidently existing in the thing and which are in its place,

---

to imagination." The alternate Arabic translation has علي ما في التوهم (ibid. [1954]); "according to what is in the imagination." Sensible images of things are received in the imagination according to Aristotle. Cf. *De Anima* 3.3, 429a2–3.

45. The Greek διαλεκτικῶς, "as dialectical," is missing from the text here but found in the other Arabic translation as بالاتفاق (Aristotle, *De Anima* [1954]); "by agreement" or "by convention." Remarks in the *Middle Commentary* seem to indicate Averroes' lack of acquaintance with this phrase here: "Therefore, any definition from which one cannot easily proceed to knowledge of the accidents of a thing is not a definition, but a sort of indeterminate discourse." *Middle Commentary* (2002), 5, lines 21–22. Cf. *Middle Commentary* (2002), 153–154, n. 22.

46. Arabic fragments correspond to Book 1, 11.22–23: وهو المسير من المتقدم الى المتأخر. (*Long Commentary* Fragments [1985], 31).

47. Arabic fragments correspond to Book 1, 11.27–30: مثل ذلك ان معرفة ماهية ⟨الخط⟩ وكذلك معرفة ماهية ⟨المستقيم⟩ وماهية ⟨السطوح في علم الهندسة⟩ هي مبدأ معرفتنا ان زوايا المثلث مساوية لقائمتين بل وعكس هذه الطريقة (*Long Commentary* Fragments [1985], 31).

the essential proximate attributes, either all or most [of them]. It is as if he says: We are not provided with the knowledge of the substance through the knowledge of the attributes except when we know either all or most of the essential proximate attributes. For then it will happen that we advance a better definition of the substance.[48] Next he said: **For the starting point of every demonstration is [the account of] what something is.** This refers to the point at which the account began, that the knowledge of the definition is useful in regard to knowledge of the attributes.[49] Next he began {16} to explain that this happens for every definition and that every definition which is such that one does not acquire knowledge of the attributes through it is called a definition only equivocally, either because something false is contained in it or because it is composed from extrinsic or accidental causes. He said: **Therefore definitions which**, etc. His account concerning this is self-evident.

12. **Concerning the affections of the soul questions arise as to whether all are common [to the body as well] and besides this belong to this in which they exist, or [whether] there are also some which belong to the soul in particular. For it is necessary to know this, but it is not easy. We see that for several of these it is impossible for them to exist outside the body as activity or as affection,[50] e.g., anger and desire, daring, and sensing generally.[51] But what seems proper to it is understanding. But if this is also imagination or cannot exist without imagination, then it is impossible that even this exist outside the body.** (403a3–10)

When he had listed the things which must be sought out in this science, he also began to say something very useful and much desired in regard to the soul, namely, whether we find all activities and affections of the soul to exist only through the body's involvement, besides the activities and affections in

48. Arabic fragments correspond to Book 1, 11.43–47: ‹معرفة جوهر› ‹وليس يتهيأله بالوقوف على أعراضه إذ لم يكن لنا علم بجميع أعراض الشيء الذاتية أو أكثرها. فانه حينئذ يمكنّنا ان نأتي بحدّ تام ‹للجوهر›› (*Long Commentary* Fragments [1985], 31); ". . . that we give a complete definition."

49. Arabic fragments correspond to Book 1, 11.49–50: أي ان معرفة ‹الحدود› نافعة للوقوف على الأعراض (*Long Commentary* Fragments [1985], 31). Ivry finds the corresponding passage of the *Middle Commentary* dependent on Themistius, *De Anima Paraphrase* (1899), 5.19; (1996), 19. See *Middle Commentary* (2002), 153, n. 21.

50. Here *actio* and *passio* correspond to the Greek ποιεῖν and πάσχειν respectively: "the soul can act or be acted upon." Aristotle, *De Anima* (1984).

51. The Arabic text was apparently much less clear than the Greek. "If we consider the majority of them, there seems to be no case in which the soul can act or be acted upon without involving the body; e.g., anger, courage, appetite, and sensation generally." Aristotle, *De Anima* (1984).

things existing in the body, or we find that among them there is something which does not involve the body and does not require something existing in a body for [its] proper activity and affection. For it is obvious that most of them involve the body but there is doubt, as he says, concerning understanding. He said: {17} **whether all are common**, etc. That is, whether all its activities and affections involve the body and besides this are activities and affections in things existing in the body. He meant this when he said: **and besides this belong to this in which they exist**, i.e., involving the body and existing in that which is in the body. It is possible for something which does not involve the body to be existent in things existing in the body and it is possible for an activity of something involving the body not to be existing in one of the things which are in the body.[52] This careful investigation concerning the soul is extremely useful and is necessary for knowing the precise nature of the soul's separation [from the body]. We ought to keep our eyes right on this. For this reason he said: **For it is** necessary to know **this.**

His statement that most of the affections of the soul seem to involve the body and that those parts of the soul which have those affections are constituted through the body, such as anger and desire, is self-evident. [This is] chiefly so in [regard to] the affections attributed to the concupiscible soul, as we will argue below,[53] and then in the affections of sense, though it is more obscure in them. For, while sensing, no obvious affection is apparent in the first instrument of sense, as is the case with anger, shame, and other affections. Understanding, however, is altogether unclear and involves a great deal of uncertainty. For it has been thought that its proper affection does not involve the body. But, as he said, if to understand is to imagine, or it involves imagining, then it is impossible that it exist without the body, i.e., that it exist outside something in a body.[54] He said this because there are, as we said, two questions concerning each of those powers. {18} First, whether or not it is pos-

---

52. A contemporary treatment of Aristotle's psychology which gives a naturalistic account somewhat similar to what Averroes suggests here is found in Wedin (1988).

53. Cf. Text and Commentary, Book 1, 14, {20–21}.

54. Arabic fragments correspond to Book 1, 12.47–50: فان كان ‹فعل العقل› تخيّلاً أو كان مشتركا مع التخيل فليس يمكن ان يكون هذا الفعل خلوا من البدن (*Long Commentary* Fragments [1985], 31). "If <the activity of understanding> is imagining or it is something which has something in common with imagination, then it is not possible for *this activity* to exist outside the body." Portions of the corresponding text of the *Middle Commentary* are identical: فان كان هذا الفعل تخيلاً أو كان لا يمكن أن يكون دون ;تخيل فليس يمكن أن يكون هذا الفعل خلوا من البدن "if this function is imagination or cannot exist without imagination, then it cannot exist without the body." *Middle Commentary* (2002), 6.9–10. As this example makes clear, the text of the Fragments would be better reconstructed by use of the *Middle Commentary* here.

sible that their activity involve the body. Next, if it does not involve the body, then whether their activity is through and in things involving the body or it is something which does not involve [anything else] at all. For this reason he said: And **what seems proper to it is understanding.** That is, understanding is something which seems to be an affection or activity of the soul without need of a corporeal instrument. But if this is the imagination or [takes place] with the imagination, it is impossible for that activity to exist outside something involving the body, though the intellect does not have any involvement with it. This is his opinion concerning the material intellect: it is separate from the body and it is impossible that it understand anything without the imagination. He did not mean by this what appears superficially [to be the case] from this account, that if understanding comes to be only with imagination, then the material intellect will be generable and corruptible, as Alexander thought from [this account].[55] His account is [something which can be] understood in its own right, but you should observe what we have said.

13. **Let us therefore say that, if some activity or affection of the soul is proper to it, then it is possible for [the soul] to be separate. If there is nothing proper to it, it is impossible for it to be separate. But the case is the same for this as it is for the straight. Insofar as it is straight, there are many [attributes] which accrue to it, e.g., that it touch a sphere of copper at one point.[56] Nevertheless, it is impossible for straightness to be separate per se, since it is always in some body.** (403a10–16) {19}

He showed that one should seek out first whether some activity or affection of the soul exists outside the body, and, if there is [one or more], whether what is outside the body is outside everything existing in a body. Then he began to show here that if there is some affection proper to the soul, i.e., without the body, it is possible that [the soul] be separate in such a way that this affection or activity is not in the things existing in the body. If it does not have some activity proper [to it], it is impossible for it to be separate, although its activity is in things which do not exist in a body. He said: **Let us therefore say,** etc. That is, if some activity or affection of the soul does not need a corporeal instrument, it is possible for that activity or affection to be separate. For if it is not in things existing in a body, it must be separate; and if it is in things existing in a body, it must be inseparable. For example, if understanding was without a corporeal instrument and was not existing in things existing in a body,

55. Alexander, *De Anima* (1887), 90.10–11; (1979), 119.

56. The Text of Averroes here omits οὐ μέντοι γ' ἅψεται οὕτω χωρισθὲν τὸ εὐθυ; "though straightness divorced from the other constituents of the straight thing cannot touch it in this way." Aristotle, *De Anima* (1984).

e.g., as is the case with the understanding of intentions[57] which are imaginable, then it must be an eternal and separate activity.[58] If it is impossible that it exist without imagination, then its activity will not be separate from the body, though the intellect be separate from it. It is obvious, as Themistius says, that for hypothetical connective propositions in which the consequent may possibly be, given the antecedent, it is always necessary that we negate the antecedent and conclude the opposite of the consequent, contrary to the nature of propositions which are such that their consequent follows the antecedent necessarily. For this reason nothing impossible happens for Aristotle inasmuch as he denied the antecedent. For example, if this visible thing is an animal, then it is possible for it to be a human being; but it is not an animal; therefore it is impossible for it to be a human being.[59] Next he said: **But the case is the same for this as it is for the straight.** That is, but if the soul does not have an activity proper [to it], {20} then the affections which are attributed to it will be just as the many things which are attributed to things existing in matter insofar as they happen to be in matter, not insofar as they are separate from matter.[60]

57. *Intentiones*. That is, forms.

58. That is, if understanding can take place without use of the body and does not itself exist in what is in a body (in contrast to the way that the understanding of imaginable intentions exists in a body), then it must be an operation which is eternal and separate.

59. Themistius, *De Anima Paraphrase* (1899), 6.11–33; (1996), 20–21. That is, when the antecedent of a hypothetical proposition can give rise to the consequent but the consequent is negated, then the antecedent is necessarily negated (*modus tollens*). When the antecedent can give rise to the consequent and the antecedent is affirmed, then the consequent necessarily follows (*modus ponens*). Here, however, it is a question of an argument which does not carry this necessity. When the consequent is possible given the antecedent but the antecedent is negated, then the consequent is also negated. If the soul has an operation proper to it without the involvement of the body, then the soul or part of it will be separate from the body. But let us say that we find no operation proper to it without the involvement of the body. Then we conclude only contingently that the soul or part of it is not separate from the body. For it may well be the case that the soul or part of it is separate but sufficient evidence for this has not been obtained.

For Themistius the point here is that Aristotle's conclusion, that the soul or a part of it cannot be separate from the body if there is no evidence of an operation or affection proper to it, is not a necessary conclusion but rather a contingent one. The text of Averroes is far less clear than that of Themistius on this point.

60. Arabic fragments correspond to Book 1, 13.41–45: بل ان كانت النفس ليس لها
فعل خاص وكانت الانفعلات التي تنسب لها تجري مجرى كثير من الأشياء التي ⟨ينسب لها
انفعال⟩ لا من جهة ما هي انفعال . وان كان يعرض لها أنها في هيولي ⟨غير أنّها⟩ لا توجد
خلوا من المادة ، فان الأمر في ذلك كمثله في المستقيم ، فانه بما هو مستقيم قد يعرض له
أن يماس كرة على نقطة الا أنّه ليس يمكن ⟨ـ⟩ الاستقامة على انفرادها وذلك أنها غير مفارقة

[Take] for example the true contact which a line has with a sphere. This is found outside the soul insofar as the line is in a body and the spherical figure [is] in a body, e.g., insofar as the line is in the wood and the sphere is in the copper. For it is impossible for the line to touch the sphere insofar as each of them is separate from matter, unless the contact is mathematical, not natural.

14. **It also seems that all the affections of the soul are in the body, such as anger, kindness, fear, pity, courage, joy, sorrow,[61] hate, and love. For the body is affected by these in such a way that sometimes the affections become strong and apparent, while of these neither anger nor fear occur to the human being. And sometimes affections small and weak will move [a human being] when the body is so disposed. It is more obvious when we see that some human beings are very fearful though nothing fearful befalls them. Hence it is obvious that the affections of the soul are intentions in matter.[62]** (403a16–25)

When he had related that most affections and activities of the soul seem to involve the body, he began here to make known the genus in which this appears in an obvious way. He said: **It seems that all**, etc. He means by **affections of the soul** the dispositions attributed to the concupiscible power.[63] {21} Next he said: **For the body is affected by these**. That is, alteration and change appear in it.[64] For every affection brought about by alteration and change is necessarily in a body or arises from a power in a body. Since this proposition is true, and also because all the attributes of the concupiscible soul come about through change, he concludes necessarily that this soul either is a body or is a power in a body. But because the major proposition is obvious but the minor

وان كان ذلك فمع جسم ما (*Long Commentary* Fragments [1985], 31); "But if the soul does not have a proper activity, the affections which are attributed to it would be just as is the case for many of the things to which an affection is attributed but not insofar as it is an affection. If it is in matter but without it being the case that it does not exist outside matter, then in this case the state of affairs is just as it is for what is straight. For inasmuch as it is something straight, it touches a sphere at a point. However, the straightness cannot exist apart from it. For it is not separable, and if this is so, it is in a body." For وكانت الانفعلات I read فكانت الانفعلات.

61. As Ivry notes, "sadness," *tristitia*, الحزن, was added to Aristotle's original list. *Middle Commentary* (2002), 154, n. 26.

62. τὰ πάθη λόγοι ἔνυλοί εἰσιν: "are enmattered accounts." *De Anima* (1984).

63. Arabic fragments correspond to Book 1, 14.16–17: «انفعالات النف» ـب ويعني ... س الحالات التي تنسب الى القوة الشهوانية (*Long Commentary* Fragments [1985], 31).

64. Arabic fragments correspond to Book 1, 14.18–19: «فان البدن ظاهر من قال ثم ... أمره انه ينفعل...» يعني انه يظهر فيه تغير واستحالة (*Long Commentary* Fragments [1985], 31).

to some extent obscure, since it is possible that some affections occur which do not arise from the body's being affected by sense, he began to explain this in another way. He said: What indicates this is that **perhaps**, etc. That is, it signifies that [the soul] uses the body as if it were an instrument and that the body is affected by [affections] even if it is not affected by sense, since [the soul's] activity differs according to the diversity of the dispositions of the body. For many things happen to a human being which naturally should cause strong motion but which move him only weakly, e.g., something fearful or something provoking anger happens to a human being and these move him only a little.[65] Or, on the contrary, when the body is disposed, as he said, and it is disposed so as to be angered. For an irascible [human being] will very easily be moved by something trivial provoking anger. It is more obvious, as he says, because we see many human beings fearful without a cause of fear.[66] All these indicate that that activity does not come about without the body. Next he said: **It is obvious that the affections**, etc. That is, it is therefore obvious that the forms coming to exist in that soul by affection and motion are forms in matter.[67] {22}

15. **Thus [their] definitions ought to be so. For anger is a motion of some part of that body or of some power belonging to it, from such a thing and on account of such a thing. For this reason it belongs to the natural scientist to consider the soul, either every sort or this sort.** (403a25–28)

Since he has explained that those affections are material forms, matter must appear in their definitions.[68] The motion which those forms follow is a material motion such that the body should be included in the definition of that motion, e.g., anger is a motion of a part of the body. Since matter appears in the definitions of those powers, it is obvious that consideration of the soul belongs to the natural scientist,[69] either of every soul, if every soul is of this sort, or of the

---

65. Arabic fragments correspond to Book 1, 14.34–36: مثال ذلك انا نرى بعض الناس يعرض لهم أمور ﴿مفزعة﴾ أو مغضية فلا ﴿يتحركون﴾ عنها الا ﴿قدرا﴾ يسيرا (*Long Commentary* Fragments [1985], 31).

66. Arabic fragments correspond to Book 1, 14.39–40: ... وذلك أنا نرى كثيرا ﴿من الناس﴾ يفزعون من غير ان يعرض لهم أمر مفزع (*Long Commentary* Fragments [1985], 32).

67. Arabic fragments correspond to Book 1, 14.42–44: ثم قال «ومن البين ان هذه الأنفعالات...» الخ ... يعني انه ﴿من البين﴾ ان الصور الحاصلة لهذه النفوس عن الانفعال والحركة انما هي صور في هيولي. (*Long Commentary* Fragments [1985], 32).

68. Arabic fragments correspond to Book 1, 15.6–8: ولما بين ان هذه الأنفعالات هي ﴿صور هيولانية﴾ فيجب ان تظهر في حدودها الهيولي (*Long Commentary* Fragments [1985], 32).

69. Arabic fragments correspond to Book 1, 15.10–13: مثل ذلك أن الغضب هو حركة ما لجزء ما من البدن. وبما ان الهيولي تظهر في حدّ هذه القوى فمن البين أن النظر في النفس للطبيعي (*Long Commentary* Fragments [1985], 32).

souls which are established to be material. This is what he meant when he said: **For this reason** consideration **of the soul belongs to the natural scientist.**[70]

16. **What the natural scientist offers as a definition of any one of these differs from what the dialectician**[71] **offers. For example, what anger is. For the dialectician says: anger is a desire for revenge, and so forth. But the natural scientist says that it is a bubbling up of the blood or of heat in the heart. The natural scientist therefore gives the matter, while the dialectician gives the form and the intention. For the intention of something is a determinate particular and a determinate particular must be in matter.**[72] **[Take] for example, a house: one gives the intention by saying that it is something covered {23} which provides protection from showers and rains, cold**[73] **and heat. But another says that it consists of stones, bricks, and wood. And yet another gives the form existing in this on account of those. Who among these is the natural scientist? Is it the one who attended to the matter and ignored the intention, or is it the one who attended only to the intention? Or is it better to say that it is the one who brings both together? To whom, therefore, would both of the others be attributed?** (403a29–b9)

When he had shown that he ought to include matter and form in the definitions of those powers, he began to raise questions about the customary practice among natural scientists and those who consider [things] separately [from matter], namely, dialecticians. For natural scientists differ from dialecticians in regard to the method of definition. For the dialecticians give definitions according to the form alone and say that anger is an appetite for re-

---

70. Arabic fragments correspond to Book 1, 15.15–16: «فان النظر في أمر النفس هو من نظر صاحب العلم الطبيعي». (*Long Commentary* Fragments [1985], 32). The *Middle Commentary* also has this phrase, هو من نظر صاحب العلم الطبيعي, but such phraseology is formulaic and need not indicate any relationship between the commentaries. *Middle Commentary* (2002), 7.16.

71. Both *sermocinalis* here in the Text of Aristotle (for the Greek διαλεκτικὸς) and *disputator* in the Comment of Averroes are translated as "dialectician" without distinction.

72. ὁ δὲ τὸ εἶδος καὶ τὸν λόγον. ὁ μὲν γὰρ λόγος ὅδε τοῦ πράγματος, ἀνάγκη δ' εἶναι τοῦτον ἐν ὕλῃ τοιᾳδί, εἰ ἔσται: "the other the form or account; for what he states is the account of the fact, though for its actual existence there must be embodiment of it in a material such as is described by the other." Aristotle, *De Anima* (1984). The alternate Arabic translation has قال بالصورة والمعنى for τὸ εἶδος καὶ τὸν λόγον and renders the sentence satisfactorily. See ibid. (1954), 6. In the *Middle Commentary* Ivry renders the Arabic معان في هيولى "intentions in matter." *Middle Commentary* (2002), 8.

73. *Et frigore.* This is apparently added to the text of Aristotle. It is found in the alternate Arabic translation as والبرد (Aristotle, *De Anima* [1954], 7) and in the *Middle Commentary* (*Middle Commentary* [2002], 8; also see 155, n. 32).

venge. But natural scientists [give definitions] according to the matter and say that it is a bubbling up of heat and blood in the heart.[74] Next he said: **For the intention of something is a determinate particular.** That is, as it seems to me: for the intention of something, inasmuch as it is a being, is a determinate particular.[75]

Next he said: **and it must be in matter,** etc. That is, that intention, inasmuch as it is a determinate particular, must exist in matter which has such a disposition, i.e., which is also a determinate particular and [which] exists through some intention existing in [the matter] by virtue of which it was suited for that thing to exist in it and not in something else. He indicated agreement by [giving] this account, for, just as the intention must exist in matter inasmuch as it is a determinate particular, so the way it is included must be [reflected] in its definition. If not, the intention will be included in a way different from the way it exists. For one who {24} includes matter in the definition and leaves form out does so leaving something out. But one who includes form and leaves out matter is thought to leave out something which is not necessary. But this is not so, for the form ought to be included in the definitions according to the dispositions by which it exists. The rest of the account is obvious.

17. **Let us therefore say that one who intends to consider the affections of matter which are inseparable from it, insofar as they are inseparable, is none other than the natural scientist who considers all the activities and affections of that body and of that matter.[76] What is not of this sort should**

---

74. Arabic fragments correspond to Book 1, 16.24–29: وقد كانت حدود أصحاب العلم الطبيعي ... تخالف حدود الجدليين وذلك ان حدود أصحاب الجدل مأخوذة من الصور فقط. فكانوا ‹مثلا› يحدون الغضب بأنه شهوة للانتقام. وأما حدود أصحاب العلم الطبيعي فانها مأخوذة من المواد فهم يحدونه بأنه غليان ‹الحرارة› والدم الذي في القلب (*Long Commentary* Fragments [1985], 32).

75. That is, insofar as a form is a being existing in the world, it must be "a this" or a determinate particular being. Averroes' comment here is based on a faulty rendering of the Greek text of Aristotle. See n. 72. On his understanding of the notion of a "this" (*hoc*), Aristotle's τόδε τι, see n. 25.

76. The Text here varies from the Greek: "Must we not say that there is no type of thinker who concerns himself with those qualities or attributes of the material which are in fact inseparable from the material, and without attempting even in thought to separate them? The physicist is he who concerns himself with all the properties active and passive of bodies or materials thus or thus defined." Aristotle, *De Anima* (1984). The alternate Arabic translation does not capture the sense either: وأما المتقدمون فليس منهم أحد يدخل في حده الأعراض المغيرة للهيولى لا الزائلة منها ولا اللازمة الثابتة ، ما خلا حد الطبيعي فانه يأتي على جميع ما هو للجرم بما فيه من الكيفية وما للهيولى من الأفعال والأعراض (ibid. [1954]); "None of the ancients includes within the scope of this study the changeable and the non-transitory accidents belonging to matter which [also] are

be considered by someone else. In some cases a craftsman such as the carpenter or the physician ought to deal with them. The mathematician deals with the things which are not separate in reality[77] but are affections of body and [does so] considering them as separable. The First Philosopher, however, deals with things which are separate in reality. (403b9–16)

After he had raised questions about definitions, he began to show here which arts use form and matter in definitions and which [use] only form. He said: **that** one **who intends to consider the affections of matter** which are inseparable **from it, insofar as they** are [**inseparable**], etc. That is, the one who intends to consider the forms consequent upon the affections of matter which are not separate from matter insofar as they are not separate, [that one] is the natural scientist[78] who considers all the affections of the body and the nature of that matter and its affections.

Next he said: **What is not of this sort**, etc. That is, what {25} among those forms and affections is not by nature but by will should be considered by productive craftsmen such as the carpenter and physician.[79] Next he said: **The things which are not** separate, etc. That is, mathematicians ought to consider the attributes [which are] inseparable from body and consequent upon it, [though] not insofar as it is changeable but insofar as it is a body only and a

---

not necessary and subsistent, except the natural philosopher, for he treats of all that belongs to body insofar as it has quality and insofar as it has matter with activities and accidents."

77. *In rei veritate.* This phrase, here and in the following sentence, has no precise correspondence to any phrase in the Greek text. See Book 2, Texts 65, 418a25, {227} and 156, 428a {368}, and the notes there. In his Comments throughout this work, the phrases *secundum rem, in re, in rei veritate,* and related constructions are consistently found to indicate what exists in reality (in actual being) and in the world, whether in the material realm or in the immaterial realm, as opposed to what exists only in the beliefs or convictions of people. This may render the Arabic phrase في الحقيقة, which is found, for example, at *Middle Commentary* (2002), 8.16.

78. Arabic fragments correspond to Book 1, 17.18–21: ان النظر في ⟨الصور الحاصلة عن⟩ الانفعالات ⟨الهيولانية⟩ التي هي غير مفارقة للمادة من جهة ما هي غير مفارقة لها ⟨انما⟩ هو لصاحب العلم الطبيعي (*Long Commentary* Fragments [1985], 32).

79. Arabic fragments correspond to Book 1, 17.21–26: لأنه ينظر في جميع افعال البدن وانفعالاته. وأما الأفعال المنسوبة الى الافادة فهي منسوبة الى الصناعات ⟨العملية⟩ مثل النجارة والطب (*Long Commentary* Fragments [1985], 32); "because he investigates all the activities and affections of body. As for the activities related to utility, they are related to the productive sciences such as carpentry and medicine." Note that the Latin translator read ارادة, *per voluntatem,* rather than افادة, "utility, benefit."

magnitude (these are those which the intellect understands in separation from matter, although in fact they are not separate). But the First Philosopher considers the forms which are separate in reality, i.e., in being and understanding.[80]

18. But we must return to our account in which we said that affections of soul are not separate from the natural matter of the animal. The things which are such as this in reality[81] are anger and fear [which are] not as the line and plane. (403b16–19)

Because this is more proper to the logician, let us return to what we said, that the affections of the concupiscible soul are separate from the body neither in definition nor in being. [Take] for example, anger and fear, which are not separate even in definition as [are] the line and the plane.

19. In the inquiry concerning the soul we must[82] mention first the opinions of the ancients. We will be helped by these and will adopt what is true and said properly, and we will avoid what {26} was said improperly. We also ought to mention first what things are properly thought to be natural [to the soul]. We assert this principle when we say that what has a soul seems to differ in its own right from what is not ensouled in two ways, in reference to motion and in reference to sense. These two ways [of distinguishing] regarding the soul we take from the ancients. (1.2, 403b20–28)

Since he had explained in the *Posterior Analytics*[83] that the consideration leading to perfect certainty in things investigated in any of the genera comes about only by considering the principles proper to the genus in question, he began to show [here] that one must consider the soul in this way with reference to [its] principles.[84] He said: In inquiring about the soul we ought to mention first the propositions and principles which seem to be proper to the soul insofar as it is soul and let us set forth those propositions as the starting point of

80. Themistius, *De Anima Paraphrase* (1899), 8.29–31; (1996), 23. Arabic fragments correspond to Book 1, 17.32–34: وهذه هي التي ينظر فيها صاحب علم التعاليم ، ومنها أيضا
.صور هي مفارقة في الحقيقة أي بالوجود والحد وهذه هي التي تنظر فيها الفلسفة الأولى
(*Long Commentary* Fragments [1985], 32). Corresponding to the Latin text's "understanding," *intellectum*, the Arabic has the more cogent الحد, "definition."

81. *In rei veritate*. This phrase has no precise correspondence to any phrase in the Greek text. See n. 77.

82. The Text here omits 403b20–21, "while formulating the problems of which in our further advance we are to find solutions." Aristotle, *De Anima* (1984). The alternate translation does not suffer from omission. See ibid. (1954).

83. Aristotle, *Posterior Analytics* 1.9, 75b37ff.

84. That is, according to the principles proper to the genus.

[our] consideration.[85] He made it known that with respect to the soul such [starting points] are two, sense and motion. For what is a living animal differs from what is not a living animal only in sense and local motion.[86] He said: **what has a soul**, etc. Here he means [to indicate] certitude by **seems**, for he uses such words in lieu of certitude in places in which certitude is customary. The remaining account is obvious.

20. **For some of them say that what is proper and prior for the soul is to move. Because they thought that everything which is unmoved cannot move another, they thought the soul to be something in motion. For this reason Democritus said that it is fire and heat. For he said that {27} it is composed of bodies and shapes[87] infinitely divisible and that those which are spherical are fire and soul, for example. Similar to this are the bodies existing in air called indivisible particles,[88] which are in the rays of the sun entering through windows. He says that the elements of all natural things exist in these by virtue of a collection of particles. Leucippus held a similar position. The spherical ones are soul because such shapes are able to pass into a thing wholly, and they move all things because they too are in motion. For they think that the soul gives motion to living things.** (403b28–404a9)

After he had made it known that the ancients considered the soul only by reference to motion or sensation, or both, he began first to list the opinions of people who consider the soul by reference to motion. He said: **For some of them**, etc. That is, since some of them held the opinion that what belongs to the soul in the first place is that it moves something else and held the opinion that what moves something else ought to be moved, they thought that the soul is something eternally moved. Next he said: **For this reason Democritus said that it is fire** or **heat**, that is, either fire or something fiery.[89] Next he said: **For he says**

---

85. Arabic fragments correspond to Book 1, 19.17–19: وينبغي ان نقدم في بحثنا عن ⟨أمر النفس⟩ المقدمات والمبادئُ التي يظن انها⟩ موجودة للنفس وأنها خاصة بها ⟨من جهة ⟨عنها⟩ أنها نفس⟩ ونجعل من هذه المقدمات مبدأ الفحص (*Long Commentary* Fragments [1985], 32). The *Middle Commentary* is substantially the same: وينبغي ان نقدم في بحثنا عنها الأشياء التي يظن أنها موجودة بالطبع للنفس وأنها خاصة بها ونجعل مبدأ الفحص منها. (*Middle Commentary* [2002], 9.3–4).

86. Arabic fragments correspond to Book 1, 19.21–22: فان المتنفس ⟨لا⟩ يخالف الغير المتنفس الا بالاحساس والحركة ⟨المكانية⟩ (*Long Commentary* Fragments [1985], 33).

87. ἀπείρων γὰρ ὄντων σχημάτων καὶ ἀτόμων·: "his 'forms' or atoms are infinite in number." Aristotle, *De Anima* (1984).

88. ξύσματα. "motes." Aristotle, *De Anima* (1984).

89. Arabic fragments correspond to Book 1, 20.22 and 25–27: فقال ... اعتقدوا ان النفس لها حركة دائمة فقال » ولذلك قال ديمقراطيس أنها نار أو شى حار« ⟨يعني⟩ أنها نار أو نارية (*Long Commentary* Fragments [1985], 33). The *Middle Commentary* uses a dif-

that it is **composed of bodies and shapes**, etc. That is, for he held the opinion that, because it moves something else and is [itself] moved, it is composed of indivisible bodies having infinite shapes and that among these [the soul] is composed of the spherical [atoms] alone. Because the spherical are fire or something fiery, they believed that the spherical ones among them are either fire or soul. Next he gave examples of these bodies according to Democritus. He said: **Similar to** these **are the bodies existing in air.** That is, those bodies {28} according to him are similar to indivisible particles which appear to be moved in the rays of the sun. When he had made it known that Democritus held the opinion that the soul is composed of indivisible bodies which according to him are similar to [those] indivisible particles, he made known what are the parts from which, according to Democritus' view, the soul comes to be, and [he made known] how [Democritus] held the opinion that these elements belong to other composite things. He said: **He says that in these by a collection of particles**, etc. That is, these are the bodies about which Democritus says that by a collection of particles in them they are fit for different beings to be composed from them, even though they are of the same nature. He means by **particles** their diversity in shape, in place, and in order.[90] For the diversity of parts in these three ways is the cause of the diversity of the things composed of them, as writing is different owing to the diversity of letters in these three [ways].[91]

After he had related that they hold the opinion that the soul is fire or something fiery because they hold the opinion that soul is spherical and that fire is spherical, he gave the reason why they held the opinion that the soul is spherical. He said: The spherical among them is **soul**, etc. That is, Democritus and Leucippus held the opinion that the spherical indivisible bodies are soul only because they held the opinion that such bodies are things which are able to pass through other things and move them, although they are themselves eternally in motion. This is the disposition which they thought to be proper to the soul since it moves the body and is [itself] always in motion.

21. **For this reason they said that respiration is the definition of life. For when the surrounding air brings together bodies and binds [them] together**

---

ferent phraseology: أنها نار او شيء حار ;"that it is fire or something hot." *Middle Commentary* (2002), 9.14–15. Translation slightly modified. This is very close to the alternate Arabic translation, which has إن النفس نار و شيء حار (Aristotle, *De Anima* [1954]); "that the soul is fire and something hot.".

90. Arabic fragments correspond to Book 1, 20.46–47: انها تختلف بعضها عن بعض (*Long Commentary* Fragments [1985], 33). بالشكل والوضع والترتيب.

91. Arabic fragments correspond to Book 1, 20.48–49: كالحال في اختلاف الألفاظ المركبة (*Long Commentary* Fragments [1985], 33). لاختلاف الحروف في هذه.

from those shapes which give animals motion, because [these bodies] are never at rest at any {29} time, they say that [these] are sustained by inhaling from outside other forms similar to these. [This is] because these also prevent what has already entered inside animals from exiting and likewise exhale with these what brings them together and binds them together. [This is] because life exists so long as the animal is able to do this.[92] (404a9–16)

Everyone who predicates one thing of the quiddity of another works to make that [attribute] fit all the sensible [appearances] and to provide the cause of that sensible [appearance] from what has been given by it in its substance. But those who held that the soul consists of indivisible spherical parts worked to give the cause of breathing in this way by saying: For this reason, because the soul consists of spherical parts which are always in motion, breathing was the definition of life or consequent upon life. When the surrounding air brings bodies together, there will be bound together many spherical figures which are inside bodies and which give motion to animals because they are always in motion. These bodies, then, will be moved to exit and that is the exit of breath. The animal, then, will be sustained by inhaling other spherical bodies from outside and this is by inhaling breath. This, however, was due to three things: first, replacement of what exited; second, prevention of most bodies [already] inside from exiting; and third, helping them also to expel what binds and brings them together. They say: For this reason life is found so long as the animal is able to do this.[93]

---

92. This text is a rough approximation of the Greek: "for they prevent the extrusion of those which are already within by counteracting the compressing and consolidating force of the environment; and animals continue to live only so long as they are able to maintain this resistance." Aristotle, *De Anima* (1984).

93. Arabic fragments correspond to Book 1, 21.16–30: فنقول ﴿ولهذا السبب﴾ أعني كون النفس أجزاء كرية دائمة الحركة كان التنفس هو حدّ الحياة أو لازم من لوازمها والتنسف يحصل للنفس بحركة التنفس التي من داخل الى خارج. وذلك ان الهواء المحيط بنا إذا جمع الاشكال الكرية التي داخل البدن ﴿و﴾ التي يعطي للحيوان الحركة ضغطت على الأبدان كثيرا من قبل انها في حركة دائمة فتتحرك هذه الأجسام لتخرج فيكون ذلك هو إخراج النفس وعند ذلك ﴿يستنشق﴾ الحيوان بأن يدخل أجساما كرية أخرى من خارج – وهو إدخال النفس – وذلك لثلاثة أمور : أولا أن يخلف بدل ما خرج منها ثانيا ان يمنع أيضا بدخولها كثيرا من الأجسام الداخلة من أن تخرج ، ثالثا أن يعينها أيضا في دفع ﴿الشيء﴾ الذي يضغطها ويجمعها للخروج . قال : ولذلك كانت الحياة ما دام الحيوان يمكنه ان يفعل هذا الفعل (*Long Commentary* Fragments [1985], 33); "so we say <for this reason>, namely, since it is the case that the soul is eternally moving fine particles, respiration is the definition of life or one of its necessary properties, and respiration occurs in the soul by the motion of respiration which is in and out. For with regard to the air contained within us, if the fine shapes which enter the body <and> which give motion to the animal are gathered together, they exert a great deal of pressure on the bodies. In this way they are always

22. **Perhaps the account of the Pythagoreans is of this sort. For some of them say that the soul is an indivisible particle {30} existing in air, but others [say that it is] what moves the indivisible particles. They said this because these seem to be eternally in motion, even when there is no wind at all. Those who say that the soul is something self-moving are very similar to these [on this matter]. For they all seem to hold the opinion that motion belongs to the soul and that all things are moved only by soul, while soul is moved per se. For it seems that nothing causes motion unless it moves itself as well.** (404a16–25)

Perhaps the opinion of Pythagoras on the soul is also similar to the opinion of Democritus and Leucippus. For some of the Pythagoreans said that the soul consists of indivisible particles of air and some [say that it] is what moves indivisible particles. They held this opinion because they believed that the indivisible particles were always moved and the soul is always moved. Next he said: **Those who say [that the soul is something self-moving]** are similar to these, etc. He has Plato in mind. They all, therefore, agree in this, that motion is proper to the soul, but they differ in regard to what it is. Some of them think that it is indivisible bodies or fire or something fiery, but others [think it to be] indivisible particles.[94]

23. **Anaxagoras also said similarly that the soul is a mover, and besides this he said that the intellect moves everything. Still, Anaxagoras meant**

---

in motion and move these bodies to go out, and so this is the soul's expulsion and in this way the animal <inhales> other fine bodies from the outside—this is the soul's entering. This happens for three reasons. First, it replaces the equivalent of what went out from it; second, by their entering it prevents many of the bodies entering from exiting, and third, it also helps in the expulsion <of the thing> which it compresses and concentrates for expulsion. He said: For this reason life continues for the animal so long as it is able to carry out this activity."

94. Arabic fragments correspond to Book 1, 22. 11–21: ويشبه أن يكون ما اعتقده

‹فيثاغورس› في النفس قريبا مما اعتقده ‹ديمقراطيس ولوقيبوس› وذلك ان بعضا من الفيتاغورين قالوا ان النفس هي الهباء نفسه ، وبعضهم قال انها الشيء المحرك للهباء. والذى قادهم لهذا انهم اعتقدوا ان الهباء يتحرك دائما من ذاته وان النفس في حركة دائمة . . . ثم قال » وشبيه بهذا الرأي ما قيل . . . «وهو يعني هاهنا أفلاطون. فهؤلاء كلهم مجمعون في ذلك أعني كون الحركة أخص الأشياء للنفس ، ولكنهم مختلفون في حد ماهيتها. وذلك أن بعضهم اعتقد انها جسم غير منقسم او انها نار أو شيء ناري ، وبعضهم أنها الهباء نفسه (Long Commentary) Fragments [1985], 33). Part of the corresponding passage of the Middle Commentary is identical to the opening remarks of this fragment: ويشبه أن يكون ما اعتقده فيثاغورش في النفس قريبا من هذا الاعتقاد، وذلك ان بعضهم قال ان النفس هي الهباء نفسه، وبعضهم قال انها الشيء المحرك للهباء; "It seems that the Pythagoreans held a similar belief concerning the soul, for some said that it is the very motes, while others said that it is that which moves the motes." Middle Commentary (2002), 10.11–13.

something different from what Democritus meant. For Democritus said simply that the soul is the same as the intellect, for he says that truth is whatever appears to be the case. For this reason Homer said, and he spoke the truth, that Acteon [Hector] swooned and was without {31} intellect.[95] For he did not use "intellect" as if it were some power; rather, he said that the intellect and the soul are the same. (404a26–32)

Anaxagoras also holds a similar opinion since he said that the soul is a mover and he said that the intellect moves everything. But by this Anaxagoras did not mean what Democritus [meant]. For Democritus put forth the notion that the soul and intellect are the same. He said that truth as discerned exists only in what is apparent to sense alone.

For this reason the poet Homer spoke well when he reported concerning someone who was without sensation that he was without intellect.[96] Democritus, therefore, does not mean that the intellect is some power in animals different from the power of sense, but says [rather] that the intellect and soul are the same.[97]

24. **Anaxagoras spoke more obliquely about these matters since he frequently said that the intellect is the cause of discovery.[98] He said in another place that the intellect and the soul are the same. For in his view intellect exists in all animals great and small, noble and base. But we do not see this intellect existing in a similar way in all animals nor even in human beings.** (404b1–6)

However, when Anaxagoras put forth the notion that the intellect and the soul are the same, he put forth the notion more obliquely than did Democritus since he frequently says that the intellect is the cause of rectitude and soundness.[99] From this his opinion appears to be that the intellect is different from sense. But in other places he seems to hold the opinion that intellect and soul

95. "Democritus roundly identifies soul and mind, for he identifies what appears with what is true—that is why he commends Homer for the phrase 'Hector lay with thought distraught.'" Aristotle, *De Anima* (1984).

96. Cf. Themistius, *De Anima Paraphrase* (1899), 9.39–10.2; (1996), 24.

97. Arabic fragments correspond to Book 1, 23.12–19: فان ديمقراطيس كان يعتقد ان النفس والعقل شيء واحد وان الحقيقة المدركة انما هي الأمر الظاهر للحس ⟨فقط⟩ ولذلك أصاب أوميروش الشاعر حين قال أن من فقد الحواس إنه فقد العقل. وان ديمقراطيس ليس يعتقد (Long Commentary Fragments [1985], 33). ان العقل قوة ما في الحيوان غير قوة الحس ، بل يقول انهما واحد ments [1985], 33).

98. *Causa in inventione.* The Greek has "the cause of beauty and order." Aristotle, *De Anima* (1984). See n. 99 regarding this.

99. In the Text, τὸ αἴτιον τοῦ καλῶς καὶ ὀρθῶς τὸν νοῦν λέγει, "he tells us that the cause of beauty and order is thought" (Aristotle, *De Anima* [1984]), corresponds to

are the same. For he says that the intellect exists in all animals, {32} great and small, noble and ignoble.[100] [But] it is not as he thought because we do not see intellect existing in the same way in all human beings, [and] much less does it exist in all animals.

25. **Those asserting that the principle of the soul is motion thought that the soul is more fit to cause motion than all [other] things. Those asserting that the criterion in this is knowledge and sensation of all beings say that the soul is [itself] the principles. Therefore some of them asserted that these principles are more than one, while others asserted it to be one.[101] So Empedocles, for**

---

multotiens dicebat quod intellectus est causa in inventione, "he frequently said that the intellect is the cause of discovery." The precise nature of the problem here is far from obvious. The Latin *inventione* may render the Arabic إدراك , which appears in the alternate translation, although not in the corresponding passage in the *Middle Commentary*. Part of this passage in the Comment, "the intellect is the cause of rectitude and soundness," corresponds precisely with the *Middle Commentary*: سبب الاستقامة والصواب هو العقل (*Middle Commentary* [2002], 11.9). In the alternate translation, however, it appears to be something added since it corresponds to nothing in the Greek. This Arabic text has العقل علة إدراك حقائق الأشياء وصحتها (Aristotle, *De Anima* [1954]); "the intellect is the cause of the perception of the truth and soundness of things." But in his Comment here Averroes quotes the text of Aristotle correctly, without إدراك, *inventio*. Perhaps the Text of the Latin translator's Arabic manuscript was corrupt and the Comment more precisely reflects the text of Aristotle which Averroes had before himself. That Averroes does not mention that there is a textual problem here, as he oftentimes does when one arises, supports this view.

100. Arabic fragments correspond to Book 1, 24.9–15: وكذلك انكساغورس فانه كان يعتقد ان العقل والنفس شيء واحد ، غير ان اعتقاده كان أخفى من اعتقاد ديمقراطيس لأنه قال في ‹غير ما موضع› ان سبب الاستقامة والصواب هو العقل. وهذا يدل من قوله على ان العقل غير النفس الا أنه قال في موضع آخر ان العقل والنفس شيء واحد ، وقال ان العقل في ‹كل حيوان ‹كبير كان أم صغير شريف كان أم حقير› (*Long Commentary* Fragments [1985], 34). As indicated in the previous note, سبب الاستقامة والصواب هو العقل is also found at *Middle Commentary* (2002), 11.9. Note that the Latin version, with "From this his opinion appears to be that the intellect is different from sense (*aliud a sensu*)," differs from this fragment, which has "He indicates this by his saying that the intellect is different from *the soul* (غير النفس)."

101. The reading *unam* probably reflects the Arabic واحدة, a feminine adjective. That the reading should be *unam* and not *unum* is clear from Averroes' quotation and explanation of the former in the Comment. Aristotle, *De Anima* (1954), 9, notes corruption in the manuscript and reconstructs the text of the alternate translation. In the *Middle Commentary* Averroes writes, "Those who said that the principles are one made the soul one: while of those who said that the principles are more than one, some made the soul more than one, and some made it one, that is, united by the principles." *Middle Commentary* (2002), 11.20–22.

example, asserted that the soul is composed of all the elements, but nevertheless asserted that each of the elements is also a soul. He said that we understand earth only by earth, water by water, air by air, fire by its like, namely,
fire, strife by strife, and friendship by friendship. (404b7–15)

When he had finished the account of those considering the soul in reference
to motion, he also began to express the opinions of those who consider it in
reference to knowledge and discernment, saying: **Those asserting that the
principle of the soul is motion**, etc. That is, those asserting that the criterion
of soul and [also] knowledge of its nature is owing to motion, on the basis of
which they judged that the soul is more fit in reference to motion than all other
things, as we said. But those asserting that the criterion for the consideration
of what is alive is in reference to its acquisition of knowledge and discernment
in regard to all beings hold the opinion that the soul is the principle of everything {33} or composed of the principles of everything. Therefore, those asserting these principles to be more than one asserted that the soul is more than
one, and those who hold the opinion that the principle is one asserted that the
soul is one. For example, because Empedocles asserts that the soul came to be
from the elements,[102] he also asserts that it is six in number according to the
number of elements in his view. For **he said that we understand earth only
by earth**, etc. When [Aristotle] said: **Some of them asserted that these principles are more than one**, he meant: some of them, because they asserted these
principles to be more than one, held the opinion that the soul is more than one,
as [does] Empedocles.[103] But he was content to state the fact in lieu of the consequent. When he said: **while others assert that the soul is one**, he means:
some who assert that there is one principle, assert that there is one soul.[104] But
he was content here with the consequent in lieu of the fact, contrary to what
he did in the first place. The rest of the account is obvious enough.

**26. In a similar fashion Plato asserted in the *Timaeus*[105] that the soul is
something composed from elements, since in his view nothing is known**

102. Arabic fragments correspond to Book 1, 25.22–25: والذين جعلوا المبدأ أكثر من واحد
، جعلوا النفس أكثر من واحد ، والذين اعتقدوا ان المبدأ واحد ، جعلوا النفس واحدة. وعلى هذا
المثال جعل انبدوقليس النفس من المبادئ (*Long Commentary* Fragments [1985], 34).

103. Arabic fragments correspond to Book 1, 25.27–31: وذلك انه يقال «انا ندرك الأرض
بالأرض الخ ...» ثم انه قال «والذين جعلوا هذا المبدأ أكثر من واحد ...» يريد : الذين وضعوا
هذا المبدأ أكثر من واحد فاعتقدوا ان النفس أكثر من واحد كما ‹فعل ذلك› انبدوقليس
(*Long Commentary* Fragments [1985], 34).

104. Arabic fragments correspond to Book 1, 25.32–34: «ومنهم من جعل
النفس واحدة» يريد ان بعضهم من جعل المبدأ واحد فجعل النفس واحدة (*Long Commentary*
Fragments [1985], 34).

105. *Timaeus*, 35Aff.

except by its like and all things come to be only from their principles. He earlier came to a similar determination in *On Philosophy*, namely, in his lectures.[106] It is obvious that the book *Timaeus* takes its point of departure from these [lectures][107] and that animal absolutely considered is composed from the form of the one and from the first length, first breadth, and first depth, and that it is so for other things. (404b16–21) {34}

In a similar fashion Plato asserted in the *Timaeus* that the soul is something composed from the substance of elements. For he also held what he who asserts the soul to be composed from principles holds, that all things are known only by their like and are known only by knowledge of their principles. Because principles are known through their like, the result is that principles are known through principles. When we join to this the notion that the soul knows things through their principles, the result of this is that the soul is [itself] the principles, for these are convertible properties.[108] Next he said: **He earlier came to a similar determination**, etc. That is, he came to a similar determination in his *On Philosophy* and in his lectures, for he said this in a different way in the *Timaeus*. He said there that animal absolutely considered in itself, which is the genus of the particular animals and of their principles, is composed from the one; from first length, which is composed from the first twoness; from breadth, which is composed from the first threeness; and from depth, which is composed from the first fourness: these are the principles of the rest of [all the] composite numbers. He held the opinion that length is composed from twoness because the line comes to be from two points, breadth from threeness because it comes to be from three points with length, and density from fourness because it comes to be from four points with length and breadth. Since he held the opinion that numbers are the principles of all things, it was necessary for him that the principles of numbers be the principles of the gen-

106. Ross (Aristotle, *De Anima* [1961], 177) points out that there is some uncertainty as to whether Aristotle is here referring to lectures on philosophy by Plato (perhaps the famous unwritten account, "On the Good" or to his own dialogue, *On Philosophy*. He indicates that he is following Cherniss (1944), 565–580, in considering the reference to be to this work by Aristotle. Averroes, however, seems to understand it differently. The alternate translation is also unclear on this.

107. "It is obvious . . . from these [lectures]" in Averroes' Text is an interpolation with no corresponding Greek. This is also not found in the alternate translation.

108. Arabic fragments correspond to Book 1, 26.11–20: ان افلاطون وضع في كتاب طيماوس ان النفس شيء من جوهر الأسطقس وذلك انه يجعل انها من طبيعة المبادئ كون ان النفس هي مبادئ وذلك انه إذا وضع ان الأشياء تعرف بمبادئها – لأن المبادئ تعرف بشبيه أو بشبيهها – يلزم أن المبادئ تعرف بالمبادئ وإذا أضفنا الى هذه ان النفس تعرف الأشياء بمبادئها لزم عن ذلك ان النفس هي المبادئ لأن هذه هي خواص منعكسة (*Long Commentary* Fragments [1985], 34).

era of sensible being and that the other numbers which are composed from the principles also be principles of particular things. [This is] so that the principle {35} of the simple animal is the first oneness, the first twoness, the [first] threeness, and the [first] fourness, while the principles of the other living things are other numbers. For this reason he said it goes this way for other things, that is, the principles of other particular animals are other numbers. Because they held this opinion concerning the principles of beings and they held the opinion that the soul is composed from principles on account of knowledge, they held the opinion that the soul is the number which is the principle of [all] numbers. Next he said: **It is obvious that** the *Timaeus* **takes its point of departure from these [lectures].** That is, as it seems to me, what was said concerning principles in the *Timaeus* is different from what was said in the lectures. [It is] as if the diversity [of views] of people in regard to the soul is only due to their diversity [of views] in regard to the principles. For all agree that [the soul] must be from principles and say that the opinion of Plato in the *Timaeus* concerning the soul is that the soul is a middle nature, between the separate indivisible forms and the sensible forms which are divisible according to matter. Themistius, however, says that of all the parts of the soul Plato meant by that middle nature the intellect, since its being is between the material forms and the separate [forms]. Generally, we can understand the opinions of the ancients [only] with difficulty because we do not know them [directly].[109]

27. **This is also said in another way, namely, that understanding is one and science two, since per se it is toward one,[110] and that opinion is the number of the plane and that sense is the number of the solid. For numbers**

109. That is, their works are not available, so their opinions can be known only indirectly. Averroes' remarks in this Comment are not based on the Arabic text of Galen's summary of the *Timaeus* but instead follow the commentary of Themistius. See Themistius, *De Anima Paraphrase* (1899), 10.23–11.38; (1996), 25–26. Arabic fragments correspond to Book 1, 26.54–62 and apparently contain additional lines not found in the Latin: فنقول ان الذي كان أفلاطون يرى في طيماوس من أمر النفس انما طبيعة متوسطة بين الصور – أي الغير المنقسمة ولا المتجزئة وبين الصور المتجزئة من قبل الهيولي ، وثامسطيوس يرى أن أفلاطون انما عني بهذه الطبيعة المتوسطة العقل ، من بين سائر أجزاء النفس اذ كان وجوده متوسط بين الصور آلهيولانية والمفارقة . وبالجملة آقول ان فهم هذه الآراء وغيرها من آراء القدماء على التحصيل عسير لأن هذه الآراء هي غير معلومة عندنا الا ما نلفى من إشارات في كتب هذا الرجل ، وانما اكتفى بالاشارة اليها لأنها كانت مشهورة في زمانه . (*Long Commentary* Fragments [1985], 31). The Arabic continues with the following in addition to what we have in the Latin: "except for allusions we find in that man's books. He was content with allusions to [those views] only because those were well-known in his time."

110. Apparently the Greek μοναχῶς γὰρ ἐφ᾽ ἕν was not clearly understood by the Arabic translator. Aristotle, *De Anima* (1984), has "because it goes undeviatingly from one point to another." The difference between these understandings is all the more

are said to be forms and {36} principles in existing things, and numbers are one of those elements.[111] But all things are open to consideration, some by understanding, some by science, some by opinion, and some by sensation. Those are numbers which are the forms.[112] (404b21–27)

They also held in another way the opinion that the soul is [itself] the principles of numbers. For they say that understanding is the number one. He means by **understanding** the primary propositions. They said that it is one because it belongs to one science to know [primary] propositions.[113] He means by **science** the conclusion. They said this is twoness because it is a procession from one,[114] that is, from propositions, to one, that is, [to] the conclusion, hence twoness arises. He meant this when he said: **for it is** individually **toward one**. They said that opinion is the number of the plane, that is, threeness. For it is from one, namely, [from] the propositions, to two, for in [opinion] some conclusions are false and others true. Hence a twoness arises there. They also said that sense is fourness. For they held the opinion that sense discerns body and that the form of the body is fourness.[115] Next he said: **For numbers are said to be forms**, etc. That is, they said this because they held the opinion that the principles of numbers are separate forms and that the principles of beings are one of their elements. Because certain things are considered, that is, known, by understanding, certain by science, certain by opinion, and certain by sense, and nothing is known except through its like, those comprehensive powers of the soul must be the principles of numbers which are the forms and elements {37} of beings, namely, of oneness, twoness, threeness, and fourness. Of these,

---

apparent with Averroes' Comment. The alternate translation has "the intellect is singularity and science is duality as two united things" (متوحدان). Ibid. (1954).

111. "The numbers are by him expressly identified with the Forms themselves or principles, and are formed out of the elements." Aristotle, *De Anima* (1984).

112. The Greek adds: τῶν πραγμάτων, of things. The alternate Arabic translation renders the Greek precisely: فصور الأشياء (Aristotle, *De Anima* [1954]).

113. "It is comprehension (νοῦν: understanding) that grasps the first principles." *Nicomachean Ethics*, VI 6, 1141a7, Ross and Urmson (trans.) in *The Complete Works of Aristotle*, Barnes (ed.) (1984). Greek and my alternate translation added.

114. Arabic fragments correspond to Book 1, 27.14–18: يعتي بـ «العقل» المقدمات الأول. وقال ان العقل هو الوحدة من قبل ان المعرفة بالمقدمات هي معرفة واحدة. ويقصد بـ «العلم» النتيجة وتسمى اثنينية لأنها ناتجة من شيء واحد (*Long Commentary* Fragments [1985], 34).

115. Arabic fragments correspond to Book 1, 27.24–26: وقالوا ان «صورة» الحس هي رباعية وذلك لأن الحس عندهم كان يدرك الأجسام ، وصورة الجسم «الأول» عندهم رباعية (*Long Commentary* Fragments [1985], 34). There is no need to add «الأول» here. Cf. Themistius, *De Anima Paraphrase* (1899), 12.5–13; (1996), 27.

understanding must be oneness, science twoness, opinion threeness, and sensation fourness.[116]

28. **Because it is thought concerning the soul that it is a mover and a knower, some wanted to bring these two together and judged that the soul is a self-moving number. But there is great diversity [of thought] in regard to the principles, what and how many they are, and it chiefly occurs among those who assert them to be bodily and those who [assert them] not to be bodily. These also differ from those who mix them and assert the principles to be from both. There is also diversity in regard to the number of principles. For some say there is one principle and others that there are many.** (404b27–405a3)

Because it was thought, that is, established, that to move and to know are principles of the soul, some intended to bring both together in the soul by saying that the soul is a self-moving number,[117] a number because it knows and self-moving because it is not moved by another.

He made known the groups which differ in regard to the definition of the soul and that there are three. First, [there are] those who define it by motion or by characteristics consequent upon motion; second, [those who define it] by knowledge; and third, [those who define it] by both. All agree that the soul is composed from principles.[118] He then began to make known the ways by which they differ from one another generally, although they agree in the fact that [the soul] is from principles. He said: **There is great diversity [of thought]**, etc. That is, they differ in regard to the substance of the soul because they differ in regard to the principles, that is, in regard to their nature and number. The greatest difference[119] in regard to the nature {38} of the principles is among

---

116. Arabic fragments correspond to Book 1, 27.29–38 and apparently contain an additional line not found in the Latin: لما كان بعضهم يعرف بالعقل وبعضهم بالعلم وبعضهم بالظن ،بعضهم بالحس ، وانما يعرف الشيء بشبيهه فواجب ان تكون هذه القوى للنفس المدركة هي مبادئ الأعداد التي هي صور واسطقسات الأشياء الموجودة أي الوحدة والاثنية والثلاثية والرباعية ⟨وجب⟩ ان يكون العقل الوحدة والعلم الاثنينية *والظن الثلاثية و ⟨الحس⟩ الرباعية حتى يكون مجموع هذه القوى – جميع الموجودات. (*Long Commentary* Fragments [1985], 34). The Arabic adds "so that the sum of these powers is the whole of existing things." الاثنينية is surely a typographical error for الاثنية.

117. Arabic fragments correspond to Book 1, 28.12–15: ⟨لما كانت الحركة والمعرفة هي مبادئ للنفس⟩ جمع قوم لها الأمرين جميعا فقالوا ان ⟨النفس⟩ عدد محرك لذاته (*Long Commentary* Fragments [1985], 35).

118. Arabic fragments correspond to Book 1, 28.17–20: أولا من حدها من قبل الحركة ، ثانيا من حدها من قبل المعرفة ⟨ثم⟩ من حدها من قبل الأمرين جميعا. وكلهم مجمعون على ان النفس من المبادئ. (*Long Commentary* Fragments [1985], 35).

119. Arabic fragments correspond to Book 1, 28.22–24: ثم قال : «وأكثر ما وقع الخلاف ... » يريد : ان اختلاف الجميع في ⟨جوهر⟩ النفس انما هو من قبل اختلافهم في

those asserting that the principles are bodily and those asserting them not to be bodily, since these two natures differ the most. Next he said: **These also differ from those who mix them and assert the principles to be from both**, that is, from the bodily and from the non-bodily. Next he said: They differ **also in regard to the number of principles**. That is, they also differ in regard to the soul because they differ in regard to the number of principles.[120]

29. **They proceed to define the soul in a way that follows upon these views. For what they figure, that [it is] the nature of principles to be a mover, is not beyond truth.[121] As a result, some thought it is fire, for fire is among the smaller parts among the elements and [is something which] seems more not to be a body. It is moved and it moves other bodies in a primary sense.[122]** (405a3–7)

When he had made known the opinions of the ancients concerning the soul, he began to praise them insofar as they speak truly and draw true consequences. He said: **They proceed**, etc. That is, those who hold the opinion that the soul is from principles because it is moved per se and defined it in this way proceeded in this matter in a correct way following the principles. For to hold the opinion that [it is] the nature of principles to be a mover per se is correct.[123] Next he said: For this reason **some thought**, etc. That is, because they

المبادئ) أعني في طبيعتها وفي عددها. وأكثر ما وقع الخلاف (Long Commentary Fragments [1985], 35). Note that I correct Ben Chehida's > to < at 35.9.

120. Arabic fragments correspond to Book 1, 28.27–30: وثم قال: «وقد وقع الخلاف بين هؤلاء وبين الذين خلطوا ‹بين المذهبين› فجعلوا المبادئ من الأمرين جميعا – أعني أجساما وغير أجسام » ، ثم قال «والخلاف وقع أيضا بينهم من قبل عدد المبادئ » يريد ان اختلافهم في طبيعة النفس انما هو من قبل اختلافهم في عدد المبادئ (Long Commentary Fragments [1985], 35). I take منن to be a typographical error for من.

121. "They assume, naturally enough, that what is in its own nature originative of movement must be among what is primordial (τῶν πρώτων)." Aristotle, De Anima (1984). Greek added. There is no mention of the soul as principle by virtue of cognition here in the Long Commentary, but in the corresponding passage of the Middle Commentary Averroes mentions knowing or cognition: "It is a principle by virtue of motion or cognition (المعرفة)." Middle Commentary (2002), 14.2. See Ivry's note on this at 158. This is in accord with the beginning of Text 28, 404b27.

122. *Prima intentione*: πρώτως, "in the primary sense." Aristotle, De Anima (1984). The alternate translation has بالذات لا بالعرض (ibid. [1954]); "essentially and not accidentally."

123. ‹ثم قال› : « وهؤلاء كلهم : « وهؤلاء الذين اعتقدوا ان النفس شيء من المبادئ من قبل انها يسلكون ... الخ ...» يريد: تحرك ذاتها ‹وجعلوا لها حدا على هذه الجهة› فهم يسلكون في تحديدها المسلك ‹الصواب› واللازم لهذا ‹المبدأ› وذلك ان من اعتقد أنها من ‹طبيعة› المبادئ من قبل انها تحرك ذاتها لم يخرج عن الصواب (Long Commentary Fragments [1985], 35).

held the opinion that [the soul] is among the principles, some thought that it is fire, because they figured fire[124] to be the element of the rest of the elements and one of the more simple parts and that it seems more not to be a body. [This is] because they hold the opinion that the principles are such as this, namely, simpler than the rest and more distant from bodily nature.[125] All those [were combined] with the fact that it seemed to them to be moved and to move other things in the primary sense, as does the soul.[126] {39}

30. **Democritus spoke more obscurely[127] about this and he judged what the cause is in each case. He said that soul and intellect are the same and that this is composed from the first indivisible bodies. He attributed it to motion on account of the smallness of its parts and on account of shape. He said that among shapes the spherical is more amenable to motion and that intellect and fire have such a shape.** (405a8–13)

His intention in this chapter is to show that the ancients spoke well insofar as they were in agreement on the notion that the soul is from the principles on account of motion and to compare their accounts concerning this. He had already spoken about the opinion of one who said that the soul is fire. He began now to speak about those who hold it to be composed from indivisible parts, saying: **Democritus**, etc. That is, when Democritus spoke about the nature of the soul with respect to motion, he gave a more obscure account than that saying [the soul] is fire. It is more obscure because he judged the reason why in regard to each power and said that it is the same and that the nature of each

124. Arabic fragments correspond to Book 1, 29.16–17: ولذلك توهم قوم انها نار〉 (*Long Commentary* Fragments [1985], 35).

125. Arabic fragments correspond to Book 1, 29.18–20: اذ توهموا ان 〈النار〉 من المبادئ وهي بهذه الصفة ، وهي أيضا 〈أبسط〉 الأشياء وأبعدها شبها من طبيعة الأجسام (*Long Commentary* Fragments [1985], 35); "They hold the opinion that <fire> is among the principles and it has this characteristic, and it is also <the most simple> of things and the most distant from likeness with the nature of bodies."

126. *Et omnia ista cum eo quod visa est ab eis moveri et movere alia prima intentione, sicut anima.* This text is grammatically problematic. *Visa est* requires a feminine subject grammatically, but the context seems to require the masculine *ignis* for sense. While it might make good sense for the referent to be the feminine *anima*, in that case *sicut anima* would be needlessly redundant. The manuscripts contain no variants to the reading *visa est.* The correct reading may be that of manuscript A, which omits *sicut anima.* I have chosen to leave the problem in place and to render the subject as "it."

127. *Dixit in hoc sermonem magis latentem.* Both of the Arabic translations available to Averroes fail to reflect the sense of Aristotle's text, since each asserts that Democritus spoke obscurely (*latentem*, غامدا; Aristotle, *De Anima* [1954]). The Greek, however, describes Democritus as speaking γλαφυρωτέρως, "more ingeniously" (ibid. [1984]) or "more precisely."

is the same, that is, [the nature] of intellect and of the moving and sensitive soul. For he said that soul and intellect are the same and that its nature is so because it is one of the indivisible spherical parts.[128]

Next he said: **He attributed it to motion**, etc. That is, he attributed it to the motion proper to the soul. That is, he asserted it to be the cause of the motion of the soul owing to the smallness of its parts, since it is indivisible, and owing to its shape. For he holds the opinion that that shape has a smoother[129] motion than all the [other] shapes, and for this reason he holds the opinion that that shape, besides being in soul, is also in fire. This account is obscure for {40} two reasons: first, because of the opinion he held, namely, that soul and intellect are the same, and [second, because] it is an indivisible part. But it is uncertain whether there is any indivisible part; that there is fire, though, is obvious.

31. **Anaxagoras seems to say that the soul is different from the intellect, as we said above, but he still uses them as if these things may be of the same nature. But he asserts that intellect is more fit than all other things to be the principle, for he said that the intellect alone of all beings is simple, un-stained, and pure. He attributes both, i.e., knowledge and motion, to it, saying that intellect moves everything.** (405a13–19)

When he had compared the opinion of the one saying that the soul is fire with the opinion of the one saying that it is a spherical part from among the indivisible parts, he began to compare the opinion of Anaxagoras with [that of] Democritus. He said: **Anaxagoras**, etc. That is, Anaxagoras seems apparently to say that the soul is different from the intellect. But, although this appears to be the case from his account, still he asserts them to be of the same nature, that is, of the same genus. Moreover, he asserts that the intellect is

---

128. Arabic fragments correspond to Book 1, 30.20–21: وقال ان النفس والعقل هما شيء (واحد من قبل ان طبيعتهما من ⟨الأجزاء⟩ الكرية الشكل التي لا تتجزأ) (*Long Commentary* Fragments [1985], 35); "He said that the soul and the intellect are both one thing insofar as their nature is composed of spherical parts the shape of which is indivisible." While Averroes does not call special attention to this passage, Avicenna regards Aristotle's remarks on Democritus as foundational for the teaching on the soul: "Already in the first book, in the course of his argument with Democritus on the subject of the soul, he Worked Out Corollary Principles in a concealed fashion, and offered to those who have an understanding of this matter the Fundamental Principle, namely, that the thing in which the universal intelligibles are conceived is indivisible. He thus precluded the possibility that it is a corporeal substance which receives the [universal] intelligible concepts. What receives them, therefore, is a substance subsisting by itself, neither divisible [itself] nor [existing] in something divisible on account of which it could become divisible." Avicenna, *Letter to Kiyâ*, Gutas (trans.), in Gutas (1988), 61.

129. *Levioris*: lighter, less encumbered.

more fit to be the principle of all things and he places it before all other things. For he says that the intellect alone is simple, unstained, and pure,[130] that is, separate from matter and unmixed with it. He attributes both, namely, motion and knowledge, to it in all parts of the world,[131] for he holds the opinion that intellect moves all things and is [itself] unmoved. It is obvious that this account is more near to the truth and to the opinion of Aristotle, that the intellect {41} is among the principles and that it is the cause of knowledge and motion. For this reason he will praise him a great deal later on and will make known what else he had to say about the intellect.[132]

32. Melissus[133] seems, as is reported about him, to say that the soul is something which is a mover, since he said that a stone[134] has a soul because it moves iron. Diogenes and many others, however, hold the opinion that the soul is air because they thought that nothing is more subtle than air, and owing to this the soul knows and causes motion. For, insofar as it is the principle of other things it knows, but insofar as it is more subtle than all other things it causes motion. Empedocles[135] also says that the soul is a principle, since he says that it is the vapor from which he constitutes all things. He asserts that [this vapor] is altogether removed from bodies and always fluid [in nature], and[136] many others [also assert] that all beings are

---

130. Arabic fragments correspond to Book 1, 31.13–19: قوله من فالظاهر انكساغوراس أما
ان النفس عنده غير العقل ، وان كان قد ينزلها ، على ما هو ظاهر من قوله ، بمنزلة طبيعة
واحدة ﴿أعني تحت جنس واحد﴾ وذلك انه جعل العقل ﴿أشرف مبادئ الأشياء كلها﴾ وجعله
اسطقس جميع الأشياء وذلك انه يقول : ان العقل هو وحده بسيط خالص (*Long Commentary*
Fragments [1985], 35). The corresponding passage of the *Middle Commentary* is closely
related: فإما انكساغوريش فالظاهر من قوله ان النفس عنده غير العقل ، وان كان قد.
يستعملهما في قوله بمنزلة طبيعة واحدة . وذلك انه جعل العقل مبدأ التحريك لأشياء كلها
وجعله اسطقس جميع الأشياء وبالجملة فوصفه بالأمرين جميعا، أعني المعرفة والتحريك. وذلك
أنه يقول ان العقل هو الذى حرك الكل عند ما ميزه وإن وحده بسيط خالص "As for Anax-
agoras, it is clear from his remarks, as we have said, that in his opinion the soul is other than the intellect, even though he sometimes treated them in his argument as one nature. For he posits the intellect as the principle of motion for all things and posits it as an element [in] all things. In general, he attributes both things to it—namely, cognition and motion—for he says that it is the intellect which moves everything as it discerns it and that it alone is simple and pure." *Middle Commentary* (2002), 14.12–17.

131. That is, everywhere.

132. See 429a19 and 429b24.

133. Thales in the Greek.

134. That is, a lodestone.

135. Heraclitus in the Greek.

136. Here Averroes' Text omits τὸ δὲ κινούμενον κινουμένῳ γινώσκεσθαι, "that what is in movement requires that what knows it should be in movement." Aristotle,

in motion. Perhaps someone else[137] also seems to hold such an opinion in regard to the soul. For he says that [the soul] is immortal because it is like immortal things and that this characterizes it because it is always moved. He said:[138] for all the gods, the moon, the sun, and the stars are forever moved with continuous motion. Others, who are more deserving of derision, judged that it is water, such as Zeno.[139] They seem to incline toward this opinion on account of seed since it is one of the more moist things. For on this basis he responds to the one saying that the soul is blood by saying that the seed is not blood and the seed is [nevertheless] the first soul. Others said that it is blood, as [did] {42} Critias, since they thought that nothing such as sensation is consequent upon [the presence of] soul and that sensation is [instead] from the nature of blood. For each of the elements, aside from earth, has someone judging in its favor, but earth has none. What was said concerning it is that it is composed of all the elements or [it is] all the elements. (405a19–b10)

He wants to list all the opinions of the ancients on the soul and to give a reason for each.[140] His account is obvious. Melissus held the opinion that the soul is a principle [which is] a mover per se since he said that the magnet has a soul because it moves iron. Diogenes held the opinion that the soul is air, for air is more subtle than the rest of the bodies and [is] their principle. Therefore, insofar as it is a principle, knowledge will be attributed to it, and insofar as it is more subtle than all other bodies, motion will be attributed to it. These two are proper to the soul. Heraclitus[141] held the opinion that the soul is a principle

---

De Anima (1984). This may be an omission by a copyist of Averroes' work, however, since the missing text is found reflected both in the *Middle Commentary* as "and that moving things are known only by a thing in motion" (*Middle Commentary* [2002], 15.8–9) and in Averroes' Comment below. The alternate translation has والمتحرك إنما يعرفه متحرك مثله (Aristotle, *De Anima* [1954]): "Only something in motion like it knows a thing which is in motion."

137. Alcmaeon in the Greek. This name is corrupt in the *Middle Commentary*. See *Middle Commentary* (2002), 15.12 and 158, n. 25.

138. "He said" is added to the text of Aristotle.

139. Hippo in the Greek.

140. Arabic fragments correspond to Book 1, 32.30–31: أرسطو جميع <ـ> وفي هذه آراء القدماء في النفس ويعطي لكل منها جهة من الاقناع ونحوا من الصواب (*Long Commentary* Fragments [1985], 35). "In regard to these Aristotle <sought to provide(?)> all the opinions of the ancients on the soul and to give for each of them something of what they found persuasive and the way of reasoning."

141. Although the Text incorrectly has Empedocles, Averroes correctly understands that Aristotle here is mentioning the view of Heraclitus. Perhaps Averroes made use of his alternate translation, which correctly has Heraclitus ايراقليطس (Aristotle, *De Anima* [1954]) or the *Paraphrase* of Themistius which also has Heraclitus (Themistius,

and that that principle is a fluid vapor which is moved, because he held the opinion that the constitution of [all] other things is from vapor and that it is altogether removed from body; these two are in the principle.[142]

Next he said: he holds the opinion with many others that all things are moved and he believes that common to them all is the proposition that like is known by like. Because according to him all things are moved, it was necessary that what knows be moved.[143] Hence he judged the soul to be vapor. In a similar fashion one who asserts it to be of the nature of the stars, the sun, and the moon[144] seems to hold the opinion that it is moved per se. But [anyone] who says that it is water ought to be laughed at, for no one said that water is the [basic] element {43} for all other things. But still he gave a reason for this, namely, because male seed, which is the principle of generation, is extremely moist, and it was thought that male seed is the soul since it forms the embryo.[145] Next he said: **For on account of this he responds to the one saying that the soul is blood.** That is, he asserts that the male seed is the first soul because he asserts that the male seed is not blood. Perhaps then he judged that the soul is water only because he sees that the male seed is the soul and water rather than blood.

Next he said: For **each of the elements, aside from earth, has someone**

De Anima Paraphrase [1899], 13.26; [1996], 28). The corresponding Fragment has *Tâlîsîs*, طاليسيس. See n. 144.

142. That is, these two characteristics, its nature as a moving fluid vapor and vapor's nature as distinct from body, are both in the principle, namely, in the soul.

143. Cf. n. 136 above.

144. Arabic fragments correspond to Book 1, 32.32–48: وقد كان طاليسيس يعتقد ان النفس ﴿مبدأ متحرك بذاته﴾ إذ قال ان لحجر المغنطيس نفسا لأنه يحرك الحديد. فأما ديوجانيس فانه ظن ان النفس هواء ﴿وذلك لأن﴾ الهواء هو ألطف الأشياء كلها ولأنه مبدؤها. وبعضهم قال انه الهواء هو المبدأ ومن قبل ذلك صارت النفس تعرف ، وبعضهم قال انها من ألطف الأجسام كلها ومن قبل ذلك صارت تحرك ﴿وهذين الأمرين خاصين بالنفس﴾. وان ايرقليطس أيضا قد ظن ان النفس مبدأ وان ذلك المبدأ هو البخار السائل المتحرك لاعتقاده ان البخار قوام سائر الأشياء وانه أبعد من ان يكون جسما ، وهذان الصفتان هما صفة للمبدأ ... ثم قال : ان جميع الأشياء متحركة وكان يرى فيه أيضا ان القضية المشتركة لكلهم وهي ان الشبيه يعرف بشبيهه ولما كانت هذه الأشياء متحركة فوجب ﴿أن﴾ يكون العارف لها متحركا. فلمكان هذه الأشياء ﴿حكم﴾ الرجل على ان النفس بخار ... وكذلك الذين جعلوا النفس من طبيعة الكواكب﴾ كالشمس والقمر (*Long Commentary* Fragments [1985], 35–36). The Arabic is generally well reflected in the Latin except in the following: "As for Diogenes, he held the opinion that the soul is air, because air is the most subtle of things and because it is the principle of them. Some of them said that it is air that is the principle and in virtue of that the soul comes to be knowing, while some others said that it is the most subtle of all bodies and in virtue of that it comes to move."

145. Arabic fragments correspond to Book 1, 32.53–55: لأن المني الذي منه مبدأ الكون هو أرطب الأشياء أي من طبيعة الماء وقد يظن أن المني نفس إذ كان مصور للجنين (*Long Commentary* Fragments [1985], 36).

judging in its favor, etc. That is, the ancients judged that each of the elements is such that soul is [composed] from it except earth. For no one held the opinion that the earth is the [basic] element of [all] the others, but only that it is composed from some of the elements or is all the elements, i.e., from all the elements.

33. **They generally define the soul in three ways, by motion, by sense, and by lack of body, and each of those is reduced to principles. On account of this those who defined it by knowledge also asserted it to be an element or to be from elements. What some say in regard to this is similar to what some others say, except for one [person].**[146] **For they say that like is known only by like. Since the soul knows all things, they held that it is constituted from all the principles.** (405b11–17)

When he had shown that those considering the soul in reference to motion ought to hold the opinion that it is constituted from principles, he began to show generally that all the things said in the definition {44} of the soul are reduced to the principles. He said: **They generally define,** etc. That is, the ancients generally proceed to define the soul and to know its substance in three ways: in reference to motion and in reference to sense, that is, knowledge, since these two seem to be proper to the soul, and third, in reference to its not being a body. For several of them held the opinion that this [third] exists for soul no less than the other two. Each of these ways leads them to hold the opinion that the soul is constituted from the principles. He meant this when he said: **and each of those is reduced to principles.** Next he began to show the way in which one who judged that the soul is constituted from principles by way of knowledge proceeded. He said: **On account of this those asserted it to be**[147] **an element,** etc. That is, because they all held the opinion that it is constituted from principles, those who defined it by way of knowledge said that it is an element or constituted from elements. The way in which they proceeded in this is the same or similar, except for one of them, Anaxagoras. Next he showed this way. He said: **For they say that like is known only by like.** That is, this was necessary in their view because they held three propositions: first, that every thing is known by its like; second, that all things are known only through their principles; and, third, that the soul knows all things. From these it follows that the soul is all the principles or constituted from the principles of all things.[148]

---

146. This is Anaxagoras, as Averroes notes below and as Aristotle explains at 405b20–22.

147. Crawford's insertion of *esse* is unnecessary.

148. Arabic fragments correspond to Book 1, 33.31–35: مقدمات : أولا ان الشيء يعرف بشبيهه ، ثانيا : ان الشبيه يعرف مبادئها ، ثالثا : ان النفس تعرف جميع الأشياء فيلزم ان

34. The one, therefore, who said that the principle and element is one thing[149] asserts that the soul is also one thing, either fire or air. The one who asserts that the principles are more than one asserts that the soul is more than one. Anaxagoras alone, however, {45} said that the intellect does not undergo affection and that there is nothing in it which it has in common with something else. But he did not say how and in virtue of what it knows by this disposition, nor is this[150] something which is apparent from his account. (405b17–23)

When he had made it known that the opinions of those in regard to the substance of the soul are consequent upon the opinions they hold in regard to the substance of the principles, he began also to show that their opinions in regard to the number of souls is also consequent upon the opinions they hold in regard to the number of principles. He said: **The one who said that** there is one principle **asserts that soul is** of one thing, that is, of one nature from that principle, either fire or air. The one who said that the principles are more than one holds the opinion that the soul is more than one.

Next he began to explain the opinion of Anaxagoras and that he proceeded in another way. He said: **Anaxagoras alone, however,** said **that the intellect does not undergo affection**, that is, it is not material, and that it does not have **anything in common** with anything else. That is, none of the things which it understands is in it in such a way that it would be common to both in some form. That is, it is neither a determinate particular nor in a determinate particular; it is neither a body nor a power in a body. No one said this except Anaxagoras. For this reason he will praise Anaxagoras later.[151] Next he said: **But he did not say how.** That is, but he did not say how it happens for it that it understands all things, whether insofar as it is in act or insofar as it is in potency. Nor did he even say how it understands things which are not intellect in act. This is what he will complete later when he will speak about the intellect.[152] {46}

النفس هي مبادئ جميع ﴿الأشياء﴾ أو من مبادئها (*Long Commentary* Fragments [1985], 36). The Arabic varies from the Latin: ". . . second, that like is known by its principles."

149. αἰτίαν καὶ στοιχεῖον ἕν is the Greek behind the Latin *principium et elementum est unum*. The alternate Arabic translation renders the Greek: العلة واحدة والعنصر واحد (Aristotle, *De Anima* [1954]).

150. I read *nec hoc* with manuscript A in lieu of *hoc*.

151. See 429a19 and 429b24. In the *Middle Commentary* Averroes does not relate the teaching of Anaxagoras specifically to his own doctrine of the material intellect as he does here. Cf. *Middle Commentary* (2002), 17.2.

152. This is a general reference to the discussions of intellect in Book 3. See *De Anima* 3.4–5.

35. Those who assert [the existence of] contrariety in the principles also constitute the soul from contraries. Those, then, who asserted that the principle is one of contraries, such as hot and cold and their like, also held the opinion that the soul is one in this way. We also see them following [the meanings] of words.[153] **Some of them say, then, that the soul is hot since the word life in Greek is derived from this intention. Some say that it is** *algidum,*[154] **that is, cold, because of respiration. And the cooling which comes from respiration is called** *ysargi,*[155] **that is, respiration. We therefore take this [much] from the ancients concerning the soul. Those [considerations] led them to say this.** (405b23–30)

He reported in this chapter the consequences of the opinions they hold in regard to the substance of the soul in relation to what they hold in regard to the principles, to the extent that one who holds the opinion that the principles are contraries says that the soul is from contraries. Those, therefore, who say that the principles are hot or cold or some other [pair] of contraries say that the soul is likewise one of those contraries. In the other translation we find this added: "Those who hold the opinion that the principles are one of a pair of contraries say that the soul is from this pair of contraries."[156] This is [just] what he said: **Those who assert [the existence of] contrariety in the principles,** etc. Next he said: **We see them pursue the words,** etc. That is, we also find {47} that they reason about this, i.e., the notion that one of the contraries is a principle and that the soul is from it, from the derivation of the word life and [the word] soul. One who therefore says that it is hot reasons by virtue

153. That is, they base further considerations on etymology.

154. Perhaps this is a corrupt form of الجامد, "freezing," in the original. The *Middle Commentary* uses بارد "cold" (*Middle Commentary* [2002], 17.9 and .11), as does the alternate translation (Aristotle, *De Anima* [1954], 12.28).

155. The Latin translator's Arabic manuscript is corrupt here. "Those who identify soul with the hot argue that ζῆν (to live) is derived from ζεῖν (to boil), while those who identify it with the cold say that soul (ψυχή) is so called from the process of respiration and refrigeration (κατάψυξις)." Aristotle, *De Anima* (1984). The alternate Arabic translation has والذين سموا النفس شيئاً بارداً زعموا أنها إنما سميت بهذا الاسم من أجل أن التنسم والتنفسس إنما يكون بالبرودة وتفسير اسم النفس باليونانية : الشيء المبرد (ibid. [1954]). "And those who call the soul something cold allege that it is called by this name only insofar as respiration and breathing are only in virtue of coldness, so the interpretation of the word 'soul' in Greek is 'the cold thing.'"

156. This may be something "added" in the other translation, though it is more likely another version of the opening lines of Text 35. والذين جعلوا في الأوائل تضاداً قالوا إن النفس من أشياء متضادة (Aristotle, *De Anima* [1954]); "Those who believed contrariety to be in the principles said that the soul is from things which are contraries."

of the fact that this word life in the language of the Greeks is derived from hot, and similarly in the case of the word motion.[157] One who said that it is cold reasoned[158] by virtue of the word respiration, which is derived from [the word] cold. Next he said: **We therefore take**, etc., that is, in regard to the substance of the soul. Those are the reasons which led them to say this— reasons taken from the distinction [of contraries] and motion—and that the soul is not a body.

36. **We ought therefore to investigate motion first. For it seems that this is not only false, that its substance is of such a disposition as those report who say that the soul is something self-moving or something which is able to move itself, but that it is even impossible that the soul be motion. I say also that it is not necessary that a mover be moved. This was also said earlier.**[159] (1.3, 405b31–406a4)

After he had completed the accounts of the ancients concerning the soul, their reasons [for their positions], and what truth is contained in these, then he began in this part to respond to what was falsely said by them, and this is the third part of this book.[160] The first is the prologue, the second is the listing of their opinions, and the third is [his] response to them.[161] He began by responding to those who defined [the soul] in reference to motion. He said: **We ought to investigate**, etc. That is, we should investigate those considering {48} its substance[162] in reference to motion. For not only have we seen that the account of those who define it [as they do] because it is something self-moving or able to move itself is false; [we have] also [seen] that the notion that the soul is moved per se—so that it is constituted through motion, as [are] several more

---

157. In the *Middle Commentary* Averroes writes, "He said: We find some people inferring the substance of the soul from the nouns [used], some saying that it is something hot, because the noun 'life' in their language is derived from the noun 'heat.'" *Middle Commentary* (2002), 17. Why Averroes mentions motion in this context is unclear. Could it be that he is asserting an etymological relationship obtains between حرق, "to burn," and حرك, "to move," like that of ζῆν and ζεῖν in Greek?

158. *Ratiocinatur.*

159. 403b29–30. Ross does not regard this as a reference to *Physics* 8.5. Aristotle, *De Anima* (1961), 186. Averroes, however, believes the reference to be to *Physics* 8. See below.

160. That is, this is the third part of Book 1.

161. Arabic fragments correspond to Book 1, 36.11–13: أولا وهو العناد الأرائهم وهو الثالث من هذه المقدمات لأن الأول هو كمثل الصدر والثاني تعدد آرائهم التي قدمنا من هذه أرائهم عناد هو والثالث، الأراء (*Long Commentary* Fragments [1985], 36).

162. Arabic fragments may correspond to Book 1, 36.15–16: وابتدأ من ذلك البحث عن اعتقاد من اعتقد فيها (*Long Commentary* Fragments [1985], 36).

beings such as the winds and rivers[163]—is false. This is what he means when he said: **but that it is impossible that the soul be motion.** That is, but the account of the one saying that the essence of the soul is constituted through motion is impossible. Next he said: **I also say that it is not necessary,** etc. That is, it was explained earlier in the *Physics* that it is not necessary that something move itself.[164] He now began to explain that [the soul] is not moved per se.

37. **Everything moved is moved in one of two ways, either by another or per se. It is called "by another" when something is moved because it is in or on something else which is moved, such as a passenger on a ship. For his motion is not the same as the motion of the ship, since the ship is moved per se and the passenger is moved because he is on what is moved. This is obvious in the case of the parts of the body. For the motion proper to the feet is walking and this also belongs to the human being [involved]. But [motion] is not found in that disposition in the passengers on the ship.** (406a4–10)

He explained that falsity is found not only in the notion that the soul moves itself, as was explained in general accounts,[165] but also in that they say that the substance of the soul is constituted through motion, as [are] the winds and rivers.[166] {49} Here he began to explain that this too is impossible. He began first to distinguish the ways in which it is said that something is moved. He explained first that motion is attributed to something in two ways, either essentially, when something is moved in its own right, or accidentally, when [something] is moved through the motion of something else, when it is in or on the moved thing. He said: **Everything moved is moved** in one of two ways, **either by another or per se.** Next he gave the example of passengers on a ship. Then he said: **This is obvious in the parts of the body.** That is, the motion of the ship is not attributed to the passengers in an essential way. This is obvious from the motion of the parts of the body on the basis of which motion is attributed in an essential way to a human being and to an animal, namely, [the motion] of the feet. For motion is attributed to a human being essentially only

163. This seems to be a general reference to *Meteorology* 1.13, 349a12–b1.

164. *Physics* 8.5. Themistius mentions that Plato held this in the *Laws* and that Aristotle discusses it in the *Physics*. See Themistius, *De Anima Paraphrase* (1899), 14.28–15.17; (1996), 29–30.

165. Averroes' mention of "the general accounts" here and elsewhere in this work refers to the general accounts of natural philosophy found in Aristotle's *Physics, On Generation and Corruption, De Caelo, Meteorology,* and other works in which basic philosophical principles of the natural sciences are set forth. At *De Anima* 2.5, 417a1–2, Aristotle refers to *On Generation and Corruption* with ἐν τοῖς καθόλου λόγοις.

166. Arabic fragments correspond to Book 1, 37.13–14: قال ان جوهر النفس متقومة بالحركة مثل الرياح والأنهار (*Long Commentary* Fragments [1985], 36).

on the basis of these parts of the body, while that [sort of] motion is not found in the passengers on the ship. Therefore, essential motion is not found in [the passengers]. You ought to realize that there are two ways in which something can be said to be moved because it is in something else moved: one is the way which is such that it is [still] possible for it to be moved in its own right, such as the passengers on the ship who are moved by the motion of the ship; the other way is what [is such that it] is not possible [for it to be moved in its own right], such as whiteness, which is moved by the motion of a white body.[167]

38. **Because there are two ways in which something can be said to be moved, we now ought to investigate with respect to the soul whether it is moved per se or in virtue of another. Because the motions are four, local motion, alteration, increase, and diminution,[168] [the soul] must either be moved by one of those motions or be moved by more than one or be moved by all these motions. If then [the soul] is moved in a way that is not accidental, then motion is in it in a natural way. {50} If that is so, then it also has place. For all the motions of which we spoke are in place. (406a10–16)**

After he had divided motion into two, essential and accidental, he began to investigate whether it is possible for the soul to be moved per se. He said: **Because there are two ways in which something can be said to be moved**, etc. That is, after it was explained that there are two ways in which something is said to be moved, it should be investigated whether the soul is moved per se or moved only accidentally. Next he put forth three propositions here. First, that motions are three in kind, but he himself said four taken in a broad sense, as if listing addition and diminution as two. The second is that if the soul is moved, it is moved either by one of those motions or by more [than one] or by all. The third is that if it is moved by one of those motions, it must be a body. For if the soul is moved, it is moved by one of those motions, and then it is [something] composed. If the soul is moved essentially, it is necessarily moved by one of the essential motions or by more [than one] or by all. Every motion is either one of place or one of alteration or one of increase. Therefore if the soul is moved, it is moved

167. Passengers present in or on a ship and moved accidentally by the ship's motion can still move themselves about the ship by motion which is essential to them. However, whiteness, which is present in a subject, a white body, does not have any essential movement and is not separate from the subject in which it is present. Cf. Themistius, *De Anima Paraphrase* (1899), 15.18–24; (1996), 30–31.

168. *Diminutionis*: φθίσεως, "diminution." Aristotle, *De Anima* (1984). Later, at 413a25 and elsewhere, Smith and Barnes render φθίσεως and related forms by the more traditional, albeit less accurate, "decay" (ibid.). Like the Greek, at times forms of *diminutio* seem to have the sense of diminution or decline rather than decay. Here the Latin will be rendered by "diminution" throughout.

either locally or in reference to growth or by alteration. When we have joined to this the notion that everything moved by one of those motions is a body, as was established in the Sixth Book of the *Physics*,[169] we will conclude that if the soul is moved, it is a body and in a place, since every body is in a place. This, therefore, we can understand about what he said: **If then [the soul] is moved in a way that is not accidental, then the motion** belongs to **it in a natural way.** If {51} therefore it is so, it has place. For all the motions mentioned are in place. Therefore if it is moved naturally, and every natural motion is[170] one of those three [sorts] and each and every one of those is in a body and every body is in a place, then the soul must be in a place. Since it is in place, it will necessarily be moved by local motion. For everything which is moved by one of those two motions is moved locally, but the converse is not the case.[171] But in these words there is some ambiguity since he said, **for all the motions mentioned are in place.** He did not say, for all the things moved by those motions mentioned are in place, but **all the motions mentioned.** But this even taken in its apparent sense is not truly said concerning those three motions, that they are in place, if this word "mentioned" refers to those three motions, for the motion of alteration is not in place. For this reason from his statement, **If then [the soul] is moved in a way that is not accidental, then motion** belongs to it **in a natural way**, that is, on account of itself and not on account of something else external, we can understand that it is necessary that it be moved with local motion. Thus he means by **the motions mentioned** all the modes of local motion. For that motion exists in the thing by nature and it is necessarily in a place. According to this, his account will be that **motion belongs to it in a natural way,** as if it were another condition added to what belongs to it essentially. For alteration can in a way be called something which is essentially in the thing altered.

It can be said that it is in it accidentally in another way. For whiteness is moved[172] to blackness only because it is in something divisible, the body, not because it is divisible in itself. Thus here there will be another sort of accidentally moved things {52}, different from the sort described. What he will say [immediately] below verifies this exposition.

39. **And if the substance of the soul is such that it moves itself, then motion will not belong to it accidentally as [it does] to whiteness and the three-**

---

169. This seems to be a general reference to the discussion of the spatially continuous (body) and change. Aristotle's discussion of this begins at *Physics* 6.1, 231a21. At 6.4, 234b10ff., he discusses the necessity that anything which changes be divisible.

170. I read *naturalis est* with manuscripts A and B in lieu of *naturaliter est*.

171. As he explains immediately below, alteration does not involve place. These two motions, then, are local motion and growth.

172. That is, changed.

cubit length. For those are moved, but accidentally; but what is moved is the body in which these two things exist. For that reason they do not have place. The soul, however, does have place since by nature it involves motion. (406a16–22)

After he had shown that if something is moved essentially, it must be moved according to one of three motions, he began to show that [the soul] cannot be moved by alteration or increase. For it is impossible to find a mover in relation to them since this is not found except in local motion alone, since what is moved in quality is also moved in one of the ways belonging to things which are said to be moved accidentally. He said: **And if the substance of the soul**, etc. That is, and if the substance of the soul is something self-moving, as the ancients describe it, then it is impossible for it to be moved in quality, as something white [changes] into something black, nor in quantity, as something which is three cubits changes into something four cubits. For if one of those were said to be moved, it will be said to be so only accidentally since what is moved in those cases is only the body. This is, as it were, the reason why nothing self-moving is found in [the cases of] these two motions. But it is obvious that we attribute motion to whiteness and blackness {53} only owing to the body in which these two qualities exist. But it is difficult to imagine how addition and diminution in quantity are attributed to the thing which can increase or dimin-ish accidentally. For what has increased essentially is moved in place, but in-sofar as there is motion in the parts, not in the whole; therefore, we attribute motion to the whole accidentally. Motion, then, we attribute in an accidental way to what can suffer alteration or increase, to what can suffer alteration ow-ing to the body which is its subject, and to what can be increased and dimin-ished owing to the bodily parts which can be increased and diminished. It is in reference to these two notions that we should understand his own account in which he said: **but what is moved is the body in which these two things are.** That is, the body in which these two [motions] in quality exist is a body which is an underlying subject, while in the case of increase they are the parts of the body in which that motion[173] is found. In this way we can solve all the difficulties which arise with regard to this account.[174]

40. **Furthermore, if it can be moved by nature, then it can also be moved by force, and if by force, then [it can be moved] by nature. It is similarly so with regard to being at rest, for something comes to be at rest by nature in that toward which it is moved by nature; and similarly it comes to be at rest by force in that toward which it is moved by force. What, then, are those**

173. That is, the motion of quantitative increase.
174. Cf. Themistius, *De Anima Paraphrase* (1899), 15.18–31; (1996), 30–31.

motions and rests which occur to the soul by force?[175] **Furthermore, if it moves upward, it is fire; if downward, it is earth. For those two motions belong only to these two bodies. The account concerning intermediate bodies is the very same.**[176] (406a22–30) {54}

If it can be moved by nature, that is, per se with respect to place, it must be able to be moved by force with respect to place. This is necessary for what can be moved in place by rectilinear motion. Next he asserted the converse. He said: if it can be moved by force, it can also be moved by nature. It is also necessary that what can be moved by force also ought to be moved by nature, for motion which is by force can only be understood by reference to natural motion. Next he said: **It is similarly so with regard to being at rest.** That is, it ought to be this way for rest, namely, that everything moved by nature be at rest by nature. Everything which is at rest by nature is at rest by force, and everything at rest by force is at rest by nature. If, then, the soul is moved by nature, it is at rest by nature; and if it is at rest by nature, then it is at rest by force. When he had recounted that what can be moved by nature can have forced rest, he recounted in what place it has forced rest. He said: for it has rest by force where it is moved by nature. That is, in the place in which it is moved by nature it is [also] at rest by force. For example, fire, which is[177] moved downward by nature, is at rest there [only] by force, while for earth it is the contrary. This was determined in the Fifth Book of the *Physics*.[178] After he had proved that if the soul is moved by nature and per se, it must be moved by force or be made to be at rest by force, with these propositions confirmed, he said: **What, then, are these motions**, etc. That is, for no one can say anything in regard to this, for this is not imagined at all in regard to the soul, and still less is it necessary. The strength of that account is the strength of two hypothetical syllogisms. {55} The first is that if the soul is moved by nature, then it is moved by force; but it is not moved by force; therefore, it is not moved by nature. The second is that if the soul is moved by nature, it is at rest by nature, and if it is

175. The Text omits οὐδὲ πλάττειν βουλομένοις ῥάδιον ἀποδοῦναι, "it is difficult even to imagine" (Aristotle, *De Anima* [1984]); ولو أردنا الإدعاء والتجنى (ibid. [1954]).

176. περὶ τῶν μεταξύ: "the intermediate movements, *termini* and bodies" (Aristotle, *De Anima* [1984]); الحركات اللاتى بين هاتين (ibid. [1954]).

177. Although there is no evidence for it in the Latin manuscripts, the sense of the text requires the addition of a negation: "fire which is <not> moved downward by nature." See the following note.

178. "And again, fire moves up naturally and down unnaturally; and its natural motion is certainly contrary to its unnatural motion. Similarly with remaining: remaining above is contrary to motion from above downwards, and to earth this remaining comes unnaturally, this motion naturally." Aristotle, *Physics* (1984), 5.6, 230b13–17.

at rest by nature, then it is at rest by force; but it is not at rest by force; therefore, it is not at rest by nature;[179] and if it is not at rest by nature, then it cannot be moved by nature. This [argument] is composed of two connective hypothetical syllogisms in each of which the consequent is negated and the opposite of the antecedent is concluded. Next he gave another syllogism which follows from those propositions, and in it he explained that the soul is not moved by nature. He said: **If it moves** by nature **upward, it is fire; if downward, it is earth.** That is, if it is moved by nature in place or is moved upward or downward, since every motion in place is one of these kinds. This is true in the case of rectilinear motion. If, then, it is moved upward, it is fire; if downward, it is earth; if in an intermediate way, it is one of the two intermediate bodies, either water or air. He meant this when he said: **The account concerning intermediate bodies,** etc. He dismissed, as it were, an impossible consequent, because it is obvious. It is that if it is fire or one of the elements, it is in the body by force. If it is one of the elements, it ought not to be moved in the body except by one motion by nature, either upward or downward, not by opposite motions. But we see that it is moved in place by opposite motions; therefore, it is not one of the four elements.

41. **Furthermore, if we see it move the body, it must move it by the motions by which {56} it is [itself] moved. If this is so, then when that account is converted, it will be true, namely, that the motion by which the body is moved is also the motion by which the soul is moved. The body is moved by local motion; hence the soul must be changed in place by change in place belonging to the body and is carried in place either as a whole or in virtue of its parts. If this were so, it would be possible [for soul] to return and exist in some place after it had left it. So it would be possible for dead animals which have died to return and to live.** (406a30–b5)

Furthermore, if we see it, etc. That is, there is also another way to think about this. For if we assert that [the soul] moves the body insofar as [the soul] is moved, it must move it by the kind of motion by which it is [itself] moved. If [the soul] is carried, it must carry [the body], and if [the soul] is changed in place, it must change [the body] in place. After he had asserted this, he said: and the contrary as well, namely, the [soul] must be moved by motion of the very same kind as the motion by which the body is moved by the soul. Having asserted this, if we assert that the body is moved by the soul by local motion, it will then be necessary that the soul be moved in the body either as a

---

179. Arabic fragments correspond to Book 1, 40.40–43: وقياس آخر : ان كانت تتحرك
طبعا فهي تسكن طبعا ولو تسكن طبعا تسكن ⟨قصرا⟩ لكنها لا تسكن قصرا فلا تسكن
طبعا (*Long Commentary* Fragments [1985], 36).

whole or in reference to its parts. It will therefore be in the body as a body is in a place. Because it is naturally constituted to move the body in different places, it is also possible for it to be moved in different places. Since this is so, it is possible, as he said, for it to return and enter the body after it has left it. Hence, it follows, as he said, that a dead animal would return and live. But that contradiction is in the account of the speaker, not in {57} reality.[180] For we do not assert that every mover is moved by that kind of motion or by local motion, unless the mover is a body, as was explained in the *Physics*.[181] Since some thought that this contradiction exists in reality, they raised questions about this proof of Aristotle's which says that every body is such that it does not move unless it is moved, and they say: We see here many things which move and are not moved by that kind of motion, such as a rubbed stone,[182] for when it becomes hot it moves straw by local motion, though it is not itself moved. But this is not the place for that difficulty; its solution was already mentioned in the eighth book of the *Physics*,[183] where he was required to assert this proposition.[184] But the question would be proper for this place if the contradiction were real, because we see many things cause change [which], nevertheless, are not [themselves] changed. Therefore, we find ourselves between these two alternatives: either we ought to assert that the contradiction is real, and then it will be true only in the case of local motion, which [is a position which] the words of Aristotle do not reflect; or [we ought] to assert that the contradiction is in the account of the speaker, not in fact. Indeed, that contradiction is con-

180. *Non secundum rem in se.*

181. *Physics* 8.6, 258b24–25. Cf. 8.10, 267a23ff.

182. The text in Crawford's edition (*Long Commentary* [1953]) has *retitus,* as does *Aristotelis Opera Cum Averrois Commentariis* (1562). I correct this to *retritus* from *retero,* "to wear down by rubbing." *Oxford Latin Dictionary* (1982), 1641A. The stone is rubbed until warm or hot and then causes motion in the straw (by static electricity). This might be rendered "a threshing stone." I would like to thank Dr. Norman Zacour for his thoughtful suggestions on this text. The Arabic merely has "the stone which draws straw." See below for the Arabic text in the corresponding fragment.

183. *Physics* 8.10, 266b27ff. Cf. *Physics* 8.5, 256a21–b3. Also see *Long Commentary on the Physics* (1962), Text and Comment 35, 373H–375B, and Text and Comment 82, 429H–431I. Alonso finds these references in the *Long Commentary on the Physics* and infers that Averroes' discussions of this issue in these two passages indicate the *Long Commentary on the Physics* must be prior to the *Long Commentary on the De Anima*. Alonso (1947), 95–96, cited in Puig (2002a), 352, n. 98. That inference is not necessary since Averroes need only to have known of Aristotle's discussion of the magnet in *Physics* 8.10 to account for his remarks in the present passage. Moreover, Averroes' own words, as cited by Glasner (2004), 58–59, seem to require the reverse. See the introduction, p. xvi, n. 3.

184. From consideration of the Arabic fragments, there appears to have been a significant omission here in the Latin version. See the following note.

firmed only by conceding the first proposition by which he began to speak, namely, that if the soul moves the body insofar as [the soul] is moved, it must move the body by the kind of motion by which [the soul] is [itself] moved. The ancients concede this or it follows from what they concede. When this is conceded, its converse follows necessarily, which is that every motion by which the body is moved must be a motion by which the soul is moved. This is obvious. Therefore, that contradiction in this passage should be understood in this way.[185] {58}

42. [The soul] is moved by motion in an accidental way only by something else, namely, when the animal is pushed by force. For it is necessary that something whose substance is able to be moved per se be moved by another only in an accidental way. To this extent it is not correct that what is good per se be good in virtue of something else, nor that what is desirable per se be desirable in virtue of something else. (406b5–10)

After he had refuted [the notion] that the soul is moved per se, he began to explain that it is not impossible for it to be moved in an accidental way, rather it is perhaps necessary. He said: **[The soul] is moved by motion in an accidental way**, etc. That is, it can be moved by an accidental motion, since such a

185. Arabic fragments correspond to Book 1, 41.29–59: الا أن ذلك محال ، فهذه المقدمات

هي بحسب القول القائل لا بحسب الأمر نفسه. فان نحن لم نضع أن كل ما يحرك فواجب
أن يتحرك بذلك النوع ⟨من⟩ حركة النقلة ولا يتحرك الا أن يكون المحرك جسما على ما تبين
في ⟨كتاب⟩ السماع. ولما توهم قوم أن هذه المعاندة بحسب الأمر في النفس شككوا على
أرسطو في هذا الموضع أعني في المقدمة القائلة أن كل جسم فانما يتحرك عن محرك فقالوا أنا
نجد أشياء تحرك ولا تتحرك ⟨–⟩ يحركها مثل الحجر الذي يجذب التبن
فانه إذا سخن الحجر جذب التبن حركة نقلة ولا ينتقل الحجر ، وهذا الشك ليس وضعه
⟨. .⟩ تعرض أرسطو لهذا ⟨في الثامنة من السماع⟩ بوضع هذه المقدمة ، وانما الذي يضع أن
كل متحرك فله محرك بذلك النوع من المحركات بأن يتحرك ، فواجب أن يتحرك بنوع ما يحرّك ،
ثم وضع أن البدن إذا كان ينتقل عن متحرك بذاته فقد يجب أن يكون ذلك المتحرك ينتقل
وهذا أمر لازم لا اعتراض فيه وانما كان يلزم الشك لهذا الوضع لو ⟨كانت⟩ بحسب الأمر نفسه
لأنا قد نجد أشياء كثيرة تحيل من غير أن تستحيل وتنتقل من غير أن تنتقل فنحن إذاً بين
أحد أمرين : اما أن نضع المعاندة بحسب الأمر في نفسه ، وانما تصح هذه المعاندة إذا سلمنا
المقدمة الأولى الذي استفتح بها الكلام وهي أن النفس كانت تتحرك حركة البدن من جهة
ما تتحرك بذاتها فقد يجب ضرورة أن تحرّك ذاتها الحركة التي تتحركها ، وهذا شيء ألزمهم
لما يسلمون من قولهم أن النفس تحرك البدن من جهة ما تتحرك بذاتها وإذا سلم هذا لزم عكسه
ضرورة وهو أن الحركة التي تحرك البدن فقد يجب أن تكون النفس متحركة بها⟨ . . .⟩ وذلك
الأمر بين بنفسه ، فعلى هذا ينبغي أن تفهم هذه المعاندة هاهنا (*Long Commentary* Fragments [1985], 36–37). At line 43 the following was omitted in the Latin version: "What he sets forth is that everything moved has a mover with this sort of motion insofar as it is moved. For it is necessary that it be moved by way of what moves. Then he set forth that if the body is altered by what is moved per se, then it is necessary that what is moved [per se] be altered. And this is a necessary statement to which there is no rebuttal."

motion is only in virtue of the motion of the thing in which [the soul] exists. This happens to it when the body in which it exists is moved forcibly by something external. When he had set forth that kind of motion as possible, he explained that it should not be necessary that what is moved by its own substance be moved by something else. For just as what is good per se is not good in virtue of something else, so too what is moved per se is not moved in virtue of something else.

43. Of all the accounts mentioned concerning the notion that the soul is moved, the better one is that it moves sensible things.[186] **But if it moves itself, it is also moved. Hence, because every motion is a going forth of the moved in accord with the character of its own motion, the soul must also go forth from its substance, if it does not move itself accidentally but motion belongs to its substance per se.**[187] (406b10–15) {59}

He had explained that it follows, for those saying that the soul moves only insofar as it is moved, that it is moved by the kinds of motions by which it moves. But the soul seems to move in several ways, such as by local motion and the motions of sensible things. He had already presented them with an impossibility if it is moved by local motion which is the kind by which it causes motion. [Now] he showed here that a more adequate account is that the soul moves by that kind [of motion] by which it causes motion so that it is moved by motion which it causes in relation to sensible things. He said: **Of all the**

186. *Et melior sermo omnium sermonum dictorum in hoc quod anima movetur est quod movet sensibilia.* "If the soul *is* moved, the most probable view is that what moves it is sensible things." Aristotle, *De Anima* (1984). The Arabic Text of Aristotle in Averroes' alternate translation accurately renders the Greek: يقول إن النفس قد تحركها الأشياء المحسوسة (ibid. [1954]). Averroes' Comment below seems to be on this faulty text, and there is no indication that he did not consult the alternate translation. Still, corruptions in the Latin translator's Arabic manuscript are the likely explanation for the problem in the Text as well as that in his Comment. It is possible that the suffix ها- may have been missing in the Latin translator's Arabic Text, with resulting confusion for the Latin translator. The *Middle Commentary* has "The most suitable factor to consider [as being] responsible for the soul's movement is its apprehension of sensible objects. This movement is thought to go out to sensible objects which are separate from the senses, in order to apprehend them—the sensible objects in this way being responsible for the soul's movement. If so, however, they move the soul only as a final cause, as prey falling in a net moves the hunter. The soul, accordingly, is moved toward sensible objects per se, and if this is so, it moves itself." *Middle Commentary* (2002), 20.10–16.

187. That is, if every motion involves a going out and away from something, then the soul's motion which arises from its substance must be a going out and away from its substance, if its motion is not accidental motion.

accounts ... the better one, etc. That is, a more adequate account is to say that the soul is moved with the sort of motion which it has in relation to sensible things. He meant this when he said: **that it moves sensible things**, etc. That is, that it is moved by the kind of motion by which it moves sensible things. For, although the senses are moved by sensible things, they nevertheless are thought to move and be moved by them at one and the same time.[188]

Next he began to mention another impossible consequence for them all. It is that if the substantial activity of the soul by which it is sustained, as it were [its] form, is motion, but motion is a change of the thing in its substance, then the soul must be changed in its substance and must not be in its final perfection, that is, in act.[189] For the being of motion is a changeable being and it is composed of being in potency and being in act. For this reason several of the ancients thought that it did not exist. He said: And **if it moves itself it is also moved**, etc. That is, but if the soul moves itself, as the ancients assert, it is also moved in its own right and in its substance. Because every motion is a change of what is moved in accord with the character of its substance insofar as it is moved, the soul must also be changed by its substance. Next he said: **if it does not move itself accidentally.** That is, as it seems to me, if motion is not something posterior in relation to the soul as an accident for it, {60} namely, so that the soul is included in the definition of motion, not motion in the definition of the soul as the ancients do. He meant by this exposition: if it does not move itself in such a way that motion is an accident following upon its substance. Perhaps he understands the aforementioned intention as concerning accident, that is, as concerning what is opposed to essence.[190]

44. **Some, such as Democritus, said that the soul also moves the body in which it exists in the way by which it is [itself] moved. He gave an account similar to the account of Chilus,[191] for he says that Daedalus made the statue of Hermafroditus[192] move by putting quicksilver in it. Democritus speaks**

188. See n. 186 above.

189. Arabic fragments correspond to Book 1, 43.24–27: والحركة صورة لها وكانت الحركة
تغير الشيء عن جوهره فيلزم ان تتغير في جوهرها وإلا توجد على كمالها الأخير أي بالفعل
(*Long Commentary* Fragments [1985], 37).

190. Arabic fragments correspond to Book 1, 43.35–42: يريد فيما أحسب هذه ان لم
تكن الحركة أمرا متأخرا عن النفس أعني كونها عرض من أعراضها وذلك ان تكون النفس
توجد في حد الحركة الموجودة لها لا الحركة في حد النفس الذي وضعه القدماء أعني ⟨...⟩ ان
لم تكن تحرك ذاتها على أن الحركة عرض تابع لجوهرها أو يريد المعنى الذي تقدم مما ⟨قاله⟩
⟨بالذات⟩ لما المقابل وهو (*Long Commentary* Fragments [1985], 37).

191. Philippus. The Greek adds τῷ κωμῳδοδιδασκάλῳ, "the comic dramatist" (Aristotle, *De Anima* [1984]), which is preserved in the alternate Arabic translation: فيلبس معلم هجاء الناس (ibid. [1954]).

192. Aphrodite.

in a similar way, for he says that the indivisible particles are always moved because it is their nature not to rest at any time, and in this way they draw with them and move the whole body. We ask him whether this also causes rest. But it is difficult, rather even impossible, to say how it does this. We never see the soul move the animal in this way, but [rather it moves it] voluntarily.[193] (406b15–25)

He had explained that it follows, for those saying that the soul is moved in its own right, that it is moved from place to place in its own right insofar as the body is moved from place to place, and he had provided them with many impossible consequences. He began here also to say that there are several people who say this. He said: some say **that the soul also moves the body**, etc. That is, some, such as Democritus, hold the opinion that the soul moves the body by local motion, even [while the soul is itself] moved. For [Democritus] holds the opinion that {61} the indivisible parts always move the body by their own motion, as Chilus said that Daedalus made the statue of Hermafroditus move, by putting quicksilver in it. For he held the opinion that just as it is for quicksilver with the statue, so is it for the soul with the body in regard to motion. Next he said: **we** therefore **ask him**, etc. That is, if in his view that is the cause by means of which the soul moves the body, we should ask him how the soul causes rest, if it causes motion insofar as it is always moved. Next he explained that it is not only difficult but rather impossible to give a cause by means of which it makes [something] to be at rest insofar as it is moved. He said: And **it is difficult . . . to say**, etc. Next he said: **We never see the soul**, etc. That is, that if the motion of the body were from the soul as the motion of the statue from the silver, then the motion of the body would not be voluntary but necessary. This is obvious.

45. **It is similarly the case with what Timaeus[194] said in [providing] a natural account, namely, that the soul moves the body. For he says that the soul moves the body only when [the soul itself] has been moved, because it is commingled with it. For the constitution of the soul is from the elements and it is divisible according to the division of composite numbers,[195] so that**

193. The Greek behind *voluntarie* here is διὰ προαιρέσεώς τινος καὶ νοήσεως, "it is through intention or process of thinking." Aristotle, *De Anima* (1984). The *Middle Commentary* has: "We see that the soul moves by way of choice and deliberation"; نراها إنما تحرك من جهة الاختيار والروية (*Middle Commentary* [2002], 21.13–14). The alternate translation renders the Greek well: وإنما يكون بضرب من ضروب الاختيار والعزم (Aristotle, *De Anima* [1954]).

194. *Timaeus*, 36Aff.

195. That is, it is divisible according to the divisions characteristic of harmonic ratios.

it has a sense consonant for the harmony and the universe might be moved
by consonant motions.[196] He said:[197] for this reason he bent the straight line
and formed it into a circle, and he divided the one into two circles separate
in two places;[198] then he divided one circle again into seven circles in such
a way that he made the motions of the heavens just as the motions of the
soul. (406b26–407a2) {62}

After he had explained that Democritus holds the opinion that when the soul
has been moved from place to place, it moves the body by local motion, and had
provided the impossibility which results from his opinion, he also began to
explain that what was said in the *Timaeus* is similar to the opinion of Democritus. He said: **This is** [199] **similar**, etc. That is, it was said in a similar way in the
Timaeus that the soul moves the body by local motion; indeed the soul is even
moved from place to place, because it is commingled with [the body], and when
[the soul] is moved from place to place, the body is moved from place to place.[200]
After he had explained the similarity between this opinion and the opinion of
Democritus, he also began to say what is specific to this opinion and to respond
to it specifically. He said: **For the constitution of the soul**, etc. (This had been
said in the *Timaeus*.) That is, the constitution of the soul is from the elements of
the world. But [the soul] is something which understands because it is composed
of elements in a composition which is musical and spherical. It discerns harmony
because it is harmonically composed. According to him this is the nature of
celestial bodies. For celestial bodies have been composed in this sort of composition according to him and their shape is of this sort. When he had said that
the constitution of the soul is from the elements, he meant from the elements
from which the world is composed according to him. Next he said: **and it is
divisible**, etc. That is, it has been composed harmonically since it can sense
harmony by this sort of proportion of composition. He meant this when he said:
so that it has a sense. Next he said: **and the universe might be moved by**

---

196. *Motibus convenientibus*: συμφώνους φοράς, "in movements well-attuned" (Aristotle, *De Anima* [1984]). The alternate translation renders the Greek somewhat better:
ولتتفق حركات الكل (ibid. [1954]); "let the movements of the whole be in harmony."

197. "He said" is added to the text of Aristotle.

198. The Greek text has διρσαχῇ συνημμένους, "united at two common points." Aristotle, *De Anima* (1984). Averroes' alternate translation faithfully renders the Greek as
تلتقيان على قطبين (ibid. [1954]).

199. I follow manuscripts B and D and omit *etiam*. This is likely a corruption which
took place early in the Latin tradition.

200. Arabic fragments correspond to Book 1, 45.19–22: ‹أي ان النفس› تحرك البدن حركة
نقلة بان تنتقل هي أيضا من جهة أنها مخالطة له ‹. .› إذا انتقلت هي انتقل البدن بانتقالها
(*Long Commentary* Fragments [1985], 37).

consonant motions, that is, because it has a harmonic number. Next he said: **for this reason {63} he bent the straight line.** That is, he means that Timaeus held the opinion that the soul acts only insofar as it is spherical, and it discerns harmony and is moved by harmonic motions, that is, by consonant [motions], insofar as it is composed from the elements in a harmonic way. For this reason, reporting about the Creator,[201] he said that when he composed the soul from the elements, first he composed it with the correct magnitude in a harmonic way. Then he bent the line and made it into a circle, so that it may have thought, and he made that circle so that it had width. Then he divided that circle into two, one of which he divided into seven, namely, the orbits of the wandering stars and the orbit of [fixed] stars, in such a way that he made the motions of the heavens the same as the motions of the soul, that is, that the actions of the heavens are the same as the actions of the soul.[202]

46. **Let us therefore say first that it is not correct to say that the soul is a magnitude. For it is obvious that one who meant the soul of the universe to be such as what is called an intelligence, for instance, did not mean the sensitive soul or the desiderative [soul], since their motion is not circular.** (407a2–6)

He says that it is not correct to hold the opinion that the soul is a body, since intellect is understood by "soul." It was explained that this is what was meant in the *Timaeus* by this word, soul. For this reason they made the body spherical, for the action of the intellect is similar to circular motion. By soul as used there we understand neither the sensible nor the desiderative [soul], for their motion and action are not {64} likened to circular motion as according to them the action of the intellect is likened to a circle because it reverts upon itself and understands itself. For this reason Aristotle likens it to a sphere.[203]

47. **For the intellect is one and continuous, as also is what is understood. What is understood is the things understood,[204] and these are one by suc-**

---

201. In Galen's summary of the *Timaeus* in the Arabic text, the Demiurge is termed الخالق, "the Creator." See Galen, *Galen's Compendium of Plato's Timaeus* (1951), Arabic 6.9. This and what follows immediately are quite similar to *Middle Commentary* (2002), 21.22–22.6.

202. Cf. Galen, *Galen's Compendium of Plato's Timaeus* (1951), Arabic 7.10–17.

203. Arabic fragments correspond to Book 1, 46.9–16: طيماوس باسم النفس ان أرادوا العقل ولذلك اشترط في الجسم ⟨المستدير⟩ ان فعل العقل يشبه الدوران ولم يرد باسم النفس هناك لا النفس الحسية ولا الشهوانية فان حركة هذه وفعلها لايشبه الدوران كما يشبه فعل العقل وإنما اشبه فعل العقل عندهم الدوران لأنه يرجع الى ذاته ولذلك شبه ⟨أرسطو⟩ النفس بالخط المنعطف (*Long Commentary* Fragments [1985], 37).

204. *Intellectum est res intellecte*: ἡ δὲ νόησις τὰ νοήματα, "thinking is identical with thoughts" (Aristotle, *De Anima* [1984]); والفهم هو المعنى (ibid. [1954]); "The thinking is

cession, as a measure without magnitude.[205] For this reason the intellect is also not continuous in this way but either is indivisible or is something continuous [though] not as a magnitude. For there is no way that we can say how it understands in virtue of one of its parts, [since] any given part is the same.[206] Understanding through some part will take place either through a magnitude or through a point.[207] The point is infinite, so it is obvious that [intellect] does not traverse it in some period of time. If it understands with a magnitude, it understands[208] many times over and infinitely; but we see that understanding can occur [only] once. If, therefore, it is sufficient for it

---

the intention." To render the Greek the Latin should be *intellectus est res intellecte*, but the reading *intellectus* is preserved only in manuscript G. The simplest explanations for the difference would seem to be either a corruption in the Latin tradition of the translation or a faulty Arabic text with المفهوم for الفهم or المعقول for العقل. What is clear is that Averroes read the Text in accord with the sense of Aristotle's Greek, as is evident in his Comment: *intelligere est ipse res intellecte*. I translate the Latin as it stands in the edition of Crawford.

205. ταῦτα δὲ τῷ ἐφεξῆς ἕν, ὡς ὁ ἀριθμός, ἀλλ᾽ οὐχ ὡς τὸ μέγεθος. "These have a serial unity like that of number, not a unity like that of a magnitude." Aristotle, *De Anima* (1984). Averroes recognized that the Text is corrupt here and proposed that we understand "without magnitude" as "without continuity"—that is, without the continuity of discrete parts which must characterize any material continuity. This suggestion is Averroes' own attempt to make sense of the corrupt Text, which was also faulty in the alternate translation: وهذه من جهة التوالى شيء واحد كمثل العدد ، وليس مثل العقل (ibid. [1954]); "These are a single thing by succession, like number, and it is not like intellect."

206. *Nullo enim modo possumus dicere quomodo intelligit per aliquam partem partium eius, quecumque pars sit idem* πῶς γὰρ δὴ καὶ νοήσει, μέγεθος ὤν; πότερον ὁτῳοῦν τῶν μορίων τῶν αὐτου, "How, indeed, if it were a magnitude, could thought possibly think? Will it think with any one indifferently of its parts?" (Aristotle, *De Anima* [1984]); وإلا فكيف يدرك الجسم وهو جسم؟ ولا بد من أن يكون إدراكه إما بجزء من أجزائه (ibid. [1954]); "But how does a body apprehend qua body? It must be that its apprehension is with one of its parts."

207. *Et intelligere per aliquam partem aut erit per magnitudinem aut per punctum.* "In this case, the 'part' must be understood either in the sense of a magnitude or in the sense of a point (if a point *can* be called a part of a magnitude)." Aristotle, *De Anima* (1984). The Text supplies the subject *intelligere* (just as the alternate translation supplies يكون إدراكه " "its perception is either . . .") and omits the parenthetical εἰ δεῖ καὶ τοῦτο μόριον εἰπεῖν (which the alternate translation has). ولا بد من ان يكون إدراكه إما بجزء من أجزاءه (إن جاز أن نقال إن له جزءا ما) (ibid. [1954]); "It must be that its apprehension is with one of its parts (if it is permitted to say that it has some parts)."

208. τὸ αὐτο at 407a15 is not explicitly rendered in Averroes' Text, though it seems to be understood in the context. The alternate Arabic translation, however, renders it explicitly as بعينه (Aristotle, *De Anima* [1954]).

to touch with one part, whatever part it be, why does it need to move in a circular way, and generally why does magnitude come about from this? (407a6–17)

And **the intellect is one**, etc. That is, the intellect is said to be one and continuous in [just] the way it is said that it is one[209] and continuous in its thought. Next he said: **understanding is the things understood**, etc. That is, understanding is itself the things understood, which are not said to be one except as {65} successive things are said to be one, namely, as number. He meant this when he said: **as a measure without magnitude**, that is, without continuity. For this reason it is impossible to say that the intellect is one and continuous except in the way this is said for successive things, namely, in regard to discrete quantity.[210] The intellect, therefore, is not a body because it is not continuous in reality. Next he said: **but it is either indivisible or continuous [though] not as a magnitude.** That is, since the disposition in the intellect is consequent upon the disposition in the object of understanding, we must say that the intellect either is indivisible as one point or [it is] continuous. But [it would] not [have] the continuity of a magnitude but the continuity of a composite, that is, of a discrete quantity.[211] Next he said: **For there is no way we can say**, etc. That is, since we have been speaking about it insofar as it is a continuous magnitude, then it will understand only by touch, as was said in the *Timaeus*. For there is no way[212] we can say how the intellect understands with some part of it for each part is the same as the things understood. Next he said: **Understanding with some part**, etc. That is, understanding by touch, since [intellect] will be a magnitude,[213] requires either that [intellect] touch parts of the thing understood with its parts or the whole with [its] whole, or both. Next, if it under-

---

209. Arabic fragments correspond to Book 1, 47.21–22: قال فيه أنه متصل واحد من الجهة (*Long Commentary* Fragments [1985], 37).

210. That is, understanding, which is identical to the objects of understanding, is one and successive or sequential in just the way we say discrete quantities can be one and successive or sequential.

211. Arabic fragments seem to contain part of a text which may belong here. التي يقال في المعقول انه واحد ... ليس اتصاله باتصال الجسم فليس بجسم (*Long Commentary* Fragments [1985], 37). "which is said in relation to the intelligible to be one. Its contact is not the contact of a body, for it is not a body."

212. Arabic fragments correspond to Book 1, 47.38–46: وان سلمنا أنه عظم متصل ويعقل بمماسة كما قيل في طيماوس فلا سبيل اليه ... ⟨على أي جهة يعقل العقل⟩ المتصور والمعقول ⟨بجزء منه⟩ أو بكله (*Long Commentary* Fragments [1985], 37); "If we grant that it is a continuous magnitude and that it understands by touch, as was said in the *Timaeus*, then there is no way . . . ⟨how the intellect understands⟩ what has been conceived and understood ⟨by a part of it⟩ or by the whole of it."

213. That is, if intellect involves touching, it will itself have to be a magnitude.

stands by means of the contact of [its] parts with the parts of the thing, it has to be either by means of some part of it which is a magnitude or by means of some part which is a point. After he had shown this, he provided the impossibility which follows for both. He said: If **the point is infinite**, {66} etc. That is, if it understood with a point, it obviously can never understand the whole body, for the points which are in a body are infinite. Therefore, if in understanding a body a point from [the intellect] must touch all the points which are in a body (which is impossible, because the points are infinite), then it is evident that it is impossible to understand a body at all in this way. After he had explained the impossibility which follows if it understands insofar as it touches a body with points, he also began to mention the impossibility which follows if it touches by some part which is a body, not a point. He said: **If it understands by a magnitude**, etc. That is, if the intellect understands the thing by touching with some part of it which is a body [touching] all the parts of the body understood, by rotating itself about so as to touch by that part of the body all the parts of the body understood, then from this it must be the case that the intellect understands the same thing an infinite number of times when it touches the body. For one part does not differ from another part in its touch; and it is impossible for it to understand the whole body. But we see that the intellect understands the whole body at once, and that after understanding it a single time it does not need to understand it again.[214] If, then, someone says that for understanding the body it is sufficient to understand one part of it, when it touches it with its part, we will say to him: How, then, does it need the body to move in a circular way so as to touch all its parts with its [own] part or parts? Generally, why is it required that the intellect be a body if it does not understand by touch?[215] {67}

48. **If to understand it must touch with the whole circle, what does it mean for it to touch with parts? Furthermore, how does it understand the divisible by the indivisible or the indivisible by the divisible? The intellect must be that very circle. For understanding is the motion of the intellect and circular motion is the motion of the circle. If understanding is circular motion, then that circular motion will also be understanding. What then does it always understand? For this is necessary if the circular motion is always eternal. For practical understanding[216] is finite since any part of it is for the sake of something else; and theoretical understanding (and this is to define by giv-**

---

214. That is, once something has been discerned by understanding, it need not be discerned again and again.

215. Cf. Themistius, *De Anima Paraphrase* (1899), 21.4–28; (1996), 36–37; and *Timaeus* 36E–37C.

216. τῶν . . . πρακτικῶν νοήσεων: "practical processes of thinking" (Aristotle, *De Anima* [1984]); الفكر في الأعمال (ibid. [1954]).

ing accounts [of things]) is similarly so. Every account is either by definition or by demonstration.[217] But demonstrations are taken from a starting point, as something ultimate, and there are a syllogism and a conclusion. Although a conclusion is not [always] reached in these,[218] nevertheless they do not return to their starting points, but always expand in the middle or extreme [term] and proceed in a straight line.[219] A circular motion, however, returns to its starting point. Also all definitions are finite. Furthermore, if the entire motion is the same, then [it will understand the same thing] many times over.[220] Furthermore, understanding is more appropriately attributed to rest[221] than to motion; and similarly [for] the syllogism. (407a17–34)

If to understand it must, etc. That is, if to understand requires that the intellect touch the thing understood with the whole circle, and then it will understand (that is, {68} the second part of the three divisions),[222] why does it need to touch by the parts? It is superfluous for it to touch with the parts. Next he

217. *Et omnis sermo est aut per diffinitionem aut per demonstrationem.* λόγος δὲ πᾶς ὁρισμὸς ἢ ἀπόδειξις "For every account is a definition or a demonstration." (Aristotle, *De Anima* [1984]). Averroes' alternate translation renders the Greek accurately here: والقول حد وبرهان (ibid. [1954]). It may be this alternate translation which Averroes follows when he cites this text in his Comment. Alternatively, it may be that this Latin text is faulty, while Averroes' citation of the Text in the Comment is sound and in accord with his primary Text.

218. That is, in these accounts which are products of the soul's movement.

219. *Crescunt semper in medio aut extremo, et procedunt recte:* προσλαμβάνουσαι δ' ἀεὶ μέσον καὶ ἄκρον εὐθυποροῦσιν; "it goes on assuming a fresh middle term or extreme, and moves forward" (Aristotle, *De Anima* [1984]); متى ما صار للبراهين واسطة وطرف استقام مذهبها (ibid. [1954]).

220. ἔτι εἰ ἡ αὐτὴ περιφορὰ πολλάκις, δεήσει πολλάκις νοεῖν τὸ αὐτο. "Further, if the same revolution is repeated, mind must repeatedly think of the same object" (Aristotle, *De Anima* [1984]); وإذا كانت حركة العقل حركة دور غير منقطعة ، فمدرك الشيء قد يدركه بعينه مرارا كثيرة (ibid. [1954]); "If the intellect's motion were circular and not step by step, then what perceives the thing would in itself perceive it many times over." Note that the phrase غير منقطعة is misplaced here and corresponds to καὶ ἐπιστάσει (line 33), "arrest" (ibid. [1984]) of the following sentence. Averroes was aware that his Text was faulty here, as he indicated by his citation of the alternate translation. It appears, however, that the alternate translation was itself less than perfectly accurate and that even that imperfect text as Averroes had it may have had additional faults.

221. ἠρεμήσει τινι: "a coming to rest" (Aristotle, *De Anima* [1984]); بالسكون (ibid. [1954]). As indicated in the previous note, καὶ ἐπιστάσει is erroneously read with the previous line.

222. "That is, understanding by touch, since [intellect] will be a magnitude, requires either that [intellect] touch parts of the thing understood through its parts or the whole through [its] whole, or both" {66}.

said: **How does it understand the divisible with the indivisible**, etc. That is, with whatever way we assert that it touches, whether with an indivisible part or with a divisible one, or whether that divisible will be a whole or a part or both, namely, that it touches a part with a part and the whole with the whole, it is impossible for us to say how it understands with touch. For if we say that it has indivisible parts, how does it touch the divisible parts of things with indivisible parts? If we say that it has divisible parts, how does it touch with them? For what touches ought to be superimposed [on the other thing]. All those issues occur for them because they assert that the intellect, insofar as it is intellect, has parts and that it understands only with touching. Next he said: **The intellect must be that** very **circle.** That is, the intellect must be a circling body, not that it is some attribute belonging to a circling body. It is obvious, then, that it follows from this that the intellect is a circling body.[223] The syllogism is composed in this way: the action of the intellect is circular motion; circular motion is characteristic of a circling body; therefore, the action of the intellect is that of a circling body. That to which the action of the intellect is attributed is the intellect; therefore, the intellect is a circling body.[224] After he had explained that it follows necessarily that the intellect is a circling body and its action is circular motion, he indicated that if its understanding is circular motion, and also circular motion has always been in it insofar as it is {69} a celestial body, then its understanding must exist always and be infinite. He said: **If understanding is circular motion**, etc. That is, if understanding is circular motion, then also the circular motion existing in the intellect will be understanding. The circular motion will be eternal. Hence, it is obvious that understanding will be eternal and infinite.[225] Next he began to provide the

223. Cf. Themistius, *De Anima Paraphrase* (1899), 22.7–.9; (1973), 5.6–.8; (1996), 38.

224. Arabic fragments correspond to Book 1, 48.47–53: يدركه العقل وأنه دوران فيلزم ان يكون العقل جسما مستديرا والقياس يتألف هكذا : العقل فعله الدوران والدوران للجسم مستدير ففعل العقل الجسم المستدير ، فتنعكس هذه النتيجة وهي : للجسم المستدير فعل العقل وللذي له فعل العقل هو العقل ، فالجسم المستدير هو عقل (*Long Commentary* Fragments [1985], 37); "The intellect grasps it and it is moving in a circular way, so it is necessary that the intellect be a circling body. The syllogism giving this is as follows: the intellect's act is to move in a circular way and to move in a circular way belongs to a circling body, so the intellect's act is a circling body [*sic*]. This conclusion is then converted: the intellect's act belongs to a circling body and what has the act of intellect is the intellect, and so the circling body is an intellect." The argument seems to require ففعل العقل للجسم المستدير, "so the intellect's act belongs to a circling body." Ben Chehida suggests a different understanding of this. See *Long Commentary* Fragments (1985), 38.

225. This argument is as follows in the *Middle Commentary*: "This position, in addition, entails that the intellect itself be that which circles. If conceptualization is an activity of the intellect and a revolution, and [if] a revolution belongs to that which moves

impossibility which follows from this. He said: And **what does it always understand**, etc. That is, since it is necessary according to this opinion that it always understands, what can they say that it always understands? For this is necessary owing to the fact that they assert that circular motion is eternal. They can say nothing in regard to this, since to understand in activity is something finite. For every understanding in activity is understood only on account of something else, and all things [are understood] on account of the final end which is intended in that practical activity. After he had explained that understanding is finite in the practical intellect, he began to explain that it is so in the theoretical [intellect]. He said: **Theoretical understanding (and this is to define by giving accounts [of things]) is similarly so.** That is, it is similarly the case in regard to all theoretical things. Next he said: **Every account is either a definition or a demonstration.** That is, every action of the intellect is either a definition or a demonstration. After he had explained this, he began to explain that each of those actions is finite. He said: And **demonstrations are taken from a starting point.** That is, demonstrations have a starting point from which they are taken, which consists of propositions, and they have an end which is the syllogism which comes about from the propositions and conclusion. Next he said: **Although a conclusion is not [always] reached in these**, etc. That is, one who reaches some conclusion does not [need to] reach that conclusion once again, as he does in a circular {70} syllogism. Rather, he adds to it another proposition which makes it impossible that the demonstration return in a circular fashion, namely, as the starting point becomes the end and the end the starting point. But one adds to this another middle term and another major extreme and another conclusion. The motion of the intellect will then be rectilinear, not circular. Circular motion, however, which they hold to be the action of the intellect, is not understood by this intellect, that is, [by] one which proceeds in a rectilinear way, but rather [by one which] returns [in a circular way]. After he had explained this in regard to demonstration, he began to explain this in regard to definition. He said: **All definitions are finite.** That is, when the definitions of things are attained by the intellect, they are finite, as things which need to be believed. Understanding does not return to these in

---

in a circle, then it follows necessarily that intellect is a circling body, and that its activity—conceptualization—is a revolution. If this is so, and the revolution is perpetual, then it follows necessarily that conceptualization is perpetual. If the intellect's conceptualization is perpetual, then it follows necessarily that it moves from one conceptualization to another, and does not stay with any one, for such a stay would be a rest. If so, though, our conceptualizing would not end when we think of something, whereas we find that the conceptualization of practical things is limited to the purpose intended for a practical object." *Middle Commentary* (2002), 24.7–16.

a circular way, just as assent does not return to demonstrations in a circular way. Next he said: **Furthermore, if the entire motion is the same, then [it will understand the same thing] many times over.** That is, if the motion of the intellect is also its circular motion in relation to the same object of understanding, then it will discern itself[226] an infinite number of times. In the other translation it is clearer as follows: "Since the motion of the intellect is circular, not spiral, then what discerns discerns the same thing many times over."[227] For this reason it is possible that the account be as follows: If the motion of the intellect is circular motion, then it will understand all things many times over. Next he said: And **understanding is more appropriately** attributed **to rest than motion.** He means by this what is apparent. For our action with [intellect] is more perfect at rest than in motion. For this reason it is better to attribute the action of the intellect to rest than to motion, as they did. {71}

49. **Furthermore, what is not done easily but, as it were, by force, is not enjoyable. But if motion is not the substance of the soul, then [the soul] is moved only by something extrinsic to its nature. Furthermore, it is very difficult**[228] **for intellect to be commingled with the body in such a way that it cannot withdraw from [the body], if it is better for the intellect not to be joined with the body, as is customarily said and as several hold.** (407a34–b5)

Furthermore, it is evident that understanding is more difficult when involved with motion than when involved with rest. Therefore motion on the part of the soul is, as it were, by force. Therefore, it is not something in its substance nor is the soul constituted by it, but rather it is [something] extrinsic to its nature. When he had made this known, he began to provide the impossibility which results for them insofar as they say that the intellect is a body. He said: **Furthermore, it is very difficult,** etc. That is, it is highly unacceptable and very difficult to understand, as people were accustomed to say, that the intellect is a body or commingled with the body in such a way that it can never escape

226. *Ipsum.* This Latin reflexive must refer to the subject of the sentence. Averroes, although working with a faulty text, clearly sees that the point is not that the intellect will perceive or discern itself an infinite number of times but that it will repeat infinitely its discerning of the object of understanding. It corresponds with the Arabic بعينه, "in itself" or "in its own right."

227. The Latin here renders precisely the alternate Arabic except for *non spiralis*, "not spiral," which corresponds to غير منقطعة (Aristotle, *De Anima* [1954]); "not step by step."

228. *Valde difficile* hardly renders the Greek ἐπίπονον, "painful." Aristotle, *De Anima* (1984). For a possible explanation of this problem in the Text and Averroes' understanding, see *Middle Commentary* (2002), 163, n. 32. The alternate translation has "Its mixture with the body would cause it pain and harm" (وجعا وأذى) (Aristotle, *De Anima* [1954]).

from it at all, since all, or [at least] several, hold the opinion that it is better that intellect not be joined with the body, and all the more that it not be a body. For the nature of the intellect seems to be completely opposite to the nature of the body.

50. Among the things which are also obscure is the reason why the heavens move in a circular way. For the substance of the soul is not the cause of its movement in a circular way, but rather it is moved by that motion accidentally. Nor, moreover, is the body the cause of this. Rather, the soul is more appropriately [cause] {72} of this. Nor did he even say why this was better. Yet God must have made the soul move in a circular way only because being in motion is better for it than being at rest, and because what is moved in this way is better than what is moved in another way. (407b5–11)

According to this opinion [the question of] providing a reason why the heavens are moved remains obscure. For according to their position, the substance of the soul does not provide that motion, since on their view the substance of the soul is only a body consisting of the elements and that motion, namely, circular motion, belongs to it accidentally, namely, because the Creator bent it from straightness into circularity. Next he said: **Nor, moreover, is the body**, etc. That is, since the soul, which is more appropriate for being the cause, is not the cause of that motion essentially, the body, insofar as it is a body, is all the more unlikely to be the cause. Next he said: **Nor did** anyone **even say**, etc. That is, even Plato did not provide an account of why it is better for the soul to be moved in a circular way than not to be moved [at all] or than not to be moved in a circular way. Nor was he able to provide [it]. For God must have made the soul to be moved only because being moved is better for it than being at rest.[229] He made it to be moved in a circular way because such a motion is better than rectilinear [motion]. He means that all those things show that this opinion is unacceptable.

51. Therefore, if that consideration is more suitable for another discussion we should immediately set it aside. Let us say that there is another unacceptable consequence which follows upon this discussion and most discussions of the soul. [This] is that they join the soul to the body {73} and place [the soul] in it, but do not provide with this a reason why [the soul] is joined with it and what the disposition of that body is. (407b12–17)

229. Lyons, at Themistius, *De Anima Paraphrase* (1973) 8, note, finds Themistius (1899), 23.13–22; (1973), 8.10–13; and (1996), 39, reflected in Averroes' mention of Plato. But Aristotle himself mentioned the *Timaeus* in Text 45, 406b26. Hence, there is no necessity to understand Averroes as depending on Themistius in this text. Regarding the pious mention of God in the *Middle Commentary*, see *Middle Commentary* (2002), 163, n. 35.

He says that this investigation is more suitable for another science, namely, [the investigation of] why it is better for the heavens to be moved than to be at rest and why in a circular way than in a rectilinear way. For that question is appropriate to First Philosophy.[230] For this reason we must set this aside immediately and **say that there is an unacceptable consequence which follows this discussion**, etc. That is, an unacceptable consequence which follows upon this discussion and most discussions of the soul is that all those saying that it is a being, whether a body or not a body, join it to the body and do not provide a reason why it has been joined with the body, nor do they even say what is the disposition of the body which has been fashioned for being joined with it.

52. **Yet this, as I see it, is necessary. For owing to this interaction [body] acts and is acted upon, moves and is moved, and this sort of thing does not come about for just any things whatsoever. For to say this in regard to these is as if someone were to say that the art of carpentry exists in music. For just as art uses instruments, the soul [uses] the body.**[231] (407b17–19, 24–26)

The reason has to be given for their not knowing in reference to the soul [the principle] that in all things there is an interaction between agent and patient, mover and moved, and that any given thing is not acted upon by any given thing. Therefore, their saying that the soul {74} is in the body without any interaction provided between the body and the soul by which the soul is fit to cause motion and of all the bodies the animal body [is the one suited for] being moved, is similar to the account of one saying that the art of carpentry exists as a subject for music. If, therefore, the art of carpentry has its own subject and its own instruments which it employs, it must be so for the soul with respect to the body, for the body is an instrument of the soul. For this reason the bodies of animals are consonant with their souls.

53. **They seek to speak only about what the soul alone is and determine nothing about the receptive body, as [is the case with] the myth which Py-**

---

230. That is, metaphysics. See Aristotle, *Metaphysics* 12, 6, 1071b3–11.

231. The last two sentences of this Text are from 407b24–26. Text 53, which follows, contains 407b20–24. Averroes' alternate translation does not contain this transposition of Aristotle's text. See Aristotle, *De Anima* (1954). The *Middle Commentary* also follows the order found in the Greek text instead of what we find here. Since Averroes' Comment also gives witness to the order of the faulty Text, this is a likely indication that while he used the same translation of the *De Anima* as his primary Text for the *Middle Commentary* and for the *Long Commentary*, he nevertheless used different manuscript versions of that translation when composing each commentary. On this issue, see the introduction, pp. lxxvii–lxxix.

thagoras employs, namely, that any given soul may enter any given body. For we see that any given thing has its own form and created nature.[232] (407b20–24)

Those who have spoken about the soul have not investigated nor do they want to investigate anything except what it is alone, and they say nothing about the nature of the body proper to it. Because they have set this aside, it seems to be possible to them that any given soul may exist in any given body and be transported from body to body, as Pythagoras said in the myth which he put forth for correcting the souls of citizens.[233] But this opinion is false, for we see that any given thing has its own form and its proper body, that is, its proper soul {75} and its proper animal body. What he says is perfectly evident in the case of species. For members of [the species] lion differ from members of [the species] deer only in virtue of the diversity of the soul of the deer from the soul of the lion. If it were possible for the soul of a lion to exist in the body of the deer, then nature would act in vain. This is also evident in individuals of the same species, and for this reason their ways of acting are different. On the basis of this we have refuted the opinion of Pythagoras.

54. **There is another opinion with which many are content and which is no less [popular] than the opinions mentioned. For they say that [the soul] is a harmony. For a harmony is a mixture and composition of contraries and the body is composed from contraries.** (1.4, 407b27–32)

When he completed his response to what was said in the *Timaeus*, he returned to respond to the account of the one saying that the soul is a form composed from the collection and harmony proper to the elements. Because that opinion is quite reasonable, he said: Here **is another opinion** about the soul. Next he said: **For they say that [the soul] is a harmonic composition**, etc. That is, for they say that the soul is something harmonic and one of the compositions belonging to the elements in the thing composed [and] mixed from them. They said this because they hold the opinion that a harmony is a composition and mixture of contraries and that the body is composed from contraries. Therefore, there is a harmony in the body; therefore, [this harmony] is the soul. {76}

232. *Formam et creaturam propriam*: ἴδιον ἔχειν εἶδος καὶ μορφήν; "form and shape of its own," Aristotle, *De Anima* (1984). Although the Latin translator may have confused خُلُق, "makeup" or "nature," with خَلق, "creation" or "creature," the sense is not adversely affected. Cf. Book 2, {258}, n. 508, and {282}, n. 548. The alternate translation has "shape and proper form," شبح وصورة خاصية (ibid. [1954]).

233. That is, for moral purposes. Themistius, *De Anima Paraphrase* (1899), 23.31–35; (1973), 9.8–9; (1996), 40.

55. Yet a harmony is a proportion or composition among things mixed or composed; but the soul is neither of those two. Furthermore, a harmony is not naturally constituted to cause motion; but everyone agrees that this is something soul has in its own right. (407b32–408a1)

After he had mentioned this opinion, he began to respond to it. He said that the harmony which they say is the soul either is a proportion of things mixed from the elements (and it will be this if the composition of the body from the elements is of the nature of a compound) or the soul is the composition itself, if the composition from the elements is a [mere] juxtaposition [of the constituents], not a mixture, for instance, the composition of the house from stones and bricks. Next he said: and **the soul is neither of those two.** He means: as we mentioned and as we will mention later. Next he said: **Furthermore, a harmony is not naturally constituted to cause motion,** etc. That is, it is immediately apparent that a harmony is not the soul because they all agree on the fact that the soul causes motion, and cannot provide the manner by which a harmony would cause motion.

56. It is more appropriate and better to say that the harmony is a consequence of health and generally that it is a consequence of something, namely, of corporeal moral goods, not a consequence of soul.[234] **This is quite evident when one works at establishing the affections and actions of the soul [as coming about] through some harmony. For making these consonant in this is very difficult.** (408a1–5) {77}

It is better to think that the harmony belongs to bodies as a consequence of health, that is, as a consequence of the forms which are in the living thing inasmuch as it is alive, not as a consequence of the soul and not [as a consequence of] the forms which are in the soul, whether the harmony be a composition or a proportion making a mixture and a compound. Next he said: **This is quite evident,** etc. That is, the difference between the corporeal forms attributed to the elements and the forms attributed to the soul is evident from the fact that in the case of corporeal forms we can attribute the diversity which

---

234. *Armonia currit cursu sanitatis . . . non cursu anime.* ἁρμόζει δὲ μᾶλλον καθ᾽ ὑγιείας λέγειν ἁρμονίαν, καὶ ὅλως τῶν σωματικῶν ἀρετῶν, ἢ κατὰ ψυχῆς. "It is more appropriate to call health (or generally one of the good states of the body) a harmony than to predicate it of the soul." Aristotle, *De Anima* (1984). The phrase *currit cursu* probably corresponds to the Arabic phrase مجراه جرى. In the alternate translation this is rendered يشبه التأليف بصحة البدن (ibid. [1954]). The Latin translator here appears to have translated what was probably فضائل in the Arabic text as "moral goods," *bonitatum moralium,* yielding the awkward term "corporeal moral goods." The alternate translation has بالفضائل التي تعرف بالأجسام (ibid.); "goods which are known through the body."

occurs in the actions and affections of bodies to the composition made in them from the elements. In this way we can say that the action of the flesh in the hand is different from the action of the bone owing to the softness and dampness of the flesh and the hardness and dryness of the bone. But we cannot say by what compound and by what composition the actions of sense differ from the actions of intellect and the actions of the power of sensation from the actions of the motive power. What he mentioned [here] is one of the difficulties which follow for one who says that the soul is a proportion of the elements or something consequent upon a proportion.

57. Furthermore, we understand harmony to be meant in only one of these two senses, [but] truly[235] with respect to magnitudes, since they have motion and place. Their composition is then meant, when they are superimposed upon one another in such a way that nothing of its own nature can intrude between them. Derived {78} from this [understanding of the word] is [the notion of] a proportion which belongs to those things. Therefore, [this view of the soul] is not right with respect to either of those two intentions. The composition of the parts of the body can be easily determined,[236] for there are many compositions of parts of the body.[237] Of which part should intellect be thought to be a composition and how? Of which part [should] sense [be thought to be] a composition? Of which part [should] desire [be thought to be] a composition? (408a5–13)

Furthermore, we understand harmony and sense it just in two ways. One, which is really called harmony, [is] when it is a case of magnitudes having motion and place, being composed with one another and being superimposed in such a way that no magnitude of its own nature can intrude between them. Similar to this and drawn from this [sense] is the proportion which comes about in commingled things before they are commingled with one another. After he had indicated that harmony is said in these two ways, he began to explain that it is unreasonable to say that the soul is [identical with] one of those two senses. He said: **Therefore [this view of the soul] is not right** to say, etc. That is, it is unreasonable to say that the differences of the parts of the soul are provided from one of those two intentions, for instance, to say that

---

235. κυριώτατα: "the most proper sense." Aristotle, *De Anima* (1984).

236. *Compositio autem partium corporis facile potest determinari.* ἡ δὲ σύνθεσις τῶν τοῦ σώματος μερῶν λίαν εὐεξέταστος. "That soul is a harmony in the sense of the composition of the parts of the body is a view easily refutable." Aristotle, *De Anima* (1984). Averroes' alternate translation is similar to Averroes' Text: وقد الفحص يمكننا إمكانا كثيرا عن تركيب أجزاء الجسم (ibid. [1954]).

237. The Greek adds καὶ πολλαχῶς; "and various" (Aristotle, *De Anima* [1984]) or "and occurs in many ways."

the intellect is such a harmony, sense is such and such [a harmony], and desire is such and such [a harmony], as is reasonable in the case of the parts of the body. Next he began to explain this, namely, that this is reasonably said in regard to the parts of the body, but not in regard to the parts of the soul. He said: **The composition of the parts of the body**, etc. That is, {79} this was so because it is easy to establish the form of any given one of the members of the body and to provide its being by composition because it is evident to sense that their compositions are diverse and of many kinds. But to know what composition is appropriate for the intellect and what for sense and what for desire, this is [something] impossible for reason to provide. This is, as it were, another difficulty which follows for those who say that the soul is a harmony or a proportion. For the first difficulty is that they cannot establish actions and affections of the soul through composition. But [this second difficulty occurs] because they cannot establish the diversity of its substance owing to the diversity of the composition. This occurs in regard to what happens for them regardless of whether the forms of composite beings are from a true harmony or from a harmony derivative upon true [harmony].

58. **And also another difficulty**[238] **is [the question of whether] the soul is similar to a mixture. For the mixture of elements which becomes flesh and bone is not of the same proportion. Consequently, there would be many souls in the body and [they would be] throughout the whole body, since all the parts of the body would be [constituted] from the mixture of the elements and the proportion of the mixture would be the harmony and the soul.** (408a13–18)

That is the third difficulty which follows for those saying that the soul is a harmony and a mixture of the elements. For it will follow for them that they assert that each and every part of the body has a particular soul and the universal body has a universal soul. What, then, is the difference between a proportion which makes the soul and [one] which makes a part of the body? For if the soul, insofar as it is soul, is a proportion of a mixture {80} and a composition, or what comes about from the proportion of the mixture and composition, and forms of the parts of the body are either a harmony or a proportion or something made from a proportion, then it is evident that it follows from this that a soul is in any given part of the body and a soul is in the whole body. Or will they say what is the difference between the harmony and proportion which makes the soul and [that] which makes the part of the body, since all the parts of the body come about from the mixture as does the soul? That dif-

238. ἄτοπον is rendered as "absurd." "It is equally absurd to identify the soul with the ratio of the mixture." Aristotle, *De Anima* (1984).

ficulty is similar to the first, in which he asked what mixture is appropriate to each of the powers of the soul.

59. Someone ought to ask of Empedocles (for Empedocles says that any given part of the body is in some proportion): Is, then, the soul a proportion or is the soul something different but which comes about in the parts of the body? Furthermore: Is friendship the cause of any given mixture or is it only a cause of mixture in some proportion? And is friendship that proportion or something else? (408a18–23)

Empedocles should be asked about this difficulty, for he says that the form of any given part of the body exists only through a proportion made by the composition of elements in it. Since his opinion is so, we should ask of him whether the proportion which is the substance of the part of the body is the soul or **something different but which comes about in the parts of the body** from something extrinsic. He means: if then he says that it is a proportion of the parts of the body, it will follow for him that any given part of the body has soul. If he says something else, he will have to provide the difference. Next he said: We should also ask whether friendship, which he holds to be the cause of the mixture, is a cause of each and every {81} mixture. He means: if he says that it is the cause of any given mixture, it will follow that there is a part of the body and a soul from every mixture. If he says that it is a cause of some mixture, he has to provide the cause for that of which it is a mixture; and all the more so if the mixture making the parts of the body is different from the mixture making the soul. Next he said: Is **friendship that proportion or something else?** He means, as it seems to me, the following: if he says that it is a proportion, then the proportion does not exist before the mixture; but the agent must exist before the patient. If he says something else, what then will it be? [It is] as if he means to indicate that those three difficulties which follow for those who say that the soul is a compound or a composition will occur for Empedocles, and those difficulties which he mentioned specifically occur for him because he puts forth [the doctrine of] friendship and strife.

60. Those, then, are the difficulties. If the soul is something other than a mixture, why is it destroyed, if it is destroyed owing to the mixture which was found with flesh and other parts of the body in animals?[239] **Further-**

---

239. *De qua causa tollitur, si tollitur propter mixtionem que inveniebatur cum carne et aliis membris in animalibus?* τί δή ποτε ἅμα τὸ σαρκὶ εἶναι ἀναιρεῖται καὶ τὸ τοῖς ἄλλοις μορίοις τοῦ ζῴου. "Why does it disappear at one and the same moment with that relation between the elements which constitutes flesh or the other parts of the animal body?" (Aristotle, *De Anima* [1984]). فلَمَ ، مع فساد صورة اللحم ، تفسد صورة (ibid. [1954]); "Why is the form of the rest of the organs of the animal سائر أعضاء الحيوان؟

more, if any given part of the body does not have soul and soul is not a proportion of a mixture, what then is that which is corrupted when it is separated from soul? (408a24–28)

Those, then, are the difficulties which follow for those saying that the soul is a compound. Yet one saying this can give a reason for it, for if the soul is something other than a mixture and a compound, why is it corrupted {82} with the corruption of the compound? For if it is something other than the form of flesh and [other than] the form of the parts of the body and is only found in the parts of the body, why is it corrupted with the corruption of the parts of the body? Furthermore, if the soul is not a compound and a mixture, why are the parts of the body corrupted when they are separated from the soul unless there is something else corruptible in the parts of the body when the soul is separated? What then is that?

61. **However, that it is impossible for the soul to be a harmony or that it move in a circular way is evident from the things mentioned. Since it is moved accidentally, as we said, and it moves itself, this is only because the soul is moved by that in which it exists and this is also moved by the soul. But it is impossible for it to be moved in place in another way.** (408a29–34)

After he had refuted the notion that the soul is something essentially self-moving, or a harmony, or a compound, he began to give a summary and to explain that [the soul] happens to move itself only accidentally. He said: **However, that it is impossible for the soul,** etc. He means by this what he said: **or that it move** in a circuit, that is, or that it move itself essentially, as was thought concerning the celestial bodies, which move in a circular fashion. After he had explained that it is impossible for it to be moved essentially of itself, he began to explain that this is possible in an accidental way. He said: **Since it is moved accidentally,** etc. That is, since it is moved accidentally and moves itself accidentally, then it is necessary that the soul seem to be moved by that in which it exists, namely, the body, when that body is moved by [the soul]. But it is impossible for the soul to be moved in place in any other way. {83}

62. **It is [even] more appropriate to raise questions about the motion of the soul in consideration of the following things: for we say that the soul is saddened, rejoices, is brave, is fearful, and even is angry, senses, and discerns.**[240]

---

destroyed with the destruction of the form of the flesh?" The *Middle Commentary* has "If the soul were not something existing in a ratio, why would it become destroyed when the ratio [is destroyed], and vice versa?" *Middle Commentary* (2002), 28.13–14.

240. *Distinguit*: διανοεῖσθαι, "thinking" (Aristotle, *De Anima* [1984]); التفكّر (ibid. [1954]); إنها تميّز, "is discriminating" (*Middle Commentary* [2002], 29.4–5).

All those seem to be motions; hence, one thinks that the soul is moved.
(408a34–b4)

After he had explained that it is impossible for the soul to be moved except accidentally, he provided a difficulty about this. He said: But there is a consideration which compels one to say that the soul is moved essentially. This consideration is that we say that the soul is saddened, rejoices, etc. All those are considered to be motions. On the basis of these two propositions it is thought that the soul is moved. For instance, the soul is sorrowful; since sorrow is a motion, the soul is therefore moved.

63. **But this is not necessary. For, if being sad, being fearful, and discerning are motions and any given one of them involves the movement of something, then this movement is only movement because of the soul. For example, being angry**[241] **is a motion for the heart, that the heart is swelled up**[242] **and discerning is a motion, that such a part of the body follows a certain course, although it may be right that something else follows such a course.**[243] **Some of those occur because of the movement of things with respect to place, while others [occur] because of qualitative change. But what those are and how they come about belongs to another discussion.** (408b5–11)

Although we concede that those are motions, it is still not necessary that they be motions of the soul. For if being fearful and discerning are motions and any given motion among these {84} belongs to some part of the body, then those motions should be attributed only to those parts of the body and that motion is in a part of the body only because of the soul. For being angry, for instance, seems to belong in particular to the heart, because the heart is moved by this motion, that is, it swells. Similarly, being fearful seems to belong in particular to the heart, since the heart is constricted. Since it is evident that those two motions ought to be attributed to the heart, he began to ask to which part understanding is attributed, if it is a motion. He said: **and discerning** is **a motion, that such a part** traverses **such a course.** (This is the way the text was in the manuscript.) He means that if discerning is a motion, then one

241. The Greek adds ἢ φοβεῖσθαι "or fear" (Aristotle, *De Anima* [1984]); والخوف (ibid. [1954]).

242. *Scilicet quod cor inflatur:* ὡδὶ κινεῖσθαι, "as such and such movements of the heart" (Aristotle, *De Anima* [1984]); بنمو القلب وانخفاضه (ibid. [1954]); "as expansion and contraction of the heart."

243. τὸ δὲ διανοεῖσθαι ἢ τὸ τοῦτο ἴσως ἢ ἕτερον τι: "and thinking as such and such another movement of that organ, or of some other" (Aristotle, *De Anima* [1984]); والتفكر أيضا إما كهذين و إما كهذا شيء آخر (ibid. [1954]). The Text here gives an interpretive translation of the Greek.

should hold that it belongs in particular to a different part [of the body], as anger belongs in particular to the heart. He said this because he had already explained that everything moved is a body. Next he said: and it is **right that something else** follow **such a course.** (This is the way the text was in the manuscript.) He means that it is right that some part [of the body] follow such a course, either in all the affections of the soul, if they are all motions, or in some, if there is one [or more] among them in which there is no motion. Among those in which there are motions, some are moved in place and some by qualitative change. Next he said: **But what those are and how,** etc. That is, which parts of the body are the ones which are moved by each of those motions in each of the parts of the soul and how they are moved is [a topic] which belongs elsewhere. He said this because in this passage alone is it necessary that those motions be essentially in bodily and divisible things, as was explained in the general accounts.²⁴⁴ {85}

64. **But to say that the soul is angered is like saying that it weaves or builds. For it seems better not to say that the soul is pious or teaches or discerns,²⁴⁵ but rather to say that a human being does this by means of the soul. This is not because motion is in the soul, but [because] sometimes it reaches it and sometimes it arises from it. For instance, sensation arises from things but memory arises from the soul.²⁴⁶(408b11–17)**

The usual way people speak in saying that the soul is angered and is fearful leads us to be mistaken, and consequently we think that those are motions existing in the soul apart from the body and that the soul is moved essentially by them. Because of that he began to explain that this is said only in an analogous way, that those motions are similar to the motions which are [evident] in the visible parts [of the body], as [are] building and weaving, and that they are no different except insofar as the former parts are internal and the latter are external. He said: **But to say that the soul is angered,** etc. That is, just as the motion

244. It is not clear what texts Averroes has in mind here. Hicks (at Aristotle, *De Anima* [1965], 274–275) suggests Aristotle may have in mind 419a7 and 427b26 and mentions that Philoponus thinks it may be a reference to *Parts of Animals* or *Movement of Animals*. Rodier (at ibid. [1900], 135) suggests *Parts of Animals* 3.6, 669a19, and *Problems* 11, 31, 902b30. See my n. 165 regarding "the general accounts."

245. *Anima habet pietatm, aut docet, aut distinguit*: τὴν ψυχὴν ἐλεεῖν ἢ μανθάνειν ἢ διανοεῖσθαι, "the soul pities or learns or thinks" (Aristotle, *De Anima* [1984]); النفس تفرح أو تتعلم أو تفكر (ibid. [1954]); "the soul rejoices [*sic*] or learns or cogitates."

246. The Text here omits ἐπὶ τὰς ἐν τοῖς αἰσθητηρίοις κινήσεις ἢ μονάς: "and terminating with the movements or states of rest in the sense organs." Aristotle, *De Anima* (1984). Averroes' citation of his alternate translation makes it clear that he was well aware of problems with his Text.

of the weaver and the builder is attributed to the soul only accidentally, so too the motion of anger and of fear [is attributed to the soul only accidentally].

Next he said: But **it seems better not to say**, etc. That is, for this reason it is better that the expression in the case of all those actions be that the human being does this by means of the soul, not that the soul discerns, builds, learns, or is pious, but rather that the human being learns or discerns by means of the soul. Next he said: **this is not because motion is in the soul**, etc. That is, those motions do not exist in the soul, but rather the starting point of motion in some {86} of them is external and the terminus [is] in the soul. After he had explained that the starting point of some of those motions is external while the terminus is in the soul, he provided an example. But the translation which is the basis for our statements here has lost it. He means that the motion of sensation is a motion which has a starting point which is external and a terminus in the soul, and the motion of memory is a motion which has a starting point in the soul and a terminus outside. That motion of memory may or may not reach sensation, for when the power of memory moves the imagination, the imagination then may or may not move the sensitive [power]. This is evident in the other translation which is as follows: "To say that the soul is angered is as if to say that it weaves or builds. But it is better not to say that the soul rejoices or learns, but that the human being [does so] through the soul. [This is] not because motion reaches [the soul] and comes about in it, but [because] sometimes it reaches it, as in the case of sensation, which retrieves from sensible things what it retrieves for [the soul], and sometimes the starting point of motion comes about from [the soul], as in the case of memory. Then either it will remain in it and will not pass through to something else, or it will arrive at and affect the senses."[247] He means by this what he said: "not because motion" comes "to [the soul] and comes about in it." That is, the soul is not said to have that motion because it is its subject. He means by this what he said: "Then either it will remain in it," etc. That is, that motion which has its starting point from the soul, namely, memory, will perhaps remain in the brain, which is that power's instrument and will perhaps pass through to something else, so that it reaches the senses, that is, the instruments of the senses. {87}

65. Intellect, however, seems to be a substance which comes to be in a thing and is not subject to corruption. For if it were subject to corruption, it would be

247. وقول القائل إن النفس تغضب بمنزلة قول القائل إن النفس تنسج أو تنبى. و عسى أن يكون الأصلح ألا يقال إن النفس تفرح أو تتعلم أو تفكر ، بل يقال : إن الإنسان يفعل كل ذلك بالنفس ؛ وليس ذلك لأن الحركة تصير إليها فتصير فيها، بل مرة تنتهى فتبلغها كمثل الحس الذى يؤدى إليها عن الأشياء ، ومرة تكون الحركة منها إبتداء مثل التذكر للشىء : فإنه يكون منها : فإما بقى فيها فلم ينفذ إلى غيرها ، وإما أتى على حركات الحواس فغيرها (Aristotle, *De Anima* [1954]).

more appropriate for it to undergo corruption in the feebleness which accompanies old age. But we see that what occurs for this in the case of the senses [also occurs] in the case of the body. For if an old person were to receive a young person's eye, he would see as a young person does. Thus old age is not a disposition in which the soul suffers something but rather a disposition in which the soul finds itself just as it is when it is drunk or ill. (408b18–24)

After he had conceded that the soul is moved accidentally, that is, owing to the subject in virtue of which it is constituted, and for this reason is generable and corruptible, he began to explain that of the parts of the soul the material intellect seems not to be movable, not even accidentally. For it is not generable and not corruptible except with respect to that [part] of the body in which it acts or with respect to that [part of the body] by which it is affected.[248] [This is] because it does not have a bodily instrument which is corrupted by [the body's] corruption, as is the disposition in regard to the other powers of the soul. He said: **Intellect, however, seems to be a substance**, etc. He means here by **intellect** the material intellect which discerns the intentions of all beings.[249] Next he said: for **if it were subject to corruption**, etc. That is, for if it were subject to corruption, it would have a bodily instrument, since it would be a power of a body. If it were to have a bodily instrument, what occurs to the senses would occur to it in old age and then it would understand the intentions of intelligible things feebly. But this is not so. Then it must not have an instrument. Since {88} that intellect is not subject to corruption, then what is subject to corruption in its own right is its affection or action, through the corruption of that by which it is affected, since that by which it is affected is inside the body, as will be explained later.[250] Then he said: **But we see that what oc-**

248. That is, the material intellect can in a sense be said to be generable and corruptible only insofar as the part of the body with which it is associated is generable and corruptible.

249. Here in the *Long Commentary* Averroes does not hesitate to explain that the intellect called a substance is the material intellect, since he has come to hold that the material intellect is a separate substance in its own right. See {385–413}, {450ff}. In the *Middle Commentary*, however, he calls this intellect شيء ما يكون في النفس, "a certain thing which comes to be in the soul." *Middle Commentary* (2002), 30.9. Ivry makes the important remark (164, n. 10) that Averroes declines to call it a substance in spite of the fact that it was so named in the text of Themistius (*De Anima Paraphrase*: οὐσία τις [1899], 29.25; جوهرا ما [1973], 21.12; [1996], 46) and was surely called substance in his Arabic text of the *De Anima*. As indicated in the introduction, pp. xxxiii–xl, the doctrine of intellect in the *Middle Commentary* holds the material intellect to be only an immaterial disposition of the individual soul accounted for by its special relationship to the agent intellect, which is a separate substance.

250. This is the cogitative faculty, which is bodily. See the introduction, pp. lxix–lxxv.

curs for this in the case of the senses, etc. That is, but because we see that what occurs in the case of the senses from feebleness in old age can be attributed to the sensitive power in this way, not because the power has been changed and become old, but because feebleness occurs to those [parts of the body] through which it understands.[251] [Consider,] for instance, the craftsman whose action becomes feeble because of the feebleness of the instrument, not because of himself. Since that account is sufficient in the case of the senses, how much more is it for the intellect! Next he said: **old age,** therefore, **is not a disposition,** etc. That is, the occurrence of old age and becoming old on the part of a human being, for this reason, is not a disposition in which the soul is affected by way of corruption, but rather the disposition which occurs to [a human being] in old age is similar to the disposition which seems to occur when he is drunk or ill. For we think that the soul in these two cases does not suffer corruption, and especially in the case of drunkenness.

This last account is sufficient though not demonstrative. But Aristotle's custom is to present accounts which are sufficient either after demonstrative ones or in places in which he cannot present demonstrative ones.

66. To understand and to contemplate are distinguished when something else inside undergoes corruption, but it is in itself {89} affected by nothing.[252] **Discerning, loving, and hating are not the being of the [intellect] but rather**

251. *Intelligit.* The argument requires *sensit* (senses) here. It may be that some lines of argument have dropped out due to homoioteleuton.

252. *Et intelligere et considerare diversantur quando aliquid aliud corrumpitur intus; ipsum autem in se nichil patitur.* καὶ τὸ νοεῖν δὴ καὶ τὸ θεωρεῖν μαραίνεται ἄλλου τινος ἔσω φθειρομένου, αὐτὸ δὲ ἀπαθές ἐστιν. "Thus it is that thinking and reflecting decline through the decay of some other inward part and are themselves impassible" (Aristotle, *De Anima* [1984]); كالذى ترى من حال الفكر والفهم في أوقات الأمراض السُكر : ([1984]) فإنهـما يضعفان. وليس ذلك لفَساد الشيء الذى داخل ، فإن ذلك لا يألم ولا يتغير .ibid) [1954]). The Text as rendered in Latin is confused, but in his Comment Averroes makes no mention of any difficulty and even provides remarks quite in line with the Greek. It appears, then, that the problems here may be primarily the result of a faulty rendering by the Latin translator. *Diversantur* may result from an incorrect text or an incorrect understanding of a form of the verbal root kh-l-f, where form V has the sense of falling behind or away, while VII has the sense of being different or diverse. The Latin translator seems to have read the latter in his manuscript. In addition to this, it is not clear in the Latin just what the referent of *ipsum* could reasonably be here. Themistius quotes 408b18–30 in his commentary and so would be available to Averroes to consult for the correct reading if his primary Text were faulty. See Themistius, *De Anima Paraphrase* (1899), 29.24–35; (1973), 21.12–22.6; (1996), 46. The *Middle Commentary* has والتصور بالعقل إنما يفسـد بان يفسـد داخل البـدن شيء آخر "Conceptualization perishes only as something else within the body perishes." *Middle Commentary* (2002), 30.17–18.

of this [whole human being], namely, what has [them] insofar as it has [them]. Furthermore, for this reason, when this is corrupted, we will not remember or love others. Therefore, it is not part of the [intellect] but of this which is common, which was left behind. However, it is more appropriate for the intellect to be something divine and impassible. However, it is evident that it is impossible for the soul to be moved. If it is not moved in any way, it is evident that it is also not moved by itself. (408b24–31)

After he had asserted that the intellect, which understands intelligible things, is neither generable nor corruptible and [that] understanding, which is an action of that intellect, seems to be generable and corruptible, he began to provide the way in which this occurs. It is that what understands is inside the body and is generable and corruptible. He said: **To understand and to contemplate are distinguished**, etc. That is, it happens that understanding is sometimes in potency and sometimes in act, not because intellect is generable and corruptible but because something else inside the body in which understanding takes place is corrupted. Next he said: **But** nothing happens to it in itself, . . . namely, the imaginative intellect. Later he will explain that this is the thing imagined or understood. It is this which he calls in the third book the passible intellect.[253] After he had provided the way of the solution {90} of the question in which it is asked how the understanding intellect is not generable or corruptible and understanding which is its action is generable and corruptible, he began also to explain about the powers because, although they are attributed to the intellect, they seem to be generated and corrupted because those powers are [those] not of an eternal intellect.

He does this so that no question may arise concerning what he said in regard to the material intellect in the third book, namely, how the intellect is ungenerable and incorruptible and after death we neither love nor hate nor discern.[254] Next he said: **Discerning, loving, and hating**, etc. That is, discerning, which is attributed to the cogitative power,[255] loving and hating, which are attributed to reason, namely, which are receptive of the action of reason. For it seems there is something susceptible to reason in this part of the soul because it is obedient to intellect in good people. Therefore, those are not ac-

---

253. 430a24–25, Book 3, Text 20, {443}. Cf. {446}.

254. 3.5, 430a22–26.

255. It seems odd that Averroes has يتذكر, "recollection," in lieu of "discerning" in his paraphrase in the *Middle Commentary*. It should be noted that cogitation (*cogitatio*, *virtus cogitativa*, or *pars cogitativa*, فكر) is not mentioned at the corresponding passage of the *Middle Commentary* and that recollecting, loving, and hating are attributed to العقل العملى, "the practical intellect." *Middle Commentary* (2002), 31.1. On the important and new role of cogitation in the *Long Commentary*, see the introduction, pp. lxix–lxxv.

tions of that intellect but rather they are actions of the powers possessing this action insofar as they possess that action. He adds this condition, namely, **insofar as** they have [them], because it is impossible for those powers to exist except with understanding. But if they were attributed to it, it would not be an attribution in accord with the way they are. Next he said: **Furthermore, for this reason, when this is corrupted, we will not remember or love.** That is, because these actions are in us by generable and corruptible powers different from the power which is the material intellect, namely, that which discerns universal intentions, no one can raise questions and say that if the intellect is ungenerable and incorruptible, why do we not remember {91} or love or hate after death? For these actions belong to powers different from that power. Next he said: **However, it is more appropriate for the intellect to be something divine and not passible**, that is, it is not something changeable owing to a mixture with matter. Next he said: **However, it is evident that it is impossible**, etc. That is, it is therefore evident from this account that it is impossible for the soul to be moved. In regard to certain parts, namely, in regard to the intellect, [it can be moved] neither essentially nor accidentally, while in regard to certain other parts [it can be moved] accidentally [but] not essentially. Since it was explained that it is not moved at all, [then] it is not moved in its own right, because it is necessary in everything moved in its own right, which is proper to animals, that it move in its own right essentially, and not the converse.[256]

67. **The most unreasonable account is the one which says that the soul is a self-moving number. For many impossible things follow for one who says this, first [all] the things which follow for one who says that the soul is moved and [then also] in particular those things which follow from saying that it is a number. For we do not know how to understand a unit as moved and by what and how it is moved. For it must have different parts.**[257] (408b32–409a3)

256. In the corresponding section of the *Middle Commentary*, Averroes writes, وقد بينا هذا المعنى على التمام فى شرح كلامه فى هذا الفصل. Ivry renders this as, "We have, however, already discussed this matter completely in the *Long Commentary* to his discussion of this chapter." *Middle Commentary* (2002), 31.4–5. While this is possible, I am more inclined to render this, "We have already explained this notion fully in the comment on his discussion in this section."

257. The Text here omits several key phrases, but Averroes' Comment shows no recognition of it. The Greek has πῶς γὰρ χρὴ νοῆσαι μονάδα κινουμένην, καὶ ὑπὸ τίνος, καὶ πῶς, ἀμερῆ καὶ ἀδιάφορον οὖσαν; ᾗ γάρ ἐστι κινητικὴ καὶ κινητή, διαφέρειν δεῖ. 409a1–3. "How are we to imagine a unit being moved? By what agency? What sort of movement can be attributed to what is without parts or internal differences? If the unit is both originative of movement and capable of being moved, it must contain difference." Aristotle, *De Anima* [1984]). Averroes' alternate translation follows the Greek

After he had completed the response to those using motion alone in the definition of the soul, he began to respond to those who use number besides motion. He said: **The most unreasonable**, etc. That is, that account concerning the soul is less adequate than all the [other] accounts, namely, the account of one who says the soul is a self-moving number. {92} For many impossible things follow for him. First, those things which follow for the one who says that the soul is something self-moving, and [then] in particular the things which follow because they assert that it is a self-moving number. Next he said: **For we do not know**, etc. That is, for we do not know how to understand an eternally moved unit. For everything moved has a position and a unit does not have a position. Similarly, it is also impossible to understand what moves it to the extent that it is divided into something moved and something causing motion, inasmuch as what moves itself [must] be divided. For a unit in itself is not divided. Similarly, it is also impossible to understand how it is moved, since what is not divided is not moved, as was said. Next he said: Therefore **it must have different parts.** That is, if there is some way in which it is moved and something else according to which it moves, those ways must be different from one another, and so it will be divisible in intention. But a unit is not divided in any way.

68. **Furthermore, since they say that when a line is moved it makes a surface,**[258] **then a point [makes] a line [when it is moved].**[259] **For a point is a unit having position, just as they number the soul in position and it has position.**[260] **Furthermore, if a number or unit is subtracted from a number, another number will remain. Plants and many animals will remain alive when cut up and, nevertheless, it is thought that the soul belonging to these segments is the same soul in species.** (409a3–10)

After he had given the ways in which that account happens to contradict itself, he also provided other impossibilities. He said: **Furthermore, since they say that**, etc. That is, it is the custom of the mathematicians {93} to say that

more precisely, although it omits καὶ κινητή, "and capable of being moved." See ibid. (1954).

258. That is, the line describes a surface when it is moved.

259. The Text omits καὶ αἱ τῶν μονάδων κινήσεις γραμμαὶ ἔσονται, "the movements of the units must be lines" (Aristotle, *De Anima* [1984]); فحركات الآحاد تصير خطوطا (ibid. [1954]).

260. *Sicut numerant animam in situ, et habet situm:* ὁ δ ἀριθμὸς τῆς ψυχῆς ἤδη πού ἐστι καὶ θέσιν ἔχει; "for a point is a unit having position, and the number of the soul is, of course, somewhere and has position." Aristotle, *De Anima* (1984). The translator may have read in his Text the Arabic عدد in عدد النفس (ibid. [1954]), "number of the soul," as a verb instead of a noun.

when the line is moved, it makes a surface, and when a point [is moved], it makes a line, but if units are moved, it is necessary that they have position, and every unit having position is a point. Consequently, the units which they assert to be the number of the soul must be points. If they are points and are moved, then they must make lines, not actions of the soul. Next he provided another impossibility. He said: **Furthermore, if a number or unit is subtracted,** etc. That is, furthermore, the kinds of numbers differ from one another as greater and lesser. For if a unit is subtracted from fourness, then it becomes threeness, and if it is added, then it becomes fiveness. We see in the cases of every living plant and several animals that although a part is taken from them, what remains remains identical to the first in species. Hence, the action of the soul seems to be in the category of quality, not quantity. If the action of the soul were in [the category of] quantity, then it would follow that the soul which remains in plants would be different in species from the earlier one.

69. **One can say that there is no difference between units and small bodies. For [on that assumption] points come to be from the small particles of Democritus and there remains quantity alone, as if there were something moved and something moving in it, just as there is in a continuum. For it is not because they are different in greatness and smallness that what we said happens, but rather because [they have] quantity. For this reason it is necessary that there be something which moves units. Therefore, if there is something which is a mover in living things, there is also [a mover] in numbers.**[261] **Hence, the soul must not be mover and moved, but only a mover.** (409a10–18) {94}

We can say that there is no difference between asserting that there are self-moving units and asserting that these units are small bodies. For by asserting them to be self-moving, we assert that they are bodies. If not, then how are the units thought to be self-moving? Next he said: **For [on that assumption] points come to be from the particles of Democritus.** He means, as it seems to me: likewise, anyone who asserts that it is possible for the point to move concedes that it follows for him that the point be a body. For this reason we can rightly say that the particles of Democritus which are self-moving are so small that they are called points. For a point, according to this view, is nothing but a body.

After he had reported this, he provided the reason why it is possible con-

---

261. εἰ δ ἐν τῷ ζῴῳ τὸ κινοῦν ἡ ψυχή, καὶ ἐν τῷ ἀριθμῷ: "If in the animal what originates movement is the soul, so also must it be in the case of the number" (Aristotle, *De Anima* [1984]; وإذا كان المحرك الموجود في الحيوان هو النفس ، فهى إذا محرك العدد (.ibid) [1954]).

cerning such points to imagine that there is something in them, as it were, moving and something, as it were, moved. He said: **and** quantity alone **remains**, etc. That is, as it seems to me, that since they are moved, quantity alone will remain in them, even if one removes from them the different [sorts of] quantities. Since the nature of quantity remains in them, it is possible to understand that there is something moved and something moving in them, as in bodies. For this happens to a body only insofar as it is body, not insofar as it is large or small, namely, that it is self-moved and that the mover in it is different from the moved. He meant this when he said: **just as there is in a continuum**, etc. That is, that the thing is not said to be self-moved even so that the mover in it is different from the moved on account of the body being large or small, but rather solely on account of {95} its being a body and a continuum. For this reason everyone who asserts that there is a self-moved unit or point has to assert that they are small bodies. So one who asserts that the soul is self-moving units or points is no different at all from Democritus, who asserts that it is small particles. Next he said: **For this reason it is necessary**, etc. That is, since the units are self-moving and in the thing the mover is different from the moved, then what moves the units has to be different from the units. Therefore, if the soul is the mover in everything which is moved, the soul is also a mover in the units, not the moved units, which are number. Hence, it is necessary that the soul be only a mover, not a mover and something moved at the same time. Next he said: **Therefore if** the soul is a mover, it is therefore also [a mover] in number.[262] That is, if, therefore, the soul is a mover of matter, it is also a mover of number. Hence, the soul must not be mover and moved by number, but only a mover.

70. **How is it possible for it to be a unit? For it must have a difference in virtue of which it differs from other units. Therefore, what diversity can occur between a point and a unit, if it is not in position? Therefore, if points and units were in the same place, [it would be] because [the units] occupy the place of the point,[263] although nothing would [then] prevent two points from being in the same place and points [from being] infinite. But things whose place is indivisible are also such as this.** (409a18–25)

262. That is, if the soul is a mover in animals, then it is also a mover in numbers, on the assumption that the soul is a number.

263. The Text omits the beginning of this sentence. The Greek has εἰ μὲν οὖν εἰσὶν ἕτεραι αἱ ἐν τῷ σώματι μονάδες καὶ αἱ στιγμαί, ἐν τῷ αὐτῷ ἔσονται αἱ μονάδες· καθέξει γὰρ χώραν στιγμῆς. "Thus if, on the one hand, these units within the body are different from the points, the units will be in the same place; for each unit will occupy a point." (Aristotle, *De Anima* [1984]); وإن كانت آحاد أُخَر في الجسم ، فستجتمع الآحاد والنقط في مكان. وليس من مانع يمنع أن يجتمع منهن إثنان أو ما لا عدد له ؛ (ibid. [1954]).

How is it possible according to them for the soul to be something composed from units? For it is necessary to provide the difference by which the units which are in the soul differ from numerical units. If not, then number would be {96} alive. When he had stated that it is necessary for them to provide the difference between the two kinds of units, he said: And **what diversity can occur**, etc. That is, there is nothing in virtue of which these two units differ, insofar as each is indivisible, unless someone may say that the unit which is in the soul has the position of number, or it does not have position. In this way the units which are in the soul will be points, for it was said that the point is a unit having position. After he had explained that they must say that the units which are in the soul are points, he began to explain that it follows that they say that they are the same as points existing in bodies. He said: **Therefore, if points and units were in the same place**, the units which are in the soul and the points which are in the body would have to be the same. But he left out the consequent because it obviously follows from what precedes [it]. Next he began to explain the antecedent. He said: **because they occupy the place of the point.** That is, they must be in the same place because the place of the units which are in the soul must be the place of [only] one of the points which are in the body. Since the place of the units having position which are in the soul is the place of one of the points of the body, they must be in the same place. Next he began to explain that the place of these must be the place of one point. He said: **although nothing would [then] prevent**, etc. That is, nothing prevents there being two points, even infinite points, in the same place; rather, this is necessary. For with respect to all the things of which the place is indivisible, when they are superimposed upon one another, none becomes divisible.

71. **If the number of the soul is the points which are in the body, or the soul is in a number which is [composed] from the points {97} which are in the body, why do not all bodies have soul? For they hold the opinion that there are points in all bodies, even an infinite number of them. Furthermore, how is it possible for the points to be separated from the bodies when lines are not divided into points?**[264] (409a25–30)

From the preceding account it is necessary that the units which are in the soul be points which are in the body or [that] the soul be something existing in a number which comes about from the points which are in the body (since in the case of two points they must be superimposed upon one another so that

---

264. *Non dividantur in puncta?*: μὴ διαιροῦνται αἱ γραμμαὶ εἰς στιγμάς; "lines cannot be resolved into points?" (Aristotle, *De Anima* [1984]); إلا أن تتجزأ الخطوط والنقط؟ (ibid. [1954]).

they become the same). Why, then, are not all bodies alive, since there are infinite points in every body? Rather, any given part of it must be alive, which is impossible. Next he provided them with another impossibility, that the soul cannot be separated from the body, with the result that it is impossible for the animal to die except through corruption of its body. He said: **Furthermore, how is it possible for the points to be separated from the bodies**, etc. That is, furthermore, it follows for them according to this opinion that the soul is not separated from the body nor does it die. For, if the soul is points and it is impossible for points to be separate from bodies (since it was explained that lines are not composed from points nor surfaces from lines nor body from surfaces, but points are not separate from the line because they are its endpoints, nor are lines or surfaces [separate] from body), then it is impossible for soul to be separate from body. But, nevertheless, separation is possible in the case of points if lines were composed from them, which is impossible, as was explained in the *Physics*.[265] {98}

72. **It follows in a way, as we said, that their account is similar to the account of one asserting that it is a body made up of fine parts. But in another way, as Democritus says concerning motion, there is an impossibility peculiar to these [people].[266] For if the soul is in the whole sensible body, there must be two bodies in the same place if the soul is a body. For those saying that it is a number, there must be many points in the same point or every body must have a soul, unless there happens to be another number which is different from the points existing in bodies.** (1.5, 409a31–b7)

The impossibility which follows for those who say that the soul is a body composed of fine parts follows in a way for those giving this account. In another way they also incur for themselves the impossibility happening for Democritus insofar as he asserts that the reason for motion is that the particles which are the soul are self-moved. For there is no difference between asserting that the cause of the motion of the soul is the body which is self-moved

265. *Physics* 6, 1, 231a17ff.

266. *Ut dicit Democritus in motu, propria est eis impossibilitas*: ὥσπερ Δημόκριτος κινεῖσθαί φησιν ὑπὸ τῆς ψυχῆς, ἴδιον τὸ ἄτοπον; "entangled in the absurdity peculiar to Democritus' way of describing the manner in which movement is originated by the soul" (Aristotle, *De Anima* [1984]); لمن قال بقول ذيمقراط وأتباعه ، لأنه إن كان النفس في (Aristotle, *De Anima* [1984]); جميع الجسد الحاس (ibid. [1954]). Both the Text used by Averroes and his alternate translation are faulty here. Note that the Arabic behind the Latin plural *eis* may refer to the plural وأتباعه, "and his followers," in a faulty Arabic manuscript. Since Averroes shows no recognition of a problem here and his alternate Arabic text is faulty, it is likely that his Arabic Text was also faulty. The problem, then, seems to be with the Arabic translation of the *De Anima*.

units or [that it is the body] which is self-moved particles. Next he began to make known what impossibility they share with those who say that the soul is a fine body. He said: **For if the soul is in the whole sensible body**, etc. That is, the impossibility is common [to both] because for those saying that the soul is a body there must be two bodies in the same place. For it will be necessary for the soul to be in the whole body, because the sensible body senses in all its parts. Hence, there must be a part of the soul in every part of [the body] and the whole soul must be {99} in the whole body. In this way bodies are superimposed upon one another and penetrate one another, namely, the body which is the soul and the body in which it exists. In this way two bodies will necessarily be in the same place. For those who say that the soul is a number many points which the intellect discerns must be in the place of the same point of the body. This is similar to the account of one saying that it is possible for many bodies to be in the same place. For besides the fact that they assert them to be in the same place, if they will not assert them to be distinct, as was explained,[267] the consequence for them will be that the points which are the soul will be the points of the body itself. Thus, every body will be alive, if they will not concede that the other points in the body are different from the points which are in the soul. But if they were to concede this, the consequence for them would be that there are many points in the place of one point. This is similar to the account of one who says that there are many bodies in the same place. This impossibility follows for one saying that the soul is a body composed of fine parts.

73. **It follows for them that a living being is moved only by number, as we said concerning the opinion of Democritus. For there is no difference between those saying that they are small parts and those saying that they are units insofar as they are moved.[268] For in each case the animal must be moved only by those things which are moved.** (409b7–11)

Here he wants to explain the impossibility specific to them and to Democritus. He said: **It follows for them**, etc. That is, it follows for them, insofar as they say that an animal is moved {100} only by self-moved units, [just] what follows for Democritus when he said that an animal is moved only by self-moving particles. Next he provided the way in which these two opinions are similar. He said: **For there [is] no difference**, etc. That is, for there is no differ-

267. Text and Comment 71, {96–97}.

268. *Nulla enim est differentia inter dicentes partes parvas et dicentes quod unitates sunt secundum quod sunt mote.* τί γὰρ διαφέρει σφαίρας λέγειν μικρὰς ἢ μονάδας μεγάλας, ἢ ὅλως μονάδας φερομένας; "For what difference does it make whether we speak of small spheres or of large units, or, quite simply, of units in movement?" (Aristotle, *De Anima* [1984]); ولا فرق بين من قال إن المحرك للنفس أجسام صغيرة مستديرة ، و بين من; قال إن الآحاد العظيمة تحركها (ibid. [1954]).

ence between saying that what moves is a small body or [saying what moves consists of] small units, since it will have been asserted that each moves the body only insofar as it is moved. For it follows that these two, namely, units and parts, move only insofar as they are self-moved. He meant: since it is so, the impossibilities following for Democritus also follow for this opinion.

74. **Therefore, those who bring together number and motion in the same thing also have these impossibilities and many others like them. For it is impossible for the definition of the soul to be such as this nor [is it possible for this combination to be] one of its accidents. This is evident if someone wishes on the basis of this to establish the actions and affections of the soul, such as cogitation,[269] sense, pleasure, and sorrow. For this, as we said above, is not easy, not even by conjecture.** (409b11–18)

He says that these impossibilities mentioned earlier and many more follow for those who define the soul at the same time by number and motion. This is obvious, for none of them can give the causes for the actions and affections in the soul by means of {101} number, not even if one conjectures by saying that one number makes sensation, another cogitation, and another pleasure. For if the causes of different things are different, and their causes are units and numbers, then the units and numbers of the cause of those things must be different. His account in this section is plainly evident.

75. **We have spoken of the three sorts of definitions of the soul (for some judged it to be self-moved and some judged it to be a very fine body or a body very far removed from the other bodies), and we already have been seen to have brought up the difficulties which follow for these two accounts. It, therefore, remains [for us] to ask whether it is composed of the elements, since this might be said because we sense beings and know each of them.** (409b18–25)

The ancients define the soul in three ways: one that it is self-moved; another that it is a very fine body or far removed from bodily nature; and some define it as being from the principles and elements because it is, as it is said, something which discerns and knows. We already responded to the opinion of those who define it through motion and those who define it {102} through fine body. Hence, we should now respond to the opinion of those who say that it is composed from the elements. You ought to know that his response to those

---

269. *Ut cogitationem et sensum et voluptatem et tristitiam:* οἶον λογισμούς, αἰσθήσεις, ἡδονάς, λύπας, "reasoning, sensation, pleasure, pain." Aristotle, *De Anima* (1984). The *Middle Commentary* has مثل الفكر والحس واللذة والأذى, "like cogitation, sensation, pleasure, injury." *Middle Commentary* (2002), 34.14–15.

saying that it is a body is grouped under the response directed toward those saying it is a mover because it is moved. For it follows for all those that they say that it is a body, and it makes no difference whether they assert that what is self-moved is small particles, as [does] Democritus, or units, as [do] those saying that it is a self-moving number or a heavenly body, as in the *Timaeus*.[270] Similarly grouped is the response to those saying that it is a compound or harmony, and generally a composite body. Therefore, it remains to respond to the opinion of those who conjecture that it is composed from the elements, owing to knowledge and sensation.

76. **But a great many impossibilities follow upon this account. For they assert that like is known only by like, and, as it were, assert that the soul is those things. But those are not the only things existing here, but [there are] a great many more; rather, it seems that things which are composed from them are infinite. (409b25–29)**

They justify that account by saying that the principles are all the things which come to be from those principles. The principles are not the things which come to be from the principles in all ways, but those which come to be from the principles are more [in number] than the principles. Rather, it seems correct that those things which come to be from the principles are infinite. Since the things which come to be from the principles in all the ways are different from the principles in a way, then it does no good for them to say {103} that the soul is from the principles, since, insofar as it is different, there is no similarity there. Since there is no similarity there, there will be no knowledge, since the knower knows only through the similarity which he has with the thing known.[271]

After he had explained that the things which have come to be from the principles are not the same principles in [their] forms and beings, he began to explain the impossibilities following upon this when we say that nothing is known except through its like.

77. **It may be asserted, therefore, that the soul knows and senses those things from which any given thing comes to be. Then it neither knows nor senses the whole, for instance, what God is, what a human being is, what flesh**

270. *Timaeus*, 34Cff., esp. 36D–37C.

271. That is, they hold that the principles are the same as the things which come to be from the principles. But the principles from which things are derived are not completely identical with the derivative things, since the derivative things are greater in number than the principles. But insofar as soul is not completely and in every respect identical with the principles from which it arises, it is different from them and dissimilar. But if such is the case, there will be no knowledge since knowledge is possible only because of similarity.

is, what bone is, and likewise other composite things. For the being of any one of those is not just [the same] as the elements may be in any given disposition, but in a certain disposition and proportion, as Empedocles had recounted in regard to the generation of bone. For he says that the large [quantity of] earth which is in things containing bone has an eighth part from paleness and four parts from fire, and in this way bones were made white.[272] For it is useless for the elements to be in the soul unless there is proportion and composition in them. For then it will know something through a similarity and it will not know bone or human being if these two are not in it. That account does not require a response. For no one thinks that the stone or a human being is in the soul, and likewise living and non-living.[273] (409b29–410a12) {104}

It may be asserted, etc. That is, it may be asserted, according to their opinion, that the soul knows and senses elements from which any given thing is composed because it is [itself] composed from the elements. For them, therefore,

272. The Greek text has in verse form, "The kindly Earth in its broad-bosomed moulds/ Won of clear Water two parts out of eight/And four of Fire; and so white bones were formed." Aristotle, *De Anima* (1984). As Ivry notes, Averroes follows his faulty Text in the Comment in the *Long Commentary*, but in the *Middle Commentary* he follows a different tradition, probably via Themistius reaching back to Simplicius and Philoponus. Ivry also notes that the translation from Arabic by Zeraḥyah (Aristotle, *De Anima* [1994]) is not in accord with the Text in Averroes' *Long Commentary* but in accord with the *Middle Commentary*'s account, which has "it is composed of eight parts: two parts of earth, four of fire, and two of water and air, it being therefore white." *Middle Commentary* (2002), 35.22–23, and p. 167, n. 4. This supports the view that Averroes likely used one manuscript version of his primary translation of the *De Anima* when composing the *Long Commentary* and a different manuscript version of his primary translation when composing the *Middle Commentary*. See the introduction, pp. lxxvii–lxxix.

273. *Vivum et non vivum.* The Greek Text has ὁμοίως δὲ καὶ τὸ ἀγαθὸν καὶ τὸ μὴ ἀγαθόν, "the good and the not-good." Aristotle, *De Anima* (1984). It would seem that the Arabic may have been الخير واللاخير, as Badawi conjectures to fill in an omission in his edition of the text, Averroes' alternate translation. See ibid. (1954), 24. The corruption of الخير واللاخير into الحي واللاحي ("the living and the non-living") would not be surprising. What is uncertain, however, is whether (i) this corruption was in the Arabic Text in front of Averroes at the time of his composition of the *Long Commentary*, or (ii) the texts were corrupted after the original composition of the work and in both the Text and Comment of the Arabic manuscript used by the Latin translator, or (iii) the texts were illegible in the Arabic and read as forms of حي by the Latin translator. In the Comment we find *vivum* used suitably several times {105} in the discussion, but this is insufficient to decide the case. In his *Middle Commentary* Averroes seems to evidence familiarity with a correct translation when he writes of the soul's "knowing something as good or not good (علمها بما هو خير وما ليس بخير), for good and bad things do not exist in the soul." *Middle Commentary* (2002), 36.9–10.

it follows that it does not know the whole of the composite thing and that it does not sense its form, for form exists above [the level of] the elements in the composite. It will follow, therefore, that it does not know God nor a human being nor flesh nor bone. For the being is not one of the elements nor [is it] composed from the elements, and this is necessarily the case in regard to all composite things. Next he said: **For the being of any one**, etc. That is, both the beings and the forms of things must be added to the elements, because any given being composed from the elements is composed in some determined proportion and composition of its own by which that being is what it is. Empedocles concedes this, for he provides a proportion in the generation of bone and says that bones are white because in them there is some earth, which has blackness and paleness, [that is] an eighth part, and some fire, which has whiteness, [that is] four parts. Next he said: **For it is useless for the elements to be in the soul**, etc. That is, for it is useless for the soul's knowledge of the forms and beings of things that [the soul] be composed from the elements unless, in addition to its being composed from the elements, the proportions and compositions which belong to the beings of things were in [the soul]. For then it would be possible for it to know any given thing. Next he said: **and it will not know bone** nor **a human being** unless **these two** are **in it.** That is, since it knows the thing through a likeness, it must not know bone or human being unless there is a composition of bone and human being in it. Next he said: **That account does not** {105} **require**, etc. That is, that account is utterly impossible, for no one is uncertain whether or not the stone is in the soul.[274] It is universally the case that no one understands that living and non-living are in the soul in such a way that it knows living by the living part which is in it and non-living by the non-living part [in it].

78. **If being is said in many ways (for it designates a determinate particular,[275] quantity, quality, and the other categories), then is the soul composed of all of these? But it is not thought that all things have elements. Is it only from the elements of substance alone? But if that is so, how does it know any one of the others? Or might they say that any of the genera has its own elements and principles from which it is constituted? The soul will, therefore, be a quality, and a quantity, and a substance. But it is impossible for a substance to be composed of the elements of quantity and not be a quantity. Therefore, these and other similar things follow for those who say that it is composed of all things.** (410a13–22)

274. Cf. *De Anima* 3.8, 431b28, and Text and Comment 38 {503–504}.

275. *Hoc*: τὸ ... τόδε τι. Aristotle, *De Anima* (1984), has the literal "a 'this,'" to which the translators add, "or substance." آنية الـشيء وجوهره (ibid. [1954]); "the being and the substance of the thing." The *Middle Commentary* uses جوهرا, "substance." *Middle Commentary* (2002), 36.18.

After he had explained the impossibility which follows for them due to the knowledge of the forms of things, since the forms are neither an element nor composed from elements, he began to explain that other impossibilities follow for them, even if we concede that it knows composite things owing to its principles, that is, because it is composed of their principles.

He said: Also **if being is**, etc. That is, also, how can they say that the soul knows things owing to its own principles? For being sometimes designates a determinate particular and sometimes the other nine categories. {106} Thus we should ask whether the soul knows any of those genera because it is composed of all their principles, if they all have principles, or [because it is] composed of principles of some, if they do not all have the principles. Next he said: **But it is not thought**, etc. That is, but if they assert it to be composed of principles of some, we should ask of them whether the soul is composed of the principles of substance alone, since of all of them this category alone may be thought to have principles. It will be said to them: How does it know any of the other categories?

Next he said: **Or might they say that any of the genera**, etc. That is, or they will be forced to the first division. This is that any of the ten categories has its own principles and that the soul knows them only because they are composed of its principles. Therefore, from this position another impossibility follows for them. This is that one part of the soul is substance and another part quality and another part quantity, since it is impossible for the substance to be an element of the other categories, for the principles of non-substances are not substances. Next he said: **Therefore, these and other similar things follow for those who say that it is composed of all things**, etc. That is, therefore, these impossibilities and other similar ones follow for those saying that the soul is composed of all the principles of things.

79. **It is also unacceptable to say that like is not affected by like and that like senses its like and that like knows like, when holding the opinion that sensing is being affected and being moved, and likewise discerning and understanding. That the account which Empedocles voiced, that any of the things knows bodily elements only {107} by likeness, has many difficulties is shown from what we will say here. This is that the bodies of living things in which simple earth[276] exists, such as bone,[277] as it seems, sense nothing.**

276. *Simpla terra*. In the Greek this is ἁπλῶς γῆς, "wholly of earth" (Aristotle, *De Anima* [1984]) or "simply of earth."

277. The Greek adds νεῦρα τρίχες, "sinews, and hair" (Aristotle, *De Anima* [1984]); عقبـا أو ظفرا (ibid. [1954]); "tendon or nail." The *Middle Commentary* omits these. See *Middle Commentary* (2002), 37.8 and p. 167, n. 8.

Therefore neither do they sense things which are like, although this will be necessary [on their account]. (410a23–b2)

After he had provided the impossibilities which follow from this opinion, he began to respond to the proposition on which this opinion is based, namely, to the proposition saying that like is discerned only by its like. He said: **It is also unacceptable to say**, etc. That is, what the ancients hold is also unacceptable, [namely] that like is not affected by its like and that contrary is affected only by contrary, and they hold along with this that knowing and sensing come about through like. Nevertheless, knowing and discerning are being affected and being moved. He meant that what follows on this opinion is contrary to the first. For what they assert, that sensing and understanding come about through like and that they are being affected, compels them to say that like is affected by its like. They do not concede this because they already asserted that like is not affected by its like. This is also impossible in itself. Next he said: **That the account which Empedocles voiced**, etc. That is, that the account which Empedocles voiced (namely, that each one knows all the bodily elements only by likeness; that is, that we know earth only by the earth which is in us and water by the water [in us], and air by the air [in us], and fire by fire [in us]) is false is shown by the multitude of difficulties which follow for him in this passage. {108} For what in the bodies of living things is nearer to simple earth, such as bones, senses nothing. Since bones do not sense earth, although earth predominates in them, like does not sense like. He meant this when he said: **Therefore neither do they sense like things.** Next he said: **although this** is necessary [on their account]. That is, that if like ought to sense like, then it would be necessary for bones to sense earth. But they are seen to lack sensation.

80. **Furthermore, each of the principles would have more ignorance than knowledge. For any of them knows only one thing and does not know a great many. It follows that Empedocles attributes the greatest ignorance to God, for he alone does not know this one of the elements, namely, strife. But a mortal animal knows all these things, for every animal comes to be from all those.** (410b2–7)

Furthermore, universal impossibilities follow for them, namely, that any of the principles has more ignorance than knowledge. For, according to them, each of these principles knows only the things from which it is composed, and these are the things which they are like. Next he said: **It follows that Empedocles attributes**, etc. That is, there follows for Empedocles another particular impossibility, namely, that God, according to him, is in the utmost of ignorance such that a mortal animal has more knowledge than [God]. For it follows for him according to his account that of the elements, which are six according to him, [God] knows only five, namely, the four elements and friendship, and that he does not know strife. But a mortal animal knows six, because {109} it is composed of them all according to him. He holds the opinion that God is composed from five alone, that is, not from strife. Therefore, it follows for him that [God] does not know strife. For this reason a mortal animal will have more knowledge than [God]. The gods whom Empedocles holds to be composed from the four elements are the celestial orbs, for he holds the opinion that the celestial orbs are gods and composed of the four elements and friendship. For this reason he surmised [God] to be immortal, for strife is the cause of corruption. Yet he had already explained that he held regarding the world that it already was corrupted and already generated.[278] But perhaps he did not hold this opinion except in regard to the things which are under the orb [of the moon], although he seems to hold this opinion in regard to all parts of the world.

81. In general, why do not all things have soul, since all things either are an element or composed of one element or many or all? For they must know one or some or all things. (410b7–10)

In general they must provide the reason why not all things have a discerning soul. For it follows for them that all things are able to have comprehension, for if the principles and elements are things which know and every being either is composed of an element or [is] an element, then all things must have knowledge. For every thing must know either one of them, if it is an element or composed from one element (since then it will know only what is composed from that element), or it must know several things, if it is composed of several, or all things if of all things. He meant this when he said: **For** it is necessary to know either **one or some or all things.** {110}

82. One ought to raise questions about what gave being to those.[279] **For the elements are similar to matter; but what binds is noble in the greatest degree. Therefore, it is impossible for there to be anything more noble and**

278. That is, it has already been corrupted and regenerated and will continue in this cycle repeatedly.

279. The Greek text has ἀπορήσειε δ᾽ ἄν τις καὶ τί ποτ᾽ ἐστὶ τὸ ἑνοποιοῦν αὐτά᾽. "The problem might also be raised, What is that which unifies the elements?" Aristotle, *De Anima* (1984). The alternate Arabic translation has ما الذي يؤلف : ويجوز لسائل أن يسأل العناصر؟ (ibid. [1954]); "It is possible for someone to ask, What is it which brought the elements together?"

dominant than the soul. It is completely impossible for something to precede the intellect, for that [intellect] must be naturally prior to what acquires nobility through it. But the elements are the principles of beings.[280]
(410b10–15)

One ought to seek that in virtue of which the elements exist, namely, the
form. For the elements seem to be similar to matter. But it is obvious that
something else more noble than these binds and brings them together in the
composite. This is what is in them as form and end. Next he began to explain
that it is necessary that this be the soul, and chiefly the intellect. He said: for
what binds is called **noble in the greatest degree**, etc. That is, what is seen to
be more noble than the elements must be the soul. For everything which is
called more noble than something is less worthy than the soul in nobility. The
soul, therefore, precedes all the elements in causality and nobility, but the elements [are prior] in time. Next he said: **It is** [even] more **impossible for something to precede the intellect.** That is, if the soul were composed of the elements, then the elements would precede it in nobility and causality, which is
impossible. It is [even] more impossible to hold the opinion that one of the elements precedes the intellect in nobility and as final cause. Next he gave the
reason for this. He said: **for it must be,** etc. That is, {111} for the intellect must
precede in being all things attributed to it and which acquire nobility from it,
such as the elements. Next he said: **But the elements are the principles of beings.** That is, they differ greatly, for souls and intellects are the principles of
beings in reference to end and form, but the elements [are the principles] in
reference to matter.

83. **All those who make the soul out of the elements on the basis of
knowledge and sensation and on the basis of motion do not speak of every
soul. For we do not see all things capable of sensation to move, since some
animals[281] seem to be permanently in the same place, although it seems that
the soul moves animals by that motion alone.[282] Also of a similar sort is the
situation of those asserting that the intellect and the power of sensation are**

280. The Text (as well as the alternate translation; see Aristotle, *De Anima* [1954], 25)
has dropped the Greek φασι, "their statement," in "But it is impossible that there should
be something superior to, and dominant over, the soul (and *a fortiori* over thought); it
is reasonable to hold that thought is by nature most primordial and dominant, while
their statement is that it is the elements which are first of all that is." Ibid. (1984).

281. *Animalia*: τῶν ζῴων, "animals." Aristotle, *De Anima* (1984). The parallel passage
in the *Middle Commentary* has الحيوان, "animals." *Middle Commentary* (2002), 38.16.

282. The *Middle Commentary* seems to quote these initial lines of this Text almost
verbatim. See *Middle Commentary* (2002), 38.12–17.

from the elements. For plants seem to live but have no part of local motion.[283] And many animals are not able to understand.[284] (410b16–24)

All those asserting that the substance of the soul is composed from the elements because it knows and because it is self-moved speak about the substance of the soul only in reference to certain souls, not universally as one who wishes to speak of it in reference to its nature ought to. He began to explain this. He said: **For we do not see all things capable of sensation** to be moved. That is, the definition of those who defined it through motion is inadequate.[285] For many things which are capable of sensation and alive do not move in place, such as the sea sponge, although on their view that motion is characteristic of soul. If it were so, then every thing which is alive would move in place. Therefore, those who think that that motion {112} is characteristic of the soul capable of sensation are in error. When he had explained the inadequacy which follows for those defining the soul on the basis of motion, he began to explain the inadequacy which occurs for those asserting it to be composed of the elements on the basis of knowledge. He said: Also **of a similar sort is the situation of those asserting that the intellect**, etc. That is, it is likewise so for those who assert that the intellect and the substance of the soul are composed of the elements because it knows. For plants seem to have life, but neither sensation nor motion in place. We see that many animals capable of sensation are not able to understand. If that were so, every living thing would be capable of sensation, and everything capable of sensation would be able to understand, as several of the ancients held. But it is not so. Therefore, all those who define the substance of the soul on the basis of knowledge or motion do not advance in a way which leads to the knowledge of the substance of the soul.

84. **If one will have conceded this and asserted that the intellect is a part of the soul, and likewise also the power of sensation, nevertheless with this [those doing so] have spoken neither universally about every soul nor about one soul taken as a whole. It occurs in a similar way for the account which is said to have been found in the verses attributed to Archoiz.[286] For he says that the soul enters inside from the universe in respiration, because the**

283. The Greek has [φορᾶς οὐδ] αἰσθήσεως, "or perception" (Aristotle, *De Anima* [1984]); ولا حس (ibid. [1954]).

284. *Non intelligunt*: διάνοιαν οὐκ ἔχειν, "are without discourse of reason" (Aristotle, *De Anima* [1984]); ليس له فكرة (ibid. [1954]); "do not have cogitation." The *Middle Commentary* follows the Text closely but has ليس له تمييز, "do not have a discriminating capability." *Middle Commentary* (2002), 38.23.

285. *Est diminuta*. That is, the definition is insufficiently broad, too limited in scope.

286. In the Greek this is Orpheus.

winds carry it. This, then, does not occur in plants nor in certain animals, since not every animal has respiration. (410b24–411a1)

If one will have conceded to them that every animal is able to understand and will have asserted that the power of intellect and sensation is the same, nevertheless with this also they have not spoken about every soul. {113} For one who has spoken about it on the basis of knowledge does not speak of the soul which does not have knowledge, while [one who has spoken of it] on the basis of motion does not speak of the soul which does not move. Thus, the account of both does not concern the same soul. For the nature of the soul which is moved is different from the nature of one which knows. Therefore they do not speak of soul as universal, and thus some of them speak concerning one sort of soul and others concerning another sort. Next he said: **It occurs in a similar way**, etc. That is, this same thing happens for Archoiz, namely, that he speaks of a particular soul and thinks he is speaking of universal soul, imagining that the nature of the soul is what enters the body from the surrounding universe in respiration. For he does not speak of every soul because plants have soul and yet do not have respiration, and likewise for several animals. For what has respiration is an animal which walks and has blood, as was said in *Parts of Animals*.[287]

85. **Those who think this, namely, those asserting that the soul is composed from the elements, did not know that there is no necessity requiring them to assert that it is from them all. For one of the contraries is sufficient for judging it and its opposite. For it is by the straight that we know the straight and the curved, for the [straight-edged] ruler judges each by its straightness. But by the curved we know neither it in itself nor the straight.** (411a1–7)

They do not know that they do not need to assert that the soul is composed from all the contraries existing in the elements. For it sufficed for them to assert that it is from one of two contraries, namely, from that which has, as it were, the disposition and form. {114} For such a contrary is sufficient for judging itself and its opposite. For we know the straight line by the straight ruler insofar as it is straight, and likewise the curved. But by the curved we know neither it nor the straight. The reason for this is that we ought to judge only through a contrary which is primary over the contrary which is secondary.

86. **Some said that the soul is in the universe. And perhaps from this passage Melissus[288] thought that all things are full of god. But in this passage**

---

287. *Parts of Animals* 2.16, 659a4–5.
288. In the Greek this is Thales.

there is a difficulty. For one should ask, since the soul exists in air and fire, why it does not make animals [there] while it does do this in what is mixed, although it was thought that the soul which is in those [elements] is more noble. One ought to respond [to the question of] why the soul which is in the air is better than the soul which is in animals and [why it is] more immortal.[289] (411a7–13)

He means, as it seems to me, that some said that the soul exists in the universe, that is, in the elements and the composites. From this Melissus thought that all things are full of god. Next he said: **For one should ask,** etc. That is, the first of the difficulties following upon this opinion is why the soul, inasmuch as it is in air and in fire, does not make animals in them, that is, why these simple bodies cannot have sensation and comprehension. For since the soul has the same proportion to the elements and to the composite, it is necessary, if one of them is alive, that the other also be alive. Next he said: although **it was thought that the soul which is,** etc. That is, although it was thought that the soul which is {115} in the elements is more fit for making the elements alive. For it was thought to be more noble than the soul which is in what is mixed from the elements. Next he provided a second question. He said: **One can respond [to the question of] why the soul which is in the air,** etc. That is, it follows for someone holding this opinion to respond to one asking why the soul which is in the elements is more noble than the soul which is in animals. For the soul which is in the elements is not mortal according to them and the one which is in animals is mortal.

87. **Each account happens to be unacceptable and irrational. For to say that fire and air are animals is like [giving] a foolish account. But also not to say that these are animals and [yet] to say that they have souls is unacceptable.** (411a13–16)

After he had explained that it follows for those saying that soul is in the elements that the elements are alive, he said: **Each account happens to be,** etc. That is, [it happens] on this assertion of theirs that the elements are alive or on this assertion of theirs that the elements have soul and are not alive. For to say that fire and air are alive is like an account given by fools. To say also that they have soul and are not alive is completely unacceptable, because there will be no difference between the soul existing in what is alive or [in what is] not [alive].

88. **They seem to think that the soul exists in those things because the form of the whole of these is the same as the form of parts. Therefore, they**

---

289. *Magis immortalis*: ἀθανατωτέρα.

must say that the form of the soul is also the same as the form of its parts, since {116} the animal has soul only because there is something from the surrounding air contained in it. If, then, air, when separated, has a similar form and soul when separated does not have similar parts, it is obvious that part of it will be a being and part non-being.[290] Then either it must have similar parts or it must not exist in any given part of the whole. It is obvious both that knowing does not exist in the soul because it is composed from the elements and that it is not rightly said to be moved. (411a16–26)

After he had enumerated the impossibilities which follow upon this opinion, he provided the reason why they thought that the elements are alive and he refuted it. He said: **They seem to think**, etc. That is, they seem to hold that soul is in the elements because the whole and the part in what receives the soul have one judgment [made about them]. Next he said: **Therefore they must say that**, etc. That is, but since they assert that the whole and the part in what receives the soul have the same judgment [made about them], they must assert that the nature of the universal soul and its form is just as the form of the parts, namely, that the judgment concerning its nature in regard to the universal and [that] in regard to the particular are the same. After he had explained this, he gave the reason why they held the opinion that a part of the elements is alive and that on account of this the whole ought to be alive. He said: **since the animal has soul**, etc. That is, they held the opinion that a part of the elements is alive because they saw that the animal becomes alive only when {117} some of the surrounding air enters the body in respiration. For this reason they held the opinion that that part of air which is in the body of animals is alive. Because the nature of the part is such as this, the nature of the whole must be such as this. The order of words ought to be this: They seem to think that the soul exists in those, that is, in the elements, because the form of the whole and of the part are the same. But the part is alive because the animal becomes alive only through air which is contained in it. For this reason

---

290. *Si igitur aer, cum separatur, est consimilis forme, et anima, cum separatur, non est consimilium partium, manifestum est quod aliquid eius erit ens et aliquid non ens.* Here the Text is ambiguous and confused. *Forme* is added to the Text here and not found in the Greek. As for the rest of the sentence, the Greek has τὸ μέν τι αὐτῆς ὑπάρξει δῆλον ὅτι, τὸ δ'οὐχ ὑπάρξει. "Clearly while some part of [soul] will exist [in the inbreathed air], some other part will not." Aristotle, *De Anima* (1984). I bracket "soul" here since it is supplied by the translators. Averroes' alternate translation reflects the Greek more precisely: فهو بَيّنٌ أن بعضها موجود وبعضها غير موجود (ibid. [1954]). The Latin appears to be a rendering of an Arabic text much like this one, although some of the sense of the argument seems to be lost. Averroes' Comment does not reflect this problem.

they must say that the form of universal soul is like the form of the particular, that the nature of the universal soul which is in the elements and [that] of the particular which is in animals is the same. After he had explained this, he began to explain the way in which this follows for them. He said: **If, then, air when separated**, etc. That is, then, when air is divided, it has a similar form, because the nature of the part and the whole is the same; and when the soul which is in the elements is divided by the division of the elements, it does not have similar parts (since what exists of it in the part, namely, in the animals, is mortal and what exists of it in the whole is immortal[291]). If that is the case, then it is obvious that the part of it which exists in the whole is different from [the part] which exists in the part. Therefore, either the soul which is in the whole must be similar to the soul which is in the part, if we assert that the whole and the part have the same judgment [made about them] in regard to the receiving of the soul, or we must assert that the judgment about the whole and about the part in receiving the soul is not the same. This is what follows from their position, that the soul which is in the whole is more noble than the one which {118} is in the part. After this was put forth, their argument is refuted inasmuch as the soul existing in the whole [is] the one which exists in the part. For since the nature of the soul is of different sorts, the nature of the recipient will be different. Hence it must be, as was said, that not any given part of it receives a mortal soul but rather appropriate parts. Therefore, the judgment about the whole and the part is not the same. You ought to know that this follows necessarily for those who say that the elements are not alive and that what is from these in animals is alive. It follows for them to provide the reason why it was so, just as this follows for those who say that the elements are alive but in virtue of a soul more noble than the soul existing in animals. But the reason given by those saying that the elements are not alive cannot be given by those who say that they are alive, namely, the mixture and the compound. For this reason, we have seen that for those who assert that the first perfections of the soul are made from a mixture and compound, not from an external cause, it follows that the elements are alive through a soul equal to the soul existing in animals. Alexander seems to hold this opinion concerning the first perfections of the soul, and this is contrary to Aristotle and truth itself.[292] In this regard first and final perfections do not differ at all. For this reason we see that that opinion is similar to the opinion

---

291. Cf. Themistius, *De Anima Paraphrase* (1899), 36.17–20; (1973), 36.11–14; (1996), 53.

292. Alexander argues at length that the soul is the material form of the body and that its characterization as the first perfection of the body is consequent upon the mixture and proportion of material elements in the body. See Alexander, *De Anima* (1887), 8.25ff.; (1979), 10ff.

of those who say that chance exists and deny the efficient cause. Next he gave a summary as a reminder of what he said above. He said: **It is obvious both that,** etc. That is, it is obvious, therefore, from what we said that it is not necessary for [the soul] to be composed from the elements on the basis of {119} the fact that it knows and has sensation, nor also is it true to say that it moves itself.

89. **Because the soul has the ability to know, to have sensation, to form opinions and also to have appetite, to will,**[293] **and generally [to have] the [various] kinds of desires, and also an animal has motion in place through the soul and also growth, maturity, and diminution, does each of those belong to the whole soul? Does it understand, have sensation, move and cause and undergo other motions and actions through the whole of itself? Or is it the case that it does or suffers different actions and affections only through different parts? Is life in one of those [parts] or [is life itself] in more than one or in all, or do they have a different cause?** (411a26–b5)

After he had responded to the accounts of the ancients concerning the soul, here he began to explain that first one should consider the soul with respect to the number of its actions which are different in genus; then next whether all arise from one power, namely, from the soul, or [whether] each of its actions differing in genus comes from powers different either in definition and subject or in definition alone. He said: **Because the soul,** etc. That is, because the soul has five actions or affections different in genus, one of which is to know and to form opinions, a second to have sensation, a third to desire and will, a fourth to move in place, a fifth to be increased and decreased and to take nutrition, do any of those actions which differ {120} in genus belong to the whole soul in such a way that by the same nature it understands, has sensation, is moved in place, desires, takes nutrition, and generally acts and is affected by each of the different motions? Or does it act or is it affected by each of them only in virtue of different powers and different bodily parts and common bodily parts belonging to them? This, then, is the opinion of Aristotle. For he does not hold the opinion that it does different actions by different powers and single bodily parts only, nor by single powers and different bodily parts only, nor even by different powers and different bodily parts only. Rather, he holds the opinion that it acts by different powers and single bodily parts, namely, principal ones, and different bodily parts. He meant this when he said: through different powers and **different bodily parts,** that is, with the

293. *Velle.* In the Greek this is βούλεσθαι, "wishing." Aristotle, *De Anima* (1984). In the alternate translation this is الإرادة, "will" (ibid. [1954]), as it is in the *Middle Commentary* (2002), 40.20.

fact that it acts with fitting bodily parts, for if this is not understood in this way, it will be the same as the account of Plato.[294] Next he said: **Is life in** one of those, etc. That is, we should investigate, besides this, whether what is called life is in one of these five powers or in more than one or in all.

90. **Some say that the soul is divisible and that it understands in virtue of one [part] and desires through another. What then holds the soul together if it is naturally divisible? For this is not a body, since one should think that the case is the contrary, namely, that the soul holds the body together. This is shown because, when [the soul] leaves [the body], [the body] will decay.** (411b5–9) {121}

He refers to Plato, who holds the opinion that the soul is essentially divided in the body according to the division of the bodily parts in which it carries out its different actions and that it does not have some bodily part in common, so that [on his view] the understanding part is in the brain alone, the desiring part is in the heart alone, and the part that takes nutrition is in the liver.[295] He said: **Some say**, etc. That is, some say that the soul is essentially divided by the division of the parts of the body in such a way that it understands by a bodily part and a power different from the bodily part and from a power by which it desires. Next he said: **What then holds the soul together**, etc. That is, if we assert that the soul is divided essentially by the division of the bodily parts in which it exists, and it is self-evident that the soul which is in single individuals is unitary for [each of] us, what then unites the parts of the soul in such a way that it can be said to be one? For no one can say that this is the body, since it is more correct to say that the body is one because the soul is one, not the contrary. He meant this when he said: for **one should think that the case is** the contrary, etc. That is, for the opinion which we naturally have concerning this is contrary to this opinion, namely, that it is more fitting for the soul to be the cause of the uniting of the body and of its unity in number than that the body be the cause of the uniting of the soul. For everything which is is not one and continuous through its matter, but rather through its form. But because that argument is, as it were, implicit in this passage, he gave a clear explanation. He said: **This is shown because when [the soul] leaves [the body], [the body] will decay,** that is, it will be divided. {122}

91. **If then there is something else which makes it to be one, that is un-doubtedly the soul. But one should ask concerning that whether it is one or**

---

294. Hicks (Aristotle, *De Anima* [1965]), 300, cites the *Republic*, 434–441, 442C, and 444B, and the *Timaeus*, 69Cff. Averroes has his eyes on the commentary of Themistius. Cf. Themistius, *De Anima Paraphrase* (1899), 37.2–23; (1973), 37.14–39.5; (1996), 54.

295. Cf. Themistius, *De Anima Paraphrase* (1899), 37.2–6; (1973), 37.14–38.2; (1996), 54.

has several parts. If then it is one . . . and divisible,²⁹⁶ then one should ask what is that which unites it. Its principles will be infinite.²⁹⁷ (411b9–14)

If, then, the body does not make [the soul] one and continuous, and someone says that there is something else which makes it one, we will say that that is the soul, and the investigation will begin again, namely, whether that in itself is one or many. If one, this is what we want. If many, the question will begin again, what unites that by which the soul is united? And so forth into infinity, and there will be no principle of first continuity there. He meant this when he said: **the principles** of that **will be infinite**. That is, the principles of continuity and unity existing in a human being will be infinite. Hence, there will be no unity.

92. **One ought to raise questions concerning its parts and to ask which power provides body for any given one of these.²⁹⁸ For if the whole soul unites the whole body, each one of the parts will have to bind together each one of the parts of the body. But that account is like an impossible one. For it is difficult even to imagine saying what part the intellect unifies and how.** (411b14–19) {123}

296. The Text suffers from an omission here. The Greek has εἰ μὲν γὰρ ἕν, διὰ τί οὐκ εὐθέως καὶ ἡ ψυχὴ ἕν, εἰ δὲ μεριστόν . . . "If it is one, why not at once admit that *the soul* is one? If it has parts, . . ." (Aristotle, *De Anima* [1984]; emphasis by Smith and Barnes). Averroes' alternate translation does not suffer from omission: ، فإن كان واحداً مفرداً (ibid. [1954]). In his Comment, وإن كان ذا أقسام ، فلأية علة لم تجعل النفس واحدة مفردة؟ however, Averroes shows no awareness of the omission. In fact, his paraphrase of the Text in question, "If one, this is what we want," would seem to indicate that there was no omission in the Text which he had before himself. The omission then seems perhaps to have been either in the Arabic manuscript which the Latin translator used or early in the Latin transmission of the Text. The *Middle Commentary* seems to indicate that Averroes knew the full text of Aristotle: فإن كان هاهنا شيء ما غير البدن يصير البدن واحدا ، فذاك الشيء هو النفس ضرورة "If, then, there is one thing here besides the body which renders it one, it is the soul, necessarily." *Middle Commentary* (2002), 41.12–14.

297. *Et erunt principia eius infinita*: καὶ οὕτω δὴ πρόεισιν ἐπὶ τὸ ἄπειρον; "and so *ad infinitum*" (Aristotle, *De Anima* [1984]); ثم تذهب العقول على هذا المجرى إلى ما لا غاية له (ibid. [1954]). The alternate translation is more faithful to the Greek.

298. *Que virtus dat cuilibet earum corpus*: τίν᾽ ἔχει δύναμιν ἕκαστον ἐν τῷ σώματι; "What is the separate rôle of each in relation to the body?" (Aristotle, *De Anima* [1984]), or: "What function does each have in the body?" أية قوة لكل واحدة من هذه التي ذكرنا في الجرم؟ (ibid. [1954]). Averroes' *Middle Commentary* (2002) offers no assistance on this precise point. His Comment below has nothing to contribute to a definitive answer as to whether the corruption was in his Arabic Text or in the Latin translator's manuscript or was a result of a problem in the Latin tradition of the translation. The Text as it stands is clearly corrupt.

After he had explained that it follows for those who say the soul is divisible in all ways that it is one insofar as it is soul and divisible insofar as it has different actions, he provided a difficulty about this. He said: **One ought to raise questions about its parts**, since it was thought that [the soul] has parts in this way, namely, so that it is divisible in one way and unitary in another way, and to ask what power gives continuity to each of those parts of the body. For if the whole soul unites with the whole body, insofar as it is in it as a whole, so that each of its parts is in each part of the body, it will have to unite with that insofar as it is in it. Next he said: **But that account is like an impossible one**, etc. That is, to assert that any given part of it unites with each part of the body and exists in it seems almost impossible. For it seems impossible for the intellect to be attributed to some part of the body. You ought to know that that difficulty follows here only because it is not determined whether it is unitary in subject and many in powers (such that the division of the soul into its parts is like that of a fruit into odor, color, and taste) or is one on account of one common nature and many because that nature has different powers (in such a way that the division of the soul into its parts is like the division of the genus into species). For in this way the difficulty mentioned above follows. For when we assert [the soul] to be unitary in subject alone, this does not follow. For the subject of its parts will be one alone and some of them will be a subject for others. {124}

93. **We see that plants also live when divided, and likewise some worms, as if the soul in them is one in form even if it is not one in number. For we see that each part has sensation and moves in place for a while.** (411b19–22)

After he had provided the impossibility which follows for the account that the whole soul is in the whole body and the parts in the parts (he had already given the impossibility also following for the account that the soul is divided by the division of the bodily parts, without the fact that there is in [the soul] a universal power uniting with the body), here he began to respond to these two opinions. He said: **We see that plants**, etc. That is, what indicates that the parts of the soul do not exist in the parts of the body is that we see plants and several [kinds of] animals, such as worms, [are such that] when they are divided, each part causes motion and sensation in animals, and growth and nutrition in plants, as [if the part has become] a whole. If a part of the sense were in part of the body other than that in which motion exists, then, when the living worm was divided, it would move or have sensation by that part, but its part which moves would be different from that which has sensation. Likewise, if the nutritive part in plants were in a part different from the part responsible for growth, then it would be impossible, when many plants are divided, for them to live, and when they are planted, for them to live. Next he said: **as if the soul in them is one in form [. . .] not [. . .] in number.** For, if it were one in number, it would follow that it would be corrupted in the division of the body, as happens for many animals and some plants. But if the parts of the soul were in the parts of the body, {125} when the body is divided into those parts, it would follow that any of them would perform its specific action such that the part causing motion would be different from the part able to have sensation, and the nutritive from the part responsible for growth. Since this is so, as he said, the soul in the whole animal must be one in subject and many in powers such that one of the parts is the subject for others, such that the nutritive is the subject for the sensible power of touch and the power of touch is subject for the other senses, and likewise some for others, as will be explained later.[299] Since the soul is such as this in every animal, either it is one in number, namely in animals having organs a part of which does not live after division, or in them it must be, as it were, one in species, namely, in these which are such that their part lives after division. They are those whose bodily parts are similar to one another.

94. It is not unthinkable that they continue in existence,[300] for they have no organs by which they might conserve their nature. But, nevertheless, this does not mean that in each of the parts all the parts[301] of the soul exist,[302] and they are similar in species to one another. However, it is of the whole soul, because it is divisible.[303] (411b22–27)

299. Book 2, Text and Comment 17 {155–156}.

300. The Greek has "That this does not last is not surprising, for they no longer (οὐκ) possess the organs necessary for self-maintenance." Aristotle, *De Anima* (1984). Averroes' Comment seems to indicate that he read the Text without the negation and nevertheless made sense of it by changing Aristotle's intention and meaning. His alternate translation did not omit it: ولكن إن لـم يكن ذلك منها دائماً ، فليس تبطل الحجة من أجل أنه ليس لها آلة حافظة طباعها (ibid. [1954]). The *Middle Commentary* is in accord with the Greek and the alternate translation. See *Middle Commentary* (2002), 42.3ff.

301. I read *partes* with Latin manuscript C in lieu of *res*.

302. Crawford adds *non* to the Text although it is missing from all of his manuscripts. I read the Text without this negation. The corresponding Greek has ἀλλ' οὐδὲν ἧττον ἐν ἑκατέρῳ τῶν μορίων ἅπαντ' ἐνυπάρχει τὰ μόρια τῆς ψυχῆς; "But, all the same, in each of the parts there are present all the parts of the soul" (Aristotle, *De Anima* [1984]); ولا يمنع ذلك من أن تكون جميع أجزاء النفس في كل واحد من أقسام ذلك الحيوان التي جزئت (ibid. [1954]). There is no evidence to indicate that the negation was in Averroes' primary Arabic Text. Averroes' Comment also indicates that he read the Text without the negation.

303. The Text is here translated as it stands in Latin, although it has several omissions and related difficulties. The Greek has καὶ ὁμοειδῆ ἐστιν ἀλλήλοις καὶ τῇ ὅλῃ, ἀλλήλων μὲν ὡς οὐ χωριστὰ ὄντα, τῆς δ' ὅλης ψυχῆς ὡς οὐ διαιρετῆς οὔσης; "and the souls so present are homogeneous with one another and the whole—the several parts of the soul being inseparable from one another, although the whole soul is divisible." Aristotle, *De Anima*

It is not unthinkable that the parts of those animals and plants may continue to carry out the actions of the whole. For the reason for this is that that kind of animal does not have different organs which are responsible for different actions of the soul with a common bodily part assigned with a distinct function in which all the actions of the soul exist in potency, as is the heart with the other bodily parts, as was explained in the Book {126} *Parts of Animals*.[304] But any given bodily part among the bodily parts of that animal is suited for all the actions of that soul, and likewise any given part of the parts of one bodily part. The reason for this ought to be understood in this way: since the definition of the part of the bodily part assigned with a distinct function is not the definition of the whole, since it is impossible for the soul to exist in any animal proper to that soul unless it has the principle, its part must not be suited for what has the whole for receiving the soul. For instance, if the heart has the nature for receiving the soul because it has such a shape, it is evident that its part does not receive the soul because it does not have that shape. Hence it is necessary for animals of which the bodily parts are similar to have the contrary judgment, namely, that what the whole receives the part receives, since they have the same definition. Next he said: **But, nevertheless, this does not mean,** etc. That is, but because that kind of animal neither has a body assigned with its own distinct functions nor has bodily parts assigned with their own distinct

---

(1984). (οὐ, "not," is omitted before διαιρετῆς, "divisible.") Averroes' alternate translation, which he may have consulted in preparing his Comment, has ولكن إن لم يكن ذلك منها دائماً ، فليس تبطل الحجة من أجل أنه ليس لها آلة حافظة طباعها، ولا يمنع ذلك من أن تكون جميع أجزاء النفس في كل واحد من أقسام ذلك الحيوان التي جزئت. والأجزاء مساوية بعضها بعضا في الصورة ومساوية لكلتيها، وإنها مساويات بعضها من أجل أنها ليست مباينة ولا مفارقة، ومساواتها لكلية النفس من أجل أنها ذات أقسام (ibid. [1954]); "However, if this among them does not continue [in existence], the argument is not groundless, for they do not have organs to conserve their nature. But this does not prevent all of the parts of the soul from being in every one of the divisions of that animal which is divided into parts. The parts are homogeneous with one another in form and homogeneous with the whole of [the soul] [reading لكليتيها instead of الكلتيتها]. And they are homogeneous [reading مساواة with the manuscript instead of مساويات] with one another because they are not different and they are not separate and their homogeneity with the whole of the soul is because [the soul] has divisions." In his Comment Averroes makes it clear that he understands the Text in a way quite similar to what is found in the Greek. If Averroes did make use of the alternate translation for his Comment, it is surprising that he did not mention his awareness of the difference as he regularly does elsewhere. Hence, it may be that the Arabic Text used by Averroes was not faulty but this part of the Text in the Latin translator's manuscript of the *Long Commentary* was faulty.

304. *Parts of Animals* 2.1, 647a30.

functions, it is not out of the question for the soul which is in any given part of it to be similar to the others in species and similar also to the soul which is in the whole. Rather, because its bodily parts do not have their own distinct functions, it is necessary that it be so. Next he said: **However, it is of the whole soul, because it is divisible.** That is, it is the case that the soul which is in things is similar in species because it is divided in act, and each of them carries out the action of the other. However, the similarity between the soul which is in the parts and the soul which is in the species (namely, the whole soul) is according to potency and divisibility, not according to act. For when it is divided, the whole then will not remain whole. But he dismisses this because he rejected the second of the two divisions, {127} because this particle, however, shows the division. As if he says: the similarity, however, which exists in species among the parts is because it is divided in act. But [it is] of the whole because it is divisible.

95. **It seems also that the principle existing in plants is a kind of soul, for plants and animals share in this alone. This is different from the sensitive principle and nothing has sensation without it.** (411b27–30)

After he had provided the reason in the account given earlier of the fact that the soul is not essentially divided by the division of the subject on the basis of what appears in plants—and that account has been accepted by reason only for one who concedes that plants have soul—he [now] began to explain how this is. He said: **It seems also that the principle,** etc. That is, it also seems that the principle by which plants are nourished and grow is the soul. For they are thought to share this principle with the animals with respect to life. For this reason we call dead only an animal which lacks the principle of the plant, not the principle of sensation and motion. After he had explained that animals share this principle with plants with respect to life, he began to explain what plants do not share with them and that the sharing of sensation and motion with nutrition is necessary. He said: **This is different from the sensitive principle,** etc. That is, in plants the principle which belongs to nutrition, growth, and generation is distinct from the principle of sensation. {128} But the principle of sensation is not distinct from that [in the case of animals] since every animal is nourished and grows. But you ought to know that the necessity of being able to be nourished and to grow is not like the necessity of being hot or cold or wet or dry or heavy or light, and that its being able to grow and to be nourished belongs to it insofar as it is living, and to be heavy or light is insofar as it is a natural body. For, if it is not determined in this way, it is not necessary for sharing the sensitive principle that the principle be soul.

Book 2

{129} 1. **This, then, is what we have received from the ancients concerning the soul. Now, however, we will begin in another way to determine what the soul is with a definition which is more comprehensively inclusive.** (2.1, 412a3–6)

After he had responded to the opinions of the ancients, he began now to inquire concerning [the soul's] substance. He said: **This, then, is what we have received**, etc. That is, this, then, we said in response to the opinions which we have received concerning the soul. Next he related that we must begin by knowing its substance and [that we must] contemplate this until we know a definition which is more universal and more comprehensively inclusive of all the parts of the soul. He said: **Now, however,** let us begin, etc. That is, now, however, let us begin to speak about the soul as does someone who finds nothing useful about the soul in the ancients. First we ought to find a definition which is more universal for all its parts. For universal knowledge ought to precede knowledge which is proper [to a specific kind of soul]. His account is [something which can be] understood in its own right.

2. **Let us say, then, that substance is one of the [various] genera of beings. Of substances, one kind is substance as matter, which is not a determinate particular**[1] **per se. Another is form, by which it is said** {130} **of a thing that it is a determinate particular. And there is a third, which is what is composed from both of these. Matter is that which is in potency, while form is actuality. Form exists in two ways,**[2] **one is like knowing and the other is like theoretical understanding.**[3] (412a6–11)

Since he wished to know a universal definition for all the parts of the soul, and it was, as it were, clear that it is located in the genus of substance, he began

1. That is, a determinate particular entity. See Book 1, n. 25.

2. The translator rendering the text from Greek into Arabic apparently took καὶ τοῦτο διχῶς, "and actuality is of two kinds" (Aristotle, *De Anima* [1984]), with τοῦτο to refer to form, while the Greek referent seems rather to be ἐντελέχεια, as in ibid. The alternate Arabic translation has the ambiguity of the Greek: وذلك على جهتين (ibid. [1954]); "and that is so in two ways."

3. τὸ δ ὡς τὸ θεωρεῖν; والآخر كالتفكر; (Aristotle, *De Anima* [1954]). At 412a23 τὸ θεωρεῖν corresponds to the Latin *aspicere*, "pondering," and at 412a26 τῷ θεωρεῖν corresponds to the Latin *scire*, "knowing." In the alternate Arabic translation the text at 412a23 is corrupt, while at 412a26 the Greek is rendered by التفكر (ibid.)

to distinguish in how many ways substance is said and in what way it is soul. He said that substance is one of the [various] genera of beings, that is, of the beings having priority in being, of which soul is one. For to assert that the soul is an accident is unacceptable in view of what primary natural knowledge[4] provides us. For we hold the opinion that substance is more noble than accident and that the soul is more noble than all the accidents existing here. After he had related that substance must in general be asserted as the genus of beings such as those, he began to distinguish its kinds. He said: **Of substances one kind is substance,** etc. That is, all the things of which substance is said exist in three ways, one of which is as prime matter, which per se is unformed and not something in act per se, as was said in the first book of the *Physics*.[5] The second is form, by which an individual becomes a determinate particular. Third is what comes to be from both of those. That form exists and is substance is clear, for it is [known to exist] because it is apprehended by sensation, and it is substance because it is part of the [entire] substance and, likewise, when part of this substance is destroyed, the [entire] substance is destroyed. Likewise, prime {131} matter is substance because it is one of the parts which is such that when it is destroyed, the [entire] substance is destroyed, namely, the individual. Next he began to describe substance which exists as matter and [substance] which exists as form. He said: **Matter is that which is in potency,** etc. That is, matter is substance which is potentially, while form is substance by which this substance which is form potentially is actualized. That form is found in two ways. One is insofar as it is in act, [although] nevertheless there does not arise from it an action which is naturally constituted to arise from it, just as [no action arises] from a knower who does not make use of his knowledge. The second is insofar as that action arises from it just as it is in the case of a knower when he knows. The first form is called the first actuality, while the second is called the final [actuality].

3. **Bodies are the things which are properly called substances, and chiefly natural bodies, for they are the principles of the other bodies. Among natu-**

---

4. *Prima cognitio naturalis.* It seems likely that Averroes is following Themistius, who remarks that there has already been sufficient discussion of these matters in the accounts on the principles of nature generally. Themistius, *De Anima Paraprhase* (1899), 39.5–6; (1996), 56. In the Arabic it is remarked that this is على ما لخص في مبادىء الطبيعة بأسرها (ibid. [1973], 43.1–2); "according to what has been summarized in regard to the principles of nature generally." If that is correct, he is here stating that the principles of natural philosophy or physics assumed in this science of psychology (which is a subdivision of natural philosophy) include the doctrine of substance and accident and preclude consideration of the soul as an accident.

5. *Physics* 1.7, 191a8–12.

ral bodies some have life and some do not. To speak of life is to speak of being nourished,[6] growing, and suffering diminution. Hence, every natural body which shares in life must be a substance and it is a substance insofar as it is composite. (412a11–16)

After he had shown us the number of substances, he began to explain to us which of these deserves more to have this name. He said: **Bodies [. . .] which are properly called**, etc. That is, composite bodies have {132} this name substance more properly insofar as it is more commonly used [of them] and chiefly [for] natural bodies, for they are the principles of artificial bodies. Next he said: **Hence, every natural body which shares in life must**, etc. That is, a natural body must be a substance; indeed it deserves more to have this name **substance**. Next he expounded [the meaning of] this name **life**. He said: **To speak of life is to speak of being nourished**, etc. That is, I understand by life the principle which is common to everything alive, namely, to be nourished, to grow, and to suffer diminution in an essential way. This is what is characteristic of plants. For this name, life, was said in the Greek language of everything which is nourished and grows.[7] Animal, however, is said of every body which is nourished and has sensation. In Arabic they seem to signify the same thing, yet only an animal which lacks the principle of nutrition and sensation at the same time, not just the principle of sensation and motion alone, is called dead. He said in an essential way[8] because we do find in addition to what is living something which is similar to growth and diminution and [which nevertheless] is not living.[9] After he had explained that it is necessary for every body having life to be a substance, he explained what sort of substance. He said: **and it is a substance insofar as it is composite.** That is, a living body must be a composite substance, and it is this individual.

---

6. τὴν δι᾿ αὐτοῦ τροφήν. See n. 8 below.

7. Cf. Themistius, *De Anima Paraphrase* (1899), 39.30–31; (1973), 44.13–14; (1996), 57.

8. *Essentialiter*. There is nothing in the Latin of the Text of Aristotle corresponding to this word. In the *Middle Commentary* (2002), at 43.17–18, however, Averroes says, "and I mean by 'life' that which has nutrition, growth, and diminution, and that essentially— that is, by means of an internal principle." وأعني بقولنا حياة ما له تغذ ونمو ونقص وذلك بالذات ، أى بمبدأ فيه. The corresponding Greek text has, "by life we mean self-nutrition (τὴν δι᾿ αὐτοῦ τροφήν) and growth and decay—that is, by means of an internal principle." My translation. *Essentialiter* may indicate the presence of the Greek δι᾿ αὐτοῦ as بذاته in Averroes' Text as he possessed it, while the Latin translator's Arabic manuscript may have been faulty, dropping this from the Text but retaining it in the Comment.

9. Cf. Themistius, *De Anima Paraphrase* (1899), 41.30–42.2; (1973), 49.7–50.1; (1996), 59. There natural growth in living things is contrasted with 'growth' in the side of a stone by addition.

**4. Because the living body is a body and is of a certain sort, it is impos-
sible for the soul to be a body. For a body is not one of the things which are
in a subject. Rather, {133} it is as subject and matter. Hence, the soul must be
substance insofar as it is the form of a natural body having life potentially.**
(412a16–21)

After he had explained that the living body is a substance insofar as it is a
composite of substance as matter and substance as form, he began to inquire
concerning the soul whether it is a substance which is composite, namely, a
body, or [whether it is substance] as form. For to say that the soul is matter is
unacceptable, and this is self-evident. He said: **Because the living body**, etc.
That is, the soul is not substance as composite. For a composite body having life
is not a living body insofar as it is just body, but insofar as it is a body of a certain sort. It is, then, living by something existing in a subject, not by something
not existing in a subject. But the body is substance insofar as it is a subject.
After he had provided the propositions from which it follows that the soul is
not a substance insofar as it is body but insofar as it is form, he said: **Hence,
soul must be substance insofar as it is the form of a natural body having life
potentially**, etc. That it is not a substance as body will be shown in the second
figure[10] through those two propositions mentioned earlier, namely, that the soul
is in a subject and the body is not in a subject. For that [the soul] is substance
as form is clear from the fact that it is a substance in a subject. For this is characteristic of form, namely, that it is a substance in a subject. It differs from accident, since an accident is not part of this composite substance, while form is
part of this composite substance. Moreover, it is said in an equivocal way that
form is in a subject and accident is in a subject. For the subject of an accident
{134} is a body composed of matter and form and it is something existing in act
and does not require the accident for its being. But the subject of form does not
have being in act, insofar as it is subject, except through form, and it requires
form in order to exist in act. This is chiefly the case for the first subject, which
is not altogether free of form.[11] Because of the similarity of those,[12] several of

---

10. That is, the second figure of the syllogism.

11. That is, the corporeal form. "In medieval Arabic and Jewish philosophy three
views were held concerning the nature of this corporeal form. Avicenna was of the
opinion that the corporeal form is identical with the predisposition for receiving corporeal dimensions, but not with the dimensions themselves. Algazali agreed with
Avicenna that the corporeal form is not identical with the dimensions, but he identified
it with cohesion. Averroes, disagreeing with both, maintained that the corporeal form
is identical with the indeterminate three dimensions." Arthur Hyman in Averroes' *De
Substantia Orbis* (1986), 41, n. 7. Also see Hyman (1965).

12. Namely, of substantial form and accidental form.

the theologians erred and said that the form is an accident. On the basis of this it will be explained fully that the soul is not substance as matter. For matter is substance insofar as it is a subject, while soul [is substance] insofar as it is in a subject. He said: **having life potentially,** etc. That is, the soul must be substance insofar as it is the form of a natural body having life to the extent that it is said to have that form potentially, so that it carries out the actions of life through that form.

5. That substance is actuality; it is, then, actuality of such a body. Because actuality is said in two ways, one as knowing and the other as pondering,[13] it is clear that this actuality is like knowing, since the being of the soul is present in that.[14] Wakefulness is similar to [the exercise of knowledge in] study, while sleep is similar to the disposition of a thing when it can act but is not acting. (412a21–26)

After he had explained that the soul is substance as form and [that] forms are the actualities of things having forms and [that] they are of two sorts, he began to show that actuality is in the definition of soul as a genus. He said: **That substance is actuality,** etc. That is, because substance which exists as form {135} is an actuality of the body having form—and it was already explained that the soul is form—it is necessary that soul be the actuality of such a body, that is, the actuality of a natural body having life potentially, insofar as it is made actual by the soul. After he had explained that the soul is an actuality, he explained in how many ways actuality is said. He said: **actuality** is **in two ways,** etc. That is, because actuality is in two ways, one as knowledge

13. Note that *scire* corresponds to ἐπιστήμη and *aspicere* to τὸ θεωρεῖν, which are translated respectively as "knowledge" and "reflecting" in Aristotle, *De Anima* (1984).

14. *Quoniam apud ipsum est esse anime* is a corrupt text which corresponds to the Greek ἐν γὰρ τῷ ὑπάρχειν τὴν ψυχὴν καὶ ὕπνος καὶ ἐγρήγορσίς ἐστιν, "for both sleeping and waking presuppose the existence of soul." Aristotle, *De Anima* (1984). The alternate translation has mention of sleep and waking but is also faulty in its own way and appears to omit the underlined text (omitted apparently by homeoteleuton either in the Greek tradition or on the part of the translator from Greek): αὕτη δὲ λέγεται διχῶς, ἡ μὲν ὡς ἐπιστήμη, ἡ δ᾽ ὡς τὸ θεωρεῖν. φανερὸν οὖν ὅτι ὡς ἐπιστήμη· ἐν γὰρ τῷ ὑπάρχειν τὴν ψυχὴν καὶ ὕπνος καὶ ἐγρήγορσίς ἐστιν. "Now there are two kinds of actuality corresponding to knowledge *and reflecting. It is obvious that the soul is an actuality like knowledge;* for both sleeping and waking presuppose the existence of soul." Ibid.; emphasis added. والانطلاشيا على جهتين : أحدهما كعلم بوجود ، لأن النوم واليقظة إنما يكونان بوجود النفس (ibid. [1954]); "Actuality is of two sorts, one like knowing with existence because sleep and wakefulness are only with the existence of the soul." Aristotle, *De Anima* (1954). The *Middle Commentary* (2002), at 44.10–12, may be dependent on Themistius. Averroes' quotation in the Comment below indicates the problem was in his Arabic Text.

existing in the knower when he does not use his knowledge and another as knowledge existing in a knower when he is using it. Next he began to show in which of those two ways it is said that the soul is an actuality. He said: **it is clear that this actuality is as** knowledge. That is, because it was already explained that the soul is the actuality of a natural body, and actuality is said in two ways, then it is clear that the actuality by which it is alive and by which [the body] differs from a body which is not alive is existing in it as knowledge [exists] in the knower. Next he provided the reason for this. He said: **since the being of the soul is present in that.** That is, since the soul is found in the being of that actuality in the thing which is alive, not in the being of the other actuality.[15] After he had shown that the actuality taken in the definition of soul, which is the substance of the soul, is that which is just as knowledge existing in a knower when he does not use it, he provided an example of this. He said: **Wakefulness is similar to**, etc. That is, when an animal is sleeping, the soul will then be in it as the first actuality. This is like the being of knowledge in the knower at a time at which he does not exercise it in study and not like the being of ignorance in one who does not know. For it is clear that in sleep an animal has a sensitive soul but is not using sensation, just as one who knows has knowledge but is not using {136} it. The disposition of the soul during wakefulness in animals is like the knowledge in the knower when he uses it. This is in the sensitive soul. The nutritive soul, however, is never found in animals except as a final actuality, unless someone asserts that there is some kind of animal which is not nourished at some time, namely, at a time at which it remains in stones, such as large frogs, which store nothing and remain in stones for the whole winter, and likewise for several [kinds of] snakes.[16] Accordingly, this will be common to the sensible and nutritive soul with the same intention. If not, then the actuality taken in these will be by equivocation. Whatever way it may be, when one understands there to be difference between the being of both of those, then there will be no harm in taking this in an indefinite way in this definition, since it is impossible to do otherwise. He said: and **sleep is similar to the disposition of a thing**, etc. That is, the disposition of the soul in sleep in animals is similar to the disposition of a thing at the time at which it can act but does not act. This is a description of the first actuality and from this we can understand the description of a final actuality. [This final actuality] is the disposition of a thing by which a being acts or is acted upon at the time at which it acts or is acted upon.

6. **In the same person knowledge is prior in being [to its exercise]. For this reason the soul is the first actuality of a natural body having life potentially.**

15. That is, the second actuality.
16. Averroes here refers to various species of hibernating animals.

And [this] is insofar as [the body] is something having organs. The parts of plants are also organs, but they are very simple, for example, the leaves are coverings and garments for the fruits, while the roots are similar to a mouth, for food is absorbed in those two ways. (412a26–b4) {137}

After he had explained that the soul's genus is [that of] actuality which is like knowledge existing in a knower when he is not using it, he began to relate that this actuality precedes the second actuality in being and that because of this one ought to add in the definition that the soul is the first actuality of a natural body having life potentially. He said: **In the same person knowledge,** etc. That is, in the individual the actuality which is like knowledge precedes in being the actuality which is like [the exercise of knowledge in] study. After he had related this, he began to relate that because of this we ought to state this intention in the definition, so that by this it may be distinguished from the final actuality. He said: **For this reason the soul is the first actuality,** etc. That is, for this reason it should be stated in the definition of the soul, etc. Next he said: **And [this] is insofar as [the body] is something having organs.** (Here there is a blank space in the manuscript.)[17] It is a body insofar as it is something having organs, and a body having life potentially is first and foremost a body having organs. After he had related that every living body is something having organs, which was clear in animals but not immediately evident in plants, he began to show that organs also exist in plants. He said: **The parts of plants are also organs,** etc. His account concerning this is clear. What he said concerning plants is clear, for the leaves are for plants like the hide in animals and the roots are like the mouth, since each takes in food. He meant this when he said: **for food is absorbed in those two ways,** namely, the roots and mouth and other openings which pass through to those. {138}

7. **If, then, something universal should be said in regard to every soul, we will say that it is the first actuality of a natural body having organs. For this reason we should not investigate whether the soul and the body are the same, just as we should not investigate this in regard to the wax and the shape nor the iron and the shape**[18] **nor generally in regard to the matter of anything and in regard to what has that matter. For since one and being are**

---

17. *Ita cedidit in scriptura locus albus.* Since there is no problem in the Text on which Averroes comments, this seems to be a remark on the part of the Latin translator.

18. *Neque in ferro et figura* has no corresponding Greek text. The alternate Arabic translation has كان الموم و طبعته شيئا واحدا, "the wax and its shape are one thing," where Badawi corrects the manuscript's القوم و صنعتهم apparently with الموم وطبعته to agree with the Greek. This addition in the Text of Averroes, however, may be related to the manuscript text which Badawi corrects in his edition of the alternate text. See Aristotle, *De Anima* (1954).

said in many ways, the actuality is that of which this is said in the primary intention. (412b4–9)

If, then, something universal, etc. That is, if, then, it is possible to define the soul by a universal definition, no definition is more universal than that one nor is any more appropriate for the substance of the soul. It is that the soul is the first actuality of a natural body having organs. He put forth this account in the form of a difficulty, when he said: **If, then, [. . .] it should be said**, etc., to excuse himself from the difficulty which occurs in regard to the parts of that definition. For actuality in the rational soul and in the other powers of the soul is said in an almost purely equivocal way, as will be explained later.[19] For this reason one can raise questions and say that the soul does not have a universal definition. For this reason he said: **If, then**, etc. As if he is saying: if, then, it is conceded to us that it is possible to find a universal account which includes all the parts of the soul, this will be that account. Next he said: **For this reason we should not investigate**, etc. That is, it had been explained that the soul is the first actuality of a natural body and that something which is alive has this being only from the fact that it has soul. Hence, we should not raise questions {139} as to how the soul and body, although they are two, become [one and] the same, just as we should not raise questions about this in the case of the wax and the iron with the shape existing in them, and generally in regard to the matter of anything whatsoever and a thing which exists in that matter. For, although these names, one and being, may be said in many ways, nevertheless the first actuality in all those, namely, the form, deserves more to have this name, one and being, than what is compounded of matter and form. For a compound is called one only by the unity existing in the form, for matter is not a determinate particular except through form. If matter and form were existing in act in the composite, then the composite would be said to be one only in the way in which that is said for things which are one by contact and by being bound together. Now, because matter differs from form in the composite only potentially and the composite is not a being in act except through form, then the composite is said to be one only because its form is one. By this he hinted in a way at the question which follows for those who say that the soul is a body, [the question of] how it is that what is compounded from soul and body becomes one.

8. **We already said, therefore, what the soul is universally. It is a substance in this intention, namely, insofar as this body is what it is.**[20] **For, if some tool**

---

19. See below {405} and {397}.

20 . The corresponding Greek, οὐσία γὰρ ἡ κατὰ τὸν λόγον. τοῦτο δὲ τὸ τί ἦν εἶναι τῷ τοιῳδὶ σώματι, is rendered, "It is substance in the sense which corresponds to the account of a thing. That means that it is what it is to be for a body of the character

were a natural body, such as an axe, then the sharpness of the axe[21] would be its substance and soul in this intention. For this reason, when that [sharpness] has been taken away, it {140} will not be an axe later on except equivocally. Now [the axe] will be an axe later on, for the soul is not the quiddity and intention of a body such as that, but it is of a natural body which is such that it has [in it] a principle of motion and rest. (412b10–17)

Since he had earlier said that the soul is a substance, [and then] next explained that it is form and actuality, he began here to set out the way in which one can be certain that natural forms are substances. This is necessary in this passage. He said: **We already said, therefore**, etc. That is, it was therefore explained from what we said what the soul is universally. According to what we said in this definition, the soul is substance in the intention in which we say the thing by which this natural body exists is substance, not in another way. Next he provided an example from artificial bodies and spelled out the difference between natural and artificial bodies in this. For the beings of artificial things are accidental. For this reason some thought that it was so concerning natural bodies. He said: **For, if some tool**, etc. That is, the forms and beings of natural bodies are substances. Since for if some tool were a natural body, such as an axe (that is, if we imagine it to be a natural being), then the axe's sharpness would be its substance. Next he provided the reason[22] for this. He said: Likewise when that [substance] is taken away,[23] etc. That is, it is necessary in the case of the axe, if it were a natural being, that its sharpness be its substance. For the only thing called an axe is what is compounded from {141} matter, namely, iron, and form, which is the sharpness. If the sharpness is removed and the axe were a natural body, then

---

just assigned" (Aristotle, *De Anima* [1984]); ففي الجملة قد قيل ما النفس وأنها الجوهر على ما في الحد ، والحد هو الدليل على ما هو الشيء في آنيته ، فأنه في جرم صفته كذا وكذا (ibid. [1954]); "For we already said what the soul is universally and that it is the substance according to what is in the definition. The definition is the indication of what the thing is in its being. Then <we said> that it is in a body whose nature is such and such." The *Middle Commentary* (2002), at 45.1–4, has, "This discourse has now clarified the fact that the soul is substance qua the perfection which is the form. For in that it is the soul by virtue of which the body is what it is—that is, the soul is predicated of the body as quiddity, and that which is so predicated is substance, so the soul is substance."

21. The Text here provides an interpretation of the corresponding Greek text, which merely has τὸ πελέκει εἶναι, "being an axe." Aristotle, *De Anima* (1984). This may be based on Themistius (*De Anima Paraphrase* [1899], 42.22; [1973], 51.5; [1996], 60), as Ivry indicates. See *Middle Commentary* (2002), 171, n. 11.

22. *Rationem*.

23. *Et similiter ista cum abstracta est* corresponds to the Text's **Et ideo, cum istud est abstractum** but takes the subject to be *substantia*, not *acumen* (sharpness).

the axe would not exist because the matter and form would not exist, unless it were called an axe equivocally. The substance is what is such that its removal results in the destruction of this substance for it is part of it. But part of the substance is substance. Next he said: **Now [the axe] will be an axe later on**. That is, now, however, because the axe is an artificial body, even though sharpness has been taken from it, nevertheless later on it will be called an axe because of its shape, for the shape proper to it is the same in it both with and without sharpness.[24] What he said will be evident from what I say. For it is self-evident that this name axe, whether it be natural or artificial, is said of that compound from that which is, as it were, a form in it and from that which is, as it were, matter [in it]. Furthermore, it is clear in itself that axe is said of one of the individuals possessing substance. In this way this name which is said of it insofar as it is an individual possessing substance must be said of it according to matter and form at once. Hence, each must be substance, for the parts of substance are substance. In this way, when form has been taken away, this name must be removed from it, namely, the name which indicates it insofar as it is an individual. Or might we say that this name is said of it only as matter alone, for instance, insofar as it is an iron body? Then the form will be an accident in it, and then, if the form is removed, it will be necessary for this name, which is said of it insofar as it is called an individual substance, to remain. But because the matters are removed and no being remains except equivocally when the forms of natural things are removed, {142} then, when we assert the axe to be a natural body and the sharpness which is in it as form is removed, the matter must be removed and no being must remain. When, therefore, the form is removed according to this intention, immediately this name axe is removed, which indicates it insofar as it is an individual possessing substance. For by the removal of the form the matter is removed; and when the matter and form are removed, nothing remains of these which are indicated by this name insofar as it indicates one of the individuals possessing substance, unless it be a different individual, and then it is called an axe only equivocally. Natural forms, therefore, are substances because, when they are removed, the name which indicates the being insofar as it is an individual possessing substance is removed. Likewise the definition which is according to that name [is removed], for the genus and difference of which one indicates the matter and the other the form are removed. For instance, when sensation is removed from flesh, the flesh remains only in an equivocal way, as the flesh of something dead. Because when an artificial form is removed, the matter is not removed but remains in name and definition (since when the shape

---

24. The corresponding text of the *Middle Commentary* seems to presuppose an explanation such as is found here in the *Long Commentary*. See *Middle Commentary* (2002), 45.8–10.

of the axe is removed, it remains the same iron as before in name and definition), then it is necessary and right that its name remain, namely, axe, which indicates this instrument insofar as it is an individual possessing substance, although sharpness is removed. This was because the name is said in natural things first from form and second from the compound. In artificial things, it is to the contrary, namely, because [it is] first [said] from matter and second from the compound. In artificial things, then, it indicates the individual possessing substance according to its first signification because it signifies matter. In individual natural things possessing substance it indicates it according to its first signification since {143} it signifies form. For this individual is a determinate particular only through its form, not through its matter.

For matter has no being in act in natural bodies insofar as it is matter, and being is not in act except as having form. This is quite clear in the forms of simple things, since when the form is removed, nothing remains. In artificial things nothing is a determinate particular except by its matter, not by its form. In this way the difference between natural and artificial things will be explained to you and you will understand what Aristotle says, and the difficulty which induces the belief that forms are accidents is removed. Next he said: **For the soul is not**, etc. That is, concerning the soul it is the contrary of what is the case for sharpness, for its name is removed from something alive by the removal of the soul, and [the name] remains in the axe, although the sharpness is removed. For the soul does not belong to the same sort of body as that in which the sharpness exists, namely, to a body of an artificial instrument but to a natural one.[25] He meant this when he said **such**. What he called **a principle of motion and rest** is the disposition of a natural body.

9. **One should consider what is said concerning this in regard to the members [of the body] also. For if the eye were an animal, then vision would be its soul. For that is the eye's substance, what it is according to its intention. The body of the eye is the matter of vision, which, when [vision] fails, is called an eye only in an equivocal way, just as is said regarding a stone eye.**[26]

---

25. *Anima enim non est talis corporis in quo est acuitas, scilicet corporis artificialis organici, sed naturalis.* While there are no significant variants for this entire sentence indicated by the editor, the thought would seem to require that *organici* be taken with *naturalis*, yielding a contrast between an artificial body and a natural organic body. The problem, however, is more satisfactorily resolved by reading *organi* with manuscript C in lieu of *organici*. In the *Middle Commentary* (2002), at 45.4–5, Averroes explains that the axe is "an artificial instrument," آلة من الآلات صناعية.

26. The Greek adds καὶ ὁ γεγραμμένος: "the eye of a statue or of a painted figure." Aristotle, *De Anima* (1984). The alternate translation retains the Greek as أو مصورة في الحائط (ibid. [1954]); "or painted on the surface." Note that Averroes evidences knowledge

What is said concerning the part should be taken in regard to the whole body, for the relation of part to part is just as [that] of the whole sensory power to the whole of that which is able to have sensation. (412b17–25) {144}

After he had explained that the soul is with respect to the body just as form in matter (for in natural bodies form more appropriately has this name substance than does matter) and that the individual is an individual only through form (because it is an individual only insofar as it is a being in act, and it is a being in act through its form, not through its matter), and had explained this with argument, he now wants to show this by way of example. He said: **One should consider what was said [. . .] in regard to the members [of the body].** That is, what was said in regard to the soul, that it is substance because when it is removed, the name is removed from the thing which is alive, is confirmed in the members [of the body] to which the particular powers of the sensitive soul properly belong. Next he provided the eye as an example of this. He said: **For if the eye were an animal**, etc. That is, since the relation of vision to the eye is just as the relation of the soul to the body, if we imagined the eye to be an animal, vision would necessarily be its soul. For vision, then, would be the substance of the soul with respect to what it is[27] and the eye would be the matter of that soul. Next he said: **which, when it fails**, etc. That is, [this is] because it is clear in the case of vision that when it fails, the eye does not remain [in existence] afterwards except in an equivocal way, just as the eye made of stone or fashioned on a wall, which does not have any of the intention of the eye except for the shape alone. And because vision is the substance of the eye, it is clear that the soul ought to have such a disposition with the body, namely, that, when it is removed, the name is removed from the thing which was alive and it does not remain alive except in an equivocal way. For instance, when animality is removed from some individual, the animal does not remain an animal except in an equivocal sense; hence soul is substance. Because he had already asserted first {145} that it is so for the part just as for the whole and that it is possible for us to have certainty concerning the whole by considering

---

of the correct text when he paraphrases this passage in his Comment: "just as the eye made of stone or fashioned on a wall." Cf. Themistius, *De Anima Paraphrase* (1899), 43.2; (1973), 52.8; (1996), 60–61.

27. *Secundum illud quod est*—that is, with respect to form. This passage is very close to what is found in the *Middle Commentary*: مثال ذلك أن العين لو كانت حيوانا لكان البصرنفسها وصورتها ، ولكان هذا هو جوهرها الذى به العين هى ما هى. ولكانت موضوع قوة البصر هى هيولى هذا الحيوان; "The eye, for example, were it an animal, would have sight as its soul and form, for [sight] is [the eye's] substance through which the eye is what it is. Accordingly, the subject of the faculty of sight would be the matter of this animal." *Middle Commentary* (2002), 45.14–15.

this in regard to the parts, he began to show in this passage the way in which judgment about the whole and [judgment] about the part are the same. He said: **for** the comparison **of part to part**, etc. That is, it must be for the whole just as it is for the part in regard to this intention, since the relation of some member according to its particular sensitive form in being the substance of that member is the relation of the whole of the sensory power to the whole sensitive body. What he said is clear. For the relation of vision, which is part of sensation to the eye, is just as the relation of the whole of the sensory power to the whole body. Because the relation is the same, and vision is [the eye's] substance, the soul will therefore be substance.

10. **What has the potency to live is not that from which the soul has been removed, but that which has soul. But seed and fruit are body of such a sort potentially. For just as cutting and seeing are actualities, so too is being awake. Just as vision is a power belonging to an instrument, so too is soul. The body, however, is that which is in potency. Just as the eye is vision and a member [of the body],[28] so too the animal is soul and body.** (412b25–413a3)

Because in the definition of soul he had included potency, which is said in an equivocal way, he began to explain what intention he means and to complete the explanation of that and of the first and the second intention by this same sort of explanation from which he began, namely, by way of example. He said: **What has the potency to live**, etc. That is, when we say of the body, {146} that it is what has the potency to live, we do not mean by this just what we say in regard to what does not have a positive disposition and form by which it is able to act and be acted upon (as we say that the seed and the fruit have the potency to live and that the menstrual blood has the potency to have sensation or to be moved). Rather, we say this in regard to what has in act a soul by which it acts or is acted upon, but at that [particular] time neither is acting nor is being acted upon, such as a sleeping animal. After he had shown this concerning the potency which is the first actuality, he provided the difference between that and the potency which is not the soul in its own being. He also began to show by example the difference between the first and the second actuality in things having forms. He said: And just as cutting and seeing, etc. That is, just as cutting in the axe and seeing in the eye are final actualities of those things, so too wakefulness is the final actuality of a sensitive animal. He

---

28. ἡ κόρη, "the pupil," is given in the Greek and reflected in the alternate translation: وكما أن الحدقة هي العين و البصر (Aristotle, *De Anima* [1954]). Note that while the Greek says "the pupil *plus* the power of sight constitutes the eye" (ibid. [1984]), the Arabic has "the pupil is the eye and the power of vision."

said this because it is clear that the relation of cutting to the instrument when it cuts and of vision to the eye when it sees is just as the relation of the action of the senses to the animal while awake. For wakefulness is the use of the senses. Just as that disposition is the final actuality of the eye, so too wakefulness is the final actuality of an animal. Next he said: **Just as vision is a power belonging to an instrument,** so too **is soul.** That is, just as vision, when an animal does not make use of it, is said to be a potency by which the eye sees, so too we say that the soul is the potency by which an animal lives, when the animal is not acting by those actions of the soul. Next he said: **The body, however, is that which is in potency.** That is, the body of the animal, however, is that which receives that potency or that which is said to have that power. It is called potency because {147} sometimes it acts and sometimes it does not; it is [also] called potency at the time in which it is not acting. Next he said: **Just as the eye is a member [of the body] and vision, so too the animal is soul and body.** That is, just as this name eye is said of that member which is a composite body and of the power of vision which is in it, so animal is said of soul and body. His account in this chapter is clear.

11. **It is not unapparent that neither the soul nor a part of it, if it is naturally constituted so as to be divided, is separate from the body. For it is the actuality of certain parts.**[29] **But nothing prevents it from being the case in regard to certain parts, because they are not actualities of some thing [which is] part of the body. Besides, it was not explained whether the soul is related to the body as the pilot to the ship.**[30] **This, then, is how we should reach this [definition] concerning the soul, according to example and description.**[31] (413a4–10)

After he had included in the universal definition of the soul that it is the actuality of a natural body, he began to explain how much is apparent from

29. The Greek is much clearer: "From this it is clear that the soul is inseparable from its body, or at any rate that certain parts of it are (if it has parts)—for the actuality of some of them is the actuality of the parts themselves." Aristotle, *De Anima* (1984).

30. *Gubernator.* The Greek has πλωτήρ, "sailor." Aristotle, *De Anima* (1984). Alexander has κυβερνήτης, "pilot," at Alexander, *De Anima* (1887), 20.28ff.; (1979), 29, as does Themistius, *De Anima Paraphrase* (1899), 43.29; (1996), 60–61. The Arabic version of Themistius has الربان *al-rubbân*, indicating one in control. The alternate Arabic translation has ركاب السفينة (Aristotle, *De Anima* [1954]), indicating the one in charge of the ship. The *Middle Commentary* has الملاح, "sailor." *Middle Commentary* (2002), 46.18. The *Middle Commentary* divides the Text here. See ibid., 46.21.

31. τύπῳ μὲν οὖν ταύτῃ διωρίσθω καὶ ὑπογεγράφθω περὶ ψυχῆς. "This must suffice as our sketch or outline of the nature of soul" (Aristotle, *De Anima* [1984]); ولكن يُجْعَل أن النفس على المجاز بهذه الحال بجهة التمثيل (ibid. [1954]); "However, it is maintained that the soul exists analogously in this disposition by way of example."

this definition concerning separation or non-separation [from the body]. He said: **That the soul**, etc. That is, it is evident that it is not unapparent from what was said in the definition of the soul that it is impossible for the soul to be separate from the body either according to all [its] parts or through some part of it, if it is naturally constituted to be divided. For it is apparent that certain of its powers are actualities of parts of the body insofar as natural forms are made actual through matter. But it is impossible for such a thing to be separate from that through which it is made actual. {148} Next he said: **But** nevertheless **nothing prevents**, etc. That is, but this is not clear in regard to all its parts since it is possible for someone to say that a certain part of it is not the actuality of some member of the body or to say that although it is an actuality, nevertheless some actualities can be separate, as the actuality of the ship by the pilot. Because of these two [considerations], then, it does not seem clear from this definition that separation is impossible for all of the parts of the soul. Alexander says that from this definition it is apparent that none of the parts of the soul are separate.[32] We will speak about this when we speak of the rational power.[33] Next he said: **In this way, then**, etc. That is, just so much knowledge, then, has been provided by such definitions which have been brought forth by way of example and in accord with universal accounts, as we have done here. That is, they do not make the thing known in a perfect way such that all the characteristics which follow for that thing are apparent from that [definition]. For this reason, after we have investigated each of the parts of the soul according to the definition proper to each, this intention and the rest of the intentions which should be sought concerning the soul will then be apparent.

12. **Because what is clear—which is more near in account to what should be understood—arises from things which are [in themselves] obscure but more apparent [to the senses], we should also seek to follow that course in regard to the soul. For it is necessary not only that a defining account show what the thing is,[34] but also that the cause be found and [made] clear in [the account]. Now, however, the intentions of definitions are like conclusions, for instance, squaring {149} is finding an equilateral surface consisting of right angles equal to a rectangle. This definition is the intention of the**

32. Cf. Alexander, *De Anima* (1887), 29.22–30.6; (1979), 44–45, where Alexander argues that the soul's higher powers, which are actualities of the soul, cannot exist separate from prior powers; and (1887), 20.26–21.33; (1979), 29–31, where he rejects the analogy of the soul and the pilot as an argument for the separability of the soul as actuality from the body of which it is the actuality.

33. See {393–394} and {396–397}.

34. For "what the thing is" (*quid est res*) the corresponding Greek text has τὸ ὅτι, "the mere fact." Aristotle, *De Anima* (1984). The original translation may have been

conclusion. But one who says that squaring is finding a mean in a thing has given an account of the cause. (2.2, 413a11–20)

The knowledge acquired from this definition is not sufficient for knowledge of the substance of each and every part of the soul. This definition is universal for all the parts of the soul and [is] said of them in many ways. Such definitions are not sufficient for knowledge of the thing in a perfect way when they are universal univocally, much less when they are universals [predicated] in many [differing] ways. For we should seek afterwards to know by an appropriate knowledge each and every one of the parts which are gathered under that definition, since the definition is not said of them in a univocal way. Hence, he therefore began here to show the way to knowledge of definitions which are appropriate to each of the parts of the things not known and [to show] the reason why definitions are not sufficient in regard to such things. He said: **Because what is clear—which is more near**, etc. That is, because the natural way for knowing the proximate causes for things is to go from things obscure by nature [though] apparent to us, which is to go from things which are posterior to things which are prior in being, as was said in the *Posterior Analytics*,[35] it is necessary for us to proceed in that way in knowing the definitions proper to each of the parts of the soul. There is no way to know such definitions, namely, those which are composed from proximate causes proper to the thing, since they are unknown, except from posterior things [here] with us. Next he said: **For it is necessary not only that a defining account show**, etc. That is, the reason {150} why such universal definitions are not sufficient for knowing a thing is because it is necessary that the account which defines perfectly not only show the genus of the thing, as many definitions do, but a defining account ought to show the thing's own proximate cause existing in it in act, namely, the form, not the genus. After he had made this known, he related what sort of definition is the definition which he seeks in regard to every part of the soul and of what sort of definition is the definition mentioned earlier. He said: **Now, however, the intentions of the definitions are like conclusions**. That is, that definition which we now seek is similar to definitions which are like a principle of demonstration. But the universal definition mentioned earlier is similar to definitions which are like a conclusion of a demonstration. After he had explained this, he provided an example concerning definitions

---

quod est res. The Text here also omits ὥσπερ οἱ πλεῖστοι τῶν ὅρων λέγουσιν, "as most now do." Ibid. The alternate translation has فإنه ينبغى للحد أن لا تكون فيه دلالة على آنية الشىء فقط دون أن يبين عن علته (ibid. [1954]); "For the definition requires that there not be in it an indication of the being of the thing alone without making its cause evident."

35. *Posterior Analytics* 1.2, 71b33–72a5.

which are like a conclusion, if they are not known to be in the thing defined or it is the cause sought in regard to them, and concerning definitions which are not like a conclusion of a demonstration, but are, if they are self-evident, a principle of demonstration. And if they are not known, then it is impossible for them to be explained to be in the thing defined except by an argument. He said: **For instance, squaring**, etc. That is, an example of universal definitions which are like a conclusion of a demonstration is to respond to one asking what something squared [is] that it is a surface possessing right angles and [lines of] equal lengths [and] which is equal to a rectangle. Next he provided an example of a definition which is like a principle of demonstration. He said: **But one who says that squaring**, etc. That is, but one who defines something squared as something which is a surface possessing right angles [made up of lines] of equal length, made on the line mediate in relation to the sides of the rectangle which will be made equal to it, [this person] defines something squared by a definition which is like a principle {151} of demonstration, since he defines it by a proximate cause. When he said: **Now, however, the intentions of the definitions are like conclusions**, he did not mean that this definition brought forth for the soul is a conclusion of a demonstration, but he meant that it is of the genus of those definitions, insofar as such definitions are universal. For this reason he said: **are like conclusions**. For those definitions either are conclusions or are similar to definitions which are conclusions. Moreover, he did not mean that the definition sought here in regard to each of the parts of the soul is from among the definitions which are like a principle of demonstration, such that they are self-evident, because they are not known from our viewpoint and the method for coming to know them is from things posterior, as he said. But he meant that it is of the genus of those definitions. For such definitions either are a principle of demonstration or are similar to definitions which are like a principle of demonstration. For this reason his account ought to be read in this way: **but the cause be found and [made] clear in [the account]**. That is, the account defining the soul in a perfect way ought to be such that the proximate cause is evident in [the definition]. That definition is from among the definitions which are similar to definitions which are principles of demonstration, inasmuch as it is a proper definition.[36] However, the definition which we provided now for the soul is from among the definitions which are similar to definitions which are conclusions of a demonstration, insofar as it is general for all the parts of the soul and in it the proximate cause was not brought forth.

13. **Let us, then, begin the inquiry and say that what is alive is distinguished from what is not alive by living. And, {152} because to live is said**

36. That is, the definition is specific, not generic.

in many ways, we will say that a thing lives if any one alone of these is found in it, for instance, understanding, sensation, motion and rest in place, to take nourishment and to suffer diminution, and to grow. (413a20–25)

Earlier he had made known the definition of the soul in a universal way and he had made known how much knowledge of a thing such definitions give and that they cause knowledge in a diminished way, not perfectly, since they are universal and like a conclusion of a demonstration. [He had also made it known] that the definition which should be sought in regard to each of the parts of the soul is similar to proper definitions which are like the principles of demonstration. In the case of such definitions, since they are not clearly existing in what is defined, as happens in the case of the parts of the soul, it is necessary to proceed to the knowledge of these from posterior things which are more known to us, namely, composites. He said: **Let us, then, begin the inquiry**, etc. That is, let us say, then, that because it is known to us that what is alive differs from what is not alive only by life, but living is said in many ways, that is, on the basis of many actions which are in it, it is clear that everything of which one of those intentions or one of those actions or more than one is said is alive. He meant this when he said: **if [. . .] any of these is found in it**, etc. Next he enumerated the actions ascribed to life. He said: **For instance**, to understand, to have sensation, to move itself and to rest in place, **to take nourishment and to suffer diminution, and to grow.** That is, those actions ascribed to life are of four kinds, one is to understand, the second to have sensation, the third to be self-moving and to be at rest in place, the fourth **to take nourishment**, to grow, and **to suffer diminution.** {153}

14. **For this reason all plants are thought to live, for there exists in them a potency, a power, and a principle through which they receive growth and suffer diminution in two contrary places. For they do not grow and suffer diminution[37] upward and not downward, but rather upward and downward alike. Everything which is nourished necessarily lives and lives only so long as it can take nourishment.** (413a25–31)

Because life is more implicit in the motion of nutrition and growth and diminution than in the other actions which he enumerated, he began to explain that this action is ascribed to the soul because it is impossible for it to be ascribed to the powers of the elements from which the bodies which carry out the actions of nutrition and growth are composed. He said: **For this reason all plants**, etc. That is, because the motion of nutrition and growth and diminution was enumerated by us in the actions of a thing which is alive, we hold the

37. **Et diminuuntur** has no corresponding Greek. The alternate translation accords with the Greek. See Aristotle, *De Anima* (1954).

opinion that all plants are living in which we see existing a principle by which they carry out the motion of diminution and growth in two contrary places, namely, upward and downward. For a body simple or composed is moved toward one direction. For if it is simple, it will be moved either upward or downward; if composed, it will be moved in accord with the dominant element. Because a body which can grow seems to be moved in both directions by the same principle, namely, branches and roots, this principle must be neither [a simple nor a composite body], neither heavy nor light, and such a thing is called soul. Because growth is an actuality of the action of nutrition, it was necessary that the principle {154} which carries out nutrition be of the genus of that which carries out growth. Therefore, the principle of nutrition is necessarily the soul. For this reason every animal is said to be living so long as it is nourished.

15. **It is possible for this to be separate, but it is impossible for the others to be separate from this in mortal things. This is apparent in plants, for in them there is not even one power different from this one among the powers of the soul.** (413a31–b1)

After he had enumerated the genera of the powers of the soul, he began to show the ordering of those powers to one another. He said: **It is possible for this to be separate** from other things. That is, it is possible for this principle which exists in what is alive to be separate from the other principles of the soul which we enumerated, namely, from sensation, motion, and understanding. Next he said: and **it is impossible for the others to be separate from this in mortal things.** That is, and it is impossible in things which are naturally constituted to die for this principle, the nutritive, to be separate from the other principles of the soul, that is, from sensation, motion, and understanding. He said this because heavenly bodies clearly seem to have understanding and to be self-moving, but not to take nourishment or to have sensation. For this reason he said: **in mortal things,** since it has been explained that these are not mortal. Next he said: **This is apparent in plants,** etc. That is, it is apparent that this principle which is nutrition and growth is separate from the other powers of the soul on the basis of what is sensibly seen[38] in plants. For in those there seems to be none of the powers of the soul {155} except that one. He directed the response against those imagining that plants have sleep and wakefulness.

16. **To live, then, is said of every living thing in virtue of this principle; animal, however, [is said]**[39] **in virtue of sensation. For [even] all the things**

38. I read *sensibiliter* with manuscript C.

39. The Greek πρώτως, "for the first time" (Aristotle, *De Anima* [1984]), is omitted here. The alternate translation has وأما الحيوان فإنه يقدم على غيره من الأحياء من أجل حسه ibid. [1954]); "Among living things the animal precedes the rest by its sensation."

which do not move themselves and do not change place but only have sensation are called animals, and we are not content to call them just living. (413b1–4)

He wants to show the difference between this power and the power of sensation in virtue of the terms asserted by them. He said: **To live, then**, etc. That is, when one says that something is living in this language, namely, Greek, it is said only of things which live in virtue of this principle, i.e., nutrition and growth, and [is] not [said] in virtue of another [principle]. Next he said: **animal, however,** etc. That is, this name animal, however, is said only of everything which has the principle of sensation, inasmuch as it has this principle alone, although it may not have the principle of motion in place. The sea sponge and many of the things possessing shells which have sensation and yet are not self-moving are evidence of this. They are called animals, not just living things.[40]

17. **The first sense existing in all these is touch. And just as the nutritive can be separate from touch and every sense, so too touch can be separate from the other senses. I understand by nutritive the part of the soul in which plants also share. All animals seem to have the sense of touch.** (413b4–9) {156}

The first power of sensation which is by nature prior in being to the other powers of sensation is the sense of touch. For as the power of nutrition can exist in plants separate from touch and from every [other] power of sensation, so can touch exist separate from the other senses. That is, when it is found, it is not necessary that other senses be found [with it], but when the other senses are found, [the sense of touch] is necessarily found. It is therefore by nature prior to the other senses, as nutrition is naturally prior to the sense of touch. Next he said: **All animals seem to have the sense of touch.** That is, of all the types of senses that sense is more necessary for all animals. For every animal has the sense of touch, but not the sense of sight or some other [sense], although a perfect animal [does have all the senses]. His account is clear.

18. **The reason why each of those two occurs should be said later.[41] Here, however, it should only be said that the soul is the principle of those things which we mentioned, namely, of the nutritive, sensitive, discerning, and moving [powers].** (413b9–13)

The reason why the nutritive power seems to be separate from the other powers and to precede them by nature, and likewise touch with the other

40. Cf. Themistius, *De Anima Paraphrase* (1899), 44.28–29; (1973), 56.7–9; (1996), 62.
41. *De Anima* 3.12.

powers of sensation, should be said later, namely, the final cause. He did this at the end of this book.[42] Next he said: **Here, however,** etc. That is, here it was only explained that the soul is divided into these four genera and that its substance {157} is in those principles. Later he will be investigating other things which should be sought out.

19. **Is each of those, then, a soul or a part of soul? If it is a part of soul, is it a part insofar as it is separate in intention alone or [insofar as it is separate] in place also? That some of these things are so is not difficult to know, but in regard to some others there is difficulty.** (413b13–16)

After he had explained that the powers of the soul are more than one and had asserted this position as self-evident, he said: **Is each of those, then,** etc. That is, is then each of those principles existing in an animal a soul or not; and if it is soul, is it a soul per se or [is it] a part of soul; and if it is a part of soul, is it a part and [also] something different in being and in place from the body in what is alive? [These are questions which] ought to be investigated. He means by his having said, **Is [each . . .] a soul or a part of soul?**, is it possible for one of those to be in an animal without the soul or is it impossible for it to be in an animal without something else of which it is a part? After he had related this, he began to show their different dispositions in each kind of animals. He said: **That some of these things are so is not difficult,** etc. That is, that those powers in certain animals are the same in subject and different in definition is not difficult. In regard to certain others, however, it is difficult and involves difficulty. Likewise, whether every one {158} of those principles is in the soul or not, in regard to certain [ones] is clear and in regard to certain others, obscure.

20. **For just as there is something in plants which, if divided, lives and is separated from the other parts, as the soul which is in it is the same in species in all plants[43] but potentially many, this occurs in another way for the soul of annelidan animals[44] when they are divided, for each part has sensa-**

---

42. See *De Anima* 3.12–13, 434a22ff. Cf. below {532}.

43. *In figura in omnibus vegetabilibus.* The corresponding Greek text has τῆς ἐν αὐτοῖς ψυχῆς ἐντελεχείᾳ μὲν μιᾶς ἐν ἑκάστῳ φυτῷ, "in *their* case the soul of each individual plant was actually one." Aristotle, *De Anima* (1984). The problem seems to have arisen in the translation of the Greek ἐντελεχείᾳ into Arabic. The problem is not found in the alternate translation, which accurately renders the Greek: من أجل أن النفس التي في أجزائها نفس واحدة ، بمعنى الانطلاشيا التي هي تمام لجميعها In his Comment Averroes has no difficulty with the text and understands it in accord with the original Greek, perhaps thanks to the alternate translation.

44. For example, earthworms.

tion and locomotion. **Everything having sensation has desire and imagination, for where sensation is found pleasure**[45] **is also found. And where those
are found, appetite**[46] **is necessarily found.** (413b16–24)

After he had related that it is not difficult in the case of most animals to
explain that those powers are the same in subject but many in intention, he
began to show this. He said: **For** as there is **something** belonging to plants
which, if cut, etc. That is, we see that certain plants live as parts with a life
proper to plants although divided, after [the parts] are separated from one
another, so that the soul in that plant is as it were one in form in act in that
plant and potentially many. That is, it may be divided into souls which are the
same in form as the soul existing in it. And so the same is likewise the case for
a certain kind of animal, namely, the annelid, because after they are divided,
the parts perform those actions of life which that animal used to. After he had
stated that after {159} that kind [of animal] is divided, the parts have all the
actions which the whole had, he began to relate how this is apparent in them
all. For someone might say that a part does not have any of the actions of the
whole in the case of this animal which you have mentioned, with the sole exception of sensation and motion, not the other parts of the soul, namely, imagination and desire. He said: Since **each part has**, etc. That is, we said that all
the powers of the soul in this animal are seen to be the same in subject because we perceive that after [the animal] is divided, each part has sensation
and locomotion. Everything having sensation and motion necessarily has
desire and imagination.[47] For, where sensation exists, there necessarily exist
pleasure and sorrow in the apprehension of a sensible thing. And where there
is pleasure and sorrow,[48] there will necessarily be motion toward what is
pleasurable and motion away from what causes sorrow. But the object toward
which there is motion is not actually causing delight or sorrow. Hence, [the
object] must be imagined and desired. In every part of that animal, therefore,
there exists a sensitive, desiring, and imaginative soul causing locomotion.
For when locomotion is due to pleasure and sorrow, the two powers will necessarily be there. But, nevertheless, you ought to know that in certain animals
the power of imagination is always joined with sensation except when the object of sensation is absent. Such an animal is maimed. However, in those which
are sound [imagination] is [also] found in the absence of sensible objects.

45. The Greek text has καὶ λύπη τε καὶ ἡδονή, "pleasure and pain." Aristotle, *De
Anima* (1984). The alternate translation also omits mention of "pain," which is added by
the editor from the Greek: فهناك ⟨ألم و⟩ لذة (ibid. [1954]).

46. *Appetitus*: ἐπιθυμία: شهوة. Aristotle, *De Anima* (1954).

47. Cf. 428a9–11. Also see Averroes' Comment on this passage.

48. Cf. Themistius, *De Anima Paraphrase* (1899), 45.38; (1973), 59.9; (1996), 64.

21. **Nothing, however, has yet been explained about the intellect and the theoretical power. But, nevertheless, it seems {160} that this is another kind of soul and that it alone can be separated, as the eternal is separated from the corruptible.** (413b24–27)

After he had said that for every one of those principles we should inquire whether or not it is soul, he began to explain a power which does not seem to be soul, but in its case it is more clear that it is not soul. He said: **The intellect and the theoretical power,** etc. That is, regarding the intellect in act, as well as the power which is made actual by intellect in act, it was still not explained whether or not it is soul, as was explained concerning the other principles, since this power does not seem to use a bodily instrument in its action as do the other powers of soul. For this reason it was not clear from the earlier account whether or not it is an actuality. For everything [which is such that] it is evident or will be evident in regard to it that it is made actual insofar as forms are made actual by matters is necessarily soul. After he had explained that this is obscure in the case of the intellect, he began to show, in regard to this intention under investigation, which of those two contradictory parts is more clear in the opinion of people and how it seems, [at least] until this is explained by demonstrative argument later.[49] He said: **But, nevertheless, it seems** to be **another kind of soul,** etc. That is, but, nevertheless, it is better to say, and seems more to be true after investigation, that this is another kind of soul and, if it is called a soul, it will be so equivocally. If the disposition of intellect is such as this, then it must be possible for that alone of all the powers of soul to be separated from the body and not to be corrupted by [the body's] {161} corruption, just as the eternal is separated. This will be the case since sometimes [the intellect] is not united with [the body] and sometimes it is united with it.

22. **It is clear that the other parts of the soul are not separate as some say, but that they are different in intention. For the being of something in sensation is different from its being in cogitation. For sensing is different from cogitating.[50] And [it is] likewise for each of the other [parts] mentioned earlier.** (413b27–32)

49. Averroes' position is that the theoretical intellect is an actuality of knowing as a consequence of the presentation of the potentially intelligible intentions of imagination, cogitation, and memory to the agent intellect and the subsequent reception of the actual intelligibles in the material intellect due to the activity of the agent intellect. He holds the theoretical intellect or theoretical intelligibles are perishable insofar as they are present in perishable human individuals but eternal insofar as they are present in the material intellect. See below, Book 3, {389–390, 399–402, 407}.

50. The Greek text has αἰσθητικῷ γὰρ εἶναι καὶ δοξαστικῷ ἕτερον, εἴπερ καὶ τὸ αἰσθάνεσθαι τοῦ δοξάζειν. "If opining is distinct from perceiving, to be capable of

After he had explained that it is not clear in the case of the intellect whether or not it is separate, although it is more clear [in its case] that it is separate insofar as it is not [identical with] soul, he began to spell out that the contrary is the case in regard to the other parts of the soul and that they do not seem to be separate. He said: **It is clear that the other parts of the soul**, etc. That is, it is clear from the accounts mentioned earlier concerning the definition of the soul that the other parts of the soul are not separate. For it was explained in the cases of each of them that it is the actuality of a natural body having organs. For actuality is the end and completion of what is perfected; but the end is not separate from that of which it is the end; hence, those parts of the soul must not be separate. After he had explained that for some of these powers there is difficulty as to whether or not they are separate and that for some it is clear that they are not separate, he began to show what that is which seems to exist in a clear way in all [these powers], i.e., that these four kinds[51] {162} are different in intention. He said: But nevertheless it is clear **that they are different in intention**, etc. That is, but nevertheless it is self-evident that all those powers are different in sense and intention and that the being of the power which is constituted by sensation is different from the being of the power which is constituted by contemplation since the action of any of those is different from the action of what corresponds to it [in the other]. For sensing, which is the action of the power of sensation, is different from understanding, which is the action of the power of intellect.[52] Next he said: **And [it is] likewise for each of the other [parts] mentioned earlier.** That is, and it likewise is apparent in the diversity in intention and definition belonging to the other powers mentioned earlier, because they also differ in actions.

---

opining and to be capable of perceiving must be distinct." Aristotle, *De Anima* (1984). Averroes' alternate translation differs from the Greek as well: وذلك أن بعضها حَسّاس ، و بعضها مُرَوّ ، والفرق بين هذين بَيّن ، وكذلك سائر ما قيل منها: الواحد غير الآخر (ibid. [1954]); "For some of them are sensitive and some are capable of reflection. The difference between these is evident. And likewise for the rest of what is mentioned with them: one is different from the other."

51. That is, "the nutritive, sensitive, understanding, and moving [powers]." Book 2, Text and Comment 18, 413b13 {156–157}.

52. Averroes' meaning here is that sensing and thinking are different intentional actions, as is also the case in the *Middle Commentary*, where he writes, وذلك أن معنى أن يحس الإنسان غير معنى أن يروى ، وكذلك الأمر فى مباينة سائر القوى التى عددنا بعضها لبعض. Ivry renders this as "The intention that a person senses is other than that which he thinks; and there is a similar difference in the other faculties, each of which we have enumerated." *Middle Commentary* (2002), 50.12–13. I understand part of this passage of the *Middle Commentary* somewhat differently: "The intention of a person's sensing is other than the intention of a person's reflecting."

23. Since certain animals have all those and certain have only one,[53] both that this causes difference between animals and why should be investigated later.[54] Something similar to this also happens in the case of the senses. For certain [animals] have all the senses, certain certain [of them], and certain one. And [that one] is that which is without qualification necessary, namely, touch. (413b32–414a3)

Since certain animals have those four powers, certain have certain of those powers, and certain have only one, what kinds of animals they are, the fact that this brings about difference between animals, and why these occur in animals {163} should be said later. For what happens to animals in regard to the four powers of the soul which we have enumerated similarly happens to animals in regard to the powers of sensation alone. For certain animals have the five powers of sensation, certain only [have] certain, such as the mole, and certain [only have] one, namely, touch, such as the sea sponge. His account in this chapter is clear by itself.

24. Because that by which we live and perceive is said in two ways, we also speak likewise in regard to the thing by which something is known, of which one is knowledge and the other the soul, for by each of those we say that we know. Similarly we say in regard to the thing by which one is healthy that one is health and the other is some member of the body or the whole body. Of these knowledge and health are a certain form and an intention in act for those two recipients. For one receives knowledge and the other receives health. For it is thought that the action of the agents is only in what receives the affection and disposition. And the soul is that by which we primarily live, perceive, and discern. It is, therefore, necessary that it be an intention and a form, not, as it were, matter and subject. (414a4–14)

Now he has returned to explain that the soul is substance as form, not as matter, and not as a composite of these, namely, a body. He said: **Because that by which we live and perceive**, etc.[55] That is, because it is self-evident that the

53. The Greek text adds here τισὶ δὲ τινὰ τούτων, "some certain of them only." Aristotle, *De Anima* (1984). Averroes' alternate translation is also imperfect: ينبغى أن (ibid. نعلم أنا قد نجد جميعها في بعض الحيوان ، ونجد الواجد منها في طائفة من الحيوان [1954])؛ "We must know that we may find all of them in some animals and one of them in a group of animals." Note, however, that Averroes' Comment appears to follow what we find in the Greek, perhaps because just a few lines below, at 414a3, the triple division is again stated.

54. *De Anima* 3.12–13.

55. Arabic fragments correspond to Book 2, 24.18–19: ثم قال» ان الشيء الذي به نحس ونحيا» (*Long Commentary* Fragments [1985], 38).

actions of nutrition, sensation, knowledge, and the other {164} powers of the soul are ascribed to us for two reasons, of which one is by reason of the power itself and the other by reason of having that power. For instance, sensation is ascribed to us by reason of the sensation and by reason of the very thing which has sensation, for sometimes we say that we see by reason of vision and sometimes by reason of the eye. Likewise, in regard to knowledge sometimes we say that we know by knowledge and sometimes by the soul, which is the power possessing knowledge. It is likewise for all the powers belonging to what is alive. For instance, we sometimes say that we are healthy by health and sometimes by a healthy body or by a healthy member [of the body]. After he had asserted this proposition as self-evident and by induction, he began to assert another proposition. He said: **Of these knowledge**, etc. That is, it is apparent that one of those two, which is like knowledge with respect to the soul and health with respect to the body, is form and the other is matter. For form is among these and it is an intention which is found in the two things receiving them, namely, in the one knowing knowledge and in the one receiving health. Hence, it is necessary that every action [be] ascribed to some being owing to some two things existing in it, so that one of them be matter and the other form. But he leaves out this conclusion because it appeared well [enough] on the basis of the things which he asserted. Next he said: **For it is thought that the action of the agents**, etc. That is, we said that one of the two is form and it is that which is like knowledge and health because health, knowledge, and the like are actions of an agent, namely, of something giving and bestowing health, and the action of the agent is that which exists in the recipient, and it is form. Hence it is necessary that knowledge be something existing as form and soul as matter.[56] He had explained that for every action ascribed to some being {165} owing to two things it is necessary that one of them be matter and the other form and [that] it is clear that the action is ascribed to the being in a primary way on account of form and that the actions of the soul[57] seem to be ascribed to the body and soul but first to the soul and second to the body. Now it is concluded in a clear way from this that the soul is form and the body is

56. Arabic fragments correspond to Book 2, 24.42, 46–48: وقال : «فانه يظن ان فعل الفاعل...الخ» يعني ان فعل الفاعل الذي هو الصورة للشيء فانما يوجد في القابل ‹فيجب ان يكون العلم انما يوجد في النفس› من قبل شيء يجري مجرى المادة وشيء يجري مجرى الصورة (*Long Commentary* Fragments [1985], 38). "He said: 'It seems that the act of the agent . . . etc.' He means that the act of the agent which is the form belonging to the thing exists in the recipient. ‹So it is necessary that knowledge exist in the soul only› by way of a thing which is analogous to matter and a thing which is analogous to form."

57. I read *anime* with Latin manuscripts B, D, and G and the Arabic fragment's النفس in lieu of Crawford's *animati*. For the Arabic, see the following note.

matter.[58] He said: **And the soul is that by which we [. . .] live**, etc. But he made manifest only some of those propositions and left out some because they were clear. The syllogism is composed in this way: the actions of something alive are ascribed to the body and to the soul together; every action which is ascribed to some being owing to two things must be such that one of them is matter and the other form; therefore, one of those two, namely, body and soul, is form and the other is matter. And after we have joined to this that an action is as-cribed to a being primarily owing to form and that this is convertible and we have joined [this] to its converse that the action is ascribed to what is alive through soul primarily, then it is concluded from this that the soul is form and the body matter.[59]

25. Since substance is said in three ways, as we said, namely, matter, form, and the composite of these, and of these matter is potency and form actuality and what comes to be from these is alive, then body is not the ac-tuality of soul, but rather soul is the actuality of some body. (414a14–19)

This is an explanation different from the one mentioned earlier, that soul is substance as form, not as matter. But because this explanation gives the cause and the being,[60] but the first {166} gives only the being, he brought this forth as the cause of the account mentioned earlier. He said: we already said earlier that substance is said in three ways, matter, form, and the composite of these, and the being of matter is potentially while the being of form is in actuality and in act, and what is composed of soul and body is alive, so that by one of these there is something alive potentially and by another [something alive] in act. Hence, it is clear that soul is the actuality of body, not body of soul. For it is alive in act by soul and what is in act ought to be the actuality of what is in potency, and not the contrary. [It is] as if he meant, when he said: what is from these is alive, that is, because what is among these is alive in act by soul and

---

58. Arabic fragments correspond to Book 2, 24.48–55: كما تبين ان كل فعل ينسب الى موجود واحد من قبل شيئين فأحدهما مادة والآخر صورة ⟨. .⟩ كان ظاهر ان الذي ينسب الفعل الى الموجود نسبة أولى هي الصورة وان أفعال النفس يظهر من أمرها انها منسوبة الى النفس نسبة أولى وإلى البدن نسبة ثانية أي من قبل النفس لنتج عن ذلك ان النفس هي الصورة والبدن هو المادة (*Long Commentary* Fragments [1985], 38).

59. Arabic fragments correspond to Book 2, 24.58–68: ان ويتألف القياس هكذا: أفعال المتنفس تنسب الى النفس والبدن معا ، وكل فعل ينسب فانما ينسب الى موجود واحد من قبل شيئين ، فأحدهما مادة والآخر صورة فينتج ان الجسم والنفس أحدهما صورة والآخر مادة. فاذا أضيف الى هذه ان النفس صورة ونسب الفعل الى الموجود نسبة أولى ، وان هذه منعكسة وأضيف الى عكسها ان الفعل ينسب الى المتنفس من قبل النفس نسبة أولى أنتج عن ذلك ان النفس هي الصورة والجسم هو المادة (*Long Commentary* Frag-ments [1985], 38).

60. That is, the fact.

in potency by body, body must not be the actuality of soul, but soul [the actuality] of body.

26. **On account of this those who say that the soul is neither outside the body nor a body thought soundly. It is not body, but through body, and on account of this it is in the body and in a body of a certain sort, not as the ancients held asserting [the soul] to be in body without determination of that body, [i.e.,] what body it is and of what sort, and this [they asserted] although it is not the case that any given [body] receives any given [soul].**[61] (414a19–25)

Owing to the fact that it appeared concerning the soul that it is the actuality of a natural body, those holding the opinion {167} that the soul does not exist outside the body and is not body spoke rightly. For actuality is so, namely, it is in a body and it is not body. For body is not made actual by body, since body is not constituted by nature to be in a subject. He meant this when he said **It is not body, but** in body, etc. That it is body, insofar as it is actuality, is not possible, but it does exist in body. Next he said: **On account of this it is in the body**, etc. That is, on the basis of this way [of understanding], which we provided in regard to the substance of soul,[62] it is possible to give the reason why the soul exists in body and the body receiving it is of such a sort. This is not in the way which the ancients provided in regard to the substance of the soul, since they said that it is body and that it enters another body. They did not determine what nature is the nature of that body and why it had the characteristic of being alive while other bodies are not and [they did not determine] in what way there was similarity between these two bodies, namely, that one receives the other, since it is not the case that anything can receive anything. For it is necessary for those people to give the reason why this body receives that body which is soul. It is necessary for them to say why this body which is soul exists properly in this body and not in others. He meant this when he said: **without determination of that body, what body it is**, namely, what is

---

61. Averroes' Text omits 414a26–28, "It comes about as reason requires: the actuality of any given thing can only be realized in what is already potentially that thing, i.e. in a matter of its own appropriate to it. From all this it is plain that the soul is an actuality or account of something that possesses a potentiality of being such." Aristotle, *De Anima* (1984). This is preserved in the alternate translation: لأن انطلاشيا كل واحد من الأشياء لا يكون إلا لما فيه من قوة لقبول تلك الانطلاشيا ، بأن كان في هيولى ذلك الشيء ⟨تهيؤ⟩ لقبولها. – فقد استبان من هذه الأقاويل أن الشيء ذا القوة الموصوف بصفة كذا و كذا له انطلاشيا واحدة (ibid. [1954]). Averroes evidences no awareness of this omission here in his *Long Commentary* or in his *Middle Commentary* (2002), at 51–52. Note that what is a general principle in the Greek is in the Latin applied to the case of body and soul.

62. That is, the explanation of form as perfection and actuality.

received,[63] **and of what sort,** namely, the recipient. He said this because demonstrative definitions are naturally constituted to give the causes of all the things which are seen in what is defined, and if the definition will not be so, it will not be a definition.

27. Those powers of the soul which we mentioned are all found in certain animals, {168} as we said, and in certain others [only] certain [are found], and in [certain] distinctive kinds [only] one is found. We name the powers nutritive, sensitive, desiderative, locomotive, and discerning.[64] Of those the nutritive alone is in plants, while in others there is that and the sensitive and desiderative, for the desiderative is appetite, anger, and will.[65] All animals have at least one sense, namely, touch. Everything having sensation has pleasure and sorrow. And everything having those has appetite, for appetite is a desire for the pleasurable. (2.3, 414a29–b6)

Since he wanted to begin to speak concerning every one of the powers of the soul, he began first to enumerate which they are and [to indicate] that certain animals properly have certain of them, as the craftsman asserts the existence of the subject of his craft. For the craftsman must assert the existence of the subject of which he speaks and he divides its genera as if they were clearly existing. For the craftsman cannot demonstrate the subject of his craft nor the species of that subject. What he said in this chapter is clear. When he said **in [some] distinctive kinds,** he meant: in a few. That is, in a few animals [only] one power of the senses exists, namely, touch. Next he said: **We name the powers,** etc. That is, when we mention **powers,** the nutritive and sensitive powers should be understood. He means by **nutritive** all the principles which are active in nutrition, which are three, namely, the nutritive, that of growth, and that of diminution. He means by **desiderative** the appetite for food. For this reason he distinguished {169} it from locomotion and asserted it to be a

---

63. *Receptum.* One expects "what receives" here. Perhaps the translator mistook an active participle for a passive one in this context.

64. *Distinguentem* here corresponds to the Greek διανοητικόν in Aristotle's text and to المفكر و المميز, "cogitation and discernment," at *Middle Commentary* (2002), 52.12. The alternate Arabic translation renders this with المفكرة (Aristotle, *De Anima* [1954]); "the cogitative power."

65. *Desiderium enim est appetitus et ira et voluntas.* The corresponding Greek is ὄρεξις μὲν γὰρ ἐπιθυμία καὶ θυμὸς καὶ βούλησις (414b2), "for appetite is the genus of which desire, passion, and wish are the species." Aristotle, *De Anima* (1984). The *Middle Commentary* (2002), at 52.14, has والشوق ، منه شهوة ومنه غضب ومنه إرادة, "desire, which ... includes passion, anger and will." The alternate Arabic translation renders this وذلك أن الحاسة هي الشهوة والغضب والإرادة ، ففيه قوة شهوة (Aristotle, *De Anima* [1954]); "The appetitive power is in it, for sensation is appetite, anger and will."

genus per se, since that power is found in animals which do not move themselves. He understands by **discerning** understanding. Next he said: **Of those [. . .] in plants**, etc. That is, in plants the nutritive alone is found, while in animals sensation, which is touch, and desire, which is desire for nutrition, and this is common[66] to all [animals]. Next he said: **for the desiderative is appetite, anger, and will.** That is, we mean by desire appetite, for desire is said of appetite and of anger, and will and universally of several [of these]. He wanted to explain that appetite exists in every animal having sensation because this was not clear to sense. He said: **Everything having sensation has pleasure.** His account in this chapter is clear.

28. **Moreover, it has sensation of food since the [activity of] discerning food belongs to sensation. For every living thing is nourished only by what is dry [or] moist, warm [or] cold, and touch senses those things. But sensing other sensible things is accidental in the case of nourishment, since no contribution is made to nourishment by sound, color, or smell, while flavor is one of the tangibles. Hunger and thirst are each appetite, hunger for the warm and dry, thirst for the cold and moist. But flavor is, as it were, the cause of those.** (414b6–14) {170}

After he had asserted that every animal has the sense of touch and desire for nourishment, and [since] in explaining this induction is not sufficient, he began to explain this by argument. He said: **Moreover, it has sensation of nourishment.** That is, moreover, every animal must have a sense by which it apprehends what is fit and unfit among nourishments, so that it may spit out what is injurious and take in what is beneficial.[67] This was because what is nourishment for it does not exist potentially in many things as is the case for plants (and for this reason plants do not need sensation to discern food). That passage requires a great deal of contemplation. After he explained that every animal must have a sense for discerning food, he began to explain which sense is necessary for discerning food. He said: **For every living thing is nourished**, etc. That is, because every living thing is nourished only by dry [or] moist, warm [or] cold, since what nourishes takes the place of what is dissolved from the elements of which it is composed, the sense directed toward what is nutritious must be the sense which is naturally constituted to discern these qualities and that is the sense of touch. [It is] as if he says: because everything living is nourished only by dry [or] moist, warm [or] cold, and the sense of touch is what senses those, then touch must be the sentient power

---

66. Cf. Themistius, *De Anima Paraphrase:* κοινοτάτης (1899), 47.18; أعمّها (1973), 62.11; "most widely shared" (1996), 66.

67. Cf. Themistius, *De Anima Paraphrase* (1899), 47.26; (1973), 62.18–63.2; (1996), 66.

which discerns what is food. Therefore, an animal necessarily has touch. Next he said: **But** what senses **other sensible things**, etc. That is, but the senses which apprehend other sensible things sense food in an accidental way, that is, they are not necessary for discerning what is food insofar as it is food, since they perceive food accidentally. For things which can be sensed by these[68] {171} are not in food insofar as it is food. He meant this when he said: **since** there should **not** be **in** food, etc., that is, insofar as it is food. Next he said: **while flavor is one of the tangibles.** That is, while flavor, if it exists in food insofar as it is food, is one of the kinds of things which are tangible and the sense of taste is a certain kind of touch.[69] Because of what he said one should hold the opinion that this sense also exists in every animal, just as the sense of touch, since it is, as it were, one of its species. Later it will be explained how it is in reality. After he had recounted that cold, warm, moist, and dry exist in food insofar as it is food and that flavor exists in it insofar as it is food, he began to explain the way in which any of those exists in food. He said: **Hunger and thirst are**, etc. That is, but if flavor exists in food inasmuch as it is food, nevertheless the primary qualities exist in it first and in an essential way. The indication of this is that when an animal desires food, it desires only warm [or] cold, moist [or] dry. For hunger is an appetite for the warm and dry and thirst [is an appetite] for cold and moist. It does not desire sweet or sour. Flavor, however, is joined with those qualities. This is what he meant when he said: **But flavor is [. . .] the cause of those**, that is, the cause for the animal knowing which of those is fit and unfit. He did not mean here by **cause** the cause in being, for the primary qualities are the cause of flavor. Perhaps he understands that flavor is the cause on the basis of which an animal uses food owing to the delight joined with it.[70] {172}

29. **This should be explained later. Here, however, we are content with this determination, which is that every living thing having [the sense of] touch has desire. The case of the imagination is obscure and should be the object of inquiry later. Let us place with this having locomotion as well. And [let us also say this] in regard to other things [which possess] the ability to discern and [which possess] intellect, as in the cases of human beings and other things if the latter are of such a sort and better.** (414b14–19)

68. *Sensibilia enim eorum*—that is, the sensibles belonging to or appropriate to these other senses.

69. Cf. *Middle Commentary* (2002), 53.4.

70. The *Middle Commentary* (2002), at 53.7–8, states وأما إدراك الطعم فكأنه توطئة للغذاء وسبب لتناوله; "The apprehension of flavor, however, is like an appetizer to the food, and a reason for taking it."

Because he wants to assert here the number of those powers insofar as the craftsman asserts the subjects of his craft, he wants to assert only what is self-evident and he leaves aside other things which are not evident, until there will be investigation concerning them. For this reason he said: **This should be explained later. Here, however, we are content with this determination**, that is, what is clear in itself or nearly so, namely, that every animal lacking touch lacks desire.[71] For this is clear in itself. Next he recounted that this is obscure in the case of imagination. He said: **The case of the imagination is obscure**, that is, whether or not imagination exists in everything which has the sense of touch. Next he said: **Let us place with this having locomotion**. That is, let us assert as clear that everything which has locomotion is something which has imagination. It can be understood [in this way]: and let us assert the power of locomotion [to be] among the number of those powers which are seen to be evident and differ in definition and being. He means the concupiscible power. Next he said: **And [let us also say this] in regard to other things [which possess] the ability to discern and [which possess] intellect**. That is, let us also assert [it] as clear that the cogitative power[72] and the intellect exist in other kinds of animals which {173} are not human beings and that they are properly in some genus, as in [that of] human beings, or in a different genus, if a demonstration arises that there exist different things of this sort. This will be the case if there are things equal to or better than human beings.

30. **Let us therefore say that it is clear that by way of this example the definition of soul and the definition of figure will be the same. For according to that there is no actuality aside from the powers mentioned,[73] but it is also possible in the case of figures that there be a universal definition fitting for all figures and [that] it not be proper to any one of them. And similarly so in the cases of all the things mentioned above. For this reason it would be right that he be laughed at who seeks in their case and in the cases of others a universal account which is proper to none of them all and is not in**

---

71. *Carens tactu caret desiderio* is surprising here since the corresponding Text has *habens tactum habet desiderium*. An account corresponding with the latter, not the former, is what is found in the *Middle Commentary* (2002), at 53.9–10.

72. *Virtus cogitativa*. The corresponding term in the *Middle Commentary* (2002), at 53.12, is المميّزة, which Ivry translates "the faculty of discernment."

73. The Text seems to omit the following: οὔτε γὰρ ἐκεῖ σχῆμα παρὰ τὸ τρίγωνον ἔστι καὶ τὰ ἐφεξῆς. "For, as in that case there is no figure apart from triangle and those that follow in order." Aristotle, *De Anima* (1984). Averroes' alternate translation follows the full Greek text: لأنه ليس هناك اشكيم غير اشكيم المثلثة وما بعدها (ibid. [1954]). The problem in the Text here, however, seems not to affect adversely Averroes' understanding as expressed in the Comment.

this properly characteristic way something which is not divided, and [who] then dismisses such an account.[74] (414b20–28)

Since the genera taken in definitions are either univocal, as animal in the definition of a human being, or said in many ways, as being, potency, and act, he began to explain of what sort is the genus taken in the definition of the soul, and he said that it is neither equivocal nor univocal. He said: **Let us therefore say that it is clear**, etc. That is, let us say that it is clear from the example that what the universal definition of the soul provides from the intention common to all the parts of the soul is similar to what the universal definition of figure provides for all figures. For it is self-evident that, just as there is no actuality fitting for some part of the soul in addition to the universal actuality which {174} we include in the definition of all the powers, even if those powers are different in the intention proper to each of them, so too here there is no figure in addition to the definition of universal figure, although figures differ from one another in proper terms (for one is round, another straight, and another composed of both). This example is very similar to the definition of soul. For it is not from among the definitions of equivocal names (since, if it were so, then Geometry would be Sophistics), nor also from the genera [of things] which are said in a univocal way. This is because if it were so, then one of two things would necessarily be the case: either there would be a power one in definition and in name, in which all the powers which we enumerated share, just as the kinds of animals share in the definition of simple animality; or all the powers of the soul would be the same in definition and being. After he had explained by example that the definition of soul is similar to the definition of figure, he began to give the nature of the similarity. He said: **but it is also possible in the case of figures**, etc. That is, that definition is not univocal but [still] it is possible for all figures, although they differ, that they have a broad universal definition fitting for them all, although they differ a great deal in definition and in being. Likewise, it is possible for those different powers to have one universal definition fitting for them all, just as the definition of figure fits all figures and is specifically proper to none. Next he said: **For this reason it would**

---

74. The Text again suffers corruption. The Greek has διὸ γελοῖον ζητεῖν τὸν κοινὸν λόγον καὶ ἐπὶ τούτων καὶ ἐφ᾽ ἑτέρων, ὃς οὐδενὸς ἔσται τῶν ὄντων ἴδιος λόγος, οὐδὲ κατὰ τὸ οἰκεῖον καὶ ἄτομον εἶδος, ἀφέντας τὸν τοιοῦτον. "Hence it is absurd in this and similar cases to look for a common definition which will not express the peculiar nature of anything that is and will not apply to the appropriate indivisible species, while at the same time omitting to look for an account which will." Aristotle, *De Anima* من أجل ذاك إن نحن قلنا هذا القول الشائع في هذه وفي غيرها وهو قول ليس يختص. (1984) بشيء من الأشياء – لا على ما يليق به من معناه الأعلى ، ولا على صورة انفراده ، فمتى أضربنا عن هذا قلنا بذاك الشائع – كنا أهلا ليهزأ بنا (ibid. [1954]).

be right that he be laughed at who seeks, etc. That is, because of what we said, it would be right that he be laughed at who seeks in the case of the soul {175} and in those of other similar things one universal definition which is not specifically proper to any of them all and which is not such as the definition which we provided for soul, but rather is like the universality of the definition of simple animality fitting for the species of animal and is not also one, that is, a definition which is of one nature and which is not divisible in species. He who has dismissed such a definition as we provided [should rightly be laughed at], since those two kinds of definition are not found in such natures and only that kind of definition which we use is found in their case. For one who works at giving the first kind of definition in the case of the soul is seeking the impossible in what he works at, just as he who dismisses this definition in dismissing what is possible. For to dismiss what is possible is similar in expression to seeking what is impossible.

31. **The disposition in the case of the soul is similar to the disposition in the case of figures. For what is prior is always found potentially in what follows in the case of figures and living things, for instance, the triangle in the quadrilateral and the nutritive in what is sensitive. It is necessary, therefore, to seek in any given thing what it is according to its definition. For instance, what is the soul of a plant and what is the soul of a beast.**[75] **One should indeed seek out why they are of such a disposition with respect to those which follow, since what has the capacity for sensation does not exist without the nutritive, but what has the capacity for sensation is separate in reference to plants. Also, none of the other senses exists without touch but touch does exist without the other senses. For many living things do not have sight or hearing or smell or another sense.** (414b28–415a6) {176}

After he had explained that the definition of the soul is similar to the definition of figure, he began to explain the kind of similarity and to show what kind of definition it involves. He said: **The disposition in the case of the soul is similar,** etc. That is, the disposition in things which are contained in the definition of the soul is like the disposition in things which are contained in the definition of figure. For just as prior and posterior are found in figures, and the prior exists potentially in the posterior, so too is it the case for the powers of the soul. For instance, in figures, the triangle is prior to the quadrilateral and the triangle exists potentially in the quadrilateral. For this reason,

75. The Greek has οἷον τίς φυτοῦ καὶ τίς ἀνθρώπου ἢ θηρίου, "of a plant, man, beast" (Aristotle, De Anima [1984]), with which the alternate translation is in accord: ما نفس النبات وما نفس الإنسان ، وما نفس البهيمة (ibid. [1954]). Averroes' Comment is also in accord with these. See below.

if a quadrilateral exists, a triangle exists, and not the converse. And likewise in the case of the powers of the soul, for the nutritive is prior to the power of sensation and exists in it potentially. And if the power of sensation exists, the nutritive exists, and not the converse. After he had explained the nature of that definition and how much knowledge it gives, he said: **It is necessary, therefore, to seek in any given thing what**, etc. That is, it had been explained that this definition of the soul is of the genus of the definition of figure and, just as knowledge of figure alone is not sufficient with respect to knowledge of a figure possessing straight lines and of a circular figure, so too is it the case for the definition of universal soul. Now one should therefore seek after knowledge of that universal definition, the definition proper to each power of the soul, namely, what is the soul of plants and what is the soul of a human being which is proper to [a human being] and what [is the soul proper] to a beast. Next he said: It is necessary to seek out **why they are of such a disposition**. That is,[76] it is necessary that one investigate also why the prior and consequent are found in the powers of the soul. For it is impossible for the power of sensation to exist without the nutritive, but the nutritive can exist without the power of sensation and this is [the case] in {177} plants. It also appears that it is impossible that any of the four senses exist without touch, but touch can exist without the other senses. For several animals lack vision, hearing, smell, or taste (he meant this when he said: **or another sense.**)

That passage requires consideration. For it is thought that taste is one of the kinds of touch, as he said above. But if some animal is nourished by things lacking flavor, then the [sense of] taste of that animal will be only with respect to warm [or] cold, moist [or] dry. Or he means, when he said: **or another sense**, that is, that another sense is not distinguished ultimately, that is, in the end, from the sense of touch as it is found in perfect animals. Universally the opinion should be held that if something has the sense of touch and is nourished by its roots, as plants are nourished, as is said regarding the sea sponge, that animal has the sense of touch without taste. Perhaps he indicates kinds of animals such as those, for every animal having a mouth has some [capability for] taste.

32. **Among those that have sensation it is the case that some have locomotion and some do not. However, the completion and end is that which has cogitation and discernment.[77] For every one of the corruptible things having**

---

76. Crawford has *Idest* italicized, but this appears to be a printing error.

77. Crawford declined to follow manuscript G, which is more fully in accord with the Comment of Averroes. I follow the correct reading in G, which is *cogitationem*, not *cognitionem*, throughout this entire passage of the *De Anima*. This is confirmed by examination of the Greek text and the edition of the Hebrew by Bos (Aristotle, *De Anima* [1994]): 415a8: λογισμὸν המחשבה; a9: λογισμὸς מחשבה; a10: λογισμός מחשבה. The

cogitation has all the others.[78] However, what has one of them does not necessarily have cogitation, and some do not have imagination and some live only through those[79] alone. [As for] the theoretical and cogitative intellect,[80] the account with respect to it is different. Therefore it was explained that the account with respect to each of those powers is the account more fitting with respect to the soul. (415a6–13) {178}

It is apprehended by sense that some animals have locomotion (this is the perfect kind) and some do not. The completion and end of animals which was intended in generation, which nature has achieved when it has been able to succeed, is the kind of animals having the theoretical and cogitative power, that is, the intelligible [power]. Next he said: **For every one of the corruptible things**, etc. That is, it appears that everything among generable and corruptible things having the cogitative power necessarily has the other powers of the soul. He said this because he did not want to include the celestial bodies. For it was explained that those have only the impulse of desire and intellect from among the powers of the soul. Next he said: **what has one of those**, etc. That is, what has one of the powers which are prior by nature to the intellect does not necessarily have cogitation or intellect, but some do not have imagination, much less do they have cogitation, and some live through those which are below imagination, powers which are prior to [imagination]. He meant this when he said: **Some live through those alone.** Next he said: **the account** concerning the theoretical intellect, etc. That is, the account concerning it is such that it is outside that nature, for it is thought that it is neither soul nor a part of the soul. He indicated its nobility and its difference from the other parts, for one must hold that it is from a nature superior to that of the soul. Next he said: **For it was explained**, etc. That is, for it was explained from what was said earlier that the first thing which was intended concerning the knowledge of the

---

alternate Arabic text has فكر, الفكر, and الفكر (ibid. [1954]). On the contaminated version of the Arabic text of the *De Anima* used by Averroes, see the discussion of cogitation (*cogitatio*/فكـ/מחשבה) in the introduction, pp. lxxvii–lxxix, and in Taylor (1999a).

78. That is, all the other powers.

79. *Per ista*. In the Greek, τὰ δὲ ταύτῃ μόνῃ ζῶσιν, the referent is to the singular φαντασία, while here it is to the neuter plural *omnia alia*. In the alternate translation the referent is spelled out as imagination: وبعضها إنما معنى حياته بالتوهم وحده) (Aristotle, *De Anima* [1954]). Latin manuscript B retains the reading *istam*, but Averroes' Comment indicates that the problem already existed in the Arabic text.

80. The alternate translation renders the Greek περὶ δὲ τοῦ θεωρητικοῦ νοῦ as في العقل البحاثة النظّار (Aristotle, *De Anima* [1954]); "concerning the intellect as investigative and theoretical." *Cogitativus*, "cogitative," is added here.

soul, which is more appropriate to an account in regard to the soul, is to speak of the [sort of] soul fitting for every one of those powers. {179}

33. **One who wishes to investigate those will necessarily need to know what each one of those is; then later there will be investigation of the things consequent upon those. And if it is necessary to say what each one of those is, for instance, what the intellect is, what the sensitive part is, and what the nutritive part is, then it is necessary to say first what understanding is.**[81] **For actions and operations precede the powers in the intellect.**[82] **If it is so, and consideration of other things opposed to those**[83] **ought to precede consideration of those, [then] for that reason we must first direct our efforts toward defining those, for instance, food, what is sensed, and what is understood.** (2.4, 415a14–22)

After he had explained that the universal definition of the soul mentioned earlier is not sufficient for knowledge of its substance, he began to say what must be known concerning the soul after that definition. He said: **One who wishes to investigate those will necessarily need**, etc. That is, he who wants to acquire perfect knowledge of the soul must necessarily investigate each of the powers of the soul per se to the extent that he knows by demonstration what each of them is and what nature it has. For instance, what the intellect is and what sense is must be investigated. Next after this there must be investigation of each with respect to things which universally and properly follow upon each of those powers, for instance, whether or not the intelligible power can be separated. After he had explained what we must investigate concerning the soul, he began to show {180} the way to this knowledge and that it is among the things which are more known from our perspective and posterior in being to things which are more known by nature and prior in being. He said: **And if it is necessary to say what each one** of those, etc. That is, if it is necessary, as we explained, to know what each of those powers is, it is necessary to know first what are the actions proper to each of those powers, for instance, what it is to understand through understanding and to sense through sensing and to take nourishment through taking nourishment. For knowledge

---

81. The Greek has τί τὸ νοητικὸν ἢ τὸ αἰσθητικὸν, "thinking or perceiving." Aristotle, *De Anima* (1984). Averroes' alternate translation renders the Greek more precisely: ما الذى يفهـم ، وما الذى يحس (ibid. [1954]).

82. Or: in understanding. *In intellectu* corresponds to the Greek κατὰ τὸν λόγον, "in definition." Aristotle, *De Anima* (1984). The alternate translation captures the sense of the Greek: في الحد (ibid. [1954]); "in definition."

83. *Oppositis istis.* The Greek τὰ ἀντικείμενα is "their correlative objects." Aristotle, *De Anima* (1984). Averroes' explicit remark on this in the Comment makes it clear that he understands this more in accord with the sense of the Greek.

of the actions of those powers is prior from our perspective in our first knowledge to knowledge of those powers. After he had recounted that knowledge of the actions ought to precede knowledge of the powers, he also recounted that the knowledge of the things undergoing those actions ought to precede the knowledge of those actions, for the same reason that knowledge of the actions ought to precede knowledge of the powers. He said: **If it is so,** etc. That is, if it is so, namely, that we ought always to go from these things which are more known from our perspective to those things which are more known by nature and that consideration of things opposite to those powers (i.e., things which are passive in relation to them) ought to precede consideration of the actions and the powers, then it is necessary to know first what food is, which is the passive object of the nutritive power, what the thing sensed is, and what the thing understood is, before one may know what being nourished and sensing are. He called these opposites, for the passive and the active seem to be in some way opposites. {181}

34. **Therefore it is necessary first to speak of nourishment and generation. For the nutritive soul is prior in all living things and is more universal with respect to the powers of soul by which [powers] what is living lives. Its actions are to generate and to take nourishment. For the action which is more fitting for the nature of every living thing from among those which are perfect, do not have defect, and are not generated per se by chance is to produce another of the same kind. Therefore an animal produces an animal and a plant a plant so that it may have a share of the eternal and divine insofar as it is able. For all things desire this and [each] does what it does by nature for the sake of this.** (415a22–b2)

He had explained which of all the definitions of the soul is more universal and how much knowledge it yields and that it is not sufficient for knowing the definition of the substance of the soul in a perfect way and that one must know first any [given one] of the powers of the soul by its own definition and in how many ways those powers are different and how they are united. [Now] he began to recount that one must first begin with the knowledge of those powers, starting with the one which is clearly prior, namely, the nutritive [power], and that first one must consider the affections and actions of those powers. He said: **Therefore it is necessary first to speak of nourishment and generation,** etc. That is, since it was explained that it is first necessary to consider the actions and affections before the powers themselves, of all those actions we must first speak about food and generation, which are affection and action belonging to that soul. We must {182} first speak of the nutritive soul because it is naturally prior to the other things by virtue of which something is called living; for this reason it is the more universal among the other powers of the soul. He indicated that it must be placed first in consideration owing to its priority and universality, for the universal is more known to us than what is proper, as was said elsewhere.[84] After he had explained this, he began to list the actions ascribed to [the nutritive] since we ought to know that it is before [we know] what it is. He said: **Its actions are**, etc. That is, the actions of that power are to take nourishment, to generate, and to make use of food. We say that to generate is an action of that power since the action which most belongs to the nature of what is called living by virtue of this power is to generate something like itself in species. This comes about with three conditions: one is that it reaches the time in which it has this power, since it is not in act in every [moment of] time; a second is that with this it does not have a defect, for that impedes this action, although it may reach the time in which that action arises from [that being]; [and] the third is that this living thing is not from these things which come to be per se. Therefore, when these three are brought together in a living thing, then it will generate [something like itself in species]. He meant this when he said: Since **the action which is more fitting**, etc. Next he provided the final cause for the sake of which that power exists in animals and plants. He said: **so that it may have a share of the eternal**. That is, that power exists in something living so that what is generable and corruptible may have something in common with the eternal according to its ability. For since divine solicitude could not make it last forever individually, it showed pity in giving it the power {183} by which it can last forever in species. In this there is no doubt, namely, that it is better in its being that it has that power than that it not have [it]. Next he said: **For all things desire this**, etc. That is, this was so because all things desire everlasting permanence and are moved toward it insofar as their nature is naturally constituted to receive [it]. For the sake of this end all beings do what they do naturally.

35. **For the sake of which is said in two ways, one is [that] in regard to which it is and the other [that] of which it is.[85] Therefore, because it was impossible for it to share in eternity with the everlasting divine, because it is impossible for something corruptible to remain forever the same in number, for this reason it shares something with it insofar as it can, in some cases more, in others less. Thus it is not that same thing which remains forever but its like and not [something] one in number but one in form.** (415b2–7)

84. See {14} and {149}.
85. *Unus est in quo est, et alius cuius est.* The Greek has τὸ μὲν οὗ, τὸ δὲ ᾧ, "the end to achieve which, or the being in whose interest, the act is done." Aristotle, *De Anima* (1984). The Arabic in Averroes' alternate translation is إحداهما له ، والأخرى فيه (ibid. [1954]); "one of the two is for it and the other is in it."

After he had provided the final cause for the sake of which the generative power exists universally in what is living (and it is the assimilation of the corruptible with the eternal, insofar as it has the nature of what must be assimilated), and that all beings carry out actions toward that end, he explained according to how many ways that end is said. He said: **For the sake of which is said in two ways, one is** that which is the end itself **and the other** that in which the end is. For instance, on this account, all beings act for the sake of {184} everlasting permanence and for this reason in some we find everlasting permanence or some disposition for everlasting permanence. After he had explained this, he began to explain how generable and corruptible things can have something in common with eternal things and the reason why they are removed from everlasting permanence. He said: **Therefore, because it** is **impossible**, etc. He means by everlasting divine the heavenly body, for those heavenly bodies last forever as individuals. And when he said: **in some cases more, in others less**, he meant the generative and the non-generative. For both last forever according to species, but the generative has this always and the non-generative most of the time and in several subjects.[86]

36. **The soul, therefore, is the cause and principle of the living body in three determinate ways.**[87] **For it is that from which motion comes to be and that for the sake of which the body existed, and the soul is also the cause insofar as it is substance, which is the cause of being for all things.**[88] (415b8–13)

After it had appeared from the universal definition of the soul that the soul is the cause of the body according to form and it had appeared here that the generative power is the cause making [it] alive, he began to explain that the soul is cause not only according to form, but also a cause according to the three ways in which it is called cause, and this is in three ways. This is necessary, namely, to know this before speaking about {185} each of the parts of the soul,

---

86. *Sed generativum habet hoc semper, et non generativum in maiori parte temporis et in pluribus subiectis.* Averroes may here be referring to animals continuous in species by generation and to animals resulting from spontaneous generation, though this is by no means evident.

87. Averroes' Text here omits a line of the Greek: αἰτία καὶ ἀρχή. ταῦτα δὲ πολλαχῶς λέγεται, ὁμοίως δ᾽ ἡ ψυχή. "The soul is the cause or source of the living body. *The terms cause and source have many senses. But the soul is the cause of its body alike* in all three senses which we explicitly recognize." Aristotle, *De Anima* (1984); emphasis of the relevant text added. Averroes' alternate text renders the whole Greek text with the exception of ἀρχή. See ibid. (1954).

88. δῆλον may have been dropped from the Greek of the Arabic translator's manuscript in this passage. It is in the alternate translation as من الظاهر (Aristotle, *De Anima* [1954]).

although it was already explained universally that every natural form is of such a sort.[89] He said: **The soul, therefore, is the cause and principle of the living body.** Because these two things are said in many ways, the soul is like-wise a cause according to three determinate ways, namely, as moving, final, and formal causes, which have been determined in the general physical ac-counts.[90] Next he said: **For it is that from which motion comes to be,** namely, the cause bringing about motion. By this we can understand motion in place and generation, and motion in growth and diminution, for the soul is the cause bringing about those three motions in what is alive. Next he said: **And that for the sake of which the body existed,** namely, the final cause. For the body was only for the sake of the soul, since it was explained that the soul is with respect to the body as form to matter. It was explained in the general accounts[91] that matter is for the sake of form alone and that it is not something consequent upon matter or something which is from the necessity of matter, as the ancients used to think, not granting there to be a formal or final cause.[92] **And the soul is also the cause,** etc. That is, and the soul is also a cause of the body according to substance and form,[93] which is the cause of the being of all things.

37. **To be for a living thing is to live, and the soul is the cause and prin-ciple of that. And the actuality [of a thing] is also the intention[94] of what is a being potentially. It is evident that the soul is a cause according to that for the sake of which, since, just as the intellect does nothing except for the sake of something, so too [is it the case for] nature, and this is its end. It is simi-larly so for the soul in animals and all things, {186} for all natural things are tools for the soul, as in animals so too in plants, such that it is also cause of what is alive.[95] That for the sake of which is said in two ways, one is that on**

89. See Book 2, Comment 8 {40}ff.

90. *Physics* 1.3, 194b23–195a26.

91. See Book 1, note 165.

92. *Physics* 2.1, 193b7–8.

93. *Secundum substantiam et formam.* The corresponding passage of the *Middle Com-mentary* has the same phrase, على طريق الجوهر والصورة, which Ivry indicates (*Middle Commentary* [2002], 56.15–16; 174, n. 6) may be related to the replacement of Aristotle's οὐσία by ὡς εἶδος in the paraphrase of Themistius. Themistius, *De Anima Paraphrase* (1899), 50.29; وكالصورة (1973), 70.1; "as form" (1996), 69.

94. *Intentio*: λόγος, "its account" (Aristotle, *De Anima* [1984]); معنى (ibid. [1954]). "Further, the actuality of whatever is potential is identical with its account" (Aristotle, *De Anima* [1984]). أيضا الانطلاشيا هى بمعنى الشيء ذى القوة (ibid. [1954]); "The actuality is also through the intention of the thing existing in potency."

95. Averroes' Text here varies considerably from the Greek of Aristotle, which has, "To that something corresponds in the case of animals the soul and in this it follows

account of which and the other is that to which this belongs. **The soul is also that from which motion in place first comes to be, but that power is not found in all living things. Both alteration and growth also come to be through the soul, for sensation is thought to be some sort of alteration and nothing has sensation unless it has soul. So too is it in the cases of growth and diminution, for nothing suffers growth or diminution in a natural way unless it is nourished, and nothing is nourished unless it shares in life.** (415b13–28)

After he had asserted that the soul is a cause of the body in the three ways in which this word "cause" is said, he began to explain that those ways are in it and in the first place that it is the cause of the body by way of form. He said: **To be for a living thing**, etc. That is, the indication of the fact that the soul is the form of the body is that this living being does not have being insofar as it is living, except by virtue of that by which it lives, that is, what is the cause of that action, namely, of life. It is evident that the cause of that action is the soul; therefore this being belonging to what is living, insofar as it is living, is by virtue of the soul. And that through which the being is a determinate particular is its form; therefore the soul is the form of what is alive, since it is a determinate particular and a being only by virtue of soul. He provided a second argument for this. He said: **And the actuality [of a thing] is also the intention of what** {187} **is a being potentially.** That is, the soul is also actuality, as it was already explained; but actuality is form and the intention of that which is a being potentially; therefore soul is form.

After he had explained that it is a cause according to form, he also explained that it is a cause according to the end. He said: **It is evident that the soul is** also a cause, etc. That is, it is self-evident that the soul is a cause of the body which is alive insofar as it is that on account of which the body was alive. For just as many artifacts are brought about only for the sake of something else, so too is it with respect to nature, namely, that it does not act except for the sake of something. This is the end of nature, namely, that it acts only for the sake of something, as art acts only for the sake of something. Next he explained that that for the sake of which nature carries out natural [activities] seems to be the soul in animals, and not only in animals but in all natural things. He said: **It is similarly so for the soul in animals and all things.** That

___

the order of nature; all natural bodies are organs of the soul. This is true of those that enter into the constitution of plants as well as of those which enter into that of animals. This shows that that for the sake of which they are is soul." Aristotle, *De Anima* (1984). Averroes' alternate translation is closer to the Greek if Badawi's reading يعقل is changed to يفعل twice in this passage. See ibid. (1954).

is, just as form is the end of art in artifacts, so soul is the end of nature in animals and in all natural things. Next he explained the way in virtue of which
it appears that the soul is the end of all natural things. He said: **For all natural
things are** instruments **of the soul**, etc. That is, and we said that the soul is
the end of all natural things because all natural things seem indifferently to be
instruments of the soul in all things which are alive. And as it seems in animals,
so does it seem in plants. Next he said: **such that** it **is also a cause of what is
alive**, etc. That is, what we said concerning it is not obscure but rather is self-
evident to the extent that it appears from the fact that the soul is also the cause
of what is alive. For that for the sake of which is said in two ways: one is that
for the sake of which something is found,[96] {188} and that is the relationship
of the soul to the body; the other is that to which there belongs this for the sake
of which something is found, and that is the relationship of the soul to what
is alive. For we say that the soul and the body both are only for the sake of
what is alive.

  After he had explained it to be a cause according to form and according to
end, he also explained that it is a moving cause according to all the kinds of
motions existing in what is alive, whether they are true motions or [just]
thought to be [so]. He said: **The soul is also that from which motion in place
first comes to be, but that power** is **not in all living things**, that is, in all animals. Next he said: **Both alteration and growth also**, etc. That is, alteration
ascribed to the senses, as some hold, if we will have conceded it to be motion,
will be by virtue of the soul, and similarly [so for] growth and diminution. For
nothing is said to have this motion, namely, sensation, unless it has soul. Next
he said: **It is** similarly **in the case of growth and** in the case of **diminution**.
That is, as it appears that only something having soul senses, so too it appears
that only what shares in some part of soul with living things either grows or
suffers diminution. For nothing is diminished naturally or made to grow
naturally unless it has the power of taking nourishment, and nothing takes
nourishment unless it shares in the life ascribed to living things. For this reason the word "dead" is said of an animal only when it has lost what it shares
with plants.

  38. **Empedocles, however, did not speak rightly and truly in regard to this
when he said that the growth which occurs in** {189} **plants, with respect to
what branches out downward through roots, comes about naturally through
the motion of earth itself toward that part (and he provided this as the**

---

  96. *Invenitur.* Here and just below the corresponding Arabic was probably يجد, " to
be found" or "to exist." Hence, Averroes' Arabic here probably said that the soul is that
for the sake of which the soul exists. That is, the soul exists for its own sake, while the
body exists not for its own sake but for the sake of the soul.

cause[97]), and with respect to what branches upward, comes about because fire is likewise moved upward (and he provided this as the cause). For what he also made use of in his account concerning up and down was not rightly said. For up and down are not the same for each and every thing, but rather as the head is for animals so are the roots for plants, since it is in virtue of actions[98] that we ought to say that their organs are similar or different. (415b28–416a5)

After he had explained that the motion of growth is not from a principle which is an element, he began to explain that Empedocles erred when he held the opinion that this principle is from the elements and that growth downward in plants is due to a heavy part and upward [is] due to a light part, namely, air and fire. He said: **Empedocles, however,** etc. That is, Empedocles, however, was not thinking properly when he held the opinion that this principle is not the soul and that the growth which occurs in plants is in virtue of the nature of the elements; [and that,] therefore, what grows downward is in virtue of the nature of earth, and he asserted this as its cause. That is, he asserted the cause of its motion downward to be a heavy nature and the cause in the growth of branches upward to be a light nature, namely, fire. Next he began to give an account of how this account is erroneous. He said: **What he also** made use of **in his account concerning up,** {190} etc. That is, that account which he brings forth in giving the cause of that contrary motion which is found in what can be made to grow is not true. For what was thought, that up in the case of plants is up in the case of the world and down down, is not true, since they are similar neither in part nor in nature and potency; in part because, although we concede this in the case of plants, nevertheless that is something we cannot concede in the case of most animals, for up in [the case of animals] does not correspond to the upper part of the world. Truth does not allow this to be conceded, for the nature of down in plants is different from the nature of down in the world, but there does occur a coincidence of these in such a part by chance, and the nature of up in animals is the very same. An indication of that is that the head in animals is like the roots in plants, since their function is the same, and we ought to note similarity and diversity in parts which can grow in virtue of actions. He said: **For up,** etc. That is, the first error of Empedocles is that the upward and the downward are not the same part in each [particular thing] and in the whole, namely, the world. For, al-

97. There is no parenthetical remark in Aristotle's Greek to correspond to this or the other parenthetical remark immediately below.

98. *Actiones*: τοῖς ἔργοις, "their functions" (Aristotle, *De Anima* [1984]); والآلة وإن اختلفت فالعمل يجمعها (ibid. [1954]); "If the instruments differ, the activity unites them."

though we may concede this in the case of plants, what can we say for most animals? For up in animals does not correspond to the upper part of the world. Next he said: **but rather as the head,** etc. That is, but rather we do not concede that down in plants is down in the world according to nature and potency, nor [that] up in them [is] up in the world, although they may be in the same part. For the nature of the head in animals is the nature of the roots in plants, since they have the same actions, and it is according to the actions that we should say that the parts of animals and plants and their organs are similar or different in nature. Since the nature of a root in {191} plants is the nature of the head in animals, then up in plants is in reality down in the world. And if we had conceded that it is down, then what occurs in the case of plants, namely, that down in them is down in the world, occurs only by chance, not because they have the same nature such that a heavy part is moved downward in plants and a light upward. For if it were so, then an animal would have neither up nor down, nor would the nature of up and down in plants and animals be the same. He said that the potency of the head in animals is the potency of the root in plants because this is the principle through which an animal is an animal, namely, sensation. But this is the principle of that through which plants are plants, namely, food. For this reason if the head from an animal and the root from plants are cut off, they die.

39. **And, besides, what is it that restrains fire and earth when they are moved toward contrary parts? For they are quick to separate unless something prevents it. And if there is something there preventing this, what prevents this ought to be the soul and the cause of growth and nutrition.** (416a6–9)

If we concede that the nature of up and down in plants is the nature of up and down in the world and that the fiery part moves upward in plants and the earthen part downward, and we see that the same part moves upward and downward at once (for we see that any given {192} part asserted as sensible and any given member moves toward each part at once); and if, then, we asserted that this part is unitary, namely, what moves toward each part, then the principle by which they move with those two motions is at once a unitary principle. Therefore, that principle has the potency to move toward each part at once, which is not something in the elements, since one of their parts has only a single motion, whether it is simple or composite (since, if it is composed from them, it will move according to the dominant element). And if the parts, which move upward in that same part in the sense or in nature, are different from the parts which move downward in that part, then those parts are necessarily distinct from one another, either because they are simple or because what is dominant in the things which move downward with respect to simple bodies is different from what is dominant in the things which move upward. If that is so, what is it which restrains fire and earth, or the fiery or earthen part, since we cannot say that these two are mixed together (since if they were mixed together, they would move toward the same part, namely, of what is dominant), and if it were so, would they not immediately separate from one another, unless something prevents it? But it happens that they must say there is something preventing it there, since they seem not to be separate but to remain [together] at once so long as the plant lives. This is necessary for them. Since they have conceded there to be something preventing it there, whose potency is not the potency of the elements, we will say to them that what prevents it is the soul. In accord with this, then, we should understand his account, although it is very brief. {193}

40. **Some**[99] **think that the nature of fire taken absolutely is the cause of nutrition and growth. For of the bodies and the elements, it is fire that is nourished and made to grow, and for this reason it is thought that it does this in plants as well as in animals.** (416a9–13)

After he had refuted the account of those imagining that growth is through an elemental principle, namely, the heavy or the light, he began also to refute the account of those imagining that the principle of nutrition and growth in what is able to take nourishment is fire or a part of fire or something fiery. He said: **Some**, etc. That is, some think that the nature of fire insofar as it is fire, not insofar as it is some given fire (he meant this when he said **taken absolutely**), is the cause of nutrition and growth. They held this opinion because they saw fire change all things into its own substance insofar as it grew in virtue of that. And because according to them what is able to take nourishment is nourished by changing all things into its own substance, for this reason they thought, in virtue of two affirmative propositions in the second figure, that fire without qualification does this.[100]

41. **Let us say, therefore, that fire is not a collaborative cause except in a certain way and is not the cause absolutely, but rather the soul deserves more to be this [cause]. For the growth of fire is infinite so long as there is something able to burn. But things which are constituted by nature all have an end and limit in quantity and growth. Those are due to the soul, not fire, and they deserve the intention more than matter.** (416a13–18) {194}

99. Heraclitus.

100. What changes all things into its substance is fire. What changes all things into its substance is the cause of nutrition and growth. Therefore fire is the cause of nutrition and growth. A syllogism in the Second Figure with two affirmative propositions does not yield a necessary conclusion.

After he had explained this opinion, he began first to recount the true part and the false part in it. He said: **Let us say, therefore, that fire**, etc. That is, let us say, therefore, that fire is not without qualification the cause of nutrition and growth in animals, but rather it is ascribed to a cause as if it were one of its tools. Rather, the soul is that to which this action is ascribed without qualification. He conceded that fire is a collaborative cause insofar as something is ascribed to something whose action is completed only through that, because what is able to take nourishment seems to change[101] food only by virtue of the fiery part existing in it. For among the elements this one either is what changes the others or the ability to cause change predominates in it more than in the other elements. For this reason it was necessary that it be dominant in bodies which are able to take nourishment. After he explained that if that action were ascribed to it, it is ascribed only insofar as it is a collaborative cause, not insofar as it is itself the cause, he then explained how it is not necessary to ascribe that action to fire without qualification and that it is more deserving to ascribe it to the soul absolutely. He said: **For the growth of fire is infinite**, etc. That is, the indication that the first mover in nutrition and growth is the soul, not the fiery part, is that if that motion, namely, to change something into the substance of what is causing the change, and its growth through what causes the change were in fire alone without another power joined to it (namely, so that the first mover is a potency of fire insofar as it is fire, not a different power joined to fire), it will be found to be infinite and will not cease at some limit so long as it finds something able to burn. However, the motion of changing and growing which is found in this nature which is able to grow is always found to be finite and determinate in quantity. Hence, it is evident, in the second figure, that this motion is not of fire {195} absolutely. And since it is not of fire, it necessarily belongs to another principle, and that we call the nutritive soul. He means by limit and measure the ultimate natural things which are found in the quantities of bodies which are able to grow.

Next he said: **and they are** more deserving of **the intention than matter.** That is, and that action which is found in this motion, namely, [the motion] which began from a determinate beginning and continued through to the determinate end, is more deservingly ascribed to what is in that action as form, namely, the soul, and not to what is [in it] as matter and instrument, namely, fire. He said this because it appears that the action of growth was composed of the action of fire and of some intention in fire. For the change which is in it

101. *Alterare*: This and related terms are used here to indicate both the accidental alteration of a substance by its consumption of food and the substantial change of the food into the substance of what is altered by nutrition. Consequently, I render it by "to change" and related forms, understanding this to be a generic term for substantial and accidental change.

ought to be ascribed to fire. And because it is determinate, it ought to be ascribed to another power joined with fire, just as softening iron by fire for making some tool, insofar as it is softening, is ascribed to fire and insofar as that softening has a limit known in the case of each tool, it is ascribed to the power of the craft.

42. Therefore, because the nutritive power and the generative [power] are the same, one must necessarily first determine what nourishment is and distinguish [it] from the other powers. (416a19–21)

He had recounted earlier that he wants first to speak about the nutritive power, since it is more universal and the first of these which are apparent in it, or [since] the first of the things contemplated on the basis of this power is that it is in the soul and that its actions are growth, nutrition, and generation. He began now to determine what must first be contemplated {196} in regard to this power after it has been known to exist in the soul. He said: **because the** potency for nourishment and generation, etc. That is, because the subject of the nutritive, growth-causing, and generative potency is the same, namely, nourishment, and we already said first that the way to the knowledge of the substances of those powers is only through knowledge first of what they act upon, hence it is necessary first to begin with the determination of what food is and what taking nourishment is. After he had explained this, he began to show what food is.

43. Let us say, therefore, that it is thought that nourishment is contrary by contrary, and not every contrary by every contrary, but rather contraries which not only come from one another, but also cause growth. For many things come from one another, but not all cause growth,[102] **for instance, what is healthy from what is ill. And we also find that they are not nourishment for one another in the same way. Rather, water is nourishment for fire, but fire is not nourishment for water. In simple bodies, however, these two are properly thought to be such that one is the nourishment and the other what is able to take nourishment.** (416a21–29)

Let us say that it was thought that nourishment is that which is contrary to what is able to take nourishment, as certain people have thought. But that opinion is not in regard to every contrary but in regard to these contraries which not only come from one another, but also cause growth. For many contraries which are generated from one another do not cause growth in one

---

102. The corresponding Greek has οὐ πάντα ποσα, "where neither is even a quantum" (Aristotle, *De Anima* [1984]); وليس جميع الأشياء هكذا (ibid. [1954]); "and all things are not so."

another, for what is healthy {197} comes from what is ill, but it is not nourished by it. He meant this when he said: **and not every contrary by every contrary,** etc. His account is understandable by itself. He indicated by this the contraries which are in the substance, for those are thought to cause one another to grow and to be nourished by one another. After he had explained that this opinion is found only in the case of contraries which are in the substance, those which are such that it is possible that they be figured to be nourished by one another, he [then] also explained that this is not found equally in each contrary. For contraries themselves do not seem to nourish one another equally. He said: **And we also** see **that they are not nourishment . . . in the same way,** etc. That is, that opinion is not equally found in regard to both of the contraries in the substance, namely, so that each of them nourishes equally what corresponds to it [in the other]. For water and generally damp bodies seem to be nourishment for fire, but fire does not seem to be nourishment for something [else]. After he had explained that this opinion is weak, if it is taken without qualification, he explained that this opinion is found only in the case of the elements. He said: **In simple bodies, however,** etc. That is, to think, however, that what takes nourishment is contrary to what is able to take nourishment is [a view] found properly only in regard to these two simple bodies, one of which is fire and the other dampness, as water and air.

44. **But there is room for doubt in regard to this. For some say that like is nourished and likewise also made to grow by like. Some take the contrary position, namely, that contrary is nourished by its contrary, for like is not affected by its like,** {198} **and nourishment is changed and digested, and change in anything is toward an opposite disposition or to an intermediate one.** (416a29–34)

But [with respect to] that opinion, although it is found in the case of the elements through sense and induction, nevertheless in the very question there is room for doubt on the basis of well-known propositions. For there is one account which asserts that the nourishment is like and another which asserts that the nourishment is contrary. Next he gave the reasoning for each account. He said: **For some say,** etc. That is, for some of the ancients held the opinion that the nourishment ought to be like, because like nourishes its like and causes it to grow. For contrary changes its contrary but neither nourishes it nor causes it to grow. After he had given this reason, he also gave the reason that the nourishment is a contrary. He said: **Some take the contrary position.** That is, they said this, namely, that the contrary is nourished by its contrary, not by its like, because they held the opinion that nourishment is affected by what is able to take nourishment, and like is not affected by its like; therefore, nourishment is not something like. After they had also seen that nourishment is changed into what is able to take nourishment and is affected, and every change is from contrary to contrary, or to that which is intermediate between contraries, they concluded from this that nourishment is among the contraries.

45. **Furthermore, nourishment is affected in some way by what is able to take nourishment, but not the converse, as the carpenter [is] not [affected] by the material, but rather the material by him. The carpenter is changed only to action from inaction. Therefore, there is a difference between nourishment as what {199} is united at the end [of the process] and as what is united at the beginning. If, therefore, each is nourishment, but one is what is to be digested and the other what has been digested, then it is possible to say that each is nourishment. However, insofar as it is not digested, contrary is fed by its contrary, but insofar as [it has been] digested, like [is fed] by like. It is evident, however, that [what] each of those groups [holds] is said in a way to be true and in a way to be untrue.** (416a34–b9)

Furthermore, nourishment is affected in some way, etc. It can be understood that this account is, as it were, a figuring aiding one who says that nourishment is contrary and dispelling objections which contradict this account. For someone can say that if nourishment is contrary to what is able to take nourishment, it would be necessary that each be changed by what corresponds to it [in the other] and be affected by it. He speaks as if responding to the position that nourishment concerns what is affected by what is able to take nourishment, not what is able to take nourishment by what is nourishment. For it is not necessary that an agent be affected by every patient in the same way in which the patient is affected by [the agent]. For wood is affected by the carpenter, but the carpenter is not affected by the wood, unless someone calls that change which is from inactivity to operation an affection. Perhaps that account was placed before what he wishes [to say] in dissolution of that difficulty to show what truth was contained in each of those two opposite accounts. Since after this is known concerning nourishment and what is able to take nourishment—namely, that nourishment is what is changed {200} into the form of what is able to take nourishment, not what is able to take nourishment into the form of what is nourishment, and not each equally by what corresponds to it [in the other], and that the case of nourishment in relation to what is able to take nourishment is just as [is] the case of the carpenter in relation to wood, not as contraries which share in the same matter—it will be immediately explained that nourishment is said in two ways. For it is said of what is still not digested and not changed into the nature of what is able to take nourishment, and it is also said of what has been digested and is changed into the nature of what is able to take nourishment, because that food is like is [something which is] truly said of what has been digested and the contrary of what has not been digested. For this reason he said later: **Therefore, there is a difference between nourishment,** etc. That is, since what takes nourishment is what transforms the nourishment into its substance, it is evident that there is a great difference between the nourishment which was conjoined with what is able to take nourishment at the completion of digestion and what is naturally constituted to be united with what is able to take nourishment, but [has] not yet [been so united].[103]

Next he said: **If, therefore, each is nourishment,** etc. That is, if, therefore, this name nourishment is said of each, but one of them is nourishment in potency (since it is its nature to be digested but it is still not yet digested) and the other is actually nourishment (and that is what is already digested), [then] we can truly say each of food, namely, that it is like and unlike, without any contradiction. For these two accounts were not contraries, unless this name nourishment were said in the same way. For undigested nourishment, which is nourishment in potency, can be said truly to be a contrary. For what takes nourishment acts on it only insofar as it is contrary. Digested nourishment, {201} however, can be said to be like, for it is part of what is able to take nourishment only insofar as it is like. Next he said: **It is evident, however, that [what] each of** the two **groups,** etc. That is, it is therefore evident from this account that in the account of each of those two groups there is a part which is true and a part false.

46. **And because nothing takes nourishment unless it takes part in life, for this reason a body which is alive is something which is able to take nourishment insofar as it is alive. Nourishment, therefore, is ascribed to what is alive in a way which is not accidental.** (416b9–11)

Because nothing seems to take nourishment unless it shares some one of the intentions of which this name life is said, as was explained, for this reason a body takes nourishment only insofar as it has soul, not insofar as it is body. That action, therefore, is ascribed to the soul in an essential way, not in an accidental way, and the substance of the part of the soul to which that action is ascribed is nothing but the power which is naturally constituted to have that action. When, therefore, we come to know that action in a proper way, we will then come to know the substance of that power in a proper way.

47. **Being nourishment is different from being something which can cause growth.[104] It is nourishment, however, insofar as it is a determinate particu-**

103. That is, there is a great difference between potential nourishment assimilated as actual nourishment and potential nourishment unassimilated.

104. Averroes' Text here omits a line of the Greek: "Food has a power which is other than the power to increase the bulk of what is fed by it; <u>so far forth as what has soul in</u>

lar and a substance, and because it preserves the substance of what is able to take nourishment, since {202} it always takes nourishment.[105] And it causes generation, not because it is self-generating, but because it causes the generation of what is like what is able to take nourishment, for that has being. And nothing generates itself, but [a thing] does preserve itself. (416b11–17)

He wants to distinguish three actions of nourishment, namely, to take nourishment, to cause growth, and to generate.[106] He said: **Being nourishment**, etc. That is, for something to be nourishment or nutritive is different from its being a cause of growth. For it is called nourishment insofar as it preserves the substance of the thing which is able to take nourishment so that it does not suffer corruption, for it provides it with something in place of what is dissipated. For this reason it endures in being so long as it is nourished and when nourishment ceases, it suffers corruption. It is a cause of growth insofar as it perfects the natural quantity of that which is diminished at the start by necessity. But he said nothing about this, since the difference between growth and nourishment is evident (if perhaps there is no omission on the part of the scribe). After he distinguished these two actions, he began to speak of the third action, which is to generate. He said: It is something which causes **generation**, etc. That is, nourishment has an action other than preservation and growth, namely, to generate. Next he expounded on generation. He said: not the generation of what is able to take nourishment, **but the generation of what is like**

---

it is a quantum, food may increase its quantity [ᾗ μὲν γὰρ ποσόν τι τὸ ἔμψυχον, αὐξητικόν], but it is only so far as what has soul in it is a 'this-somewhat' or substance that food acts *as* food; in that case it maintains the being of what is fed, and that continues to be what it is so long as the process of nutrition continues." Aristotle, *De Anima* (1984); emphasis in original; Greek and underlining added. Averroes is aware that there are problems with the Text here. See below in his Comment, where he mentions that the Text may be faulty because of scribal error. The omission also affects the understanding of the line that follows, where the Greek ᾗ δὲ τόδε τι καὶ οὐσία, τροφή is found rendered *Est autem nutrimentum secundum hoc et substantiam*. For this Text Averroes' alternate translation is in different ways also imperfect (e.g., rendering ᾗ δὲ τόδε τι καὶ οὐσία as only جوهر, "a substance") and suffers omissions (e.g., ἤδη γὰρ ἔστιν αὐτοῦ ἡ οὐσία, "the substance of the individual fed is already in existence" [ibid.], which is rendered in the Latin as *illud enim habet esse*) but reflects the Greek somewhat better than what we find in the Latin. See ibid. (1954).

105. Although Averroes' Text is much less clear than the Greek, "in that case it maintains the being of what is fed, and that continues to be what it is so long as the process of nutrition continues," (Aristotle, *De Anima* [1984]), his comment shows he understands the Text in accord with the Greek.

106. Cf. Themistius, *De Anima Paraphrase*, (1899), 53.9–10, (1973), 75.8; (1996), 72.

what is able to take nourishment, that is, [like] in species. Next he said: **for that has being**. This can be understood [in this way]: for that is in every way its own being,[107] and it preserves what is able to generate so that it may endure as one in species, as we said earlier.[108] Next he said: **And nothing generates itself, but [a thing] does preserve itself.** That is, there is a difference between these two actions because to take nourishment {203} is to preserve itself and this generating is to generate another, not itself. For it is impossible for something to generate itself.

48. **This principle, therefore, is a power of the soul which is able to preserve what belongs to it as a disposition. And nourishment is that by virtue of which it is prepared for acting. For this reason, when nourishment is lacking, it is impossible for it to exist.** (416b17–20)

It was explained that those actions are different in accord with the diversity of their ends, although the subject is the same, namely, nourishment. It is also necessary that those actions be ascribed to some power belonging to the soul and, since it is so, it is necessary that this principle of soul, namely, the nutritive power, be a power which can preserve a being in its form according to a [certain] disposition, that is, according to some disposition of preservation. He said this because there are some powers which preserve being according to every disposition and all its parts in the same mode, namely, the powers of the heavenly bodies.

Next he said: **And nourishment is that by virtue of which it is prepared**, etc. That is, nourishment is an instrument through which it carries out this action [of self-preservation]. For this reason, when that power lacks nourishment, then it does not have this action [of self-preservation], just as the carpenter, when he lacks a saw, is not able to saw.

49. **They are, therefore, three: what is able to take nourishment, that by which it is nourished, and the agent which brings about nourishment. The agent which brings about nourishment, then, is the first soul; what is able to take nourishment is the body; and that {204} by which it is nourished is nourishment. And because all things must be named from their ends, and the end is to generate [its] like, for this reason the first soul is what generates [its] like.** (416b20–25)

107. That is, that nourishment is a being and material substance in its own right. This is how Averroes understands the Text. In the Greek text, however, Aristotle seems rather to be referring to that which takes nourishment and to be saying that it is a substance in its own right already prior to taking nourishment and that it does not generate itself though it does preserve itself through nourishment.

108. See Book 2, Text 35 {183}.

After he had described this principle of the soul and described nourishment, he returned to distinguish the intentions of those names which are denominated by nourishment. He said: **They are, therefore, three**, etc. That is, it is self-evident that the three are different according to the diversity of related things: one is what is able to take nourishment, the second that by which it is nourished, and the third is what nourishes. And it was already explained that what is the agent for nourishment is the soul to which this action is ascribed. Hence it is evident that the agent for nourishment is the soul, which is first among the rest of the powers which are ascribed to nourishment; and he means by first here what is prior by nature. What is able to take nourishment is the body and that by which it is nourished is food. Next he said: **And because all things must**, etc. That is, because all things must be named from their ends, since this final cause is more befitting the being of the thing than all the [other] causes, it is necessary that the nutritive soul be described through the action which is its end, and it is to generate its like, [and] not through the action of taking nourishment, which is to preserve [itself], as we said earlier. It should, therefore, be said that the nutritive soul is a power which is naturally constituted to generate from food something like in species to the individual in which it exists, since all its actions are only for the sake of this power. This is evident in plants and in animals.

50. **That by which it is nourished is twofold (just as that by which a ship is steered: both the hand and the rudder), one is mover and moved and the other is only mover. {205} It is necessary that all nourishment be capable of being digested; and what causes digestion to take place is heat; hence every living thing has heat. We, then, already said in outline what food is. Later we will give an [extensive] account of it.** (416b25–31)

After he had shown the ways of the nutritive soul's action and both described [that action] and described nourishment, he began now to explain the first instrument by which that soul acts upon food. For he had already said in a general way that the definition of the soul is the actuality of a body having organs. He said: **That by which it is nourished**, etc. That is, that by which the action of nourishment is brought to completion is twofold, namely, a first mover which is not moved while it moves, and a mover which moves and is moved. That is what is related to the first mover as subject, and the first mover [is] related to this as form.[109] Concerning what he said, some things he explained here and some in the general accounts. What was said here, then, is that the nutritive soul is the first mover in regard to the food and that it acts

109. That is, the moved mover is related to the first mover as its subject, and the first mover is related to the moved mover as its form.

upon the food by means of heat by which [the food] becomes digested. But whether it is necessary that it move and not be moved, insofar as it is a first mover, and that heat move in such a way that it is moved by a first mover, was explained in the general accounts. For there it was explained that if every first mover were bodily, it would be composed of a mover which is not moved and a mover which is moved, insofar as things are composed from matter and form.[110]

But there is a difficulty in regard to what he said. For the motion of the nutritive power is in the category of alteration, and what is self-moved, which is composed of an unmoved mover and a moved mover, is found only in local motion. {206} In the motion of alteration, however, self-motion is not found, for it is not necessary that a first bodily cause of alteration suffer alteration and then alter [something else], as is necessary in the case of the first bodily mover, namely, that it move in place only if it is moved. How, then, did he say here that one of them is mover and moved and the other only mover, while he gave an example from things moving in place? If this were said of the local motion of animals, then the example would be sound. Let us say then: that the proximate mover of food ought to be a body is evident; but that the body causing alteration is not sufficient to be the first mover causing that motion was explained earlier, when he said that heat is not sufficient to bring about the completed action of alteration, unless some power which is not a body but in a body be there. The body, therefore, which is the first cause of alteration, is composed of what causes alteration but does not suffer alteration, namely, the soul, and what causes alteration and is altered, namely, natural heat. It was explained, therefore, that that by which nourishment comes about is twofold, namely, what causes alteration but does not suffer alteration (for everything which suffers alteration is a body), and this is the soul, and what causes alteration and suffers alteration, namely, natural heat. This name motion, therefore, is taken in a broad and general way in this passage. According to this exposition, what was explained in that account is not needed, namely, that the first mover in place be composed of an unmoved mover and a moved mover. We can say that natural heat alters food only if it is first moved in place. For it was explained that local motion precedes the other motions and in particular that motion which is complete, namely, which alters the thing at one time and not at another. And also it not only alters, but it takes into itself and expels food, and this is local motion. {207} According to this exposition the disposition will be evident, but the first exposition seems more fitting. Also, the example was taken in a broad sense, for the hand is not the first unmoved mover of the ship, but rather the pilot himself. After it had been explained that the

110. See *Physics* 8.4, 255a28, and 8.5, 257a32ff.

nutritive soul is a form in the body, since the proximate cause of alteration in the body, which is food, ought necessarily to be a body, and that the form is an unaltered cause of alteration, since it is not a body, and that the body is an altered cause of alteration, he then began to explain what this body is. He said: **All nourishment** must necessarily, etc. That is, all nourishment which is already nourishment in actuality must necessarily be digested by means of a body which is a cause of alteration [and] which is an instrument of the nutritive soul. Since this body ought to be a cause of alteration and digestion, and such is a warm body (hence the ancients said that fire nourishes), everything having a nutritive soul must necessarily possess heat, not without qualification but rather natural heat. For it was explained in the fourth book of the *Meteorology*[111] that what causes digestion is heat belonging to that being, not extraneous [heat]. Next he said: **We, then, already said in outline**, that is, in a general and broad way. . . , etc. That is, the completion of the account in regard to each of their parts from which nourishment is constituted should be expounded later in an appropriate place. He said this because the account concerning nourishment and growth is realized only in several books. For in the book *On Generation and Corruption*, motion of growth and diminution was established,[112] while in the *Meteorology* the kinds of heat and [their] kinds of actions were established, such as to be boiled and {208} to be roasted.[113] In this book the first mover in those motions was also explained, while also in the book *On Animals* it was established how many instruments of that power there are in each animal, how action is brought to completion by [that power] in the case of each of them, and how many members there are and how those members serve [each animal], and what is the nature of the relationship of those to one another in that action, and so forth.[114] For this reason he said that the explanation of nourishment given here only concerned the first mover and the first instrument alone.

51. **Since we have already established those things, let us now speak in regard to all sensation in a general way. Let us say, then, that sensing occurs with motion and affection, as we said, for it is thought to be some sort of alteration. Some say that like is affected by its like and unlike by unlike.**[115]

111. *Meteorology* 4.3, 381b4–9.
112. *On Generation and Corruption* 1.5, 320b26–322a34.
113. *Meteorology* 4. Cf. 4.3, 380b13ff.
114. *Parts of Animals* 2–4.
115. These last four words are additions to the text of Aristotle, which has φασὶ δέ τινες καὶ τὸ ὅμοιον ὑπὸ τοῦ ὁμοίου πάσχειν; "Now some thinkers assert that like is affected only by like." Aristotle, *De Anima* (1984). Averroes' Comment below indicates that he read what we find in the Text. Averroes' corresponding remark in his *Middle*

We already spoke of acting and being affected and how they can come to be or not come to be in the general accounts,[116] and in this passage we have also spoken of it.[117] (2.5, 416b32–417a2)

After he had spoken of the nutritive power, he began to speak of the sensitive [power] and first of what is common to all the senses. He said: **Let us say, therefore, that sensing**, etc. That is, let us therefore say that sensing comes about through an affection and motion in the senses from sensible things, not through an action of the senses upon the sensible things. For this is what was first considered concerning sensation, namely, whether it is counted among the active or passive powers. After he had placed it in the genus of passive powers, he gave the reason for that view. {209} He said: **for it is thought**, etc. That is, we said that sensation comes about as an affection because it is thought that the senses are altered in some form of alteration by sensible things. He said **some sort of** in order to signify what is specific to it, because later it will be explained that this change is called an alteration only equivocally. Next he said: **Some say that like**, etc. That is, since we asserted that affection is the genus of sensation, consideration should be given to the things in which the affection exists, for some say that like is affected by its like and some the contrary, namely, that contrary is affected by its contrary. He meant here by **general accounts** the book *On Generation and Corruption*. What was established in that book is not sufficient for him because here the account seems to be more specific, for the subject of which he speaks here is more specific than the subject of which he spoke there. He first began to raise questions in his assertion that sensation is one of the passive powers, not one of the active ones.

52. **But it is irrational [to ask][118] why the senses do not sense themselves and why also no sense acts in absence of something external, while fire, earth, and the other elements are in them and are what are apprehended by the sense per se, and [likewise for] the accidents consequent upon them. Let us say, therefore, that the sense is not in act but only in potency and for this**

Commentary (2002), at 60.17–18, is similar: و بعضهم قال إن غير الشبيه ينفعل عن غير شبيهه; "others say that it is affected by that which is unlike it." Averroes' alternate translation, however, does not contain this addition. See Aristotle, *De Anima* (1954).

116. *On Generation and Corruption* 1.7, 323b1ff.

117. The Greek version is slightly different: "in what sense this is possible and in what sense impossible, we have explained in our general discussion of acting and being acted upon." Aristotle, *De Anima* (1984).

118. *Sed est irrationabile*. The Greek has ἔχει δ ἀπορίαν; "Here arises a problem" (Aristotle, *De Anima* [1984]), which is reflected in Averroes' alternate translation: ولنا في الحواس مسألة (ibid. [1954]); "Concerning the senses we have a question."

**reason we do not have sensation, just as what is combustible does not burn
by itself in the absence of something causing it to burn. If this were not so,
it would cause itself to burn and not need fire to be in act.** (417a2–9) {210}

After he had asserted sensation to be among the passive powers, he began
to raise questions about pressing the position that it is among the passive and
not the active powers, and this is the case if he does not mean by "it is thought"
"it is confirmed," for he often uses "thought" for "certainty." He said: **But it is
irrational [to ask] why the senses do not sense themselves.** That is, as it seems
to me, but it is irrational, since we will have asserted that the sensitive powers
are active, to say why the senses do not sense in their own right in the absence
of something external. For it is necessary, if the sensitive powers were active,
to say that the senses sense in their own right and that they do not need something external for their sensing. Next he said: Among them are **fire, earth, and
the other elements**. That is, the composition of some of the senses is ascribed
to each of the elements and those are sensible things; therefore, they must sense
themselves. He meant this when he said: **the accidents consequent upon them**,
that is, things consequent upon those sensible things from which the instruments of those senses are composed. After he had explained that it is irrational
to say why the senses do not sense in the absence of something external, if we
have asserted that the senses are among the active powers, he began to explain
the way in which there will be a response to this question. He said: **Let us say,
therefore, that the sense is not in act but . . . in potency,** etc. That is, let us
therefore say in response that sensation is not among the active powers which
act in their own right without need of an external mover in the action which
comes from them, but rather they are among the passive powers, which need
an external mover. For this reason they do not sense in their own right, just as
what is combustible does not burn in its own right without an external mover,
namely, fire. And just as {211} in the case of what is combustible, if it were combustible in its own right, it would be possible for it to burn without fire existing
in act, so too if the senses would sense in their own right, insofar as they are
active powers, then it would be possible for them to sense in the absence of
anything extrinsic. You ought to know that this is the first difference by which
the powers of the soul differ from one another and it is a starting point for the
consideration of the intellect and the other powers.[119] However, that the nutritive
power is among the active powers is evident from what was said earlier.

53. **Because there are two ways to say that something senses (for what
hears and sees in potency we say hears and sees even though it may be**

---

119. Cf. Themistius, *De Anima Paraphrase,* (1899), 54.28–55.2; (1973), 78.14–79.7;
(1996), 74.

sleeping and we [also] say this in regard to what achieves act), hence [it is that] **sensation is spoken of both in potency and in act. And similarly sensing also exists in potency and exists in act.** (417a9–14)

He had explained that sensation is one of the passive powers, not one of the active powers, and [that] those [passive powers] have a twofold being, namely, being in potency before their powers are perfected by an external mover and being in act, when they are completed and found in actuality by an external mover in act. [Now] he began to explain that these two occur in the case of the powers of the soul. He said: **Because there are two ways to say that something senses,** etc. That is, because it is self-evident that there are two ways to say that something senses, one of which is when we say in regard to someone hearing and seeing in potency that he hears and sees, as we say of one who is sleeping. He meant this when he said: **for what hears and sees,** etc. That is, for what one who hears and one who sees in proximate potency is customarily said to be is one who hears and one who sees, even though one who is sleeping is one who is more removed {212} in all the modes of potency. For what is in darkness is a seer in potency, but that potency is more near to act than a potency which belongs to the vision of one who is sleeping. Next he said: **this is said in regard to** what **achieves** act. That is, what attains sight and hearing and in general sensing of sensible things is also said to hear, to see, and in general to sense. After he had explained that this word **sense** is said of each intention,[120] he said: It is necessary that sense also be said in two ways, of potentiality and **actuality, and similarly sensing,** etc. That is, similarly sensing, which is an action of sense, must be said also in two ways, as of a disposition and a form from which sensing arises.

54. **In the first place, then, our account is not**[121] **insofar as being affected and being moved is the same as acting and moving. For motion is an action, but an imperfect one, as was said in other places. And everything which is affected and moved is affected and moved only by some agent in act. For this reason being affected is sometimes by like and sometimes by unlike. According to what we said, what is affected is unlike and, after it is affected, it becomes like.** (417a14–21)

120. Arabic fragments correspond to Book 2, 53.27–28: ولما عرف ان العادة جرت ان يطلق اسم «الحس» على هذين المعنيين (*Long Commentary* Fragments [1985], 38).

121. The Greek text has οὖν, "then," rather than οὐ, "not," where Averroes' Text has *non*, "not." "To begin with let us speak as if there were no difference between being moved or affected, and being active, for movement is a kind of activity." Aristotle, *De Anima* (1984). The alternate Arabic translation reflects the Greek suitably enough with the particle ﻓ rendering οὖν. Ibid. (1954).

After he had explained that sensation is one of the passive powers and that it exists in two ways, he said: **[In the first place,] then our account,** etc. That is, there is a great difference between the account of sensation presenting the opinion that it is a passive power and the account of it presenting the opinion that it is an active power. For the account of something insofar as we hold in regard to it the opinion that its being is to be affected and to be moved is different from the account in regard to it insofar as we hold the opinion that its being is to act and to move. After he had explained this, {213} he provided the difference between each of these two beings. He said: **For motion is an action, but an imperfect one,** etc. That is, these two kinds of being are different. For the being of one kind is of the genus of the being of motion, and it was already explained that motion is an imperfect action (for it is the actuality of something in potency insofar as it is in potency). But the being of the other kind is a perfect action. Next he provided another difference between these two beings. He said: **And everything which is affected and moved,** etc. That is, they differ also since everything counted in the genus of affection[122] has being only from another, namely, the agent, and for this reason, if the agent does not exist, this will not exist. But everything counted in the genus of action has being in itself, not from another. Next he said: **For this reason being affected is sometimes by like,** etc. That is, because the being of passive powers is a mixture of potency and act, for before it is affected, the passive is contrary to the agent, and when the affection is completed, it is like, and, while it is being affected, it is a mixture of like and contrary. For so long as it is moved part of the contrary does not cease to be corrupted in it and part of the like [does not cease] to come to be. It is evident that one who does not understand that there are passive powers in such a being [as this] will not be able to solve the question mentioned earlier,[123] nor also can one who has not conceded that the powers of sensation are among the passive powers even say whether the sensible thing is like or contrary. This is the foundation and it must be preserved as we said in regard to the other powers of the soul, and chiefly in regard to the rational power, as will appear later.[124]

55. **We must also determine potency and actuality, since in this passage we spoke of these without qualification. Let us, therefore, say what we mean when {214} we say of something, for instance a man, that he is a knower, because a human being is among those having knowledge. Sometimes we say this as we say of one who already has acquired the science of**

122. That is, what is acted upon by something else.

123. See Book 2, Text 52 {209}.

124. See Book 3, Text and Comment 3 {381–383}.

grammar that he is a knower. But the potency in each of them is not of the same sort. Rather, the potency of the first is because its genus is of such a sort,[125] while [the potency] of the second is because, when he wishes, he is able to exercise knowledge, so long as something external does not impede him. (417a21–28)

After he had explained that sense is said in two ways, namely, in potency and in act, and also that each of those is said in two ways, he began to make determinations regarding this. He said: It is necessary also to determine, etc. That is, since we know that sense is found in two ways, namely, in potency and in act, we must determine the intentions in which potency, actuality, and act are said without qualification, since in this passage we speak of them only without qualification. After he had given the reason why it is necessary to speak in this passage about potency and act without qualification, namely, that they exist in sensation without qualification, he said: **Let us, therefore, say what we mean**, etc. That is, let us therefore say that it is evident that when we say that something is such in potency, that this is meant in two ways: either as we say that a human being is a knower in potency, that is, naturally constituted to have knowledge, or as we say in regard to one who knows grammar in act that he is a knower in potency when he does not use his knowledge. After he had explained those two modes of potency, he provided the difference between them. He said: **But the potency in each . . . is not of the same sort**, etc. That is, but the intention of potency in each of them is not the same. Rather, since we say that someone ignorant is a knower in potency, we mean that his genus {215} and matter is receptive to knowledge; and when we say in regard to one who knows grammar that he is a knower in potency, it is said because he has the potency for contemplating grammar when he wishes.[126]

125. The Text here drops the Greek καὶ ἡ ὕλη, "or matter" (Aristotle, *De Anima* [1984]), which is found in Averroes' alternate translation as كهيولى (ibid. [1954]) and which reappears in Averroes' Comment.

126. That we are able to excercise our ability to think when we wish is important for Averroes' assertion that the material and agent intellects are in us. See, for example, {390}, {406}, {437}, and {438}. At the corresponding text in Themistius, *De Anima Paraphrase* (1899), 56.20–24; (1973), 82.17–83.1, we find sensation distinguished from knowledge by the fact that "knowledge has the objects of knowledge from within, in that thoughts are universal objects of knowledge that it amasses and stores for itself. And it is in its power to make them available for itself whenever it wishes, while for sense-perception there are particular (i.e. individual) objects, but these are external and the activity of nature, not of the soul. That is why it is in our power to think whenever we wish, but not in our power to perceive." Ibid. (1996), 76. Also see ibid. (1899), 99.13; (1973), 179.11; (1996), 123; (1990), 90–91.

56. But one who is contemplating is in a state of actuality and is one who really knows this.[127] Those first two, therefore, are knowers in potency, but one of them will be altered by learning and will be changed many times over by habitual activity to a contrary disposition, while the other, when he is changed from having sensation or knowledge of grammar (but he is not acting)[will be altered and changed] up to the point that he acts.[128] Therefore its mode is different. (417a28–b2)

One who knows grammar in contemplating it is a knower according to complete actuality, and such a person we say is really a knower of what he contemplates, not insofar as he knows that but does not contemplate it in act. Next he said: **Those first two, therefore, are knowers in potency**, namely, one who does not know and one who knows but does not make use of his knowledge.

Next he said: **but one of them**, etc. That is, but one of them will be changed from potency into actuality when he is altered by learning and changed many times over from one state to the contrary disposition and from the contrary disposition to a state, until this state is firm and fixed. He means by state the form of knowledge and by **contrary disposition** ignorance. Next he said: **while the other**, when **he is changed from having sensation or knowledge of grammar (but he** is **not** understanding)[129] **up to the point that he acts**. That is, the one goes out from potency {216} into act and into complete actuality when he is changed from having sensation in act or knowledge of grammar in act at a time at which he is not understanding by it, to acting by it. The mode, therefore, of that power is another mode.

57. Affection is also not without qualification, but rather one is a corruption from a contrary and another seems more to be an eduction[130] of what is in potency by what is in act and is [its] like. That, then, is the disposition of what is in potency in relation to actuality, for only one having knowledge

---

127. The Greek has τόδε τὸ A, "e.g. this A" (Aristotle, De Anima [1984]), which Averroes' alternate translation reflects with «ألف) فعلم بالحقيقة أن هذا الحرف المشار إليه (ibid. [1954]).

128. The sense of the Text is not rendered well in the Latin translation. Aristotle here is saying that the second kind of knower in potency is one who has possession of sensation or knowledge of grammar but is not actively using it and then comes to put it to active use.

129. The difference between the Text and the Comment is likely due to an error based on the similarity of يفعل, "he acts," and يعقل, "he understands."

130. Evasio. The Greek has, "the maintenance [τὸ δὲ σωτηρία] of what is potential by the agency of what is actual" (Aristotle, De Anima [1984]); my addition of Greek and underlining) and is followed by Averroes' alternate translation: سلامة (ibid. [1954]).

contemplates. And this either is not an alteration, since there will be an addition to the actuality in him, or it is another kind of alteration. (417b2–7)

This word **affection** does not signify the same simple intention but rather one is the affection which is a corruption of a patient by a contrary by which it is affected, as the affection of the hot by the cold and the moist by the dry. Next he said: **and another seems more**, etc. That is, there is also the affection which is an eduction of what is affected in potency by what is in actuality and act, insofar as what is in act is like, not contrary, namely, drawing it out from potency to act, contrary to the disposition in the first [kind of] alteration. Next he said: **That, then, is the disposition**, etc. That is, that final mode of affection is the disposition of a part of the soul which is in potency in relation to the actuality which moves what is in potency and which draws [the potency] out into act, [though] not according to the first mode of affection. {217} Next he said: **for only one having knowledge contemplates**, etc. That is, that mode of affection is from a mode which is an eduction of the patient by what is moving it in act, not its corruption. For only one who knows contemplates something after he was not contemplating. This is not an alteration according to the first intention, which is the corruption of what is affected. Next he said: **since there is an addition to actuality in it**, etc. That is, because that change is not from non-being but is an addition in what is able to be transformed and a going toward actuality without there being a corruption or change there from non-being, it is asserted as a change from ignorance to knowledge.[131] [It is] as if he means that this is more remote from true alteration in two ways. For alteration which is an eduction of the patient is twofold, namely, change from non-being to actuality and change from first actuality to final [actuality], and this [latter] is the addition which he indicates. Next he said: **or it is another kind of alteration.** That is, that mode which is an eduction of the patient either is not called alteration or it will be another kind of alteration.

58. **Likewise, it is not right to say regarding what understands that it is altered when it understands, just as it is not said that the builder is altered when he builds. In the category of understanding**[132] **that [something] is reduced to actuality from what exists in potency is not rightly called learning, but rather must be given another name. One who learns after he was in potency and acquires knowledge from one who is a teacher in actuality, must either not be said at all to have been affected or [it must] be said that**

---

131. That is, there is a change from not actively knowing to actively knowing.

132. *In capitulo intelligendi*: [κατα] τὸ νοοῦν καὶ φρονοῦν, "in the case of thinking or understanding" (Aristotle, *De Anima* [1984]); العلم والفهم (ibid. [1954]).

alteration is twofold, namely, change to dispositions of non-being and change to a state and nature. (417b8–16) {218}

Likewise, it is not right to say of what comes from ignorance to knowledge, whose disposition is called learning, that it is altered. Similarly, it is not said of what is changed by this that it does not act by a state existing in it in act to what acts by it, as the carpenter who is changed from not being engaged in carpentry to being engaged in carpentry, the example which we find in the other translation.[133] Next he said: **[In the category of understanding] what is reduced to actuality,** etc. That is, he who acquires the actuality of knowledge after potency by a reduction to that which he had already acquired in the first place, then next lost it, ought not to be called by that name by which we call one who is in the first potency always and has never acquired that which is called learning. Rather, that mode ought to have another name.[134] That mode which he indicated is called recollection. He said this because Plato holds the opinion that learning and recollection are the same. Next he said: **One who learns after he was in potency,** etc. That is, change from ignorance into knowledge by a teacher who is a knower in actuality and in act necessarily either is not called alteration or is such that it is said that alteration takes place in two ways, one is the change which comes about through an agent in dispositions which were not yet existing in a patient and the other is the change which comes about from the agent in the disposition of a state and form existing[135] in the patient. The latter is an affection which is the corruption of the patient, not an eduction. This is what he said before: **or it is another genus of alteration.**[136]

133. كما أنه لا يحسن أن يقول في البناء إذا بنى (Aristotle, *De Anima* [1954]); "just as it is not right that it be said when he builds."

134. Arabic fragments correspond to Book 2, 58.25: بل يجب ان يلقب بلقب آخر (*Long Commentary* Fragments [1985], 38).

135. Arabic fragments correspond to Book 2, 58.29–35: يعني ان كانت الاستحالة أيضا على حال خروج المتعلم من الجهل الى العلم – وهو حصول العلم بالاستكمال والفعل – فينبغي اما الا يسمى ذلك انفعالا واستحالة ، واما ان يسمى على انه معنى آخر حتى يقال ان الاستحالة ضربان : أحدهما تغير المستحيل وحصول حال ما فيه ﴿بدون انفعال عن الفاعل﴾ والآخر ﴿الاستحالة عن طريق الملكة﴾ والصورة الحاصلة (*Long Commentary* Fragments [1985], 38). "He means that the change also to be a disposition of the emergence of the learner from ignorance to knowledge—which is the coming about of knowledge in completeness and act—so it is necessary either that this not be called affection or change, or that it be so called insofar as it has another meaning. In this way change has two senses, one of the two is the forming and coming about of a certain disposition in it <without affection on the part of the agent> and the other <the change by way of state> and form coming about."

136. 417b6–7, Book 2, Text 57.

59. The first alteration of what senses is from what generates [it], such that when it was generated, immediately the ability to sense exists just as knowledge exists. And what is also in act is like contemplating. Nevertheless, they do differ because in this the agents are external, as what is seen and heard, and likewise the other sensible things.[137] (417b16–21) {219}

The first change on the part of what senses, which is like the change of a human being from ignorance to knowledge through a teacher, is the change which comes about through the agent generating the animal, not from sensible things. He indicates this difference between the first actuality which has come to be in the sense and the last. For it is held that the first actuality of sense comes from the agent intelligence,[138] as is explained in the book *On Animals*,[139] but the second actuality comes from sensible things. Next he said: **such that**

137. Averroes' Text here is far less clear than the Greek: "In the case of what is to possess sense, the first transition is due to the action of the male parent and takes place before birth so that at birth the living thing is, in respect of sensation, at the stage which corresponds to the possession of knowledge. Actual sensation corresponds to the stage of the exercise of knowledge. But between the two cases compared there is a difference; the objects that excite the sensory powers to activity, the seen and the heard, etc., are outside." Aristotle, *De Anima* (1984).

138. *Ab intelligentia agenti.* This is the first occurrence of the term *intelligentia agens* in this work. Could the distinction of *intelligentia agens* from *intellectus agens* be one made by the translator, perhaps under the influence of the thought of Avicenna? The Arabic العقل الفعال can be rendered either way. For Averroes in the present work, the referent is the same for the terms "agent intelligence" and "agent intellect." See the introduction, pp. xix–xx, n. 10, and p. xxiv, n. 20. Also see Book 3, n. 732 {390} regarding the use of the phrase "intellect which is in act," *intellectus qui est in actu*, to denote the agent intellect.

139. See *Generation of Animals* 2.3, 736b21–28. Here Aristotle is concerned with intellect and says nothing about sense. "It remains, then, for the reason alone so to enter and alone to be divine, for no bodily activity has any connection with the activity of reason." 736b27–28. Aristotle, *Generation of Animals* (1984). The corresponding passage of the *Middle Commentary* (2002), 63.8–14, does not trace sensation to the agent intellect. Since the agent intellect is not generally held to be the cause of sensation for all animals, it may be that Averroes has in mind the apprehension and processing of bodily sensation by the internal sense powers of imagination, cogitation, and memory. These taken together as the cogitative power do constitute a "kind of reason" {449} by the preparation of denuded intentions for the separate intellects. Moreover, at {450} in explaining Aristotle, he writes, "Perhaps he indicated the material intellect in its first conjoining with us, namely, [in] the conjoining which is through nature." It may be, then, that the human ability for pre-intellectual formation of pure—albeit still individual—intentions in preparation for abstraction by intellect is an ability which he understands ultimately to come from the agent intellect via our natural affiliation and connection with the material intellect.

when it was made [to be], etc. That is, such that when the first power comes to be, immediately it will have sensation unless there is some impediment or sensible things are not present. This is like the knowledge which is in the knower who does not put the knowledge to use. Next he said: and to sense is just as to know. That is, the complete actuality of sense, which is to apprehend sensible things in act and to contemplate them, is like making use of knowledge and contemplation. Next he said: **And what is . . . in act is** similar to contemplation. That is, to have sensation in act is similar to contemplating and knowing. Next he said: But **they do differ**, etc. That is, but the first actuality of sense differs from the knowledge of the knower which is in act when he is not contemplating, in that what is the cause moving the first actuality of sense and what draws it out into the second [actuality] are external sensible things, such as visible things, and what moves the knower from the first actuality into the second is something united with the soul by a uniting in being.[140]

60. **The reason for this is that sense in act apprehends particulars, while science [apprehends] universals existing, as it were, in the soul itself. For this reason a human being can exercise understanding when he wishes, but not sense, because he requires a sensible object. That disposition is also in the knowledge of sensible things, for that cause is a cause {220} of them,[141] namely, that sensibles are from particular external things. But we will speak of these and expound on them later, and it will have [its] time.** (417b22–29)

The reason for the difference between sense and intellect in the acquisition of complete actuality lies in the fact that the mover is external in the case of sense and it is internal in the case of intellect. For sense in act is moved only by a motion which is called apprehending and [is dependent] upon sensible particular things which are outside the soul. Intellect, however, is moved to complete actuality by universal things and those are in the soul. He said: those are, **as it were, in the soul**, because he will explain later that these— which are from the first actuality in the intellect as sensibles from the first

---

140. *Copulatione in esse.* For Averroes the Aristotelian notion that knowing is a way of being entails that there is some joining in being with the separate material and agent intellects as well as with intentions in the inner senses derived from sensation when the second actuality of knowing takes place. Cf. {228}.

141. The Latin *ista enim causa est causa* is based on a corrupt Arabic text, apparently due to a confusion between علم, "knowledge," and علة, "cause." In the Greek this is καὶ διὰ τὴν αὐτὴν αἰτίαν, "on the same ground" (Aristotle, *De Anima* [1984]); لعلمنا بنا من أجل هذه العلة بعينها (ibid. [1954]); "Our knowledge is by way of this cause itself." From Averroes' Comment it is perhaps likely that he read the sort of thing we find in the Latin in his Arabic Text.

actuality of sense, namely, insofar as both cause motion—are intentions which can be imagined and those are universal in potency, although not in act. For this reason he said: those are, **as it were, in the soul**, and he did not say "they are," because a universal intention is different from an imagined intention. Next he said: **For this reason a human being can exercise understanding**, etc. That is, because the things which move the rational power are inside the soul and possessed by us always in act, for this reason a human being can contemplate them when he wishes and this is called "to conceptualize,"[142] and he cannot sense when he wishes because he necessarily needs sensibles which are outside the soul. Next he said: **That disposition is also**, etc. That is, that disposition is also in us in the case of the knowledge of sensibles and we learn from them because they exist in the senses. The cause for the existence of that disposition in us for the knowledge of sensibles is the same as the cause for their existence in the senses themselves. Similarly we should understand {221} that the disposition existing in us for the knowledge of universals is in us because it is in the rational power and the reason that we are in this mode through that [disposition] is the reason why [that power] is in that mode.[143] But because the account in regard to the intellect is not evident here, he referred us to another time. He said: **But** the account concerning **those** things, that is, concerning the intellect. One can say that sensibles do not move the senses in accord with the way they exist outside the soul, for they move the senses insofar as they are intentions, since in matter they are not intentions in act, but in potency. And one cannot say that this difference occurs by virtue of the difference of subject such that the intentions come to be on account of a spiritual matter which is the sense, not on account of an external mover. For it is better to think that the reason for the difference of matter is the difference of forms, rather than that the difference of matter is the reason for the difference of forms. Since it is so, we must assert that the external mover in the case of the senses is different from the sensibles, as was necessary in the case of the intellect. It was seen, therefore, that if we concede that the difference of forms is the reason for the difference of matter, it will be necessary that the mover be external. But Aristotle was silent about this because it is hidden in the case of sensation and is apparent in the case of intellect. You ought to give this consideration, since it requires investigation.

142. *Formare*. See Book 1, {6}, n. 14.

143. Human beings are linked to the agent and material intellects insofar as humans provide the images which are the basis for the knowledge which comes about in the material intellect. That knowledge in the material intellect and the activities of the agent and material intellects are together responsible for the knowledge and rationality which particular human beings have in this world. See Book 3 {388}, {406}, {416}.

61. **Now to this extent it may be determined that what is said to be in potency is not [so] without qualification, but of one sort it is said as it is said that a boy can lead an army and of another sort it is said as it is said of an experienced man, and the same goes for sense.** (417b29–32) {222}

The whole of what was explained from this account and in this passage is this. He means by **without qualification** one intention and he said that what is in potency is not one intention, but several. He said: **but** one **is said**, etc. That is, a sense is said to be in potency just as it is said that a boy is able to lead an army. This is a first remote potency from which, when a change comes about to proximate potency, it comes about through the generating agent and not through sensible things and it is similar to the potency for knowledge in one who is ignorant. Next he said: **and of another sort it is said as it is said of an experienced man, and it is similarly so with regard to sense.** He means the potency which is the first actuality of the sense, namely, that from which there comes to be the change to the complete actuality through sensible things themselves. It is like the one who knows when he is not using his knowledge. He means by all those things to explain that the power of a sense which receives sensible things is not a pure disposition,[144] as [is] the disposition which is in the boy for receiving knowledge, and that the power of sense is a certain act, as having a positive disposition when he does not make use of his positive disposition.[145]

62. **But because their differences are not named, and we already determined in regard to them that they are different and how, we must use [the terms] affection and alteration as [if they were] the real things. That which senses is in potency just as what is sensed in actuality, according to what we said. For while it is unlike it is affected and after it is affected, it is like.** (417b32–418a6) {223}

But the differences of potency and change belonging to things existing in the sensitive soul and in things which are alive do not have names of their own. We already explained that these are different and we explained the way in which they are different. It, consequently, seemed to us that it is necessary, insofar as that intention which we have explained concerning the soul does not have a name of its own, to give the name of affection and alteration to that which is the subject of real things. For this does no harm, since we already

144. *Pura preparatio.* That is, a receptive disposition and a directed receptivity.

145. Arabic fragments correspond to Book 2, 61.20–24: يعني ان قصده من ذلك كله ان يبين ان قوة الحس التي تقبل المحسوسات ليست استعدادا محضا بمنزلة الصبي الذي فيه استعداد لقبول العلم وانما هو فعل ما بمنزلة ⟨ملكة العالم⟩ في حين لا يستعمل علمه (*Long Commentary* Fragments [1985], 39). Note that for علمه, "his knowledge," the Latin translator has *suo habitu,* "his disposition."

determined the intention by which they differ. He said: **we must** because that intention lacks a common name and the adoption of a name already in common use is easier than conjuring up another name. After this had been explained concerning what has sense, he began to describe it in an unqualified way. He said: **That which senses in potency is just as what is sensed in actuality.** That is, it is therefore evident from what we said that what has sense in an unqualified way is what is in potency to the intention. We explained this concerning the potency [actualized] through the intention of a sensible thing in actuality, that is, that which is naturally constituted to be actualized by the intentions of sensible things, not by the sensible things themselves.[146] And if [it were] not [so], then the being of color in the sense of sight and in a body would be the same; and if it were so, then there would be no apprehension of its being in the sense of sight. For that reason he said: that which is **in potency is just as what is sensed in actuality,** and he did not say: that which is sensed in potency. For, if it were so, the being of color would be the same in the sense of sight and in its matter. Next he said: Therefore, **while it is unlike it is affected and after it is affected, it is like,** etc. That is, what occurs for it is what occurs for all things subject to alteration, as was said in the general account,[147] namely, that it is affected by what is sensible while it is not like it and, when the affection is completed, it will then be like.[148] {224}

---

146. The same notion is expressed in the *Middle Commentary* by way of a distinction between the perfection of the sense (استكمال) and the sensible in actuality (بالفعل). See *Middle Commentary* (2002), 64.5–10, and 178, n. 14.

147. See *On Generation and Corruption* 1.7, 323b18ff.

148. Arabic fragments correspond to Book 2, 62.27–36: لان اللون في البصر هو بعينه وجوده خارج العين في الجسم ، ولو كان الأمر كذلك لما كان يدرك وجوده في البصر ، ولذلك قال «وهو أن الحاس بالقوة يصير كالمحسوس بالاستكمال » ولم يقل» «انّ الحاس بالقوة هو المحسوس » فان كان ذلك كذلك لكان البصر بوجود اللون فيه ملونا باللون الذي في الجسم ، ثم قال : «والحاسة تنفعل عن المحسوس من جهة ما هي متشبهة ... » يعني ويلحقه جميع الأشياء المستحيلة ، وهو أنه ينفعل عن المحسوس ما دام غير شبيه به حتى إذا انفعل وتم انفعاله صار شبيها كما يظهر ذلك في الأقاويل الكلية (*Long Commentary* Fragments [1985], 39). Note that the Arabic contains a clause at the beginning of this section corresponding to Latin Book 2, 62.27, and differs from the Latin in other ways. "And if [it were] not [so], then the being of color in the sense of sight and in a body would be the same, *because the color in the sense of sight exists in its own right external to the eye in the body [seen];* and if it were so, then there would be no apprehension of its being in the sense of sight. For that reason he said: "it is the case that what senses in potency sees insofar as the sensible is in act" and he did not say: "that what senses in potency is the sensible." For, if it were so, then the sense of sight with the existence of color in it would be colored by the color which is in the body. Next he said: "the sense is affected by the sensible insofar as it is similar," etc. That is, what occurs for it is what occurs for all things subject

63. **Before we begin to speak of each of the senses, let us speak of sensible things. Let us say, then, that sensible is said in three ways, of which two are said to be sensed per se and the third accidentally. One of the two [first indicated] is proper to any given sense and the other is common to them all. And one calls proper what another sense cannot sense and what is such that it is impossible for there to be any error in regard to it, for instance, sight with reference to color, hearing with reference to sound, and taste with reference to flavor. Sense has several modes in one,**[149] **but each of them judges those things and it does not err in regard to color as to what color it is nor in regard to sound as to what sound it is,**[150] **but rather in regard to a colored thing as to what it is and where it is and in regard to something heard as to what it is and where it is. What, then, is of such a sort is proper.** (2.6, 418a7–17)

After he had explained what sense in an unqualified way is, he wants now to speak about each of the senses. Because he already said earlier that the way to [do] this is to speak about sensible things themselves, since they are better known than the senses, he said: **Before we begin to speak,** etc. That is, because it is necessary to go from these things which are better known from our point of view to those which are better known by nature,[151] we must first speak of sensible things themselves.

Because some sensible things are universal and some are proper, he began to speak of universal ones. He said: **Let us say, then, that** what is sensed, etc. His account in this chapter is clear. And when he said: **sense has several modes,** he means that the sensible objects of each of those {225} senses are several in one mode, but each of the senses judges its proper sensed object and does not err in regard to it for the most part.[152] For the sense of sight does not err in regard to color as to whether it is white or black, nor hearing in regard to sound as to

---

to alteration, namely, that it is affected by what is sensible while it is not like it until, when it is affected and the affection is complete, it becomes like, as is apparent in the general accounts." Additional Arabic emphasized in translation.

149. *Sensus autem plures modos uno habet. Sensus* here corresponds to the Greek ἡ δ᾽ ἁφή, "touch." Aristotle, *De Anima* (1984). Averroes makes no comment on this, although the alternate translation has اللمس (ibid. [1954]); "touch." Note that Latin manuscript C has *uno modo* for *uno.*

150. The Greek has καὶ οὐκ ἀπατᾶται ὅτι χρῶμα οὐδ᾽ ὅτι ψόφος, "never errs in reporting that what is before it or colour or sound" (Aristotle, *De Anima* [1984]). Averroes' alternate translation has وليس يدرك اللمس القرع و اللون (ibid. [1954]); "touch does not perceive sound and color."

151. Cf. *Physics* 1.1, 184a16–18.

152. Note that in contrast to this remark in the Comment, the Text has "it is impossible for there to be an error in regard to it."

whether it is low or high. But those senses do err in apprehending the differences of those sensible individuals, for instance, in apprehending that white thing which is snow or the differences of their places, for instance, so that it apprehends that this white thing is above or below. Next he said: **What, then, is of such a sort** is called **proper**. That is, sensibles which are found to belong to some sense alone which does not err in regard to them for the most part, are called proper. And when he said: **but rather in regard to a colored thing as to what it is and where it is and in regard to something heard as to what it is and where it is,** he did not mean that sense apprehends the essences of things, as some have thought, for this belongs to another power which is called intellect. Rather, he meant that the senses, with their apprehension of their proper sensibles, apprehend individual intentions which are different in genera and species. They, therefore, apprehend the intention of this individual human being and the intention of this individual horse and generally the intention of each of the ten categories of individuals. This seems to be proper to the senses of a human being. Hence, Aristotle says in the book *Sense and Sensibilia* that the senses of the other animals are not as the senses of a human being, or something like this statement.[153] That individual intention is what the cogitative power discerns from the imagined form and refines from the things which were added with it from those common and proper sensibles, {226} and it deposits it[154] in the memory. This same [individual intention] is what the imaginative [power] apprehends, but the imaginative [power] apprehends it as joined to those sensibles, although its apprehension is more[155] spiritual, as is explained elsewhere.[156]

64. **Motion, rest, number, shape, and quantity are common [to all the senses]. For those are not proper to any but all [are] common to them, for motion is sensed by touch and the sense of sight.** (418a17–20)

153. *Sense and Sensibilia* 1, 436b18–437a3. Cf. {219}.

154. I follow manuscripts B and G, with *eam* instead of *ea*.

155. Arabic fragments correspond to Book 2, 63.50–60: ان يكون هذا خاصا بحواس الانسان ولذلك يقول أرسطو في ⟨كتاب الحس والمحسوس⟩ ان حواس سائر الحيوان هي كالقشور بالنسبة لحواس الانسان أو شبيه بهذا الكلام. وهذا المعنى الشخصي هو الذي تميزة القوة المفكرة من الصورة المتخيلة وتجرده ⟨مما كان مقترنا به⟩ من هذه المحسوسات المشتركة والخاصة وتودعه الى الذاكرة. وهذا بعينه تدركه المتخيلة لكن تدركه مقترنا بهذه المحسوسات. وإذا كان ادراكها لها أتم ⟨روحانية ، كما لخصه هناك⟩ (*Long Commentary* Fragments [1985], 39). In the Arabic we find an analogy not found in the Latin: "that the senses of the rest of the animals are like shells in relation to the senses of human beings, or something like this statement." The printed text has المحسوسا, which must be an error for المحسوسات.

156. Cf. {416}. This important passage explaining the mediating role of cogitation in process toward intellectual understanding is key to the doctrine of cogitation developed in *Long Commentary* and is not at all touched upon in the corresponding passage of the *Middle Commentary*. See *Middle Commentary* (2002), 64.4–17.

After he had explained the proper mode from among the two essential modes, he began to explain the common mode. He said that they are five: motion, rest, etc. What he said: **For those are not proper,** etc., does not mean that each of those five is common to each of the senses, as Themistius understood,[157] and as it appears. Rather, three of them, namely, motion, rest, number, are common to all, but shape and quantity are common to touch and the sense of sight alone. He intends this by what he said: **but all [are] common to them,** etc, that is, but all are common to the senses, not all to all senses. That these sensibles, namely, the proper and the common, are ascribed to the senses in an essential way is evident, for we cannot ascribe the apprehension belonging to the senses to these in a way different from that by which they are senses. (This [sort of attribution], then, is the intention of what exists in an accidental way, which is opposed to what exists in an essential way.) For those[158] are things which can be apprehended and which belong to the senses insofar as they are senses, not insofar as they are certain [particular] senses.[159] {227}

65. **[To be] in an accidental way is said in regard to a thing because it is sensible just as the white thing is Socrates, for he is sensed only in an accidental way, for it happens to the white thing to be him. For this reason one is not affected by a sensible thing insofar as it is so [as a particular individual]. But what are sensible things per se and proper are sensibles in reality, and they are what the substance of each sense is naturally constituted to sense.** (418a20–25)

After he had explained the two modes of per se sensibles, namely, proper sensibles and common sensibles, he began to explain the third mode, which is the per accidens sensible. He said: **[To be] in an accidental way is said in regard to a thing because it is sensible,** that is, in this mode. Next he gave an example. He said: for **the white thing** which **Socrates** is **is sensed only in an accidental way.** That is, for to judge that this white thing is Socrates is to sense in an accidental way. Next he gave the reason. He said: **for it happens** that the white thing which is sensed is that thing. That is, we say that this apprehension is per accidens because we sense by the sense of sight that this thing is

157. Themistius, *De Anima Paraphrase* (1899), 57.16 and 57.36–58.14; (1973), 85.1–2 and 86.9–87.10; (1996), 77–78. In the *Middle Commentary* (2002), at 65.3–4, Averroes, as Ivry puts it, "believes he is following Themistius" and takes a position different from the one found here in the *Long Commentary*. He writes, "That which is common is movement, rest, number, shape and size—all the senses perceiving each of these." See Ivry's note at 178, n. 15.

158. That is, the proper and common sensibles.

159. That is, it is essential to them as senses, not as this or that particular sense.

Socrates only insofar as it is colored and the fact that this colored thing is Socrates is per accidens insofar as it is something colored. But one can say that shape, number, motion, and rest similarly occur for it. How, then, have those been counted among these which are essentially sensibles? For if they have been counted because they are common, similarly also the intentions of individuals are common to all the senses. In regard to this we can mention two accounts. One is that this commonness seems to be more necessary in the being of prior sensibles, for instance, of quantity. For color is not stripped from it, and likewise heat {228} and cold, which are associated with touch. Color, however, need not be in Socrates or Plato, neither with a proximate nor a remote necessity. Furthermore, common sensibles, as will be explained, are proper to the common sense (insofar as those are proper to any of the senses) and apprehension of the intention belonging to the individual is not, although it is an action of the common sense. And for this reason oftentimes it is required in the apprehension of the intention belonging to the individual that more than one sense be used, as physicians use more than one sense, in knowing the life of what is thought to have a mass of blood vessels.[160] Nevertheless, it seems that this action is not of the common sense, insofar as it is the common sense, but insofar as it is the sense of some animal, for instance, of an intelligent animal. That, then, is also another of the accidental modes, namely, that it happens to the senses to apprehend the differences of individuals (insofar as they are individual) not insofar as they are simple senses, but insofar as they are human senses. This is chiefly the case for substantial differences, for it seems that the apprehension of the intentions belonging to individual substances, which the intellect contemplates, is proper to the senses of a human being.[161] And you ought to know that the apprehension of the intention belonging to the individual belongs to the senses and the apprehension of the intention of the universal belongs to the intellect, whereas universality and individuality are apprehended by intellect, namely, the definition of the universal and of the individual. Next he said: **For this reason one is not affected**, etc. That is, the sense of sight is not affected by a sensible intention per accidens, for if it were affected by some individual insofar {229} as it is that individual,

160. *Et ideo pluries indigetur in comprehensione intentionis individui uti pluribus uno sensu, ut utuntur Medici, in sciendo vitam eius quod existimatur habere superpositionem venarum, pluribus uno sensu.* What Averroes intends here is apparently that at times one must look at something again and again using the same sense in order to perceive the object in its full complexity. In his example he may be referring to a ganglion, a cystic lesion resembling a tumor, consisting of a tangle of blood vessels. Cf. *Short Commentary on the De Anima* (1950), 27.13–14; (1985), 42.4–5; (1987), 127.

161. Cf. Book 2 {219–221}.

it ought not to be affected by another individual.[162] Next he said: **But what are sensible things per se**, etc. That is, of the two modes of things sensible per se, the proper are those which ought first to be counted in these which are essentially and are sensibles in reality and essentially, since those are what are sensed first and essentially; the others, however, although they are sensed essentially, nevertheless are not first. Next he said: **and they are what**, etc. That is, they are what are naturally constituted to be sensed first and essentially by any one of the senses and likewise the nature and being of any one of the senses is in sensing them.

66. **That, then, with which the sense of sight is concerned is the visible. And the visible is color and [the sort of thing] which can be spoken of but [in fact] is not spoken of.[163] What we are speaking of will be more apparent later. For the visible is color and this is visible per se. That is to say per se not according to [its] intention, but [because] a cause is found in it for its being visible.** (2.7, 418a26–31)

After he had completed the general account of sensibles, he returned to the account proper for each sensible and first to the sensible belonging to the sense of sight. He said: **That, then, with which the sense of sight is concerned,** etc. That is, it is self-evident that the sensible with which the sense of sight is concerned in a proper way is the visible. The visible is color and what

---

162. Arabic fragments correspond to Book 2, 65.45–55: ان ‹ادراك› المعنى الشخصي
‹عن طريق جوهره› الذي ينظر اليه العقل انما هو شيء يخص حواس الانسان وهي المعاني التي
تدل عليها أسماء الأشخاص وينبغي ان نعلم ان ادراك المعنى الشخصي للحواس ‹وادراك المعنى
الكلي للعقل› والكلي والشخصي هما مدركان بالعقل ، اعني حد الكلي والشخصي. ثم
قال : «‹ولذلك ليس ينفعل› أي ولكون المعنى الذي به زيد المشار اليه مدرك بالبصر بطريق
العرض صار البصر لا ينفعل عن ذلك المعنى المحسوس من طريق انه زيد أو عمر وفانه لا
انفعال عن شخص ما مشار اليه (*Long Commentary* Fragments [1985], 39); "that <the apprehension> of the individual intention which the intellect considers is that which is the proper object of the human senses. *These are the intentions which individual names indicate. We must know that* the apprehension of the individual intention belongs to the senses <and the apprehension of the universal intention belongs to the intellect>, and both the universal and the particular are apprehended by the intellect, namely, the definition of the universal and of the particular. Then he said, 'For this reason it is not affected,' that is, owing to the nature of the intention by which Zayd as a determinate particular is apprehended by the sense of sight incidentally, the sense of sight does not come to be affected by that sensed intention insofar as it is Amr or Zayd. For it is not an affection from a certain specific individual." Additional Arabic emphasized. The names Zayd and Amr are commonly used in examples for any given person.

163. *Et quod possible est dici sed non est dictum:* καὶ ὃ λόγῳ μὲν ἔστιν εἰπεῖν, ἀνώνυμον δὲ τυγχάνει ὄν, "a certain kind of object which can be described in words but which has no single name." Aristotle, *De Anima* (1984).

is like [color] among the things which are seen in the dark, which do not have a collective name[164] in color, nor do they even have in themselves a name which shows for them what is, as it were, a genus, but they can be explained only {230} with a complex account. For instance, we may say that they are those things which are seen in darkness and not seen in light, such as [phosphorescent] shellfish. Next he said: **[What we are speaking of] will be more apparent later.** That is, we will explain later the way in which it is said that color and those [other things] are visible, namely, whether this may be said equivocally or according to the prior and the posterior. Next he said: For **the visible is color**, etc. That is, for the visible in reality is color; but color is that which is per se visible. This is to say per se not according to the first of the intentions by which one speaks of what is essentially (this is the way in which the predicate is in the substance of the subject), but [per se] in the second intention (which is that in which the subject is in the definition of the predicate).[165] For color is the cause that the thing is visible.[166] And when he said, **but [because] a cause is found in it**, he means: insofar as color is the cause or the cause is found in it for something to be visible.

67. **And every color is a cause of motion in what is actually transparent; and this is its nature. For this reason it is not visible without light, but any**

164. *Nomen congregans.* That is, there is no collective or comprehensive name used of all of them.

165. Visible is not a constitutive part or a cause of what it is to be color. However, color is a constitutive part or cause of what it is to be visible. This is why Averroes goes on to say, "For color is the cause that the thing is visible." Cf. *Posterior Analytics* 1.4, 73a34–39. Ivry finds the account in the *Middle Commentary* different from this one. See *Middle Commentary* (2002), 179, n. 2. But the accounts are quite compatible when read in the context of the discussions of *per se* in the *Posterior Analytics*. To make this clear, in what follows I revise Ivry's translation by indicating the uses of *per se* (بذاته , بالذات , and بذاتها): "The truly visible, then, is color, and it is color which exists *per se* outside the soul. The visible is such only in relation to the viewer; and, therefore, our remark concerning its *per se* existence ought not to be understood as it is in the *Posterior Analytics*—namely, that the predicate is in the substance of the subject, or the subject in the substance of the predicate. This [kind of existence] is in contrast to that which is accidental, but that which is in contrast to what is *per se* here is that which is predicated in relation to another. [The essences of] some things are predicated *per se* without relation to anything else, while the essences of other things are predicated in relation to something else. Color belongs to those things which exist *per se*, while the visible belongs to those things which are predicable in relationship [to others]." *Middle Commentary* (2002), 66.3–11.

166. Cf. Themistius, *De Anima Paraphrase* (1899), 58.27–32; (1973), 88.11–89.5; (1996), 78. While Themistius may be the source, this is by no means a sufficient account of his position.

of the colors[167] necessarily is visible only in light. For this reason we ought to say what light is. And this will occur in the course of saying, as it were, what the transparent is. (418a31–b4)

The substance and being of color, insofar as it is visible, is that which moves what is transparent in act. Next he said: **and this is its nature**, etc. That is, that description shows {231} its nature and substance insofar as it is visible. The indication that color is what moves what is transparent in act, not transparent in potency, is that it will not be visible without light, by which the transparent in potency becomes the transparent in act. Either this shows that he holds the opinion that colors exist in act in darkness and if light is necessary for seeing color, then it is [so] only insofar as it makes the transparent in potency into the transparent in act; or [it shows] that he holds the opinion that light is necessary for seeing insofar as colors exist in potency in darkness, and insofar as the transparent, in order to receive color, needs to be transparent in act. Ibn Bâj-jah[168] had doubts about this description of the transparent and said that it is not necessary that the transparent, inasmuch as it is moved by color, be transparent in act. For its transparency in act is its illumination and its illumination is some color, for color is nothing but the mixture of a luminous body with a transparent body, as was said in the book *Sense and Sensibilia*.[169] And everything which receives something receives it only in the way in which it is lacking it. This forces him to explain this account in a way different from what was related by the commentators and he said: this is to say that color moves the transparent in act, that is to say, it moves the transparent from potency to act, not that it moves the transparent insofar as it is transparent.[170] Light, however, is necessary for seeing because colors in darkness are in potency and [light] makes them in act so that they move the transparent insofar as the transparent lacks light or [lacks] that which comes to be from light, namely, color. This explanation is very difficult, as expressed [here].

Alexander, however, gives a reason that the transparent in act {232} is moved by color on the basis of what is apparent. For air seems oftentimes to be colored by the color which we see with the mediation of the air, so that walls and earth are colored with the color of plants after the passage of the clouds above them.

167. *Unusquisque colorum.* The Greek has πᾶν τὸ ἐκάστου χρῶμα, "the colour of a thing" (Aristotle, *De Anima* [1984]). كل لون (ibid. [1954]); "every color."

168. **Avempeche**, or Avempace: Abu Bakr Muhammad Ibn Bâjjah. The translator consistently uses this name with the exception of Book 3, Comment 5 {397}, where he twice gives Abubacher.

169. See *Sense and Sensibilia* 3, 439a13–b18, though the definition of color is not altogether the same.

170. Ibn Bâjjah, *Book on the Soul* (1960), 108; (1961), 85–86.

If, then, air were not colored with the color of those plants, then the walls and earth would not be colored.[171] And it is evident that color, although it may come to be from a luminous body, nevertheless differs from it in definition and being, for color, as it is said, is the boundary of the determinate transparent, but light is the actuality of the indeterminate transparent.[172] Hence it is evident that it is not necessary that what is moved by color should be non-luminous but necessary that it should be uncolored. For nothing receives itself or is something's cause in receiving itself.[173] That proposition is self-evident and Aristotle uses it frequently. It makes no difference whether being moved and receiving is spiritual, as air receives color, or material, as a body which is a mixture of illuminated and dark transparent receives color. Since it is possible for the transparent in act to be moved by color, it is necessary that this belong to it either essentially or accidentally, namely, either insofar as it is transparent in act or insofar as it is transparent only but it happens to it that it is moved by colors only by being transparent in act, for this is insofar as it is transparent. That is the opinion of Ibn Bâjjah.[174]

But it is self-evident that light is necessary for colors to be visible. This will be either because it gives the colors the form and positive disposition by which they act on the transparent or because it gives the transparent the form by which it receives motion from colors, or both. It is evident, when we keep [in mind] {233} what Aristotle said in the beginning of that account (and he asserted it as self-evident), that then it will be necessary that light be necessary for there to be colors moving the transparent only insofar as it gives the transparent some form by which it receives motion from color, namely, illumination. For Aristotle asserted the principle that color is visible per se and that saying color is visible and a human being is able to laugh are similar, namely, from the kind of essential proposition in which the subject is the cause of the predicate, not the predicate the cause of the subject, as when it is said: human

171. "The proof that light and illuminated transparent substances are somehow set in motion by colors is the fact that we see light itself as being colored in the same way as the various colors which it makes visible to us by carrying them along with itself. Thus light is tinged with a yellow sheen when it is in contact with gold, it looks purple from contact with violets, and has the shade of grass when the object is green. We often observe, too, that a wall or pediment seems to have the same color as <a mural> standing opposite <the wall or mounted on a pediment>; and any people who happen to be standing <in the courtyard> will appear to us colored in this same way." Alexander, *De Anima* (1887), 42.11–19; (1979), 56–57.

172. See *Sense and Sensibilia* 3, 439b11–12.

173. That is, nothing is a potency for receiving what it already has in actuality. Cf. {231}.

174. Ibn Bâjjah, *Book on the Soul* (1960), 108–109; (1961), 86.

being is rational. He meant this when he said: but insofar as **a cause is found in it for its being visible**, as we have expounded. When this has been conceded, it is evident that it is impossible to say that light is what bestows upon color a positive disposition and form by which it becomes visible. For if it were so, then the relation of sight to color would be accidental and second, not first, namely, through the mediation of that positive disposition. For it is evident that sight is something posterior to the visible and that its relation to color is not like the relation of rational to human being. It is evident, therefore, that its relation is as the relation of being able to laugh to human being. And thus color, insofar as it is color, is visible without the mediation of another form accruing to it. Since it is so, light is not necessary for there to be color which is causing motion in act, except insofar as it gives the subject proper to it the ability to receive motion from [color]. It seems that Aristotle asserted what he asserted only intending to provide a solution to that question. It is in this way that we should understand his account that colors move the sense of sight which is in potency in darkness, for light is that which makes them able to move {234} in act. Hence, he likens light to the agent intelligence and colors to universals.[175] For what is brought forth by example and in a general way is not like what is brought forth by demonstration. In the case of an example, the intention is only to make something evident, not to provide verification. And no one can say that color is found in act only when light is present. For color is the boundary of a determinate transparent; but light is not the boundary of a determinate transparent and for this reason it is not necessary for its being color, but for its being visible, as we determined. Let us return, then, and say that when he had explained that color, insofar as it is visible, moves the transparent in act and that this is its nature owing to the fact that it is visible per se, and that it is impossible for there to be sight without light, he returned to recounting what should be considered first concerning those things. He said: **but** it is necessary that **any** color, etc. That is, but because any color is visible only in light, we should first speak about light, for light is one of the things by which sight is brought to completion. Next he said: **And this** is in the course of saying what **the transparent** is. That is, and this will be brought to completion by us by saying first what the transparent is.

68. **Let us say, therefore, that the transparent is that which is visible but is not visible per se and without qualification, but rather owing to the color of something extraneous. In such a state we find air, water, and several celestial bodies.**[176] **For it is not insofar as air is air or insofar as water is water**

---

175. *De Anima* 3. 5, 430a14–17.

176. The Greek has καὶ πολλὰ τῶν στερεῶν, "and many solid bodies" (Aristotle, *De Anima* [1984]); وكثير من الأجساد الكثيفة (ibid. [1954]); "and many solid bodies." The *Middle Commentary* (2002), 66.20, has الأجسام الصلدة, "smooth bodies."

that they are {235} transparent, but on account of the same nature existing in these two and in the highest eternal body. (418b4–9)

After he had recounted that it is necessary first to consider the nature of the transparent, he began to describe it. He said: **the transparent is that which is visible**, etc. That is, the transparent is that which is not visible per se, namely, through a natural color existing in it, but rather [it is] that which is visible per accidens, that is, through an extraneous color. What he said is evident. For this reason it is naturally constituted to receive colors, since it has none of its own in itself. Next he said: **For it is not insofar as air is air**, etc. That is, because transparency is not in water alone or in air alone but [is] also in the celestial body, it was necessary that transparency not be in one of them insofar as it is that which it is, for instance, insofar as water is water or the heavens heavens, but according to a common nature existing in them all, although it may not have a name. What he said is evident.

69. **Light is the act of that, namely, of the transparent, insofar as it is transparent, but in potency it is that in which there is darkness besides. Light is, as it were, the color of the transparent, since the transparent is in actuality by fire and the like, as is the higher body, for in it there also exists that same thing. It was already said, therefore, what the transparent is and what light is, and that it is not at all fire or a body nor is it something emanating from a body. For if it were, then in this way {236} it would be a body. But there is the presence of fire or its like in the transparent. For it is impossible for there to be two bodies in the same place. (418b9–17)**

After he had explained the nature of the transparent, which is related to light as matter to form, he began to define what light is. He said: **Light is the act . . . of the transparent**, etc. That is, the substance of light is the actuality of the transparent insofar as it is transparent or the actuality of that nature common to bodies. This is what he said: **but in potency it is that in which there is** this and darkness, that is: a body transparent in potency is that in which that common nature is found together with darkness.

Next he said: **Light is, as it were, the color of the transparent**, etc. That is, light in the indeterminate transparent is as color in the determinate transparent, since the transparent is transparent in act naturally by a luminous body, such as fire and similar things from the highest luminous bodies. Next he said: **for in this there also**, etc. That is, for the nature of the transparent existing in the heavenly body is always associated with that which makes it a disposition in act. For this reason the heavenly [body] is never found to be transparent in potency, as [are] those which are [here] below, since sometimes light is present and sometimes it is not, while that heavenly nature is always illuminated. From this it was explained also that colors do not acquire a positive disposition from light, for light is only a positive disposition of a transparent body. . . .[177]

70. **It is thought that light is contrary to darkness, while darkness is the privation of a positive disposition from the transparent. It was explained from this, therefore, that light is the presence of that intention. Neither Empedocles nor anyone else spoke correctly {237} if someone said as he himself said that light travels and goes forth in a time between earth and the circumference, but [in a time] imperceptible for us. For that account exceeds truth and appearance. For it is possible that this is not perceived in a short space, but there is a very great difference [between that and the assertion] that it is not perceived [in its movement] from east to west.** (418b18–26)

After he had explained that light is the actuality of a transparent body insofar as it is transparent, he began to explain the way in which it will be proven that light is not a body but is a positive disposition and a positive state in a transparent body. He said: **It is thought that light is contrary to darkness,** etc. That is, it seems that light is opposite to darkness as privation and positive disposition. Next he said: **It was explained from this, therefore, that light is the presence of that intention.** That is, it was, therefore, explained from this, namely, that darkness is a privation of light in the transparent, that light is not a body but is the presence of an intention in the transparent in the presence of a luminous body, while the privation of this [intention] is called darkness. What he said is evident, since the subject of darkness and light is a body and it is transparent. Light, however, is a form and a positive disposition of that body, and if it were a body, then body would penetrate body. Next he said: **Neither Empedocles,** etc. That is, Empedocles said nothing at all when he said that light is a body and that it first travels and goes out between earth and the circumference [and] next travels [back] to earth, but sense does not perceive it owing to the speed of its motion. Next he said: **For that account exceeds truth,** etc. That is, for that account, namely, of Empedocles, is unreasonable. For it is possible for this not to be sensed over a short space, but [for it not to be sensed] over a great distance, namely, from the east to the west, is to retreat far from reason. {238}

71. **What receives color is what does not have color, and what receives sound is what does not have sound. But what does not have color is the invisible transparent, or that which is seen insofar as it is thought to be so**

177. Averroes' Comment here is incomplete in the Latin manuscripts. Apparently he is asserting here that light is a positive disposition of a body which is transparent in act always, such as the heavenly bodies which are always actually luminous.

from consideration of the dark.[178] **And such is the transparent, but not when it is transparent in actuality, but rather in potency, for the same nature will be perhaps darkness and perhaps light.** (418b26–419a1)

After he had recounted that color is what moves the transparent insofar as it is transparent in act, he began to give the reason for this. He said: **What receives color is** that which **does not have color**, etc. That is, color is what moves the transparent because what receives color should lack color. And what lacks color is the transparent which is invisible per se, but if it is said to be visible, it will be as if it is said that the dark is visible, that is, it is something naturally constituted to be seen, since the transparent is dark when light is not present. He meant this when he said: **or that which is seen** as **it is held to be so from consideration of the dark.** That is, or that which is visible insofar as it is said that the dark is visible. Next he said: **And** what is **such is the transparent,** etc. That is, and the transparent which is not visible per se is not the transparent which is brought to actuality by light, but the transparent which is luminous in potency.

Next he said: **for the same nature,** etc. That is, and the transparent is found according to these two dispositions because the nature receiving transparency in certain things receives both, for sometimes it is found dark and sometimes transparent. He said **perhaps** because this does not occur equally in that nature, but only in generable and corruptible transparent things. {239} The heavenly nature, however, never receives darkness, except for what is thought concerning the moon during an eclipse and in the diversity of its positions from the sun (if we will have conceded that the moon's nature is among the transparent natures, not among the luminous natures, for perhaps the moon is composed from those two natures).

72. **Not all things are seen in light, but only the proper color of any given thing. For there are some things which are not seen in light but in darkness they cause sensation, for instance, those things which seem to be fiery and to become bright. Those do not have one name, for instance, the seashell, the horn,[179] the heads of certain kinds of fish, and fish scales and eyes. But its own color is not seen in any of these. But why those are seen requires another account.** (419a1–7)

---

178. The Greek has ἄχρουν δ᾽ ἐστὶ τὸ διαφανὲς καὶ τὸ ἀόρατον ἢ τὸ μόλις ὁρώμενον, οἷον δοκεῖ τὸ σκοτεινόν. "What is colorless includes what is transparent and what is invisible or scarcely visible, i.e. what is dark." Aristotle, *De Anima* (1984). The reference here is to the potentially transparent medium which is invisible.

179. *V.g. concha, et cornu*: οἷον μύκης, κέρας, "instances of it are fungi, horns." Aristotle, *De Anima* (1984).

After he had mentioned earlier that among the visible are something which is color and something which is non-color (and it is this which does not have a common name), and that it is proper to color that it may be seen only in light, he began to say that the state of those other visible things is contrary to that of color, namely, that they are seen in the dark and not in light. He said: **Not all things are seen in light**, etc. That is, not every visible thing is seen in light, but rather only this is true, that the proper color of any given visible thing is seen in light, and it makes no difference whether that visible thing is seen in the dark or not. Next he said: **For there are some things which are not seen in light**, etc. That is, we said that it is not necessary that every visible thing be seen in light because there are some which are seen in the dark and not in light, as several [kinds of] animals, seashells, {240} horn, and other things. All those things do not have the same name. Next he said: **But its own color is not seen**, etc. That is, but although those are sensed in the dark, nevertheless the proper color of every one of these is not sensed then, but only in the presence of light. For this reason no one can say that some color is seen in the dark. Next he said: **But why those are seen**, etc. That is, the reason why those are seen in the dark and not in the light should be said in another place. It seems that those are seen at night and not in the day because in them there is [too] little of a bright nature, for it remains hidden when there is incoming light due to its feebleness, just as this occurs in weak lights in [the presence of] strong ones. (For this reason the stars are not apparent during the day.) The nature of color is different from the nature of light and what is luminous, for light is visible per se, but color is visible with the mediation of light.

73. **In this passage, however, this alone is apparent, namely, that all that is seen in light is color and, likewise, it is not seen without light. For this is also what was the essence**[180] **in the case of color, namely, that it is what moves the transparent in act; and the actuality of the transparent is light. The indication of this is evident, since if you place something having color right on the sense of sight itself, it will not be seen. But color moves the transparent just as the sense is moved by the air since [air] is continuous.** (419a7–15)

After he had explained what the visible is, namely, color, what the transparent is, and what light is, he began to state a summary of what {241} he had explained. He said: **In this passage, however, this alone**, etc. What he said is evident, namely, those two propositions, one that everything which is seen in light is color and the other the converse, namely, that every color is seen in light. For it is evident that those things which appear in the dark are not seen according to their own color.

180. *Quid est.*

Next he said: **For this is also what**, etc. That is, for this also is what led us to say in regard to the knowledge of the substance of color, insofar as it is visible, that it is that which moves the transparent in act. He means by this that this definition explains the being of color only insofar as it has been apparent to us that it is impossible for color to be seen without light and that light enters into sight insofar as it bestows upon the transparent the disposition for being moved by colors, not that it bestows a positive disposition on colors. This was explained earlier.[181] Next he said: **and the actuality of the transparent is light**, etc. That is, and light is simply the act of the transparent. The indication of the fact that light does not exist without the transparent is that if something colored were placed on the sense of sight, it would not be apprehended. For then there will be no light between the color and the sense of sight because there is no transparent there. When, therefore, the transparent is removed, light is also removed; and when there is light, there will be the transparent. Next he said: **But color moves the transparent**, etc. That is, but on account of what we said—that when color will have been placed on the sense of sight, it is not seen—it was necessary that the sight of color not be completed unless color moves the transparent which is the medium between it and the one who sees and the medium moves the one who sees by its continuity with the one who sees. [This is] just as air, since when it is united with the one who sees, it is moved by color when it is illuminated, then next it moves the sense of sight. {242}

74. **Democritus, therefore, did not speak truly in regard to his having thought that if the medium were a vacuum, then sight would be more accurate, even an ant [could be seen] if it were in the sky. For this is impossible. For sight comes about only when the sense is affected by some affection. But it is impossible for sight to be affected by color. Therefore, it remains that it is affected by the medium; hence, it is necessary that there be something in the medium. If, however, there were a vacuum, not only would sight not be accurate but nothing at all would be seen. We have, therefore, mentioned the reason why it is necessary that color be seen only in light. Fire, however, is seen in both, namely, in dark and in light, and this is necessary, for the transparent is transparent in virtue of this.** (419a15–25)

Earlier he had explained that the action of the sense of sight is brought to actuality only through a mediating transparent, by the indication that when color[182] is placed on the sense of sight, it is not seen, and also because sight is brought to actuality only through light, and light is found only in a transpar-

181. See above {232}.
182. *Color:* The argument requires "a colored object" here.

ent medium. Here he begins to reprimand Democritus, who said that if sight were in a vacuum, then it would be more accurate.[183] He said: **Democritus, therefore,** etc. That is, when it had been explained that sight comes about only through a medium, [it was evident that] Democritus incorrectly held the opinion that if sight were via a mediating vacuum, then it would be more accurate. Next he said: **For this is impossible**, etc. That is, for what he said, that sight will be more perfect in a vacuum, is impossible. The indication of this is that he had already explained that the sense of sight, insofar as it is a sensible power, is moved and affected by color and color moves {243} it. It is impossible for the sense of sight to be affected and moved by color, if the colored body is external to the sense of sight, unless [it is] such that this colored thing first moves the medium by touch and the medium moves the sense of sight. If there were a vacuum between the sense of sight and the visible object, then it would not be able to move the sense of sight. For every positive disposition existing in a body acts only by touch. If, therefore, the last thing moved is not touched by a mover, it is necessary that there be a medium between them which conveys the affection and that medium will be what is touched and what touches [something else]. The first,[184] however, will be what touches while being untouched, and the last thing moved [will be] touched while not touching [anything else]. Hence it is necessary that the sense of sight be affected by the medium, not by a vacuum as Democritus thought. This is the demonstration that it is impossible for sight to come about through a vacuum, not that it is impossible for sight to come about except through a medium. For someone may say that if the necessity for there to be a medium were due to the fact that what is sensed is distinct from what senses, then it would be necessary that when what is sensed touches the sense of sight, [the sense of sight] senses it, and this is not so. For this reason Aristotle does not mean by this account that sight needs a necessary medium, but [he means] to show that when sensible things are discerned by it, it will be impossible that [sight] be via a vacuum as Democritus thought. He was supported by the fact that the senses need a necessary medium, because when the sensibles are placed on them, they do not sense, and because there will be no sight except through light and light is found only through a medium. Next he said: **We have, therefore, mentioned** already **the reason**, etc. That is, after he had explained that {244} the sense of sight needs a necessary medium, by this the reason why color is seen only in light was explained and it is because it is seen only via a medium. This shows that he does not hold the opinion that the reason for there being light for sight is that it makes colors in act, as certain people have held. Next he said: **Fire,**

183. Cf. Themistius, *De Anima Paraphrase* (1899), 62.12–13; (1973), 97.2–3; (1996), 82.
184. That is, the visible.

however, **is seen in** them, etc. That is, fire is seen in darkness and light alike because each is brought together in it, namely, because it makes the medium transparent in act insofar as it is luminous and it moves it insofar as it is color in a body.

75. **That account is the same both for sound and for smell. For neither of these, if it has touched its sense, causes sensing. Rather, the medium is moved by smell and by sound, and by that each sense is moved. If, then, you would place either something having sound or having smell on the sense itself, they would not cause sensing at all. And it is likewise for touch and for taste, but this is not apparent. Later on we will explain the reason for this.** (419a25–31)

After he had explained that the sense of sight does not come to be except via a medium, he began to say also that by that same explanation three senses need a necessary medium. His account is evident. By his having said, **And it is likewise for touch and for taste**, he means: and our opinion in regard to the sense of touch and taste, concerning the fact that they need a medium, is just as our opinion in regard to the other senses, although those two senses seem to sense when their sensibles are placed {245} on them, and for this reason they seem not so evidently to need a medium as do those other three. Next he said: **Later on we will explain the reason for this**, that is, the cause on account of which the senses of touch and taste sense sensibles placed on them and it is not so with respect to the three other senses.

76. **The medium in the case of sound is air. In the case of smell, however, it does not have a name, for it is a certain affection common to air and water and it is with respect to smell as transparency is in regard to color, and for this reason it is found in both. For also animals living in water have the sense of smell, but human beings and all animals which walk and breathe cannot smell without breathing. Later on we will give the reason for those things.** (419a32–b3)

He says that the medium in sound is air, not water, because animals which are in water do not sense, as it seems to me, except through sounds occurring in the air outside the water. For it appears that the sound does not come about from the striking of bodies in water, though the contrary is the case for smell. Next he said: **In the case of smell, however, it does not have a name.** That is, the nature receiving the smell, namely, what is in the medium, does not have a name, while the nature which receives color in water and in air does have [one], namely, this name, the transparent. Next he said: **for it is a [certain] affection common,** etc. That is, for it appears from this that the reception of smell is not of air insofar as it is air nor of water insofar as it is water, but it

must be some affection in the nature common to these. That nature is naturally constituted to receive extraneous smells and this will be such that it does
not have a smell at all in itself, just as {246} the transparent is a nature which
receives colors and assumes extraneous things, insofar as it does not have its
own color. This shows that he does not hold the opinion that smell is a body
dispersed in the air by what is able to be smelled, but rather it is some quality
through which that nature is naturally constituted to be actualized. But the
smell is not actualized by that [nature], just as the transparent [is actualized]
by color but color [is] not [actualized] by the transparent. As color has a twofold being, one in the determinate transparent (this is that in which it is natural) and the other in the indeterminate transparent (this is that in which it is
extraneous),[185] so too smell has these two similar beings, namely, being in the
odoriferous dampness (this is natural being) and being in the non-odoriferous
dampness (this is extraneous being). Later on we will explain this, when we
will speak of this sense.[186] Next he said: **and** owing to this **it is found** from
both. That is, owing to this common nature smell is found from both these
elements, namely, water and air. For aquatic animals have the sense of smell
and there is no doubt but that this comes about with the mediation of water.
Next he said: but **all animals which walk**, etc. He meant by this to explain
that fish have the sense of smell without breathing and that this is not unthinkable, just as many non-breathing animals living in air have the sense of
smell without breathing. Next he said: **Later on the reason for** this sort of
thing will be given, that is, why certain animals have the sense of smell through
breathing and certain do not. {247}

77. **In this passage we will make some determinations first about sound
and smell. Let us say that sound is twofold, for it is in act and in potency.**

185. Arabic fragments correspond to Book 2, 76.21–30: كما ان الشفيف له طبيعة تقبل
اللون الغريب لأنه ليس لها لون يخصها هذا يدل ان الرائحة ليس جسم يتحلل في الهواء
من هذه الرائحة وينبسط. بل هي ⟨كيفية⟩ تستكمل تلك الطبيعة بها من غير ان يكون
قوام الرائحة بها ، كما ان يستكمل المشف باللون من غير ان يكون اللون قائما بالمشف ،
وكما ان اللون ⟨له وجودان ، وجود⟩ في المشف المحدود ، وهوالذي به اللون بالطبع ووجود ⟨آخر⟩
في المشف الغير محدود ، وهو الذي ⟨يدخل⟩ عليه من خارج (*Long Commentary* Fragments
[1985], 39–40); "Since the transparent has a nature which is receptive of foreign color
because it does not have a color specific to it, this indicates that smell is not a body which
is separate and spread out in air apart from this smell. Rather, it is <a quality> by which
this nature is actualized without smell subsisting in it. Just as the transparent is actualized by color without the color subsisting by means of the transparent, so too color <has
two beings, a being> in the determinate transparent which is what the color has by
nature, and <another> being in the indeterminate transparent which is what <enters>
it from outside."

186. See below, Book 2, Texts and Comments 92ff. {270ff.}.

For there are certain things which are not said to make sound, such as the
sponge and wool. And certain things are said to have sound, such as copper
and everything hard; for what is smooth can make sound; and this is able
to cause sound in act between itself and the sense of hearing. (2.8, 419b4–9)

He seems to order the consideration of the powers of sense according to
nobility, not according to nature, and for this reason he placed the account of
sight before that of the other senses, then hearing and then smell. The summary
of this account in this section is that some things have sound, such as hard
things, and some do not, such as soft things, and of those having sound some
are said to have sound in act and some in potency.

78. **Sound in act always comes to be through something and on something
and in something. For the striking is what causes [it] and for this reason it
is impossible that sound come from some one thing. For what strikes is one
thing and what is struck [is] another; hence it is necessary that what causes
sound cause sound only on something. The striking does not come about
without motion and transference.[187] As we said, sound is not the striking of
a body whatever it be. For when sheepskins of wool are rubbed together,
they make no sound at all, but copper and everything smooth and hollow
[do]. Copper, however, [does so] because it is smooth, but hollow bodies [do
so] because {248} through reverberation they make many strikes after the
first by preventing its escape. (419b9–18)**

He means by **through something** what causes a striking, by **on something**
what is struck, and by **in something** the medium, namely, air or water. What
he says in this chapter is evident and the summary of it is that sound comes
from what causes a striking, what is struck, and something in which the striking occurs. For the striking is an action; therefore it has an agent, namely, what
causes a striking, and matter, namely, what is struck. Because the striking is a
local motion, it comes about only in water and air, since it is impossible for it
to exist in a vacuum,[188] as was explained in the general accounts.[189] What is
struck, however, from which sound comes, exists in two ways: either as something smooth and hard such as copper or something hollow. Sound, therefore,

---

187. *Et translatione.* These words are additions not found in the Greek or in the
alternate Arabic translation.

188. Arabic fragments correspond to Book 2, 78.18–21: لأن القرع هو فعل فلا بد من
فاعل وهو القارع وهيولي وهو المقروع المتوسط ولأن القرع هو حركة نقلة ولا يمكن كون متوسط
وهو الماء والهواء ، ان يكون في الخلاء (*Long Commentary* Fragments [1985], 40). The Arabic
has "namely, what is intermediate and struck. Because. . . ."

189. This seems to be a general reference to Aristotle's attack on the notion of the
existence of the void in *Physics* 4, 7–9.

comes from the smooth owing to the expulsion of air at the striking from its parts equally. He meant this when he said: **Copper, however, [does so] because it is smooth**, etc. For it is so concerning sound in this intention just as [it is] concerning the reflection of rays, namely, because it appears very strongly in hard bodies because it exists equally in them, and for this reason one action is compounded in them,[190] just as people who drag something of great weight. [Sound,] however, [comes] from hollow bodies due to the frequent repetition of air in them because it cannot exit from them, and thus it is repelled just as a ball is repelled from a wall. Here he means this by **reverberation**. You ought to know that sound does not come to be in air in such a way that air which is expelled by what strikes is moved per se individually until it reaches the sense of hearing. But you ought to know that what comes to be in air from the strik-ing of bodies against one another is similar to what comes to be in water when a stone is thrown into {249} the water, with respect to motion of a circular sort,[191] namely, that a spherical figure or one nearly spherical comes to be in air at the striking, the center of which is the place of the striking through the expulsion of air from that place equally [in all directions], or nearly so. The indication of this is that it is possible to be heard in any given point of air whose remoteness from what strikes is the same, and it is a natural remoteness from the more remote of which that sound cannot be heard. For this reason every striking has a determinate sphere. It is so for smell and color, namely, that they move air from all parts according to that spherical figure.

79. **Furthermore, [sound] is heard in air and in water but less so. But nevertheless for sound air alone is not sufficient nor is water, but there needs to be the striking by solid bodies against one another or against the air. This will be when the air is fixed in place for receiving the striking and not dispersed, and for that reason, when the striking is quick and hard, it will make sound. For it is necessary that the motion of what strikes precede the dispersal of the air, just as if one were to strike a mound of sand.** (419b18–25)

After he had explained that the striking comes about through something, on something, and in something, and he had explained these through which and according to which the striking comes about, he began to explain that in which the striking comes about. He said: **it is heard in air, and in water but**

---

190. Arabic fragments correspond to Book 2, 78.27–30: وكذلك فان الصوت في هذا المعنى بمنزلة انعكاس الشعاع أعني انه يظهر له تأثير قوي في الأجسام الصلبة لكونه فيها متساوية فيجتمع له فعل واحد ⟨على جهة⟩ (*Long Commentary* Fragments [1985], 40).

191. This is a reference to the outward movement of waves in the pattern of a circle when a stone is dropped in water.

less so. That is, but water returns the sound less strongly than air. Next {250} he said: **for sound air alone** is **not** sufficient, etc. That is, air is not sufficient for the sound to come about without something struck, nor is water sufficient in this regard. Rather, there needs to be in the air a striking by solid bodies against one another and in the air itself.[192] Next he said: **This will be when the air is fixed in place**, etc. That is, the sound comes about when the striking is by solid bodies against one another and against the air itself, and the striking of the air is with a quick motion, in such a way that it precedes the motion of the air and what strikes has breadth and quantity, since the air will then resist it. For when what strikes and the striking are of such a sort, it happens that the air is seen to be fixed, as it were, and not dispersed, namely, when what strikes is not dispersed and its motion is not slow. Next he said: **for that reason, when** something is struck, etc. That is, the indication of the fact that the sound comes about only when the motion of what strikes is quicker than the dispersal, is that when something among the things which are not naturally constituted to make sound is struck quickly and forcefully, sound will come about, as happens when one will have struck a column of sand forcefully and quickly. Because of what he said, it happens that these things which are of quick motion make sound in the air, although they do not strike something else, just as the motion of a strip of leather[193] in the air.

80. **Echo comes about from air when it is one[194] on account of the vessel by which it is contained and is prevented from dispersal, when the air rebounds and is forced out from it like a ball. Perhaps an echo always comes about but not in a way that is evident. For it happens in the case of sound just as in the case of light. For light is always reflected (and if it were not so, then [light] would not be {251} everywhere, but there always would be darkness outside of the place on which the sun falls), but [this light] is not reflected as it is reflected by water, by copper and by different smooth bodies such that it also causes a shadow (and it is that by which light comes).[195]** (419b25–33)

192. Arabic fragments correspond to Book 2, 79.14–18: الماء للصوت أقل من تأدية الهواء ‹ثم قال : والهواء ليس وحده كافيا لحصول الصوت› يعني أن الهواء ‹لا يكفي› لحدوث الصوت ولا الماء أيضا دون المقروع وان يكون في الهواء قرع عن الأجسام ‹الصلبة› بعضها ببعض أو ‹عن› الهواء نفسه (*Long Commentary* Fragments [1985], 40).

193. *Corrigie*: a rein or a shoelace. The reference seems to be to the sound of a whip slicing through the air. Cf. *Middle Commentary* (2002), 70.14–17.

194. That is, made into a unified whole.

195. The Greek has ἀλλ᾽ οὐχ οὕτως ἀνακλᾶται ὥσπερ ἀφ᾽ ὕδατος ἢ χαλκοῦ ἢ καί τινος ἄλλου τῶν λείων, ὥστε σκιὰν ποιεῖν, ᾗ τὸ φῶς ὁρίζομεν, "but this reflected light is not always strong enough, as it is when it is reflected from water, bronze, and

After he had explained the things from which sound comes about and how it comes about, he began to explain the being of a certain accident of sound, which is called echo. This is the repetition of sound while preserving its pattern, as happens in empty houses. He said: **Echo**, etc. That is, echo comes about from air which comes to be one, that is, confined and enclosed, on account of what contains it and prevents it from escaping. For, when its motion is actualized by what first strikes, the air is pushed from the sides of that by which it is contained and it strikes it a second time by a strike like the first one which made the sound. And in this way the same sound is repeated, for it is heard as if responding to the first.

He likened that to a pushed sphere since when the sphere is pushed, a motion similar to the first motion comes about in it. And the echo is heard after the first sound as if responding, because it was already explained that between any two motions there is rest. From what he said, **it comes about from air when it is one**, we should not understand that it comes from one [part of] air because it is distinct from the other parts of air by virtue of motion, as [in the case of] a stone when it is thrown and a ball. Rather we must understand that he means by "one air" [something which is] one because it is confined and contained by a vessel. For when some affection and strong motion comes about in air which is so, it will come about {252} then from a striking similar to what comes about from the fall of the stone in water, namely, that this motion is not actualized on account of what confines it. Hence, it is struck a second time by the walls of the confining vessel and in this way another affection similar to the first comes about. For this reason that sound is repeated. Aristotle, therefore, likened air in this motion to a ball which, when thrown, is pushed as moved by that which it encountered,[196] when its motion is not actualized, by an expulsion similar to the first, not insofar as one part of the air is that to which that rebounding and expulsion happen a second time. Next he said: **Perhaps the echo always comes about but not in a way that is evident.** He indicates by this how the motion of the sphere comes about in the air at the striking. For such motion comes about in the air from the striking only by way of rebounding. For what strikes first pushes the air in its path toward the part toward which what strikes is moved. Unless the motion of reaction happens to the parts of the air, that motion will not come about equally or nearly so from all the parts of the thing struck, such that from this there will arise a spherical figure or nearly so, the center of which is the thing struck. He said: **Perhaps the echo always comes about**. That is,

---

other smooth bodies, to cast a shadow, which is the distinguishing mark by which we recognize light." Aristotle, *De Anima* (1984). The alternate Arabic translation is in accord with the Greek here.

196. That is, it bounces off what it strikes.

perhaps the reason why the echo comes about, namely, the reaction, [is that it] is always in the sound, but in a weak way. For when it is so strong that it will make the affection remaining in the air different in number from the first affection and similar to it in quality, then an echo will come about. Next he said: **just as** happens **in the case of light. For light is [. . .] reflected**, etc. That is, what happens in the case of sound is similar to what happens in the case of light. For light has two reflections, a strong one and a weak one. For a strong one makes a second light {253} and is a reaction which comes from polished bodies and is like a reflection which makes a second sound in air. The second [reflection], however, is a weak light on account of which things are seen in shade and is like the reaction by means of which a human being hears his own sound. It is something which does not reach the point that it is like the reaction which comes about from water and copper which makes a second light in the part opposite to the first light, just as a strong reaction makes a second sound in the air in the part opposite to the first sound. The reason why we know this reaction of light, as he said, is because we see in a place upon which the sun does not fall. For light is naturally constituted to go forth from what is bright according to straight lines to the part opposite to the bright part from the luminous body, as [explained by] those who wrote the *De Aspectibus*.[197] If, therefore, the reaction were not there, then there would be darkness in all the parts except for the part to which the rays are opposite. Likewise, if the motion of the air which makes the sound were only in the part in which it is pushed from what strikes alone, then the sound would be heard only by one who is in that part alone. But the sound is heard in all the parts of the thing struck. For this reason we know that what happens for light with respect to the spherical figure is similar to what happens for the motion of the striking in the air. Therefore, we should understand in this way the similarity between these two reflections. When, however, the body is luminous from all parts, there is no doubt but that it makes a bright sphere, and this was explained in the *De Aspectibus*.[198] The difference, therefore, between this sphere and the first is that the light in that is similar and the light in this differs according to strength and weakness. It also seems that the sphere of light made by the luminous body from one of its parts, {254} besides not being similar to itself in light, is also not of perfect roundness, namely, because the longest diameter is that which goes out from the luminous body to the circumference in the part to

197. *De Aspectibus*. This is likely a reference to the *Optics* of Ibn al-Haytham, though similar discussions are found in a work of al-Kindî known under the same Latin title. See Ibn al-Haytham, *Optics* (1983), 75 and 81; (1989), vol. 1, 15 and 20. Cf. al-Kindî, *On the Causes of Differences of Perspective* (1997), 448–449.

198. See Ibn al-Haytham, *Optics* (1983), 81; (1989), 20. Still, perhaps he has in mind what we find at al-Kindî, *On the Causes of Differences of Perspective* (1997), sec. 14, 482–487.

which the rays are opposite and the shortest in the part opposite (and it is the part which is of denser darkness than all the parts and of lesser light).[199]

81. **It was, therefore, rightly said that the vacuum plays a valuable role in hearing. For it is thought that air is a vacuum and this is what causes hearing, when it is moved as something continuous and one. But [this is] not because it is pliant. For [sound] does not come about unless what is struck is smooth, and then one echo will come about, since it comes at once from its surface, for the smooth surface is one.**[200] (419b33–420a2)

After it had been explained from this that air is the matter of sound, because it is impossible for it to come about except through [air], the one who said that

---

199. Arabic fragments correspond to Book 2, 80.59–96: فالضوء له انعكاس قوي وانعكاس
ضعيف. فالقوى يحدث ضوءا ثانيا وهو الانعكاس الذي يكون عن الأجسام الصقيلة وهو
شبيه بالانعكاس الذي يحدث في الهواء صوتا ثانيا ، وهو الصدى ، والضعيف هو الذي به
‹نرى الأشياء› في الظل ، وهو نظير الانعكاس الذي به يسمع المرء صوت نفسه ، وهو الذي
لا ينتهي الا أن يكون مثل الانعكاس الذي يكون عن الماء والنحاس ، محدث ضوء ثاني في
جهة مقابلة للضوء الأول كما يحدث الانعكاس القوي في الهواء صوتا ثانيا ، وهو المسمى
صدى ‹في الجهة المقابلة للصوت الأول›. والذي أوقفنا على هذا الانعكاس للضوء هو اننا
نبصر في المواضع التي لا يقع عليها الشمس وذلك ان الضوء من شأنه ان يخرج المضيء على
سمت مستقيم ‹ . . .› كما قد تبين أمره في ‹كتاب المناظر› فانه لا يخلو الضوء من الانعكاس
، ولولا ذلك لما كان الضوء الا في المواضع التي يقع عليها الشعاع وكانت تكون الظلمة في
سائرها. كما انه لو كانت حركة الهواء التي تحدث في الجهة التي يدفعها القارع اليها فقط لما
سمع الصوت الا من كان في تلك الجهة فقط ، لكن إذا ما سمعنا الصوت من جميع جهات
الشيء المقروع علمنا من هذا ‹ما الشيء الذي› يحدث للضوء من التشاكل بشكل كري شبيه
بما يحدث للحركة من القرع في الهواء ، فعلى هذه الجهة ينبغي ان نفهم التشابه بين هذين
الانعكاسين . وكذلك الجسم إذا كان مضيئا ‹من جميع الجهات . . .› فيحدث كرة مضيئة وقد
بين ذلك أصحاب المناظر. والفرق بين هذه الكرة والكرة الأولى أن الضوء في هذه متشابه في
تلك مختلف في القوة والضعف. وشبيه أيضا ان تكون كرة الضوء الحادث ‹عن الجسم› المنير
من أحد جوانبه مع انها متشبهة بالضوء غير تامة الاستدارة حتى يكون أطولها هو القطر الذي
يخرج من الجسم المنير إلى محورها في الجهة التي يقبلها الشعاع ، واقصرها في الجهة المقابلة
لها ، وهي الجهة التي هي أصغر الجهات ظلا وأقلهما ضوءا (*Long Commentary* Fragments
[1985], 41). At 80.74, after the reference to the *De Aspectibus*, the Arabic adds "for light is
not without some reflection." The Arabic also adds "and this is echo," corresponding to
80.62, and "and it is called echo," at 80.68. At 80.91, where the Latin has *non consimilis sibi
in luce*, "not being similar to itself in light," the Arabic has no negation. In this passage
the translator used both *conversio* and *reflexio* to render the Ababic انعكاس.

200. The Greek here has τότε δὲ εἷς γίνεται ἅμα διὰ τὸ ἐπίπεδον· ἓν γὰρ τὸ τοῦ
λείου ἐπίπεδον. "But then it becomes a single mass at the same time because of the
surface; for the surface of the smooth object is single." Aristotle, *De Anima* (1984). The
alternate translation has وإذا كان المضروب أملس كان الهواء واحداً متصلا – وكذلك حال
السطح الأملس (ibid. [1954]); "And when the thing struck is smooth, the air is one and
continuous. And the disposition of the smooth surface is similarly so."

sound comes to be through a vacuum did not err in this way when he believed that air is vacuum, even though he did err insofar as he thought that air is vacuum. [Aristotle], therefore, praised them because they spoke rightly in one way, although they erred in the opinion they held. Next he said: **But [this is] not because it is pliant**, etc. That is, air is that which causes hearing, when it is moved as something one and continuous. But that motion is not found to be one and continuous for it insofar as it is pliant alone, but only when what has been struck would be smooth body. After he had given the reason why the motion is one and continuous—[the reason] is that what is struck is a smooth body—{255} he gave the reason for this. He said: **and then one** sound **will come about**, etc. That is, and we say that it is necessary in the coming to be of sound that what is struck be smooth because one sound comes about only from one motion, when the body struck is smooth. Then, therefore, the motion which comes about in the air comes about from one striking, since the parts of air are at once pushed from its surface, for the surface of a smooth thing is one. For this reason the striking will be one; hence the sound will also be one. An uneven surface, however, is not one, but many surfaces; hence the striking will be many; hence sound will not come about there at all on account of their diversity and lack of uniformity. And because one of them is not sufficient for making sound, neither are they all at once unless there is one striking.

82. What has sound, therefore, is what moves one [body of] air in a continuous way right up to the point that it reaches the organ of hearing. The organ of hearing, however, is united with the striking because it is in air.[201] And for this reason an animal does not hear in every place [in the body] nor does air enter into every place. For the member which is moved and breathes[202] does not have this in every place, just as the disposition of what sees with liquid.[203] (420a3–7)

201. The text here suffers from omission and is a confused version of the Greek. Ross, in Aristotle, *De Anima* (1956), has ἀκοῇ δὲ συμφυὴς ἀήρ· διὰ δὲ τὸ ἐν ἀέρι εἶναι, κινουμένου τοῦ ἔξω ὁ εἴσω κινεῖται ("air is united with the organ of hearing"), while Smith and Barnes, in ibid. (1984), opt for a variant and read ἀκοὴ δὲ συμφυὴς ἀέρι, διὰ δὲ τὸ ἐν ἀέρι εἶναι, κινουμένου τοῦ ἔξω ὁ εἴσω κινεῖται, "the organ of hearing is physically united with air, and because it is in air, the air inside is moved concurrently with the air outside." The alternate translation has فذلك فعال للقرع ؛ والهواء مجانس للسمع. والقرع إنما يكون في الهواء الخارج (ibid. [1954]); "For this is an activity of the striking. The air is akin to the sense of hearing. The striking is only in the external air."

202. The Latin *anelans* corresponds to the Greek ἔμψυχον, which Ross emends to ἔμψοφον, "makes noise," following the lead of Torstrik (Aristotle, *De Anima* [1862]). Aristotle, *De Anima* (1956). The alternate translation also follows the Greek codices and renders it ذى نفس (ibid. [1954]), "possessing soul."

203. The clause *sicut dispositio videntis apud humorem*, "just as . . . liquid," is an addition to the text of Aristotle. The alternate translation has كالرطوبة للحدقة, "like the

After he had explained the dispositions by which sound comes about, namely, the dispositions of what strikes, of what is struck, and of air, he began to explain how the uniting of sound with the organ of sense comes about from those things. He said: **What has sound**, therefore, etc. That is, it is therefore necessary from what we have explained that what causes sound be what moves one [body of] air moved by one continuous motion {256} all the way until it reaches the organ of hearing. He means by his having said **one** not one on account of a distinction from the other parts of air, but one on account of one continuous motion. Next he said: And **the organ of hearing is united**, etc. That is, and the sense of hearing is united with sound because there exists in it air which is continuous with the external air. If there were not, it would sense nothing. Next he said: **And for this reason [an animal does] not [hear] in every place**, etc. That is, and it is necessary that the air in this sense be continuous with the external air on which the striking takes place. For this reason the animal is not able to hear in every place, but [only] in the places in which there is no division between the air struck and the air in the sense of hearing; nor does hearing come from every member, but from the member in which the air enters, namely, the ear. Next he said: **For the member which is moved and breathes**, etc. That is, so is it that the animal hears only from the proper member just as in the cases of breathing and vision. For the member through which there is breath is not just any member but the proper member, namely, the lung. The disposition of one who sees in relation to the gelatinous liquid [of the eye] is likewise, namely, that vision is not suited for it except through the member in which there is a transparent liquid suited for receiving colors, for instance, the gelatinous liquid [of the eye]. For this reason an animal lacking those instruments lacks those senses.

83. **This, therefore, does not itself have sound, namely, the air, because it disperses quickly. When, therefore, it is prevented from dispersal, then its motion will be sound. Air, however, which is in the ears, was positioned in them as unmoved, so that it may sense perfectly all the kinds of motion. And for this reason we also hear in water, because it does not enter upon the air which is united [with the ear], since it does not enter {257} in the ear also on account of the twist [of the tube of the ear].**[204] **When this does happen, we do not hear nor [do we hear] when damage has occurred to the eardrum,**[205] **just as the disposition of the membrane which is above the organ**

moisture belonging to the pupil of the eye." See Aristotle, *De Anima* (1954), 49, where Badawi suggests their excision.

204. That is, the Eustachian tube.

205. Here *matri cerebri* corresponds to the Greek ἡ μῆνιγξ which is also used of the dura mater or membrane enclosing the brain. Aristotle, *De Anima* (1984), has "the tympanic membrane."

of vision when damage has occurred to it. **What happens concerning the destruction of the organ of hearing by the entrance of water upon that air is the same as what happens from the entrance of external air upon [the organ of sight]. You know this.**[206] (420a7–15)

He had explained that through air it comes about that sound is united with the sense and that it is itself an element proper to that sense, just as there is also an element proper to the sense of vision. Now he began to explain the way in which air receives sound. He said: **This, therefore, does not itself have sound, namely,** the air, etc. That is, air is receptive of the proper sound because it does not have sound in itself, since there is no motion in it which causes sound. The reason for this is that it disperses quickly. This in air is similar to what is the case in the transparent. For just as the transparent would not receive colors if it had color, so too air would not receive sounds if it had sounds from itself. Next he said: **When, therefore, it is prevented,** etc. That is, when it happens in this through a different motion which prevents it from dispersal, this is the motion which comes about from what strikes in what is struck, then that motion will cause sound in it. Next he recounted that this is the reason why nature put air in the ears, not as something subject to change [in its own right], but as altogether still. He said: **Air, however, which is in the ears was [. . .] in them as unmoved, so that it may sense perfectly all the kinds of motion** made in the external air. That air placed in the ears, therefore, {258} surpasses the external air in stillness. Next he said: **And** on account of this **we [. . .] hear in water,** etc. That is, and because air is necessary for the sense of hearing, we hear in water when water has not entered upon the air which is in the ear and has not corrupted it, on account of the spiral which is in the created nature[207] of the ear. When it has entered, we do not hear, and then there happens to us what happens when the destruction of the eardrum has happened, because then we do not hear, just as when the destruction of the membrane which is on the organ of vision has happened, we do not see. He meant to explain that the relation of the air placed in the ear is just as the relation of a member proper to each thing sensed, namely, [that it is that] through which the action of that sentient being is first actualized. For this reason he likened what happens to this air with respect to destruction through the entrance of water upon it to what happens with respect to a striking taking place upon the ear and upon the organ of sight itself. What happens with

---

206. *What happens . . . You know this.* These two sentences are additions to what is found in the Greek. They are not found in the alternate Arabic translation.

207. *In creatione.* The Latin translator seems likely again to have confused خُلِق, "make-up" or "nature," with خَلْق, "creation." Cf. {74}, Book 1, n. 232 and {282}, Book 2, n. 247.

respect to the corruption of the organ of hearing through the entrance of water upon that air placed in the ears happens through the entrance of external air upon [the organ of vision].

84. Furthermore, a sign [of the presence] of hearing in the first place is constantly to hear resonance in the ear, as with a horn.[208] **For air in the ear constantly moves with some motion of its own, but sound is [from something] external, not its own. For this reason they said that hearing comes about through a vacuum capable of producing resonance, because we hear only through something in which there exists air which is separate.**[209] (420a15–19) {259}

After he had explained that this air which exists in the organ of hearing is necessary for [hearing], he began to provide evidence that there exists in the ear a [body of] air separate from the external air. He said: **Furthermore, a sign [of the presence] of hearing,** etc. That is, he shows also that this air exists in the ear because the sign of the verification [of the presence] of hearing in a human being, as the physicians say, is that he constantly hears resonance in the ears, even when uninjured. Hence, this happens for a human being when he places a horn on the ears and hears sound in it, on account of the air enclosed in the horn and the hardness of the horn. Next he said: **For air in the ear always moves,** etc. That is, the cause of this resonance which the sense of hearing belonging to one who hears well hears is that the air which is in the ear constantly moves with its own motion, but that motion is its own and the motion of sound is external; hence that motion does not impede the motion of sound. Next he said: **For this reason they said,** etc. That is, on account of that resonance which is heard in the ear due to the enclosed air, the ancients said that hearing comes about through a vacuum possessing a resonance, because they believed air to be a vacuum. They said this because we hear only through a bodily part in which air exists separate from the external air.

85. Is it, however, what strikes or what is struck that makes the sounds? Let us, therefore, say that it is both, but in two different ways. For sound is the motion of what is able to be moved in such a way, namely, as smooth bodies are reflected by some body. But not everything struck and [every-

208. That is, we hear a faint sound or tintinnabulation when we hold a horn or shell over the ear.

209. *In quo existit aer distinctus*: τῷ ἔχοντι ὡρισμένον τὸν ἀέρα, "a chamber which contains a bounded mass of air" (Aristotle, *De Anima* [1984]); حيثما كان الهواء محدودا (ibid. [1954]); "wherever the air is confined."

thing] which strikes has {260} sound, as was said, for instance, if a pin strikes a pin. But it is necesary that it be an even [surface]. (420a19–25)

Since sound comes from a striking, but a striking comes from what strikes and what is struck, he began to ask to which sound is ascribed. He said: **Is it, however,** etc. Next he said: This comes about **in two different ways. For sound is the motion of what,** etc. That is, for sound is a motion of the air which is moved as repelled from the fall of what strikes upon what is struck, just as something goes forth and is moved from a smooth body when another smooth body is struck against that body. Therefore, just as the motion of the things which have gone forth is ascribed to what strikes as agent and to what is struck as subject, so too sound, which is the motion of the air which is in such a mode, is ascribed to what strikes and what is struck. Next he said: **But not everything struck and [everything] which strikes,** etc. That is a different condition added in bodies which provide sound, namely, that they be broad. Therefore there are three conditions, namely, that they be smooth, hard, and broad, which can precede the dispersal of air through their motion.

86. **However, the kinds of things which provide sound are exhibited in sound which is in act. For just as colors are not seen without light, so flat and sharp [noises] are not sensed without sound. This is said by analogy with things which are tangible. For the sharp moves the sense a great deal in a short time, while the flat [moves the sense] little in a long time. But {261} nevertheless the sharp is not quick nor the flat slow, but the motion of the former will be as quickness and the motion of the latter as slowness. Perhaps this is similar to what is found in regard to the sense of touch with respect to the sharp and the blunt. For the sharp is, as it were, something which pricks, but the blunt pushes out, as it were, for the former moves in a short time and the latter in a long [time]. It happens, therefore, from this that the former is quick and the latter slow. (420a26–b4)**

He wants to explain in this chapter when the first kinds of sound are apprehended and what they are. He said: **However, the kinds of things which provide sound,** etc. That is, but the differences of sounds are apprehended and exhibited in the being of sound in act. Next he said: **For just as colors are not seen,** etc. That is, for just as the differences of colors are not apprehended without the being of color in act, and that will be in the presence of light, so the sharp and the flat in sound, which are the first differences of sound, are not apprehended without the being of sound in act. Next he said: **This is said by analogy,** etc. That is, to call the differences of sound the flat and the sharp is according to [the understanding of their] likeness to tangible things. For some sound moves the sense a great deal in a short time, and a sharp tangible thing is such as this, and for this reason its name was transferred to that.[210] Similarly also, because some sound moves the organ of hearing a little in a long time, it is similar to the tangible thing which moves the organ of touch a little in a long time, namely, what is blunt. Next he said: **But nevertheless the sharp is not quick,** etc. That is, but nevertheless sound which moves the organ of hearing {262} a great deal in little time is not in fact quick nor is flat sound slow. For quick and slow in fact concern dispositions of things which move; but this is called flat because it moves slowly and this [is called] sharp because it moves quickly. Next he said: **Perhaps this is similar,** etc. That is, perhaps that intention which is found in sound concerning quick and slow motion is, as it were, similar to what is found in the sense of touch with respect to the sharp and the blunt. For this reason that ordering was transferred with respect to the sharp and the blunt, not with respect to the quick and the slow. And because the blunt is similar to the flat, for this reason such a sound is called flat. Next he said: **For the sharp, as it were,** pricks. That is, for a sharp sound, as it were, pricks, as a sharp body pricks; and a flat sound, as it were, pushes out, as a blunt body pushes out, because it is likened to the flat. **It happens, therefore, from this that the former is quick and the latter slow.** That is, from this it happens to be customary to call sound which seems, as it were, to prick, sharp, and sound which seems, as it were, [to be] something which pushes out flat.

87. **This, therefore, is what we have determined concerning sound. Voice, however, is a sound in what is alive . . .[211] for instance, that pipes and other things have length, tone, and timbre.[212] They are similar because those also**

210. *Ad illud.* The sense of the passage requires that the referent here be *sonus,* "sound," even though the demonstrative pronoun should be masculine, not neuter as it is here.

211. The Greek text continues: τῶν γὰρ ἀψύχων οὐθὲν φωνεῖ, ἀλλὰ καθ᾽ ὁμοιότητα λέγεται φωνεῖν, οἷον αὐλὸς καὶ λύρα καὶ ὅσα ἄλλα τῶν ἀψύχων ἀπότασιν ἔχει καὶ μέλος καὶ διάλεκτον. "Nothing that is without soul utters voice, it being only by a metaphor that we speak of the voice of the flute or the lyre or generally of what (being without soul) possesses the power of producing a succession of notes which differ in length and pitch and timbre." Aristotle, *De Anima* (1984). Averroes evidences no knowledge of the omission in his Comment here or in his *Middle Commentary.* Yet the alternate translation has the complete text without omission: إنما لأن ما لا نفس له لا يصوت : ولا نفس له وله طنين ولحن ونغمة يقال بالتشبيه كمثل السورناى واللورا وغير ذلك مما لا نفس له (ibid. [1954]). Averroes' understanding of the passage does not suffer, perhaps due to his consultation of the corresponding remarks by Themistius. See Themistius, *De Anima Paraphrase* (1899), 66.15–23; (1973), 106.11–107.3; (1996), 86–87.

212. *Idioma* is apparently derived from the Greek ἰδίωμα, which is a peculiarity or a specific property, perhaps as a property of numbers. Hence, the Latin translator used it to render the notion of timbre. The corresponding Greek of Aristotle has διάλεκτον, as indicated in the previous note.

exist in voice. Many animals do not have voice, such as those bloodless and fish among the animals which do have blood. This was necessary, for sound {263} is a motion of air. But these things which are said to have voice, such as animals which are in the river which is called Amelus,[213] make sound only through the passages of the orifices or through similar things. (420b5–13)

After he had spoken of sound in a general way, whether with respect to what is alive or with respect to what is not alive, he began to speak concerning sound belonging to what is alive. He said: **Voice, however, is**, etc. That is, voice, however, is a sound of a living animal, in which melody, *irah*, and articulations[214] are found. For this reason many instruments are said to have voices by analogy, because these three, or something representing them, are found in them. For the pipe and other instruments are said to have voices only because they have length, that is, melody and tone, that is, *irah*, and articulations, that is, something similar to letters and words. Next he said: **They are similar**, etc. That is, those instruments in having voice are similar to animals, for these three things exist in an animal in reality, but in these instruments by analogy. Next he said: **Many animals do not have voice**, etc. That is, it rightly happens that many animals do not have voice, such as bloodless animals and fish among the animals having blood, since it was explained that sound is a motion made by what strikes and what is struck in air. Those animals lack the air which strikes them in their interiors and they lack the instruments which strike the air. After he had recounted this about those animals, he introduced the notion that perhaps some one will have some doubt regarding this sort of thing {264} on the basis of the fact that some kind of fish has voice. He said: **But these things which are said to have voice**, etc. He means by **passages** gills. He meant by this that such noise is called the making of voice only equivocally, since those three characteristics, melody, *irah*, and letters or things similar to letters, are not found in it.

88. **Voice, however, is sound belonging to an animal, but not through any bodily part whatsoever. But because every thing has sound only by striking something, namely, air, it is also necessary that those things alone have voice, namely, the things which take in air. For nature makes use of the air breathed in two actions, just as the tongue [is used] in taste and speech. But**

213. That is, the Achelous.

214. These terms seem to correspond well with what is found in the *Middle Commentary*: neuma: نغم, "melody"; irah: إيقاع, "pitch"; and dictiones: لفظ, "articulation." *Middle Commentary* (2002), 82.13. I have followed the lead of the *Middle Commentary* and Ivry's translation in rendering this Latin text. *Irah* is perhaps a transliteration of a corrupt Arabic text.

taste is necessary and for this reason is in most [animals], but speech [is necessary] for better living. And thus one uses breath in regard to internal heat and this is necessary (and we already gave the reason for this in another book[215]), and in having voice for better living. (420b13–22)

After he had explained that having voice is said in an equivocal way in regard to those things which have voice by virtue of gills and in regard to animals which breathe, he now wants to make known the genus of the animals in which true voice is found. He said: **Voice, however, is**, etc. That is, true voice, however, is a sound belonging to an animal as something proper to it, and through a proper bodily part. Next he began to explain the account of which bodily part it is and which animal is this animal. He said: **but, because not every thing has** voice, etc. That is, but because it was already explained that everything having sounds has sound only through {265} what strikes and what is struck in air, it is evident that it is impossible to find an animal having sound unless it has a bodily part from which what strikes and what is struck come; and [has] air which it draws into and expels from that bodily part; and that this bodily part has figure, quantity, and determinate place. Hence it is necessary that animals having true voice be animals which in their interiors take in and expel air, for in those one finds those three things from which true voice comes about. Next he began to explain that this function to which nature puts air in the animal which breathes is different from the function of cooling and that nature uses the same bodily part for both, of which one is useful and the other necessary, as was explained in *On Animals*.[216] He said: **For nature makes use of the air breathed**, etc. He intends by **two actions** having voice and cooling. Next he said: And **taste is necessary**, etc. That is, but of these two modes [of the tongue], taste is necessary for the being of animals and for this reason it is found in most animals. Its use in speech, however, is for the sake of better living and for this reason many animals lack it. Next he said: **And** likewise **one uses breath in regard to [internal] heat**, etc. That is, and nature uses the inhalation of breath on account of the heat which is internal and this was necessary for animals which breathe; and it uses it in reference to having voice for better living. The passage which he indicated as one in which he had spoken concerning this intention is the treatise which he wrote *On Respiration*.[217] That treatise has not reached us. And it is necessary to investigate this individually in its own right; {266} for it seems that what Galen says[218] concerning this is not sufficient.

215. *On Youth, Old Age, Life and Death, and Respiration*, ch.14 (8), 474 b20–23.
216. *Parts of Animals* 3.6, 668 b33–669b13.
217. See n. 215.
218. Averroes may be referring to Galen's *On the Use of Breathing*, which is mentioned in Arabic sources. See Ullmann (1970), 41, and Galen, *Galen on Respiration and the Arter-*

89. The windpipe[219] is the instrument of breath and voice. And the lung
[is] that for the sake of which this bodily part existed, since through this
bodily part the animal which walks on land surpasses the other animals in
heat. It needs breath in the first place for the sake of the heart. For this reason it necessarily needs air to be cooled so that it may breathe it in.[220]
(420b22–27)

After he had explained that it is necessary that no animal have voice unless
it breathe and that the animal does both through the same bodily part, he began to say [something about] that bodily part. He said: **The windpipe**, etc. He
means by **windpipe** the epiglottis and the pipe. It is evident that this bodily
part is the instrument of voice, since at the end of this bodily part there is a
body similar to the covering flap of a reed-pipe. Likewise it is evident that this
bodily part is for the sake of the lung because it is a passage to it. He said:
through this bodily part [the animal which walks on land] surpasses, etc.
That is, because this bodily part is found in animals which have blood and
walk on land, for this reason they are warmer than the animals which lack
this bodily part. Next he said: **It needs breath in the first place for the sake
of the heart.** That is, those animals need breath on account of the heat of the
heart in the first place and in the second place on account of the heat of that
bodily part.[221] Next he said: **For this reason it [. . .] needs that air be cooled**,
etc. That is, on account of the heat of the heart the animal needs to inhale cool
air in the first place and on account of the heat of the lung in the second place
it needs to exhale it. And {267} what he said is necessary. For the first action in
breath is for inhaling, the second for exhaling. The first, however, is on account
of the heart and the second on account of the lung, since if it were not for
the heat of the lung, the animal would not need to exhale the air frequently.
This is similar to what is found in the cases of many artisans, namely, because
they need to change the instrument by which they act, on account of the change
they bring about in the instrument they use. For the instrument is changed
only when it is consumed and the consumption happening to it either is on

---

ies (1984), 74. Cf. n. 222 below. On Galen in the Arabic tradtion, see *Medical Manuscripts
of Averroes* (1986), 16–36; Bürgel (1967); and Sezgin (2000). On the issue of respiration,
see Bürgel (1967), 297ff.

219. *Trachea arteria*: ὁ φάρυγξ.

220. *Et ideo indiget necessario ut aer infrigidetur, ut anelet ad interius*, "For
this . . . it in," corresponds to "That is why when animals breathe the air must penetrate
inwards." Aristotle, *De Anima* (1984). The alternate Arabic translation has this latter text
as لذلك كنا مضطرين إلى اجترار الهواء داخلا (ibid. [1954]); "For this reason we must draw
air in from the outside."

221. That is, the heat in the lung.

account of the one using [it] or on account of the use itself. If therefore the lung desires to exhale warm air, then its motion is not from the chest alone, as Galen held.[222] That intention needs investigation in its own right.

90. **It is necessary, therefore, from this that the striking of air breathed by the soul which is in those bodily parts against what is called the windpipe be the voice. For not every sound which comes about in animals is voice, as we said (for we can make a sound with the tongue as in the case of a cough), but it is needed that what strikes be alive and have some imagination. For voice is the sound of that,[223] and it is not air breathed as a cough, but through this it strikes the air which is in the pipe. The indication of this is that we cannot speak while drawing air in or exhaling, since we cause motion by means of this bodily part only when we have closed it.** (420b27–421a3) {268}

It is necessary, therefore, that the striking of the air breathed by the soul which is in those bodily parts against the pipe be what makes voice. It is necessary, therefore, that the being of voice be nothing other than the striking of breathed air against the bodily part which is called the pipe, by a voluntary exhalation on the part of the imaginative soul which is in those bodily parts, just as playing the pipe is the striking of air against the flap[224] of the pipe by the pipeplayer having a soul exhaling breath according to the imagination of

222. Averroes seems to be referring to an account such as this: "The breathing through the arteries is enough for all other members, but for the brain and the heart two special organs of breathing are provided; for the first, the nostrils; for the second, the lung. But that the lung might move, the chest was needed; and so, considered as the companion of the heart, the lung is the first organ of breathing; but insofar as it is moved by the chest, it is the second." Galen, *Galen on Respiration and the Arteries* (1984), 127. Cf. ibid., 106–109. "Galen did not accept the doctrine of Aristotle that respiration serves mainly to cool the heart. . . . Galen concluded from . . . clinical observations that the purpose of respiration could not only be to cool the heart but also to raise the lowered body temperature by increasing breathing." Siegel (1968), 162. In his *Kitâb al-Kullîyât* (2000), 86, Averroes explains that breathing in cool air and exhaling warm air is for cooling the heart and rejects the notion that it is for replenishing "the vital spirit" (الروح الغريزي). Later citing Galen, Averroes explains that more study is needed concerning Galen's understanding that the lungs expand because of the motion of the chest. He then explains that without the motion of the chest the lungs would not move and there would be death. Because these motions have different ends, he asserts that these are two related but distinct motions. *Kitâb al-Kullîyât* (2000), 88. My thanks to Tzvi Langermann for e-mail communications regarding Averroes' references to Galen.

223. *Vox enim est sonus illius*: σημαντικὸς γὰρ δή τις ψόφος ἐστὶν ἡ φωνή, "for voice is a sound with a meaning" (Aristotle, *De Anima* [1984]); وذلك أن الصوت قرع ‹له› (ibid. [1954]); "For voice is a striking indicative of something."

224. That is, the opening or the reed at the opening.

melodies. Next he said: **For not every sound**, etc. That is, we said that it is necessary for the being of voice that what strikes have an imaginative soul because not all sound made by an animal is voice (as sound which comes without will at a cough and at the motion of the tongue), but voice is sound which occurs with imagination and will.[225] For this reason he said: **alive and have [. . .] imagination**. For he indicated that this action is completed by two powers of the soul, one of which is the concupiscible and the other the imaginative. Next he said: **For voice is the sound of that**, etc. That is, the first mover in the case of voice is the imaginative and concupiscible soul. For this reason voice is the sound of that which moves first and is not the sound of what moves the breathed air, as sound which occurs at a cough, but what moves in voice is different from that mover, although it moves only through it. He meant this when he said: **but through this it strikes the air which is in the pipe.** That is, but that first mover which is proper to voice strikes the air which is in the pipe when there is voice through what moves the breathed air. Next he said: **The indication of this is that we cannot speak**, etc. {269} That is, the indication of the fact that the first mover in voice moves the air with the mediation of the first mover of air in the breath is that we cannot speak while drawing air in or exhaling. For the mover in breath does not use an instrument at that time different from the instrument of the first motion in the striking which makes the sound. But it is impossible that it use one instrument in different actions at one time. Next he said: **we do not move through** that **bodily part except when we have closed it.** That is, for this reason we do not move the air by a motion of the voice through this bodily part which draws air in and exhales except when we will have held our breath and provided it rest from that action which is breath.

91. **The reason why fish lack voice is also evident, for they lack the pipe because they do not breathe air (and one who says this to be the case is wrong[226]). The reason for this, however, should be stated in another place.** (421a3–6)

He says that the reasons why fish do not have voice are three. He first began with the more remote cause and said: because they have neither lung nor pipe.

---

225. As Ivry (1997b), 532, notes, the corresponding passage of the *Short Commentary on the De Anima* (1950), 37.15–17; (1985), 52.8; (1987), 141, links voice with imagination and desire, while the *Middle Commentary* (2002), 75.9, has imagination and will.

226. This parenthetical remark is found in some Greek manuscripts but is understood by Ross as an addition to the text of Aristotle: ἀλλ᾽ οἱ λέγοντες οὕτω διαμαρτάνουσιν. Aristotle, *De Anima* (1956). It is also found in the alternate Arabic translation: ومن قال إنها متنسمة فقد أخطأ (ibid. [1954]).

Next he gave the cause for this cause. He said: **because they** do **not** take in **air**, that is, because they do not need the inhalation or exhalation of air. Next he said: **The reason for this, however, should be stated in another place.** That is, the cause of that cause (this is the proper cause proximate to this accident) should be said in a different book, namely, in *On Animals*.[227] {270}

92. **Smell and the objects of smell, however, are more difficult to determine than those that have been mentioned earlier. For what smell is**[228] **is not clearly exhibited as [it is] in the cases of voice or light or color. The reason for this is that this sense is not accurate [in discrimination] in us, even less [accurate in us] than in many animals. For the power of smell belonging to human beings is very weak and senses nothing of the things which are objects of smell without pleasure or pain [being involved], because that sense is not accurate [in discrimination] in us.** (2.9, 421a7–13)

Having completed the account of hearing, he wants to speak about the sense of smell. He said: **smell and the object of smell, however,** etc. That is, to know what smell is and what can have smell, from which we can proceed to know what that sense is insofar as the natural scientist teaches, is more difficult than to know what voice or color is. The reason for the difficulty in regard to this is that what it is to which smell belongs and what are the differences proper to each of them are not clearly exhibited, while the differences of colors and voices are clearly exhibited. After he had explained that the reason for the difficulty in knowing what smell is is that the specific differences are not apprehended well by us, he [then] gave the reason for this. He said: **And the reason** for this **is** that this **sense is not accurate [in discrimination] in us**, etc. That is, and the reason why we do not know perfectly the differences of smell is because that sense is weaker in us than in many animals. He meant by this to show the reason why the intellect apprehends the differences of smell with difficulty. It is because that sense apprehends weakly the sensible differences of smells. For the apprehension of the differences of sensible things by the sense is the cause for their apprehension {271} by the intellect and for this reason what lacks the sense lacks the understanding of that genus of sensibles. Next he said: but it is weaker in us **than in many animals**, that is, in apprehending the differences of smells. For many animals seem to know their foods by differences of smells as do we by flavor. It is not in this alone that animals surpass us, namely, in the apprehension of the differences of smells, but [also] in apprehending them from a distance. Next he said: We do not sense the object of smell **without pleasure**

227. *Parts of Animals* 3.6, 668b33–669a8.
228. That is, the essence of smell.

or pain. That is, we do not have sensation of the differences of the object of smell unless it is something which is pleasurable or painful; that is, we do not sense anything about them except the more common differences. For the pleasurable has many modes and likewise for the painful; and the pleasurable and painful are found only in the most remote extremes.

93. **It seems that animals having hard eyes sense colors in this way and that in their cases the modes of the colors are not clearly exhibited except as pleasing or displeasing to the eyes,**[229] **as the human race senses smells. For it seems, on account of the similarity which smell has with flavor, that the kinds of flavors are just as the kinds of smells.** (421a13–18)

It seems that human beings sense the differences of smells just as animals having hard eyes [sense] the differences of colors. For just as those [animals] do not apprehend the differences of colors except in terms of what is pleasing or displeasing, so too human beings apprehend the differences of smells only in terms of the pleasurable and painful. For it is seen, {272} on account of the similarity which there is between flavor and smell, that the differences of smells are according to the differences of flavors. But the differences of flavors can be apprehended on our part and those [others] are not, since we surpass all animals in this sense, because it is touch in some way. The similarity which there is between flavors and smells is because smell is found only in what has flavor, as was explained in *Sense and Sensibilia*.[230]

94. **But taste in us is more accurate [in discrimination] because it is a kind of touch. And if that sense is very accurate [in discrimination] in human beings, in other matters [humans] are less apt than are many animals. But in touch they surpass all and for this reason are more subtle [in discrimination]**[231] **than all [other] animals. The indication of this is that in the human race also a human being is able to discriminate on the basis of that sense and a human being is not at all so on the basis of something else. For one**

229. *Conveniens oculo et inconveniens*: πλὴν τῷ φοβερῷ καὶ ἀφόβῳ, "only by the presence or absence of what excites fear" (Aristotle, *De Anima* [1984]); إلا بالخوف وغير; الخوف is Badawi's correction—following the Greek—of the manuscript of the alternate translation, which has إلا بالبحث و غير البحث (ibid. [1954]); "except in terms of searching or not searching." The *Middle Commentary* (2002), at 76.11, has something close to the Latin: إلا المألوف وغير المألوف; "other than that which is familiar and that which is non-familiar."

230. *Sense and Sensibilia* 5, 443b6–17.

231. φρονιμώτατόν ἐστι, "reaches the maximum of discriminative accuracy." Aristotle, *De Anima* (1984). The Latin of this sentence and the one which follows is a generally accurate, albeit perhaps too literal, rendering of what we find in the Greek.

with hard flesh is not discriminating and one with soft flesh is discriminating.[232] (421a18–26)

The sense of taste in us is more perfect than the sense of smell, because
taste is touch in some way and the sense of touch in us is more perfect than in
all the other animals. Next he said: **And if that sense**, etc. That is, and although that sense is more perfect in a human being than in the other animals,
nevertheless it does not follow from this that this is [the case] in regard to all
the senses. Rather human beings are less apt in these [others] than many animals. Next he said: **But in touch** we surpass, etc. That is, in the excellence of
the sense of touch, however, we surpass all [other] animals. On account of the
excellence of that sense human beings are more subtle and more discriminating than all [other] animals, namely, because the constitution {273} fitting for
the excellence of that sense is fitting for the discrimination belonging to the
intellect. Next he said: **The indication of this is**, etc. That is, the indication of the
fittingness of the constitution of that sense for the constitution of the intellect is
that also in the case of humankind, when that sense is excellent, then the human
being will be discriminating, and the contrary. Next he said: **and [a human being is] not [at all] so on the basis of something else**, etc. That is, the excellence
of discrimination does not seem to follow upon the excellence of the other senses,
for a human being of excellent vision can be without discrimination and likewise
[one] of excellent hearing, but [someone] with an excellent sense of touch constantly seems to be exercising discrimination. Next he said: **For one with hard
flesh**, etc. That is, the indication that the excellence of discrimination follows
upon the excellence of touch is that one of soft flesh, that is, having an excellent
sense of touch, constantly seems to be discriminating and intelligent, and the
contrary. What he said is true, and when you will have examined intelligent
human beings, you will always find them to be of such a disposition. For this
reason a human being has softer flesh than the rest of the animals.

95. And just as there are the sweet and the bitter in flavor, so too [are there
the same] in smells. But in some the smell and the flavor correspond, for
instance, a sweet smell and a sweet flavor, and in some they are contraries.
For this reason smell is found to be pungent, acrid, acid, or delectable.[233]
But just as we said that smells are not so evident as flavors, so too [smells]

232. *Dure enim carnis non est discretum, et mollis carnis est discretum*. The Greek
has "men whose flesh is hard are ill-endowed with intellect [ἀφυεῖς τὴν διάνοιαν],
men whose flesh is soft, well-endowed." Aristotle, *De Anima* (1984); Greek added. The
alternate translation reflects the Greek well: وذلك أن من كان جاسى للحم فلا ذكاء
لطبعه ، من كان لين المجسة في ملامسته دل ذلك على ذكاء الطباع (ibid. [1954]).
233. *Acutus et ponticus et acetosus et delectabilis*: δριμεῖα καὶ αὐστηρὰ καὶ
ὀξεῖα καὶ λιπαρά, "pungent, astringent, acid, or succulent." Aristotle, *De Anima* (1984). وفي

are called by those names only by similarity to flavors. For the smell of saffron and honey is a sweet smell, the smell of garlic[234] and the like is pungent, and so forth for the rest. (421a26–b3) {274}

He wants to explain how the differences of smells follow upon the differences of flavors. He said: **And just as there are the sweet and the bitter** in flavors, etc. That is, and just as there is a first contrariety in flavors, namely, bitterness and sweetness, from which the others are composed, so too we should hold that there is a first contrariety in smells from which the intermediates are composed. After he had recounted that these differences [in smell] ought to be the same in number as those [in flavor] and how there is a first contrariety in those [in flavor] and so also is there here in these [in smell], he then began to recount that each of those [differences found] in one of two genera does not always follow [the pattern of] its like in the other genus. He said: **But in some the smell and the flavor,** etc. That is, but in some like follows like and in some it does not, namely, because smell and flavor will not be of the same species, for instance, because flavor will be sweet and smell pungent. Next he said: **For this reason smell is found to be pungent**. That is, because the differences of smells correspond to differences of flavors, smell is found pungent, that is, its relation to smells is just as the relation of the pungent to flavors, and so forth. Having explained that we apprehend the differences of smells only on account of the similarity of these with the differences of flavors, he wants to recount that this is the reason why the names of flavors have been transferred to them. He said: **But just as we said** that **smells,** etc. That is, but as we said that the differences of smells are not evident for us in such a way that we can apprehend them without comparison and assimilation to the others,[235] as [we in fact can in the case of] flavors, this was the reason why we transferred the names of flavors to [smells] by analogy. We did not impose proper names on them because we did not understand the proper intentions in them {275} except by analogy. Next he said: **For [the smell of saffron and the smell of honey is] a sweet smell,** etc. That is, for it is evident for us that the smell of what is sweet is just as the smell of saffron or honey, that is, that the relation of the smell of saffron and the smell of honey to the other smells is just

لرائحة ‹منها ما هي› حريفة ، ومنها عفصة ، ومنها حامضة ، ومنها دهنية (ibid. [1954]).
The *Middle Commentary* (2002), at 77.4–5, has رائحة حلوة ورائحة حامضة وحريفة وقابضة, "sweet, sour, pungent and harsh." In the Latin of Avicenna's *De Anima* of his *Kitâb al-Shifâ'*, عفوصة, "acridity," is rendered by *ponticum* and *ponticitas*. See Ibn Sînâ, *Kitâb al-Nafs* (1972), 144.4, 145.9, and 146.20.

234. *Allium.* The Greek has θύμου, "thyme." Aristotle, *De Anima* (1984).

235. That is, to other smells or odors.

as the relation of what is sweet to the other flavors; and so is it for the other smells.

96. **Just as with hearing and each of the other senses, the object is in one case the audible and the inaudible, and in another the visible and the invisible, so too the sense of smell has as its object the odorous and the odorless. The odorless is called odorless because it is impossible for it to have a smell, or because it has a weak smell, or because it has a bad [smell].**[236] **The case is similar for what is called tasteless.** (421b3–8)

Here he wants to relate something common to that sense and the other senses and it is that every sense apprehends its proper sensible and its privation. He said: **Just as with hearing,** etc. That is, just as with hearing and any other of the senses it is the case that it apprehends its own proper sensible and its privation, for instance, that hearing apprehends the audible and the inaudible and sight the visible and the invisible, so too the sense of smell apprehends the odorous and the odorless. Next he began to relate in how many ways these privative names are said. He said: **The odorless is called,** etc. That is, the odorless, the invisible, and the tasteless are said in three ways: of what completely lacks that {276} sensible, or that in which it is found in a weak way, or in which it is found poorly. For instance, odorless is said of what lacks smell completely and of what has it weakly and poorly. And similarly with respect to what can be tasted.

236. *Et non odorabile dicitur non odorabile . . . aut quia habet odorem debilem, aut quia habet malum.* ἀνόσφραντον δὲ τὸ μὲν παρὰ τὸ ἀδύνατον <εἶναι> μηδ᾽ ὅλως ἔχειν ὀσμήν, τὸ δὲ μικρὰν ἔχον καὶ φαύλην. "Inodorous may be either what has no smell at all, or what has a small or feeble smell." Aristotle, *De Anima* (1984), here follows a variant. وإذا قلنا شيء لا رائحة له أو غير مشموم ، فذلك إما لأنه لا يمكنه أن تكون له رائحة ألبتة ، وإما كانت له رائحة يسيرة (ibid. [1954]); "When we say that something has no odor or no smell, this is either because it can have no odor at all or <because> it has an insignificant odor." *Malum* fails to render the Greek well here, while يسيرة , "insignificant," is an adequate rendering. This problem may be the result of a corruption in the Arabic manuscript of Aristotle's *De Anima* used by Averroes. شرير is an adjective meaning "evil" or "wicked." For the sake of comparison, note that in the Latin of Avicenna's *De Anima* of his *Kitâb al-Shifâ'*, شر is rendered by *malitia* (Ibn Sînâ, *Kitâb al-Nafs* [1972], 118.10 and .14) and *malum* (ibid. [1968], 133.32, .33, .37, .38) and شرير by *malitiosus,* (ibid. [1968], 32.37). The *Middle Commentary* (2002), at 77.13, has رائحة ردية, "a bad odor." Themistius notes that the odorless is what has no odor at all, what has very little odor, and what the organ cannot tolerate. Themistius, *De Anima Paraphrase* (1899), 69.1–2; (1973), 112.7–8; (1996), 89. Averroes' Comment would seem to indicate that this problem existed in his Arabic manuscript of Aristotle's *De Anima.*

97. **Smelling also comes about through a medium, for instance, air and water. For animals living in water are thought to sense smell (and likewise both for those having blood and those bloodless) just as animals which are in the air have sensation. For some are moved toward their food from a great distance.**[237] (421b8–13)

After he had explained here what he was able to explain, concerning smell he explains in this passage that this sense in this way also requires a medium just as the two aforementioned senses. His account is evident, but it ought to be read this way: smelling comes about through a medium and this medium is air or water. For animals living in water seem to sense a smell just as animals living in air, and in this way it seems that animals living in air and those not living [in air] sense smell. The indication of this is that many of those are moved toward their food from a distance, although they do not see [it]. For bees are moved toward nourishment from a very distant place. In whatever region they exist, they seek out the seashore every year at a certain determined time to take the vigor of their food from slime.[238] And they are animals which lack blood. It is similarly so for fish and for many water animals. The reason for what he said about the medium is the aforementioned reason, namely, that when what is odorous is placed upon the sense of smell, it will not be sensed. What he said concerning sight, that the intermediate nature which {277} serves sight is not air insofar as it is air or water insofar as it is water, but a common nature, this should be understood here in this way in regard to the nature which is the medium, namely, because it is a nature common to water and air. And [it should further be understood] that smells are extrinsic to that nature and that that nature lacks smells just as the transparent [lacks] colors, in such a way that, just as color has a twofold being, namely, being in the colored body (this is corporeal being) and being in the transparent (this is spiritual being), so too smell has twofold being, namely, being in the body which is odorous and being in the medium. The former is corporeal being and the latter spiritual, the former natural and the latter extrinsic. When some were ignorant of this and thought that the smell is not separate from the body able to bear the smell and that it has only one being alone, they said that an odorous body, which

237. *Quedam enim moventur ad suum cibum in remoto*: καὶ γὰρ τούτων ἔνια πόρρωθεν ἀπαντᾷ πρὸς τὴν τροφὴν ὕποσμα γινόμενα, "at any rate some of them make directly for their food from a distance *if it has any scent.*" Aristotle, *De Anima* (1984); emphasis added. فإن طائفة منها لمكان اشتمامها قد تنزع إلى الطعم من بعد بعيد (ibid. [1954]); "Some of them desire food, traveling to the location of the scent from a distance."

238. Or: to feed vigorously on the slime. That is, they feed on the rotting debris washed ashore.

has a subtle body and a subtle smell, is released from the body able to bear the
smell and is moved in the air until it reaches the sense of smell. This [under-
standing] is refuted in many ways. For we see that many animals are moved
to their nourishment through the space of many places[239] as is apparent in the
case of vultures and as is apparent concerning tigers which come from distant
regions to the location of an attack, which happens in the land of the Greeks.

Because we already asserted that every sensible which is apprehended
through a medium ought to be sensed equally from all parts, unless something
is impeding [this], it is thus necessary that this vaporous body always be one
and that its half-diameter be according to the length of the lines[240] {278} whence
come those animals to their food, as it is said that vultures are moved from
500,000 feet. But it is impossible for a small body to be extended up to the point
that it receives such dimensions, since it is impossible for matter to receive extension to such a great extent. For the greatest dispersal which matter receives is
the dimension of fire, then of air. If, therefore, a body which is able to have smell
is altered wholly into fire or air, it is impossible for it to receive the dimension of
100,000 feet. For the least of the dimensions which matter receives is the dimension of earth and the greatest is the dimension of fire; and between those two
dimensions + this quantity is not sensed from the diversity, namely, that the
magnitude of one handful of earth becomes [dispersed to] 100,000 feet;[241] for
this is impossible.[242] Furthermore, if it were so, then it would be necessary that

239. *Dietarum*: The Latin *diaeta* means a medical regimen or a room in a house. It is
derived from the Greek δίαιτα, a way of living or a place of living. See *Oxford Latin
Dictionary* (1982), 535A.

240. Arabic fragments correspond roughly to Book 2, 97.44–48: ولما كنا قد وضعنا
المشموم وغيره من المحسوسات التي تدرك بمتوسط من جميع الجهات ⟨انه يحس من جميع
أجزائه بدون⟩* ان يكون هناك عائق ، فقد يجب أن يكون هذا الجسم البخاري الذي ينعكس
كري وان كان ذلك فقد وجب ان نصف قطر هذه الكرة (*Long Commentary* Fragments [1985],
40). *I correct Ben Chehida's bracket here. The Arabic differs from the Latin. "Since we
have already set forth regarding smell and the rest among the sensibles which are apprehended through a medium with all its parts that it senses all of its parts when there
is nothing to obstruct this, then it is necessary that this vaporous body which is cast
back be spherical. And if that is the case, it is necessary that we describe the diameter
of this sphere."

241. As Crawford indicates with +, the text is clearly defective here. The sense of
the argument seems to be that fire allows for the greatest dispersal of matter and earth
the least dispersal. Between these is the dispersal characteristic of air and water. But,
the argument would seem to proceed, the notion that a handful of earth, the element least
amenable to dispersal, would be able to disperse an odor to a distance of 100,000 feet
is absurd.

242. Arabic fragments correspond to Book 2, 97.50–62: فمحال ان يوجد جسم كري
صغير القدر يتمدد هذا القدر ، كما انه محال ان تقبل المادة ان تتمدد الى قدر أقصى ، فان

this spherical body able to bear the smell penetrate the air completely or that the air recede from its place. Since this is impossible, it is also impossible for the smell to be in the air just as in a composite body, for simple things do not receive smells. It remains, therefore, that it is in it as color is in the transparent. But, nevertheless, it is apparent that the being of color is more spiritual than the being of a smell. For the winds seem to bring smells and this is the basis for it being thought that a smell is a body. But it is so for a smell in this intention as [it is] for sound. For sound comes from an affection in air, but it is also impeded by winds; but nevertheless it does not follow from this that it is a body. It is, therefore, as it were, necessary that in the case of these two affections, namely, of sound and smell, since they are in the air, they not be motions there in the air in one case and not in the other.[243] {279}

98. **And for this reason it appears that this is a questionable matter, namely, that all animals smell in the same way and that human beings smell only when they breathe drawing air in. But when they exhale or hold their breath, they do not smell [things], be they distant or near, nor even if what is odorous were placed on the nostril. But that the sensible will not be sensed when it is placed on the very thing which senses is common to all [the senses]. But that sensing does not come about [in the case of this sense] without drawing air in is proper to human beings. This will be evident to those who try it.** (421b13–19)

We have said that the animals living in water and the animals without blood do smell. As a consequence there arises a question when we have conceded the two following propositions: all animals ought to smell in the same way; and human beings smell when they draw air in and not when they exhale or hold their breath. For it follows from this that if there is some animal which does not breathe, then it would not smell.[244] Next he said: **But that it will not**

أقصى ما تقبل المادة بعد النار بعد الهواء فلو استحال الجسم المشموم كله نارا لا يمكن ان
يقبل قدر بعد ألف ميل لأن أصغر الأبعاد التي نقبلها المادة هو بعد الأرض وأكبرها بعد النار
من التفاوت وبين هذين البعدين ﴿لا يحس باختلاف﴾ هذا المقدار أعني ان يكون مقدار شبر
من الأرض إذا انقلب نارا صارت ألف ميل ، وهذا مستحيل (*Long Commentary* Fragments [1985], 40). The problematic portion of the Latin text corresponds to the overlined text above: "and between those two dimensions the difference of these measures cannot be sensed." Note also that the Latin has "a small body" while the Arabic has "a small spherical body" (جسم كري صغير).

243. That is, sound and odor are each affections of air and not bodies.

244. Arabic fragments correspond to Book 2, 98.12–19: وإذا قلنا ان الحيوان الذي مأواه الماء والحيوان الغير ذي الدم يشم ، ففيه موضع شك إذا سلمنا مقدمتين : أولا ان الحيوان كله يجب ان يشم كله على مثال واحد ، ثانيا ان الانسان يشم بأن يتنفس فقط ، أما إذا لم يتنفس بل يخرج الهواء أو يحصره فهو لا يشم لا من بعد ولا من قرب فيلزم عن هذا أيضا

be sensed if **the sensible is placed**, etc. That is, but that it is necessary for all the senses and for all animals that there be a medium and that sensing not come about when the sensible is placed on the very thing which senses, this is common to all. For Aristotle holds this concerning touch and taste, as will be apparent later. Next he said: **But that sensing does not come about** without **drawing air in**, etc. That is, but that it is impossible for human beings and other breathing animals to smell {280} without drawing air in is self-evident to those wishing to consider and to try it.

99. **It is, therefore, necessary from this that bloodless animals have another sense since they do not breathe. But this is impossible since they sense smell, for to smell is to sense good smell and bad smell. And we also see that strong smells which are injurious to human beings are harmful to them [as well], such as that of putrefaction**[245] **and of sulphur and the like. Hence it is necessary that they smell but not by inhaling.** (421b19–26)

After we have asserted that all animals smell in the same way, and it is evident that human beings do not smell without drawing air in, it is necessary that, since bloodless animals do not breathe and [still] seem to come to their nourishment from a distance, they have a sense different from the sense of smell. Next he said: **But this is impossible**, etc. That is, but to assert that these have a sense different from the sense of smell is impossible, since we have asserted that nothing apprehends smell except through that sense. For to apprehend good and bad smell is to smell and to smell is an action of that sense, not of another. Next he said: for **strong smells which** are harmful to **human beings are harmful to them [as well]**. This is the second argument. It is that those animals are sickened and pained by bad smells and flee them, as do human beings, and because human beings flee them on account of the sense of smell, it is necessary that it be so for other animals. Next he said: **Hence it is necessary** {281} **that they smell but not by inhaling.** That is, it is therefore necessary, from what we said—namely, that those animals smell since they seem to move toward and to flee smells, and that it is impossible for that action to be through a sense differ-

---

أن الحيوان الغير المتنفس أن يكون غير شام (*Long Commentary* Fragments [1985], 40–41). The emphasized Arabic text is not reflected in the Latin: "and human beings smell when they draw air in and not when they exhale or hold their breath, *so they do not smell from near or far. For it follows. . . .*"

245. The corresponding Greek has ἀσφάλτου, "bitumen." (Aristotle, *De Anima* [1984]); والاسفلطوس is Badawi's correction of the manuscript (ibid. [1954]). The *Middle Commentary* (2002), at 78.5–6, has مثل القفر ورائحة الكبريت وما أشبهها, "the odor of asphalt, sulfur, and the like," as is found in Themistius, *De Anima Paraphrase* (1899), 69.27–28; (1973), 113.14; (1996), 90.

ent from the sense of smell—that those animals necessarily employ the sense
of smell and it is not necessary that all animals smell in the same way.

100. **It seems, therefore, that this sense is different in human beings from
[what] it is in other animals, just as the eyes [of human beings] are different
from the eyes of animals having hard eyes. For the former have covers,
namely, eyelids, which are such that when they are not open, a human being
does not see. But animals having hard eyes do not have such a thing but see
immediately what comes about in the transparent. So it also seems to be for
the sense of smell, namely, that in some animals there is no covering, as is
the case of the eye. But in animals which take in air it does have a covering.
And when those animals draw air in, the veins and passages swell and that
[covering] is drawn away. For this reason these [animals] which breathe do
not smell in what is wet, for drawing air in is necessary for smell, hence it
is impossible to do this in what is wet. Smell is of what is dry, as flavor of
what is wet. And what senses[246] and what smells is that which is of that
disposition in potency.** (421b26–422a7)

After it had been explained that some of the animals sense smell without
drawing air in and some by drawing air in, {282} it was seen that the reason
for this is that this sense in human beings and in animals which breathe differs in creation and form from smell in other non-breathing animals, just as
the eyes in human beings and in other [animals] differ in creation[247] from the
eyes of animals having hard eyes, namely, those lacking eyelids. After he had
recounted the similarity between these in this intention, he gave the mode of
the similarity. He said: **For those** have covers, etc. That is, the eyes in human
beings and in other [animals] have eyelids with which they are covered, and
it is impossible for a human being to see until he opens his eyelids, while
animals having hard eyes do not have eyelids but immediately see the colors
which have come about in the transparent without some covering. So it seems
that the disposition of the sense of smell in animals which breathe differs
from what it is in those which do not breathe. For in those which breathe it
has a covering, but in those which do not breathe it does not have a covering.
Thus animals which breathe for smelling require breath to open the closed
passages of the sense of smell, through which it is impossible to smell before
they are opened, just as it is impossible for animals having good sight to see

246. *Et sentiens*. This is neither in the Greek nor in the alternate translation. Note
that when Averroes cites this line of the Text in his Comment, he does so without these
words.

247. *In creatione*. They differ in makeup. See Book 1, {74, n. 232}, and Book 2, {258,
n. 207}.

until the eyelids are opened. But animals which do not breathe do not require this. That will be the reason why animals which breathe do not smell in water. But there is a question in regard to what he said. For animals having hard eyes have weaker sight than other animals, but many animals which do not breathe seem to have a stronger sense of smell than do human beings, and it would be necessary, if the eyelids on the eyes were just as the nostril in animals which breathe, that the animals which breathe have a more accurate sense of smell {283} than those which do not breathe. For this reason we should investigate whether the nostril in animals which smell through the nostril is for better living, as the eyelids are in animals having eyelids, or out of necessity. If, therefore, it is out of necessity, it is not necessary that those which breathe have a more exacting sense of smell than do those which do not breathe; but if for better living, it will be the contrary. But what he said, **the veins and passages swell**, shows that this is out of necessity, not for the better living, and that animals having hard eyes are not analogous to those which smell without drawing air in except according to the diversity of creation alone, not that the function provided by the eyelids is of the same sort as the function provided by drawing air in. Next he said: **Smell is of what is dry, as flavor of what is wet.** That is, the smell is ascribed to the abundance of the dry part in what is able to have smell, just as flavor is ascribed to the abundance of the wet part in what is able to be tasted; and this will be explained in the book *Sense and Sensibilia*.[248] Next he said: **[. . .] and what smells is that which is [. . .] of that disposition**. That is, after it had been explained what smell is and how it is apprehended by sense, the sense of smell, then, is what is naturally constituted to receive smells.

101. **Taste is a kind of touch; it is that which is potentially of that disposition [but] not through a medium which is an external body, for even touch is not such as this. Taste in the body in which there is flavor is in the wetness as a thing in matter[249] and this is something tangible. For this reason, if we were in water and something sweet were in the water, {284} we would sense it not through a medium but by virtue of its mixing with the wet, just as it is for wine.[250] Color, however, is not seen by virtue of being mixed nor because something flows from it.** (2.10, 422a8–15)

After he had completed the account of smell—and the sense of taste is what ought to follow now according to the order which begins from what is for bet-

---

248. *Sense and Sensibilia* 5, 443b3–8. Cf. Themistius, *De Anima Paraphrase* (1899), 70.7–8; (1973), 114.16–17; (1996), 90.

249. *In humiditate sicut res in materia*: ἐν ὑγρῷ ὡς ὕλῃ, "in a liquid matter." Aristotle, *De Anima* (1984). See n. 251 below on Averroes' citation of his alternate translation.

250. *Sicut est de vino*: καθάπερ ἐπὶ τοῦ ποτοῦ, "just as if it were mixed with some drink" (Aristotle, *De Anima* [1984]); كالذى تراه في الشراب (ibid. [1954]).

ter living and proceeds toward what is more necessary—he began to speak of it and to explain that it is a kind of touch and that on account of this it does not need to apprehend its sensible through a medium which is an external body, but through a medium which is a part of the animal. He said: **Taste is a kind of touch and it is that which is potentially of that disposition [but] not through a medium which is an external body, for even touch is not such as this.** That is, that sense is what is not potentially of that disposition through a medium which is an external body, but through a medium which is a non-external body. Next he said: **for even touch is not such as this.** That is, for even touch does not apprehend its sensible through a medium which is an external body, as it is for the three senses mentioned earlier. He introduces, as it were, that account on the basis of the notion that taste is a kind of touch. He says, as it were: but taste is a kind of touch, since, just as touch, it does not apprehend its sensible through a medium which is an external body. This is more evident in the second translation, where he says: "But the sense of taste apprehends through touch and the reason for that is that what is sensible {285} through taste is not apprehended through a medium between what tastes and what is tasted, which is an external body; and even touch does not apprehend [its object] in this way."[251] Next he said: **[Taste] in the body in which there is flavor**, etc. That is, in another way also we say that this sense is a kind of touch. For the body in which flavor exists is able to be tasted only insofar as that flavor exists in it in a liquid related to that flavor as matter to form.[252] For this reason that sense does not apprehend flavor unless it apprehends a liquid, since it is impossible for it to exist separate from [a liquid]. To apprehend the liquid is to touch something. Hence that sense seems to be a kind of touch. Next he said: **For this reason, if we were in water**, etc. That is, because taste does not require an external medium, for this reason, if we were in water and there were something sweet found in the water, it would be sensed by us in virtue of its being mixed with the water, not because water receives the flavor separated from the matter and returns it to that sense, as it is for external media which return sensible things to the senses. For those do not receive sensibles with the bodies in which

---

251. وأما حس المذاق فإنما يدرك بالملامسة ، وعلة ذلك أن المحسوس بالمذاق لـم يدرك بالمتوسط (Aristotle, *De Anima* بين الذائق والمذوق وذلك هو جسم قريب : ولا إدراك اللـمس بهـذه الجهـة [1954]); "The sense of taste perceives only through touch. The reason for this is that what is sensed by taste is not perceived through a medium between what tastes and what is tasted: this is a *proximate* body. Perception on the part of touch is not like this." The term قريب, "proximate," was probably originally غريب, as it is in the *Middle Commentary* (2002), 78.21–22: لا بمتوسط هو جسم غريب أعنى من خارج, "not <through a medium> which is a foreign, i.e., external body." I use Ivry's translation with a minor change for clarity. Neither of these renders the Greek ἐν ὑγρῷ ὡς ὕλῃ accurately.

252. Cf. Themistius, *De Anima Paraphrase* (1899), 70.32–33; (1973), 116.3–5; (1996), 91.

they exist, but separated from matter. This shows that he holds the opinion that smell is not a body; for if it were a body, [smell] would be a kind of touch.

Next he said: **Color, however, is not seen**, etc. That is, but color is not seen because some of it is mixed with water or air, nor because something flows from it into water or air. Rather, they only receive from it the intention of color separated from matter. Hence we say in regard to this and the like that they are apprehended through an external medium. {286}

102. **But in this kind [of sensation] there is no medium. Rather, just as color is visible, so too flavor is able to be tasted. Nothing receives the sensation of flavor without wetness, but rather there is wetness in it in act or in potency; for instance, salt, for it is quick dissolving and besides it dissolves the tongue.** (422a15–19)

But that sense differs from the senses which apprehend [things] through an external medium in that it does not apprehend its sensible through a medium. Rather, just as color is visible in fact as something proper to vision, so too flavor is able to be tasted in fact as something proper to taste. Next he said: **Nothing receives the sensation of flavor**, etc. That is, nothing receives the sensation of flavor, which is called taste, unless the flavor is in a liquid and the liquid is in what is flavorful either in act or in potency, for instance, salt, which is in proximate potency to being wet since it is dissolved quickly and it dissolves liquids which are on the tongue. For this reason nature prepares the saliva in the mouth and prepares the branchial passages in human beings for collecting that wetness so that by means of it dry things may be tasted. Hence we say that flavor is flavor in act only in a body wet in act.

103. **Just as sight is of things which are visible and things which are not visible (for darkness is not visible and is also discerned by sight), it is also evident {287} in reference to what is too gleaming and bright (for this is in a way also not visible, although in a way different from darkness). Similarly hearing is of sound and silence, one of which is audible and the other inaudible. [Hearing] is related to very loud sounds just as vision is related to what is [very] bright (for just as the least sound is inaudible, so too in a way is the loudest sound inaudible). Some of what is invisible is spoken of generally in this way, just as [similar terms are used] in regard to all things which are lacking this [capacity], and another is of the sort that it is naturally constituted to be seen but is not or is but barely, as [one speaks of something] lacking a foot.**[253] **Taste is similarly of what is able to be tasted and what is unable to be**

253. *Et non visibile quoddam dicitur sic universaliter, sicut in omnibus carentibus hoc, et quoddam est innatum videri sed non habet, aut habet sed diminute, ut carens pede:* ἀόρατον δὲ τὸ μὲν ὅλως λέγεται, ὥσπερ καὶ ἐπ᾿ ἄλλων τὸ ἀδύνατον, τὸ

tasted. (This is what has a flavor weak, bad, or destructive of taste.) And it is similarly thought concerning what is drinkable and undrinkable, for they are taste in a way, but the latter is bad and injurious to taste and the former is natural. What is drinkable is common to both touch and taste. (422a20–34)

His account in this chapter is evident. Its summary is that non-sensible is said in reference to each of the senses in three ways: [1] of what lacks [the ability to apprehend] a sensed object proper to that sense from among sensible objects which it is naturally constituted to have [as its object], [2] of what is in itself an intense sensible object for that sense, or [3] of what is a weak sensible object. For instance, [these are] darkness, which is non-sensible in virtue of its being a privation in regard to vision; bright color, which is non-sensible in virtue of its intensity; and latent color, which is non-sensible in virtue of its {288} weakness. In hearing [these are] silence in virtue of privation, loud sound in virtue of its intensity, and latent sound in virtue of its weakness, while in taste the insipid in virtue of privation, the disgusting in virtue of its offensiveness, and the weak in virtue of its frailty. For all those are called non-sensibles, because each of them is a privation of some disposition naturally belonging to the sensible of that sense. Next he said: **Some of what is invisible is spoken of**, etc. That is, invisible is said generally in many ways, just as in reference to the other senses: [1] because [the thing] is not naturally constituted to be seen at all, as we say that sound is invisible and in regard to color that it is inaudible, or [2] because it is naturally constituted to be seen but it is not seen because it lacks color, or [3] because it has color but in a way different from that according to which it is naturally constituted to have [it]. That is to say, this is called invisible either on account of its intensity or on account of its weakness, as is said in regard to what has a frail foot that it does not have a foot. Next he said: **What is drinkable is common to both touch and taste**, that is, because in virtue of the wetness which is in it it is tangible and in virtue of the flavor it is able to be tasted.

104. **Because what is able to be tasted is wet, it was necessary that its [corresponding] sense not be wet in actuality and [that it] not be incapable of**

δ ἐὰν πεφυκὸς μὴ ἔχῃ ἢ φαύλως, ὥσπερ τὸ ἄπουν καὶ τὸ ἀπύρηνον, "and as one thing is called invisible absolutely (as in other cases of impossibility <*sic*>), another if it is adapted by nature to have the property but has not it or has it only in a very low degree, as when we say that something is footless or stoneless." Aristotle, *De Anima* (1984). For "impossibility," "incapacity" may be more felicitous. إما كذلك الشيء الذى ليس بمبصر لم يبصر لإنّه لا إمكان في رؤيته ، وإما لم يبصر لغاية قلّته كصغير الأرجل من الحيوان يقال لا أرجل له (ibid. [1954]); "Like the thing which is not seen, either it is not seen because it is incapable of being seen or it is not seen owing to its extreme smallness, just as animals having tiny feet are said not to have feet."

becoming wet. For taste in some way is affected by what is able to be tasted insofar as it is able to be tasted. Hence, what is such that it is possible for it to become wet (while it is still preserved intact) necessarily becomes wet, but the sense of taste is not what is wet. {289} The indication of this is that the tongue does not sense when it is too dry or too wet. For touch itself is through the first liquid, as one who earlier tasted a strong flavor then tasted another flavor and as those who are ill sense all things as bitter because they sense them through a tongue submersed in such a liquid. (422a34–b10)

After he had explained these things which are common to that sense, to the sense of touch and to the other senses, he began to speak about something proper to the bodily part of that sense, namely, the tongue. He said: **Because taste** is wet, etc. That is, because the matter of flavor is liquid, as was explained in *Sense and Sensibilia*,[254] it was necessary that what receives flavor receive a liquid along with flavor. Hence it is necessary that this sense not be wet in act nor also that it be impossible for it to receive liquid, since it is naturally constituted to receive flavor, which is impossible without the reception of liquid. He said that it is necessary that it not be wet in act because that which is something in act is not naturally constituted to receive that which is in it in act insofar as it is in it in act. For if sight were to have some color in act, it would not receive colors. Next he said: **For taste in some way is affected**, etc. That is, it is necessary that this sense be naturally constituted so as to be liquified. For the part which tastes is affected in some way by what is able to be tasted; and because what is able to be tasted is always associated with a liquid, it is necessary that what tastes be affected by the liquid which accompanies flavor. Hence it is necessary that this tasting part be in this disposition by which it is possible that it become wet. {290} This will be such that it is not wet in itself and that besides it be preserved from accidents.[255] He meant this when he said: **Hence, what is such that**, etc. That is, because it is necessary that this part become wet, it is necessary that it be naturally constituted so as to become wet, namely, so that it be preserved from excessive dryness and so that it not be wet. Next he said: **The indication of this is that the tongue**, etc. That is, the indication of the fact that the tongue, when apprehending flavors, ought to be preserved from excessive dryness and from being dominated by liquid is that it does not sense flavors when it is characterized by excessive dryness or by excessive wetness, but it only senses when it is in a natural disposition according to which it is naturally constituted to receive the wetness of flavor. Next

254. *Sense and Sensibilia* 4, 441a21ff.

255. That is, this is so that it is also preserved from being affected by other wetnesses which are accidental to it and which would disrupt taste's ability to discern the liquid proper to the particular flavor, as Averroes explains below.

he said: **For touch itself**, etc. That is, since the tongue is naturally constituted to receive flavor with its wetness, it is necessary that there be no other wetness dominant in it. For the first wetness dominant on the tongue will hinder it in its process of receiving a second wetness, just as one who has tasted some strong flavor and later on tastes another flavor. For then he will not sense the second flavor on account of the domination of the first upon the tongue. Next he said: **and as** those who are sick **sense all things as bitter**, etc. That is, and as those who are sick sense all flavors as bitter, because they sense them through a tongue which is submersed in bitter liquid, so too one who tastes some flavor and his tongue is made wet in an accidental liquid then will not apprehend the proper liquid of the flavor, except as mixed with the quality of that first liquid. And thus it will happen necessarily that he does not apprehend the flavor because he does not apprehend the matter of the flavor in the disposition according to which it is the matter of that flavor. {291}

105. **The kinds of flavors are just as the kinds of colors. The simple ones are the contraries, the sweet and the bitter. Those that follow are, in the case of the former, oily, and in the case of the latter, salty. Those that are between these are pungent, astringent, acrid, and acidic.[256] For those kinds are seen commonly to be the kinds of flavors. Hence it is necessary that what tastes is that which has that disposition in potency and what is able to be tasted is what acts.[257]**(422b10–16)

The disposition of the kinds of flavors with respect to one another is just as the disposition of colors with respect to one another. Therefore, just as the simple colors are white and black, from which the rest are composed, some of which are nearer to some of the simple, so too is it for flavors, namely, that the simple among them are contraries, namely, the sweet and the bitter. The oily follows upon the sweet and the salty upon the bitter. Among them are the pungent, the astringent, and the acidic. What he said in regard to colors is evident, but he has a question in regard to flavors. For Galen held the opinion

256. *Et que sunt inter ea sunt acutus, et stipticus, et ponticus, et acetosus*: μεταξὺ δὲ τούτων τό τε δριμὺ καὶ τὸ αὐστηρὸν καὶ στρυφνὸν καὶ ὀξύ, "between these come the pungent, the harsh, the astringent, and the acid" (Aristotle, *De Anima* [1984]); وبين هذين الحريف و العفص ، والقابض والحامض (ibid. [1954]); "Between these are the pungent, the bitter, the astringent and the acidic."

257. *Unde necesse est ut gustans sit illud quod est in potentia istius dispositionis, et gustabile sit agens.* ὥστε τὸ γευστικόν ἐστι τὸ δυνάμει τοιοῦτον, <τὸ> γευστὸν δὲ τὸ ποιητικὸν ἐντελεχείᾳ αὐτοῦ. "It follows that what has the power of tasting is what is potentially of that kind, and that what is tasteable is what has the power of making it actually what it itself already is" (Aristotle, *De Anima* [1984]); فالمذاق ما كان بالقوة ذائقا ، والمذوق هو المخرج لذلك إلى الفعل (ibid. [1954]).

that the acrid and the acidic are cold and that the pungent is warmer than the bitter.[258] If we concede that those flavors follow upon warmth and cold, it is necessary that the contrariety in them be in that which is warm to the greatest degree and in that which is cold to the greatest degree. If we concede that it is so for flavors just as for colors, namely, that the same color is from warmness or from coldness, then the impossible will not occur. It seems that the opinion {292} of Galen is erroneous. For we see that bitterness sometimes is found with coldness, for instance, that bitterness which is in fruits in the first growth exhibits coldness and the bitterness which is in things burned exhibits warmth. Likewise it is not impossible that some sweetness be cold, for it seems that plants having a bitter flavor at maturity are sweet or insipid when immature. The indication that those flavors are so is that plants having flavors are not transformed from bitterness to sweetness, in those things which are naturally constituted to be sweet in the end, except by the mediation of one of those flavors. This will be in accord with what pertains to that bitter [flavor] existing in one plant and that sweet [flavor] existing in another. [This is] just as [is the case for] white, [which] is not changed to black or the contrary except through the mediation of one of the intermediate colors. In one, therefore, it is changed through the mediation of grey and in another through the mediation of yellow,[259] for it is not necessary for the movement from extremes to be through all the intermediates. It is generally self-evident that bitter and sweet have the greatest contrariety insofar as they are flavors. Hence it is necessary that other flavors be intermediate between those two and be composed from the extremes. According to this, therefore, we ought to assert this and we ought not to turn to the account of Galen, for his account is not true in regard to the mixtures of flavors according to their natures. If we concede that everything sweet is warm and also everything bitter is warm, we ought also to say that this is only with respect to the body of a human being, not with respect to the nature of the thing. For although experience testifies to this in the case of the human body, nevertheless {293} this does not show the nature of flavors themselves.

It seems that flavor follows upon wetness and dryness rather than warmness and coldness. For it is necessary to hold that some mixture is determined from which bitterness comes and another from which sweetness [comes], and that those two mixtures are contraries in this way. The locus of this investiga-

---

258. Taste in Galen is discussed in Siegel (1970), 3, 158–173.

259. *Karopo*, "grey," is apparently a transliteration of what the translator found in the Arabic. This corresponds to the Greek χαροπός, "grey." *Kiano*, "yellow," corresponds to the Greek ξάθός, "yellow." Cf. *Sense and Sensibilia* 4, 442a21–25, where the term τὸ φαιὸν is used for grey, not χαροπός.

tion and of [that into] the number of kinds of flavors is in the book *Sense and Sensibilia*.[260] Next he said: Hence **it is necessary that what tastes is that**, etc. That is, it was therefore explained from what was mentioned earlier that this sense is what is all those flavors in potency and that flavor and taste are what act on and move that sense from potency to act.

106. **The account is the same for the tangible and for touch. For if touch is not of one genus, but of more [than one], it is necessary that tangible things also be of more than one kind. But there is a question as to whether they are one or more kinds.** (2.11, 422b17–20)

Now he wants to speak about touch. He said: **The account is the same for the tangible and for touch**, etc. That is, there is a question as to whether the tangible is one or more than one, as is the case for touch. His account concerning these is the same. He indicated by this the reason why this is obscure in the case of this sense and not obscure in the cases of the other senses. For with respect to those, because it was evident that their sensible [object] is one in genus, it was also evident that [those senses] are [each] one in genus; but in the case of this sense, because there was no knowledge about its sensibles, there was also no knowledge about its sense. Next he said: **For if touch is not of one genus**, etc. That is, the account concerning these in regard to this intention is the same. For it was noted by us that if touch {294} is not one genus but many, it is necessary that the tangible things be more than one and that if the tangible things are more than one, it is necessary that this sense be more than one. But although the consequence is evident in those two syllogisms, nevertheless refutation or assertion in reference to it is something unknown.

107. **Is the sense of touch in the flesh or in something similar or [is it] not [in flesh], but is [flesh] rather the medium, while the first thing that senses is something else internal?[261] For every sense is thought to be of the same**

---

260. 4, 442a13ff.

261. *Sensus autem tactus utrum est in carne aut in alio simili, aut non, sed ista est medium, primum autem sentiens est aliud intrinsecum?* πότερον ἡ σὰρξ καὶ ἐν τοῖς ἄλλοις τὸ ἀνάλογον, ἢ οὔ, ἀλλὰ τοῦτο μέν ἐστι τὸ μεταξύ, τὸ δὲ πρῶτον αἰσθητήριον ἄλλο τί ἐστιν ἐντός. "Is it or is it not the flesh (including what in certain animals is analogous to flesh)? On the second view, flesh is the medium of touch, the real organ being situated farther inward." Aristotle, *De Anima* (1984). وما الجزء الحاس المدرك لحس اللمس : اللحم ، أو غيره؟ أو إنما هو شيء متوسط ، والحاس الأول غيره وهو داخل؟ (ibid. [1954]); "What is the sensing part apprehensive of touch? Is it the flesh or not? Or is it something intermediate, the first thinking which senses something else entering?" While it is clear that the Text is faulty, Averroes nevertheless makes sense of it in his Comment in accord with the original Greek's apparent meaning.

contrariety, for instance, sight of white and black, hearing of flat and sharp, and taste of sweet and bitter. For tangible things, however, there are many contraries: hot and cold, dry and wet, hard and soft, rough and smooth,[262] and others of the like. (422b20–27)

After he had recounted that there is a question about whether the sense of touch is [one and] the same power or more [than one], he began to voice the accounts which are questionable in reference to this. He said: **Is the sense of touch,** etc. That is, the starting point of consideration in regard to this is whether the sense of touch is in flesh or in something similar to flesh in animals lacking flesh; or is the sense of touch not in flesh but rather flesh is, as it were, a medium? He said this because if it is explained that the sense of touch is in flesh in such a way that the relation of flesh to it is just as the relation of the eye to sight, it is evident that the sense of touch is one power, since one organ belongs only to one power. But if it is explained that this power is more than {295} one, it is necessary that flesh be, as it were, a medium, and that it is not, as it were, an organ. After he had recounted this, he began to bring forth the accounts which are questionable. He began with those which show that the power of touch is more than one because afterwards he will bring forth those which show that it is one on the basis of it being apparent that when the sensible is placed upon the flesh, [the power of touch] will sense immediately, from which it is thought that this power is one. He said: **but rather [flesh] is the medium,** etc. That is, but there is a question as to whether the sense of touch is in flesh in such a way that it is one power or it is not in flesh, but inside and is more than one power. For someone can say that flesh is the medium and that the first thing that senses, which is the organ of that power, is some internal organ and that it is more than one organ. The indication of this is that it is evident that [one and] the same sense apprehends only [one and] the same contrariety and its intermediaries. For vision apprehends white and black and the intermediaries, hearing the flat and the sharp and the intermediaries, taste the sweet and the bitter and the intermediaries. Touch, however, [apprehends] many contraries, for instance, hot and cold, wet and dry, rough and smooth, hard and soft, and other contraries. Hence, it is necessary that this power be more than one and that flesh be, as it were, the medium. What he said is evident because if there is one power which apprehends one contrariety, it happens that opposite is

262. *Et asperum et lene.* These are additions not found in the Greek text or in the alternate Arabic translation. Themistius, however, adds βαρὺ κοῦφον, λεῖον τραχύ. Themistius, *De Anima Paraphrase* (1899), 72.20; والخفيف والثقيل والأملس والخشن ibid. (1973), 119.8; "the light and the heavy, the smooth and the rough"; "heavy/light, smooth/ rough" ibid. (1996), 93. The *Middle Commentary* (2002), 81.15, has والخشن والأملس, "rough and smooth."

convertible with opposite, namely, that what does not apprehend one contrariety but many is not one power but many. {296}

108. **But there is something here by which that question is resolved. For in the other senses there are more than one kind of contrariety. For instance, in sound, with the sharp and flat, there is also loud and soft, and smooth and rough sound, and other similar things; and in color there are also other things similar to those. But nevertheless it is not evident what that one subject is [which is the subject] for touch just as sound is [the subject] for hearing.** (422b27–33)

After he had provided the account making it credible that the sense of touch is more than one, he gave another account raising a difficulty for the previous account. He said: **But there is something**, etc. That is, but someone can say that there is something by which that account proving that the sense of touch is more than one is dissolved. This is that even in the other senses the kinds of contrariety are more than one, for instance, hearing apprehends flat and sharp, loud and soft, smooth and rough. Similarly, sight apprehends many things, namely, white and black, bright and dull. For this reason it is not necessary from the fact that touch apprehends more than one [sort of thing] that it be many and that flesh be, as it were, a medium. When he had provided this doubt regarding the account proving that this sense is more than one, he began to set out the way of its weakness. He said: **But [. . .] it is not evident**, etc. That is, but that account does not follow. For, if the great contrariety which is in touch is similar to the greatest contrariety existing in each sense, it is necessary that the subject of the kinds of contrariety which is in touch be one, just as is the case for sight and hearing. For sound is the subject of those aforementioned contraries and likewise color is the subject {297} of the kinds of contrariety which can be apprehended by sight. But what is the one subject of the contraries of the sense of touch is not evident. Rather, it appears that the subject is multiplied in accord with the multiplication of the contraries. He means by **subject** here the genus which is divided into these contraries. What he said is evident. For it is necessary, if we assert that one sense apprehends many kinds of contrariety, that the subject genus for those kinds be one. For it is necessary that something be common to that multitude which is apprehended by that one sense; and if not, then nothing will exist there by which that sense could be called one, since one sense is one only through one intention. Since the contraries will be different in genera, then the powers will be different and for this reason what receives the contrariety of colors is different from what receives the contrariety of smells and from what receives the contrariety of flavors, since those contraries are different in genus. Hence it is necessary, if touch is one power, that the kinds of contraries which it apprehends be one subject genus for these and that the [subject genus] be said of them univocally such as sound, which is said univocally of the kinds of sounds, and color of the kinds of colors. But the contraries of touch do not seem to have a genus which is said of them except in an equivocal way. For quality, which is said of warm and cold, is said only in a purely equivocal way of heavy and light; and what was said concerning the equivocation in this name quality [is the same as] what is said of [its use with regard to] taste, warmness, coldness, color, and smell. For all these have been named in the category of quality, but heavy and light are in regard to the category of substance. For this reason it is necessary that the power {298} apprehending contrariety which is in the heavy and the light be in every way a power apprehending the contrariety which is in the warm and the cold, and in every way not, since that [power] which apprehends what is heavy and what is light apprehends them only through the mediation of motion, namely, because it apprehends the heavy only when a heavy or light body moves [the power]. For this reason it is necessary to hold the opinion that Aristotle wants the sense of touch to be more than one and that flesh is, as it were, a medium for it. Yet that account is contrary to the account in the book *On Animals*; but nevertheless perhaps that account was in accord with what was apparent in that context, namely, what he knew about the parts of animals at that time, for then he still did not know about nerves and he said that the organ of that sense is the flesh.[263] That account provides [the view that] the organs belong to those animals which are able to sense touch inside the flesh and this is consonant with what appeared afterwards through anatomy, namely, that the nerves have a passage for touch and motion. What, therefore, Aristotle knew by argument afterwards became apparent by sense.[264]

109. **[Regarding the question of] whether or not the sense is inside, but is the first thing that is apparent, namely, flesh, it is thought that this indication is of no value, namely, that the sense is [in act] when it is touched. For if you take a membrane and you wrap the flesh with it, then the sense will feel these in the same way as when the membrane is touched, although it is evident that what senses is not in {299} those things. If, therefore, it were**

263. Cf. *Parts of Animals* 2.1, 647a14–21; 2.8, 653b19–30.

264. The discussion in the corresponding passage of the *Middle Commentary* (2002), at 91.12–92.1, is different from what is found here. That discussion is much more brief, consisting of a precis of the Text and a short explanation of the insufficiency of the account of the unity of the sense of touch in the Text. *Middle Commentary* (2002), 92.1–8, is based on remarks by Themistius. Themistius, *De Anima Paraphrase* (1899), 72.25–36; (1973), 119.13–120.6; (1996), 93.

bonded together with it,[265] then the sensation would come about even more quickly. (422b34–423a6)

He had provided the necessary account from which it appears that the sense of touch is more than one and that flesh is, as it were, a medium, as we expounded. (Even if it is contrary to the opinion of Alexander[266] and the exposition of Themistius, although Themistius says plainly that this is the opinion of Aristotle, namely, that flesh is, as it were, a medium.[267] But they do not seem to know the reason by which Aristotle was supported in this. It is that because the sensibles of touch do not share in the same genus which would be said of them in a univocal way, it is necessary that it be more than one. We will afterwards state the argument of Alexander in regard to this and we will refute it.)[268] He also had already completed explaining and resolving a question relating to this. Hence, he returned to refute that [argument] from which it is thought that flesh is the organ of that power. He said: **Whether the sense** is **inside**, etc. That is, it is of no consequence to say, however, that what touches is not inside but rather in the first of these [parts] which is apparent, namely, in the flesh (for, when something tangible is placed upon flesh, it immediately apprehends it); namely, that this argument does not hold, that the sense of touch is [in act] when the tangible touches the flesh. Next he undermined this argument. He said: **For if you take a thin cloth**, etc. That is, for if you take a membrane which is not dense and you wrap the flesh with it and you place something tangible on it, then immediately it will be apprehended by the sense as if it were without the membrane. Next he said: **although it** is **evident that what senses is not in those things.** That is, although it is evident that the first thing which senses is not in the "skin." Hence it is not impossible {300} that the flesh have such a disposition, namely, that it be a medium, as it were, of the "skin." In regard to sensations appearing in the flesh, however, there is no doubt about these which have already been explained by argument. Next he said: **If, therefore, it were bonded together**, etc. That is, there is no difference in this inten-

---

265. *Si igitur fuerit consolidatum cum eo*: εἰ δὲ καὶ συμφυὴς ψένοιτο, θᾶττον ἔιτ διικνοῖτ ἂν ἡ αἴσθησις. If it were to correspond with the Greek, the Latin sentence would have to have a feminine subject corresponding to *membranam* (*fuerit consolidata*) and a feminine pronoun (*cum ea*) corresponding to *carnem*.

266. τοῦ δὲ τὸ μεταξύ δι' οὗ μέσου ἡ τῶν ἁπτῶν ἀντίληψις γίνεται, ἐπὶ μὲν τῆς ἁφῆς προσπεφυκέναι τῷ αἰσθανομένῳ (τοιοῦτον γὰρ ἡ σάρξ). Alexander, *De Anima* (1887), 58.5–7. "As for the intervening medium by means of which the perception of tangible objects would [then] take place, this is, in the case of touch, something that grows naturally on the sensing subject—I mean, of course, flesh." Ibid. (1979), 66–67.

267. Themistius, *De Anima Paraphrase* (1899), 75.10–27; (1973), 125.10–126.8; (1996), 96.

268. See below {311–312}.

tion whether the flesh is continuous with what senses or whether the membrane is not continuous. For if the skin were continuous, then it would report more quickly to the sense. The continuity, therefore, provides the flesh only with the ability to reach through to the sense; [it is] not that the continuity makes it possible for the flesh to be an organ of that sense.[269]

110. **For that reason that part is related to the body as air [would be] if it were affixed [so as] to envelop the body. For then we would think that we sense sound, color, and smell in virtue of the same thing and that sight, hearing, and smell are one sense. Now, however, because the air through which those motions come about, namely, to see, to hear, and to smell, is distinct, the senses which we mentioned are evidently different.** (423a6–11)

He had explained that touch is more than one sense and that on account of this flesh ought to be the media for those senses. [He had also explained] that the question [raised] about this on the basis of what is apparent to sense, which makes many people say that flesh is the organ belonging to that sense and that this sense is one, is insufficient.[270] Now he began to explain the way in which that view is common to all of them. Perhaps he is himself, in the book *On Animals*,[271] one of those who thought this. He said: **For that reason** this {301} **part is related to the body**, etc. That is, that view arises for all of them because this part, namely, flesh, is likened to air if [air] would have been affixed to the body as is flesh. For if air, inasmuch as it is a medium, were affixed to the body as flesh is, that is, [if] it were part of the body, then we would think that we sense sound, color, and smell through the same thing and that these three are one sense. This same thing occurs for the senses of touch with flesh, in such a way that it was thought that they are one sense. Next he said: **Now,**

269. This is stated more clearly in the *Middle Commentary* (2002), at 82.9–18: "As for the statement that flesh is the organ of this sense and [that it] is therefore one, as proved by the evident fact that we sense a tangible object as it is placed upon the flesh, [we say] that this fact does not prove anything. If you were now to take a membrane of leather or something else and dress the flesh with it, we would find the sense of touch remaining as vigorous as ever in the same way [as before], though it is obvious that the sense is not in this membrane. This being the case, it is not farfetched (to believe) that this is indeed the nature of flesh but that it has an additional aspect in its being affected by a tangible object, for it is attached to the sense. The contact of the sense through the medium of the flesh is thus faster than its contact through the medium of the membrane placed over the flesh, the flesh being attached to the sense and the membrane separate from it."

270. That is, it is insufficient to undermine the view being presented.

271. Cf. *Parts of Animals* 2.1, 647a14–21; 2.8, 653b19–30. See also Averroes' remarks at {298}.

however, because the air, etc. That is, but it is apparent that those three senses are different, although they are in virtue of the same medium, because the medium is not part of us. However, because flesh is part of us, this was not apparent in the senses of touch and it was thought that they are one sense. But the demonstration forces [us to say] that they are more than one sense, for it senses more than one sensible in genus.

111. **But in the case of touch this is now obscure. For it is impossible for the constitution of what is living to be of air or of water, for it needs to be solid. It remains, therefore, that it is of earth and of those things in flesh and the like. Hence, it is necessary that the bodily medium of touch be affixed and through the mediation of this the senses will be more than one.**[272] (423a11–17)

After he had explained the way in which that view follows in regard to the senses of touch and does not follow in regard to the other senses, he began to relate the cause and necessity for the fact that the medium in touch is something affixed and in the others is not affixed. He said: **But in the case of touch**, etc. That is, for touch, however, this occurs {302} in such a way that this intention is obscure in its case, namely, that it is more than one sense, from the fact that every sense needs a medium. For [their] health animals need to sense things tangible and for this reason it was necessary that the medium be part of [the animal]. It was impossible for this medium which is part of [the animal] to be water or air, for it is impossible, as was said, that the constitution of the body be of air or of water. For animals necessarily need a solid body, from which it follows that the medium in the senses of touch would be a mixed body in which earthiness would abound. This is flesh and its like in animals lacking flesh. This is how that account should be understood. He roused us

---

272. The corresponding Greek has ὥστε ἀναγκαῖον τὸ σῶμα εἶναι τὸ μεταξὺ τοῦ ἁπτικοῦ προσπεφυκός, δι' οὗ γίνονται αἱ αἰσθήσεις πλείους οὖσαι. "Consequently it must be composed of earth along with these, which is just what flesh and its analogue tend to be. Hence the body must be the medium for the faculty of touch, naturally attached to us, through which the several perceptions are transmitted." Aristotle, *De Anima* (1984). The alternate Arabic translation has والكثيف لا بد من أن يكون خلط من أرض وغيرذلك ، مما يكون جزءٍ منه اللحم . لذلك وجب بالاضطرار أن يكون الجرم متوسطًا بين اللامس والملموس ، وبه كانت الحواس كثيرة (ibid. [1954]); "The solid must be a mixture of earth and the like with that of which flesh is a part. Hence it is necessarily the case that the body is a medium between what touches and what is touched and in virtue of it the senses are many." Averroes in his Comment writes, "Next he said: through the mediation of which the senses will exist and they are more than one, that is, the senses of touch." {302}. This is a variant way of rendering the Text, not a different version.

over what is given little attention in the account by what he said: Therefore, **it is necessary that the bodily medium of touch be affixed**. That is, it is, therefore, necessary that every sense be through a medium, since the senses do not sense their sensible objects except by touching; and animals, in order to sense the sensibles which arise, need that the medium be affixed and part of the body. Next he said: **through the mediation of this the senses** will exist and are more than one, that is, the sense of touch.

112. **Touch on the part of the tongue shows that they are more than one. For all tangible things are sensed through that same bodily part, and flavor [as well]. If, therefore, another flesh were to sense flavor, then it would be thought that taste and touch are the same sense. Now, however, they are two, because they are not convertible.** (423a17–21)

Touch which is in the tongue shows that the sense of touch is more than one and [also] that this is obscure because flesh is the medium, as it were. {303} For because we sense through this part all tangible things and flavor as well, it was necessary that flesh which is in that member be a medium, as it were, not an organ, as it were. For if it were an organ of flavor, it would not apprehend what is tangible, and if it were the organ for the tangible, it would not apprehend flavor. For the same sense has the same organ. If, therefore, another flesh which is in the body were to sense the flavor as does the flesh which is in the tongue, then it would be thought that taste and touch are the same sense. Next he said: **Now, however, they are two, because they are not convertible.** That is, now, however, this does not happen because it is not convertible, namely, because every flesh which tastes is also one which touches, but not every flesh which touches is one which tastes.

113. **Among the things about which one has questions is this. Every body has depth and this is the third dimension. It is impossible for bodies which have some body as a medium existing between them to touch one another. The wet or what has been made wet does not exist without body; rather, it is necessary that it be water or something in which there is water. The things which come into contact with one another in water, since their extremities are not dry, must have between them a medium[273] and it is that in which their extremities are submersed. If this is correct, it is impossible for one thing to touch another in water. Likewise for air, for air is with these things which are in it just as water is with the things which are in water. But we are more ignorant of the things which are in air, [just as], for instance,**

---

273. *Necesse est ut inter ea sit medium*: ἀναγκαῖον ὕδωρ ἔχειν μεταξύ, "must have water between" (Aristotle, *De Anima* [1984]); يلزم بالاضطرار أن يكون منها ماء (ibid. [1954]). The Greek and the alternate Arabic translation specify the medium as water.

animals which are in water [fail to note] if a body which has been made wet touches a body made wet. (423a21–b1) {304}

After he had explained that touch needs flesh for the medium and that it is more than one [sense], he began to ask also whether that sense, besides its needing flesh, also needs an external medium or [whether] flesh is also sufficient without an external medium. That question also arises in the case of taste. He said: **Among the things about which one has questions is this,** etc. That is, regarding this there is a question as to whether touch needs an external medium, besides its needing the medium which is flesh. For every body has depth, which is the third measure of body. Next he said: **It is impossible for bodies which,** etc. That is, since every body has depth, it is necessary that there be a body between any two bodies not touching one another. Since it is so, it will happen that it is impossible for dry bodies between which there is a wet body as medium to touch one another without their surfaces being made wet by that wet body. It is impossible for the wetness to exist without that body as medium, for instance, bodies which have been made wet, since it is impossible for them to touch one another unless there is some water or something of water between them. Next he said: **The things which come into contact with one another in water, since** their **extremities are not dry,** etc. That is, since dry bodies do not come into contact while in wet bodies unless their extremities are wet, it is necessary that they not come into contact unless there is a medium between them, and this is the body in which their surfaces are submersed. Since it is so, it is impossible for a dry body to touch a dry body in water or in air unless there is a body of water or of air between them. Next he said: **Likewise** concerning **air, for air,** etc. That is, it is so for air as for water in this regard. But the wetting of the things which are in water is evident to sense, while the wetting of those[274] which are in {305} air is not sensed, but the argument concludes that it is of the same sort. For instance, [consider] an animal which is in water. For since it is evident that it is impossible for something to touch it except through the mediation of water, it ought to be so for animals which are in the air.

114. **Is the sensation of all things in the same way or is the sensation of different things different, as it is thought that taste and touch are through touching but other things [are apprehended] from a distance? Or is it not so, but [rather that] we also do not sense hard and soft except by other mediating things, as we sense what makes sound, what is visible, and what is able to have smell, but the latter are from a distance and the former two from**

274. That is, the coating of these with air, since air is considered humid too, whereas earth and fire are dry.

near by,[275] and for this reason it was not perceived? In this way we sense all things through some medium, but it is not apprehended by us in these two. For we already also said earlier that if we were to sense tangible things with a thin cloth mediating so that we would not perceive it, then our disposition would be just as our disposition now in water or in air, for now we think that we touch them and that is not [the case].[276] (423b1–12)

When what we said has been conceded, that it is impossible for dry bodies to touch one another in wet bodies unless there is between these some body from that wet thing, it should be asked whether sensing all sensibles comes about in the same way, namely, through a medium, or sensing different things is different, namely, that sensing certain things is not through a medium, {306} as is thought concerning touch and taste, and certain things through a medium and without touch, but from a distance, as hearing, smelling, and sight. Or is it not so, but [rather that] we sense all tangible things through this same medium through which we sense those last three, but they differ only in the fact that in those three the sensibles are apprehended from a distance, and in touch and taste from close by. Since it is so, we do not sense all things except through an external medium, but that medium is not perceived by us in touch, just as if we were to sense tangible things through the mediation of a membrane without our perceiving that membrane to be on us. For just as our disposition would be with this membrane through the mediation of which we sense tangible things while not perceiving [this cloth], our disposition in sensing things by the mediation of water and air would likewise be so. Namely, just as it happens that we think that we do not sense tangible things except by touching, this [membrane] not mediating, since we do not at all perceive that it exists, so too it is possible that this happens for us in water or air, namely, to think that we sense things without their mediation, but in fact we touch nothing except through their mediation.

115. **But what is tangible differs from visible things and things which make sound. For we sense those so that the medium acts on us in a certain way and we [sense] in regard to tangible things not by the medium but along with the medium, for instance, [as] one on whom a striking falls through**

275. That is, taste and touch require proximity, even contact, in contrast to sight, hearing, and smell.

276. *Modo enim existimamus tangere ea, et non est illud:* δοκοῦμεν γὰρ νῦν αὐτῶν ἅπτεσθαι καὶ οὐδὲν εἶναι διὰ μέσου; "In their case we fancy we can touch objects, nothing coming in between us and them" (Aristotle, *De Anima* [1984]); فإنا نظن أنا نماسها بغير شيء متوسط بيننا وبينها (ibid. [1954]); "For we hold the opinion that we touch them with nothing intermediate between us and them." I understand نماسها to be an error for نلمسها.

the mediation of a shield. For the shield is not that which strikes him {307} when the shield was struck, but it happens that the striking of both was simultaneous. (423b12–17)

But although it follows from this account that tangible things are [grasped] only through a medium, just as [it is for] the [other] three senses, nevertheless we should hold that the action of the medium in the case of the former is not as the action of the medium in the latter, but rather tangible things differ from colors and sounds in the way they need a medium. [This is] because sensible things in the cases of those three first act on the medium, then the medium on us, while tangible things act simultaneously on us and on the medium. But you ought to understand here by "simultaneous" not that the medium and the sense are affected at the same time by tangible things, while in the other senses it happens at two [distinct] times. (For one thinks that sight and air are altered by color in the same instant.) But [rather] he means here by priority and posteriority for those senses priority according to cause, namely, that the sensible is the remote cause in the motion of the sense and the medium is the proximate cause. In the case of touch, however, the medium and the sense are moved simultaneously by what is tangible, but the medium has no action on [the sense], but is a necessary accident, not because it is necessary in the being of the sense as the medium is necessary in the being of the other [senses]. For this reason he likened our affection by tangible things to our affection by the striking through the mediation of a shield. Therefore, just as one ought not to say that the shield is necessary for the action of striking us, such that the shield be the proximate cause and the striking be the remote cause, so too is it for air with tangible things, namely, that one ought not to say that [air] is necessary for sensing tangible things, but we say that we and the shield are simultaneously affected by the striking. By "simultaneous," therefore, we ought {308} to understand the lack of priority and posteriority in cause, not in time. He meant by this to explain that this is not a medium which is necessary for every sense in sensing. But the medium which is of this sort in the case of this sense is flesh, and if this[277] will be called a medium, it will be accidentally. This passage should be understood, therefore, in this way, not such that Aristotle was doubtful about this and did not complete [it] and did not explain the way in which it is said that tangible things are sensed only through an external medium. Nor also was Aristotle quite neglectful in this account, as Themistius and others say.[278] For they say that if we concede that tangible things are not appre-

277. *Hoc.* In spite of *aer*, "air," being masculine, the sense of the passage requires that it be the referent of this neuter demonstrative pronoun.

278. See Themistius, *De Anima Paraphrase* (1899), 75.28–76.2; (1973), 126.10–127.1; (1996), 96. But Themistius says quite the opposite of what Averroes reports.

hended in water and air except through the mediation of these, what can we say about the apprehension of the qualities of tangible things in those two media themselves? I say that the severe neglect was only on the part of the one voicing this account, although it is quite sufficient insofar as it appears. For every animal which is naturally constituted to exist in water or in air does not sense some quality of warmth or of cold in these, if they are in the simplicity which they ought to have, because it is its natural place and the place is like what is placed [in it], as was explained in the general accounts,[279] and it was already explained that the sensible is a contrary before the affection. Since that is so, the animal senses heat or coldness in air or in water only when warm or cold bodies are mixed with these; those bodies, therefore, are different from natural water and air. Since it is so, what happens from this, when we sense that air or water is made warm or made cold, is the same as what happens in {309} bodies which appear to sight to be different from air and water, namely, that we do not sense them except through the mediation of natural water and air, as was explained from the earlier account. If the air and water containing animals have the contrary quality, they then hinder the apprehension of the contrary qualities by animals. On account of what we said one should not hold that water is made warm so long as it is simply water and not that the air is cooled so long as it is simply air, but [that] this happens on account of the warm or cold bodies mixed with them. This causes questions to arise in people such that [it is thought that] coldness is not an inseparable accident of water, as warmth [is] of fire. That view arises because common folk are accustomed to call [anything] water so long as liquefaction remains in it, although in fact it is not simply water, but rather is mixed. For that quality is the best known of all its sensible qualities, as heat in the case of fire. For this reason the common folk do not simply call fire what is cooled on account of the admixture of cold bodies, and perhaps call fire warm bodies, although they are made wet by the mixture, so long as they remain warm by fiery heat. Let us return, therefore, to our [topic] and let us say:

116. **Generally it seems that flesh and tongue are as air and water in regard to sight, hearing, and smelling, and thus the disposition of the former with respect to the sense is as the disposition of each of the latter. But when [something] touches the sense itself, sensation would not occur here or there, for instance, if someone placed some white body upon the ultimate organ of sight. Let us, therefore, say {310} that it is evident that the sense of touch is inside, and, if this were not so, what happens to the others would happen to it: it would not sense when [something] is placed upon the sense.**

279. *De Caelo* 4.3, 310b5ff. Also see 1.8, 277b12–23. Averroes' mention of "the general accounts" refers to the general accounts of natural philosophy. See Book 1, n. 165 {84} regarding this phrase.

Flesh, however, senses when [something] is placed upon it; hence it follows that flesh is the medium in touching. (423b17–26)

After he had explained the way water and air are media for touch, if they ought to be called media, he returned to speaking of what is the true medium in the case of this sense, namely, that without which it is impossible for that sense to sense. [This] is flesh, which is related to that sense as water and air are related to the other three senses. He said: **Generally it seems**, etc. That is, generally we should hold that flesh and the tongue are to touch and taste as air and water are to sight, hearing, and smelling. Next he said: **and thus the disposition of the former with respect to the sense is**, etc., that is, in such a way that the disposition of flesh and the tongue in what touches and what tastes is just as the disposition of water and air in regard to the other three [senses]. Next he said: **But when [something] touches the sense itself**, etc. That is, in regard to all senses, when the sensible thing is placed on the sense itself, it will not sense at all, or if it will sense, [it does so] poorly, as happens when some white body is placed upon the organ of sight. Next he gave a different demonstration that flesh is a medium, as it were, and not an organ, as it were. He said: **Let us, therefore, say that it is evident**, etc. That is, it is evident that the sense of touch is inside the flesh and that flesh is not, as it were, the first organ for it. For, if it were so, {311} what happens in regard to the others would happen in regard to it, namely, that when the sensible thing would be placed upon the flesh, it would not be sensed by the power which is able to feel touch, just as with color, which, when placed on the organ of sight, will not be sensed. Now, however, because we see that the power which is able to feel touch senses only when a tangible thing is placed upon the flesh, it is necessary that the flesh be a medium and not an organ. What he said is self-evident. For the fact that three senses need a medium either is because it happens in the case of their sensible objects that they are at a distance from them or because it is impossible for them to receive their sensible objects unless they are first in a medium, because most seem to be contraries, namely, because they are not changed to the [opposite] extremities unless they are changed to the intermediate. If this were on account of the fact that sensibles are at a distance, it would happen that [the senses] would sense [them] when they were placed upon them, for then they would not need a medium. But they do not sense [when the remote sensible objects are placed upon them]. Therefore, they need a medium only for sensing itself. Because this accident cannot be ascribed to one of them in an essential way, since it is common to them, it remains, therefore, that this is common to them through a nature common to the three senses. But no common nature is the cause for this occurrence unless it be that they are senses. Therefore, the need for a medium for the senses belongs to them insofar as they are senses, not insofar as they are certain senses. Therefore, every sense necessarily needs a medium in which to sense, but it is not the case that the medium belongs just to those three senses, since their sensible objects are at a distance, as Alexander figures. For, if it were so, it would happen that when [the sensible objects] were placed on them, they would sense. There is nothing to what Alexander said in contradicting this opinion, namely, that, if flesh were, as it were, {312} a medium, then it would happen that under the flesh there would be another part through which that sense comes to be,[280] either one, if that sense were one, or more than one, if more than one. For it already appeared after Aristotle's time, i.e., in Alexander's time, that in animals there are certain bodies which are called nerves and they have a passage into the sense and what is moved. What, therefore, was apparent to Aristotle by argument later was evident by sense. There is nothing to what the later Peripatetics say, namely, that the nerves do not have a passage into the sense of touch.[281] For the account of Aristotle is in regard to the proximate[282] power and this is also sensible.

117. **However, the differences of body insofar as it is body are tangible things. I say the differences by which the elements are determined, namely, hot, cold, wet, and dry, are also those about which we spoke in the account of the elements. What, however, senses and touches,[283] and in which the primary sense which is called touch exists, is a bodily part which is of such a disposition in potency.** (423b27–31)[284]

And **the differences of body insofar as it is body are tangible things**. That is, and the differences existing in all bodies are, in general, tangible things, namely, those common to all generable and corruptible bodies. Next he said: I say the differences, etc. That is, I understand {313} by **the differences** universal differences from which no body escapes. They are the first differences existing in the four elements, namely, hot and cold, wet and dry, and what comes to be from them, such as rough, hard, and the other differences of tangible things, and what is joined with them, such as heavy and light. Next he said: **those about which we spoke** earlier in the account of the elements, namely, in the book *On Generation and Corruption*, for there he explained the first

280. Alexander, *De Anima* (1887), 56.14–57.14; (1979), 64–65.

281. Cf. *Short Commentary on the De Anima* (1985), sections 67–69, 64–65; (1987), 155–158.

282. In lieu of *propinquo* I read *propinqua* with manuscripts B, D, and G.

283. *Illud autem quod est sentiens et tangens*: τὸ δὲ αἰσθητήριον αὐτῶν τὸ ἁπτικόν. "The organ for the perception of these is that of touch." Aristotle, *De Anima* (1984). The alternate translation is an accurate rendering of the Greek: وحسها اللمس (ibid. [1954]).

284. Crawford has this as 423b26–31.

and second kinds of tangible objects.[285] Next he said: **What, however, senses,** etc. That is, what, however, senses these differences is a part which is these differences in potency, that is, what is naturally constituted to be actualized through these differences. We should hold that this is flesh or the nerves.

118. **For to sense is to be affected by something in some way. Hence it is necessary that what brings about its like in act brings about only what is such in potency. For this reason what is hot does not sense what is like it nor [does] the cold or the hard or the soft, but rather [there is sensation only of] these things which are more intense. For sense is, as it were, a mean[286] between the contraries in sensible things.[287] For this reason it discerns sensible things, for the mean discerns; for it is brought to actuality by both [extremes] equally.[288]** (424a1–7)

After he had said that what primarily senses is what is those differences in potency, he began to explain this. He said: {314} **For to sense,** etc. That is, for

285. *On Generation and Corruption* 2.2, 329b7ff. Themistius makes explicit mention of *On Generation and Corruption* in his corresponding account. Themistius, *De Anima Paraphrase* (1899), 76.35–36; (1973), 129.3–4; (1996), 98.

286. The term *medium* corresponds to the Greek μεσότητος and μέσον and carries two notions: (1) it is a medium which is receptive of intentions, and (2) it is a mean which allows for perception insofar as its balance is affected by contraries.

287. *Sensus enim est quasi medium inter contrarietatem in sensibilibus*: ὡς τῆς αἰσθήσεως οἷον μεσότητός τινος οὔσης τῆς ἐν τοῖς αἰσθητοῖς ἐναντιώσεως; "the sense itself being a sort of mean between the opposites that characterize the objects of perception." Aristotle, *De Anima* (1984).

288. In the *Middle Commentary* (2002), at 86.14, Averroes has, "It can, therefore, distinguish extremes," ولذلك صارت تميز الأطراف, while here in the *Long Commentary* the Text and Comment reflect the Greek of Aristotle more precisely with "it discerns sensible things." The alternate translation uses a potentially ambiguous pronoun: ولذلك يقضى عليها (Aristotle, *De Anima* [1954]); "For this reason it discerns them." The Greek *De Anima*— γίνεται γὰρ πρὸς ἑκάτερον αὐτῶν θάτερον τῶν ἄκρων, "relatively to either extreme it can put itself in the place of the other" (ibid. [1984])—is reasonably well reflected in the *Middle Commentary* (2002), at 86.14–15, وذلك أنه يتشبه بكل واحد منها ويستكمل به, "it becomes each extreme and is perfected by it." The Text of the *Long Commentary* seems to have suffered some corruption in the Arabic manuscript tradition or was misunderstood by the Latin translator. Nevertheless, Averroes' Comment at {314} seems to reflect accurately the sense of Aristotle's Text. This also seems to reflect what is found in Themistius, *De Anima Paraphrase* (1899), 77.20–21: γίνεται γὰρ πρὸς ἑκάτερον αὐτῶν θάτερον τῶν ἄκρων ἤδη καὶ πάσχει ὑφ' ἑκάτερου τῶν ἄκρων. "[In the case of touch], that is, the medium [itself] can discern the extremes because it becomes one of the actual extremes relative to the other, and is affected by each of the extremes." Ibid. (1996), 98–99; ibid. (1973), 130.14–15: وذلك أنه يصير عند كل واحدة من الغايتين الأخرى ويتفعل عن كل واحدة من الغايتين

because to sense is an affection in the way mentioned, and everything affected has an agent [of the affection], and every agent acts to bring about what is like itself in act, it is necessary that it bring about its like only from something which is like it in potency, not in act. Next he said: **For this reason what is hot does not sense what is like it,** etc. That is, because the agent does not act on what is its like in act but rather in potency, for this reason it is necessary that the sensitive part not sense a body as warm as itself nor a cold body part equally as cold, and likewise for the hard and the soft. Next he gave the reason for this. He said: For **sense is, as it were, a mean,** etc. That is, the sense of touch apprehends only the more intense among tangible things, contrary to the other senses with their [own] sensible objects, because the sense of touch is found in something which is a mean between some contrariety in sensible things, since it is impossible for some body to be stripped of tangible qualities, in contrast to other sensible qualities. I understand that it is impossible for the sense of touch to lack the hot, the cold, the dry, and the wet in an absolute way, whereas sight did lack color and hearing sound. For this reason those senses apprehend their sensibles wholly, while the sense of touch apprehends the extremes. Next he said: **For this reason it discerns sensible things, for the mean discerns,** etc. That is, for this reason the sense of touch discerns and apprehends sensible things, because it is a mean, for the mean discerns because it receives each of the extremes and is assimilated to it and is made the same with it. {315}

119. **And just as it is necessary that what is naturally constituted to sense white and black be neither, but each in potency, and likewise for the other [senses], so in the case of touch it ought to be neither hot nor cold.** (424a7–10)

Just as it is necessary that what is naturally constituted to sense white and black be neither, but each in potency, and likewise for each sense, so also it is necessary that what touches be neither hot nor cold, in the way it is possible for it, namely, that [hot and cold] are in it according to a mean or something like it, since it is impossible that [touch] be stripped of them completely, whereas it was possible for the other [senses] to be stripped from their own sensible objects. You ought to know that what follows from this in regard to the organ of that sense is the same as what follows in regard to the medium. For this reason we cannot say that the flesh is the organ of that power insofar as it is a mean between contraries, as several have thought.

120. **Just as sight is in some way of the visible thing and of the invisible, and likewise for the other [senses],**[289] **in this way touch is of the tangible**

289. *Et similiter de aliis:* ὁμοίως δὲ καὶ αἱ λοιπαὶ τῶν ἀντικειμένων "(and there was a parallel truth about all the other senses discussed)" (Aristotle, *De Anima* [1984]), or perhaps more literally, "likewise for the other senses *regarding opposites,*" as in وسائر

and the intangible. The intangible is that in which there is a very slight degree of the disposition belonging to tangible things, such as air, or a very intense degree [of it], such as [in the case of] things which are destructive. (424a10–15)

After he had made known the nature of the sense of touch and the nature of tangible things and how and through how many things touch comes to be, he returned {316} to speaking about something common to all senses. He said: **Just as sight**, etc. That is, just as sight apprehends what is visible and what is not visible in some way, and likewise the other senses apprehend the privations of their proper sensible objects, so too the sense of touch apprehends the tangible and the intangible. He said **in some way** because it does not apprehend presence and privation in the same way, for [the senses] apprehend one of the two opposites in an essential way and the other in an accidental way. Next he set out in how many ways intangible is said. He said: **The intangible is that in which there is**, etc. That is, intangible is said in two ways, one is that in which there exists very little of the qualities, just as it is for the air around us, and the other is that in which there exists something of the tangible qualities which is very intense and destructive of the sense, such as fire and ice.

121. **We have given a descriptive account of each of the senses. We should say generally of every sense that sense is receptive of sensible forms without the matter. For instance, wax receives the form of the ring without the iron or gold and it receives an impression which is [from something] of bronze or of gold, but not insofar as it is bronze or gold. Likewise each of the senses is affected by what has color, flavor, or sound, but not {317} insofar as each of them is said to be such,[290] but insofar as it is in this disposition and in virtue of an intention.[291]** (2.11, 424a15–16–2.12, 424a24)

He means by **a descriptive account**, that is, in a general way. For in *Sense and Sensibilia* he speaks of them individually. He said: **We should say [. . .] of every sense**, etc. That is, we should hold that the reception of sensible forms by any sense is a reception free of matter. For if it were to receive them with matter, then they would have the same being in the soul and outside the soul.

الحواس على ما أشبه ذلك من التضاد (ibid. [1954]), with Badawi's correction of the manuscript's القضاء to التضاد.

290. That is, not insofar as each of them is said to have such characteristics—namely, color, flavor, or sound.

291. *Sed secundum quod est in hac dispositione, et in intentione*: ἀλλ' ᾗ τοιονδί, καὶ κατὰ τὸν λόγον, "insofar as it is of such and such a sort and according to its form" (Aristotle, *De Anima* [1984]); لكنه يصير بصفة كذا ، وكذا محتمل للحد (ibid. [1954]); "but it comes to have a characteristic such as this and in this way bears the definition."

For this reason in the soul they are intentions and apprehensions and outside the soul they are neither intentions nor apprehensions, but material things which are not apprehended at all. Next he said: **For instance, wax receives,** etc. That is, that reception which is in the senses as separate from matter is similar to the reception in wax of the shape of a ring. For it receives it without the matter, since it receives it in the same way whether [the ring] be of iron or of gold or of bronze. Next he said: **Likewise each of the senses is affected,** etc. That is, in this way each of the senses is affected by the things by which they are naturally constituted to be affected, be it color or sound, but it is not affected by that by virtue of which there is color or sound. For, if it were so, it would happen that when it would receive it, it would be color or sound, not an intention. He meant this when he said: **but not,** etc, that is, not insofar as each is said [to be such], but insofar as it is an intention. For the intention of color is different from color. He said **insofar as it is in a certain disposition and in virtue of an** intention by keeping them [separate] from the intentions which the intellect receives, for the latter are universal, while the former are only these [individual intentions]. {318}

122. **What primarily senses is that in which that potency exists. They are, therefore, the same, but different in being. For what senses is a magnitude, but not insofar as it senses; nor is the sense a magnitude, but [it is] rather an intention and a power of that thing.**[292] (424a24–28)

What receives that power which is an intention separated from matter is what primarily senses. When it has received it, they are made the same, but they differ in number. For what senses is a body and it does not sense because it is a body; nor is the sense a body, but an intention and a power of that body which is what primarily senses.

292. Aristotle compresses a great deal into a few words here. The Latin of the Text accurately reflects the Greek, which is translated with clarifying expansions as follows: "What perceives is, of course, a spatial magnitude, but we must not admit that either the having the power to perceive or the sense itself is a magnitude; what they are is a certain form or power in a magnitude." Aristotle, *De Anima* (1984). Aristotle holds that what senses is a spatial magnitude and that the sense is a power existing in this magnitude. The sensation is the actualization of this power in that spatial magnitude. As such, neither the sense nor the sensation is a spatial magnitude but rather an actualization of a power which happens to exist in that magnitude. Consequently, the sense's actualization is the sensation and the two are one in actuality. In this way the affected sense becomes the actuality of the sensible object insofar as it becomes the sensible object's form or its intention. This affects the way the Latin *sensus* should be understood since at times it means "the sense" and at other times "the sensation," and yet the two are one when the sense power is actual.

123. **From this is evident the reason why intense sensibles destroy the organs of the senses.**[293] **For when the motion of what senses is stronger than it, its intention is dissolved (and this will be the sensation), just as the harmony and melodies of strings are dissolved when they are touched forcefully.** (424a28–32)

From what we said, that sensation is an intention, the reason why intense sensible objects destroy the organs of the senses will be explained. For when the motion caused in the sense by a sensible object is stronger than what the sense is able to tolerate, that intention through which what senses is something which senses is dissolved. The body will remain without that intention which is sensation, just as the harmony and melodies of strings {319} which are in an intention existing in them are dissolved when [the strings] are touched forcefully and are moved by a motion more forceful than the motion which [the strings] are able to tolerate.

124. **The reason [is clear] why plants do not sense, while there is in them a part which is alive and which receives affection from tangible things because it becomes hot and cold. The reason for this is because it does not have a mean nor a principle through which it can receive the forms of sensible things.** (424a32–b2)

In this account he worked at providing the reason why plants do not have the sense of touch, although they do have a nutritive soul and are even affected by tangible things and become warm and cold. He means by **a part which is alive** the nutritive soul. He said: **the reason for this is because it does not have a mean,** etc. That is, for the reason why is nothing more than that plants do not have a mean, as flesh, nor a principle such as that through which animals can receive sensible forms. After he explained that something which does not apprehend tangible things is affected by them, he began to relate that the contrary is the case for the other sensible objects of the senses.

125. **But what cannot smell is not affected by smells, nor is what cannot see [affected] by colors, and so forth for the rest. If, therefore, what is smelled is smell, it happens that everything which smells does so through a smell. Hence it is necessary that {320} none of these things which are unable to smell be affected by smell, and that is the account for the other [senses as well], nor also is any of them which can [be affected in fact affected], except insofar as any one of them is what can sense.** (424b3–9)

---

293. *Que sit etiam.* I omit this, following manuscript A. There is nothing in the Greek, corresponding to this, nor is there anything supporting the reading in Averroes' Comment or in the alternate Arabic translation. See Aristotle, *De Anima* (1954).

Although something which is not naturally constituted to touch is affected by tangible things, nevertheless it is not affected by smells with the affection proper to smells, that is, insofar as it is smell, unless it is what can smell. Only what can see is affected by colors with the affection proper to color insofar as it it color. And only what can hear is affected by sound. Next he said: **and so forth for the rest.** This makes one think that flavor is of this disposition. But he himself will say later that something is affected by flavor which is not naturally constituted to sense it.[294] Perhaps he did this because it is a questionable matter. Next he said: **If, therefore, what is smelled**, etc. That is, if, therefore, the nature which is able to cause smell, which exists only in what causes smell, is the smell itself, not a comparable intention which happens to the smell, it is evident that smell makes everything smelled smell. And everything in which smell acts, insofar as it is smelled, is something which smells. For, if the being of smell is only insofar as it is smelled and what is smelled is found only in what smells, it is evident that everything which is affected by smell is something which smells. Next he said: **Hence it is necessary**, etc. That is, if, therefore, everything which smells is affected by smell, and everything which is affected by smell smells, it happens by the conversion of opposites that what is not something which smells is not affected by smell. He himself did not put this forth in this account except as a later consequence, while [he did set forth] the first principle from which it was concluded, namely, that if smell is relative, that is, smelled, it is necessary that what is smelled belong to what smells. He did not put forth this proposition saying that everything which is affected by smell is something which smells, nor did he put forth {321} the conversion of its opposite. He holds, as it were, that touch is something consequent upon tangible contrary things and he does not hold that what is able to provide smell is something consequent upon smell, nor the visible [consequent] upon color, but he does hold that what is smelled is, as it were, the smell itself and the visible color itself and the audible sound itself. For this reason it was necessary for him that everything which is affected by smell be smelling, by color be seeing, and by sound be hearing. But it was not necessary that everything affected by what is tangible be touching. This needs much investigation. For he holds, as it were, that some of the senses are in the category of relation and some in the category of action and passion per se and relation [merely] happens to them.

126. **Besides it is also evident in this way. For neither light nor darkness nor sound nor smell bring something about in bodies, but the things in which [such qualities] exist [do], for instance, that air, in which there is thunder, splits wood. But tangible things and flavors do bring something**

294. 424b10ff. See Texts 126 and 127 and Averroes' Comments below.

about, for if they do not, by what, therefore, are non-living bodies affected and altered? + On the basis of that they are also affected. +[295] (424b9–14)

Besides what is evident in the earlier account, in virtue of which we explained this with reference to sensible things, this is self-evident. For it appears that neither light nor darkness nor sound nor smell bring something about {322} in bodies, but they bring things about only in things in which these senses exist.[296] Next he said: **for instance, that air, in which there is thunder, splits wood.** But sound which is thunder is not the very motion which wood receives from the motion of the air; rather, sound is an intention which is found only in what hears, and, as it were, it is in the category of relation, not quality. Likewise smell is in it, as we explained. Next he said: **But tangible things and flavors,** etc. That is, but tangible things and flavors are more in the category of action and affection than in the category of relation. For if only what has the sense of taste and touch is affected by these, then by what are the other non-living bodies affected? For it will happen that there are no action and passion, which is impossible. What he said in regard to tangible things is evident, but in the case of flavors it needs consideration. For someone can say that flavor is itself what is tasted, just as smell is itself what is smelled. But we see, as Plato says, that flavors have in non-living bodies different affections added to warming and cooling, for instance, to make rough, which is of the acrid; to make soft, which is of the oily; and many other things which are mentioned in the *Timaeus*, which Galen worked to expound.[297] Therefore, whether those actions

---

295. Crawford marks this text as faulty with +. The corresponding Greek text has ἆρ᾽ οὖν κἀκεῖνα ποιήσει. "Must we not, then, admit that the objects of the other senses also may affect them?" Aristotle, *De Anima* (1984). فلا محالة أنها ولا هى أيضا تفعل (ibid. [1954]); "So it is necessarily the case that even these are affected."

296. The notion here seems to be that the organ is affected not as body but as sense organ, that is, as a mean which exists in a body and which is such that the disturbance of it from its mean state constitutes sensation.

297. The *Middle Commentary* (2002), at 88.21–89.5, has, "If affections like roughness or smoothness, which occur to the tongue in sensations of flavor, are the cause of its perception of flavors, as Plato and Galen say, then flavors act both on the sense of taste and elsewhere. If, however, the intention of flavor is something additional, then [sensory] affection will be an intention peculiar to this sense. Now, the [flavor of] harshness which the tongue perceives is the intention of roughness which it receives from that which is harsh, and the oily flavor is the intention of smoothness which it receives from that which is oily, just as the heat which the sense of touch senses is the intention of heat which is in matter. Flavors thus act on things other than their senses, for otherwise they would act only on the sense peculiar to them; and this is what is clear to me." Cf. Plato, *Timaeus*, 65C–66C, and Galen, *Galen's Compendium of Plato's Timaeus* (1951), sec. 15, Arabic 19.15–20.10; Latin 67.01–69.16.

are of flavor or they concern flavor, as the motion of air concerns sound, needs consideration. But here he accepts that flavor is a kind of tangible thing, since it is similar to it.

127. **Let us say, therefore, that not every body is naturally constituted to be affected by sound and by smell and what is affected is not determined or permanent, {323} for instance, air, for it is wind and on account of this it is affected.**[298] **What, therefore, is the difference between smelling and being affected? Let us, therefore, say that to smell is to sense. But when the air is affected, it comes to be sensed quickly.**[299] (424b14–18)

After he had explained that nothing is affected by any of the three sensibles except the senses proper to them, he began to provide the difference between the affection they cause in bodies which are media and the affection tangibles cause in things. He said: **Let us say, therefore, that not every body,** etc. That is, if someone imagines that bodies are affected by sound and by smell and gives an argument for this from the affection they cause in air and[300] water, we will say to him that not every body is naturally constituted to be affected by sound and by smell. For they affect no bodies except what is not determined in itself, that is, which does not have shape or proper constitution of its own, for instance, air. For air is not affected by these except because it is wind and wind is a body neither determined nor fixed. But bodies which are affected by tangibles are determined and fixed. Next he said: **What, therefore, is the difference between smelling and being affected?** That is, if, therefore, someone inquired and said: Since to smell is an affection and the reception of smell from a medium is also an affection, what then is the difference between each of these affections? We will say to him that since air is affected quickly by the sensible object, this affection gives rise to the object of this sense; the sense, however, comes to be sensing through this affection, not sensible.[301]

298. The corresponding Greek has οἷον ἀήρ (ὄζει γὰρ ὥσπερ παθών τι; "as in the instance of air, which does become odorous, showing that some effect is produced on it by what is odorous." (Aristotle, *De Anima* [1984]); كالجو ، فإنه إذا ألم وتغير فاحت رائحته (ibid. [1954]); "as air, for when it causes pain and change, its odor is diffused."

299. The corresponding Greek has ὁ δ᾽ ἀὴρ παθὼν ταχέως αἰσθητὸς γίνεται, "Is it that air, when affected quickly, becomes perceptible, but that smelling is actually perceiving?" Aristotle, *De Anima* (1984). The alternate Arabic translation has إلا أن يكون الاشتمام الإدراك بالحس مع تصيير الهواء محسوسا سريعا (ibid. [1954]); "However, smelling is the perception of what is sensed quickly by the sense by way of an affection of the air."

300. For *at* here I read *et*, assuming this to be a typographical error.

301. Ivry (1995), 87–88, rightly cites this text as an example of the dependence of the *Middle Commentary* on text found in the *Long Commentary* at Book 2, 127 {322–323}.

128. **That, however, there is no other sense in addition to those five, namely, sight, hearing, smell, taste, and touch, is believed from the following considerations. For** {324} **if everything which touch is able to sense we are now able to sense (for the affections of what is tangible, insofar as it is tangible, can all be sensed by us through touch), it is also necessary, if we lack some sense, that some sensing organ be lacking in us.** (3.1, 424b22–27)

After he had completed the account concerning each of the five senses existing in a fully formed animal, he began to explain that it is impossible to find an animal having a sixth sense. He said: **That, however, there is no other sense**, etc. That is, from the demonstrations [which follow], however, there arises the belief that it is impossible to find an animal having a sixth sense in addition to those senses existing in human beings and in fully formed animals. Next he began to explain this. He said: **For, if everything which touch**, etc. That is, for it is evident that we can apprehend every sensible which the sense of touch is able to apprehend and [that] nothing is lacking to us from among the things which are naturally constituted to be apprehended by this sense. [It is because of that] likewise for each sense, namely, that we lack none of the sensibles [which are] in some animal having that sense [and] which are naturally constituted to be apprehended by it. In this way no one is able to say that some [sense of] touch can be found in an animal which apprehends a tangible object which we cannot apprehend. (For it is self-evident that all tangible qualities,

---

Since his translation of the passage from the *Middle Commentary* in the article does not differ significantly from that of his complete translation, I quote from the complete translation:

He said: If one were to assert that [all] bodies are affected by sound and smell, and [were to] claim, accordingly, that air and water are affected by them, we would respond that not every body is affected by sound and smell, but, rather, these bodies [are affected] which are not intrinsically determinate—that is, those which do not have definition, end, structure, or shape, like air and water. On the other hand, the bodies which are affected by tangible objects are those which are determinate [and] fixed.

Now, given that the smelling of a smell is an affection and that the medium's reception of odor is an affection also, if one were to ask for the differences between these two affections, we should say that, when air is affected quickly by the sensible object, it thereby becomes the sensible object for the sense—that is, its moving force—whereas the sense becomes sensate [and] not sensible, by means of this affection. *Middle Commentary* (2002), 89.6–16.

Note that Book 2 of the *Middle Commentary* ends here, as does Book 2 of Aristotle's *De Anima*. Book 2 of the *Long Commentary* continues and includes the Text of Aristotle through 3.3, 429a9. See Book 3, n. 5.

insofar as they are tangible, can be sensed by us and apprehended through touch; and it is likewise with respect to visible, audible, and olfactory qualities.) When he had asserted this account as if an antecedent, he drew the consequence. {325} He said: **it is also necessary, if we lack some sense**, etc. That is, when we have asserted that we do not—nor does any animal in which there is found the things those senses as senses are naturally constituted to grasp—lack those five senses, it is necessary, if some sense is lacking in us, that some sensing organ be lacking in us. For we already asserted that with respect to those senses we do not lack [the ability to] sense anything naturally constituted to be sensed by [such senses]. Since it is so, then if there is such a lack, it necessarily is on account of our lack of a sixth sense, since that sense which we assert to be lacking is not [thought to be] lacking on account of any of the senses [actually] existing in us.[302]

129. **Everything which we sense by touching is itself able to be sensed by us through touch which is in us. And everything which we sense through media, [and] not because we touch it, is through simple elements, for instance, through air or through water. It is so, namely, that if through one [medium] the sensibles come to be more than one which differ from one another in kind, what has that sense necessarily is what senses both, for instance, if the sensing organ is composed of air and air is [the medium] of sound and color. If one [simple sensible] comes to be through more than one [medium], for instance, color through air and water (for they are equivalent[303]), then it is evident that what has just one [medium through which it senses] senses what it senses through each [properly correlative medium].[304]** (424b27–425a3)

He had explained that if we lack some sense, it is necessary that we lack a sensing organ. It was also {326} evident from this that if we lack a sensing

302. This is much more clear in the *Middle Commentary* (2002), at 90.3–10: "He said: There is not a sixth sense beside the five senses, and that which I shall say will confirm this. Firstly, if each one of these senses is congruent with all the sensibilia which belong to that sense organ whose nature is to perceive them—for example, if the sense of touch is congruent with all tangible objects, the sense of sight with all visible objects, and so forth for each sense—then it follows necessarily that, if we lack a given sensation, we lack a particular sense organ. However, none of the senses whose nature is to have perception lacks these sensations, though—if one did, we would lack a particular sense organ."

303. *Equales*. The Greek has διαφανῆ, "transparent" (Aristotle, *De Anima* [1984]); شيء واحد لأن كليهما ذو صفاء (ibid. [1954]); "are one thing because both of the two have clearness."

304. That is, in the case of objects which are sensible through two media, they can be sensed by what has the capability of sensing through one or the other medium even if it cannot sense through both.

organ, it is necessary that we lack some sense which differs in kind from the senses of those powers, since those powers do not lack the ability to sense something from among the things which are naturally constituted to be found in them. It is clear that these two are convertible, namely, whatever was for one will be for the other, and if one is destroyed, the other is destroyed. Now he began to explain that it is impossible for there to be a sixth power, because it is impossible for there to be sensing distinct in kind from those sensory powers. This is shown with three demonstrations, the first of which is taken from the media and the second from the organs by which sensing comes about. The cause given in those two demonstrations is the material, as it were. The third is taken from the sensibles themselves and is stronger than those other two, since the cause taken in it is the final [cause]. He began from the demonstration which is taken from the medium, but he was silent about certain propositions and the conclusion. That demonstration is founded on propositions of which one is that everything which an animal senses, either it senses through contact or through the mediation of an external body. Everything which we sense through contact, we sense either through the mediation of flesh or through flesh itself, if flesh is taken to be the organ. He meant this when he said: **Everything which we sense**, etc. Everything which we sense not through contact but through the mediation of an external body, we sense through the mediation of one of those two elements or both, namely, water or air. He meant this when he said: **And everything {327} which we sense through media,** etc. Since it is as we said, it is evident that it necessarily follows from this that everything having sensation through flesh or through one of those two elements or through both is found to have of sense only what can come to be through these two, namely, through flesh and through a medium. Therefore, it is the case for all animals that they partake only of those senses which can come to be through these two, namely, through flesh or through an external medium. After he had explained that every animal necessarily senses only through flesh or through media, he began to explain that it follows from this that every animal having one of those media necessarily grasps from among the sensibles [only] those sensibles which that medium provides and yields and [grasps] no other [sensibles]. He said: **It is so, namely, that if through one [medium]**, etc. That is, it is evident that when we assert that every animal senses only through a medium which is flesh, air, or water, if through one of those media more than one kind of sensibles were to result, it is necessary that every animal sensing through that medium not partake of sensibles other than these which are naturally constituted to be yielded by that medium; if two, two; if three, three. He meant by this that since the media are determined in number, namely, flesh, air, or water, and the sensibles which those media yield are also determined in number, it is necessary that the powers be according to the number of those sensibles which the media yield for animals which are naturally constituted to sense through these media. It is evident that everything which is yielded through flesh is tangible or able to be tasted. And everything which is yielded through air, water, or both is sound, color, {328} or smell. All sensing, therefore, is tasting, touching, hearing, seeing, or smelling.[305] Next he said: **if through more than one [medium] it comes to be** the same, etc. That is, if one sensible comes about through more than one medium, as color through air or water, which are equivalent in this, it is evident that an animal having one of these [media] has sensation of these sensibles as a thing which has both. He meant by this that the animal which is in water ought to have the powers of sense corresponding to the number of powers of the sense belonging to the animal which is in air and belonging to the animal which senses in water and in air.

130. **The senses composed of simple elements are of air or of water. For the organ of sight is composed of water, the organ of hearing of air, and the organ of smell of one of those two things. Fire, however, either is not [in any] or is common to these,[306] for there is nothing which senses without heat. Earth either does not belong to any of them or properly is mixed with touch. It remains, therefore, that there is no sense without water and air.** (425a3–8)

This demonstration is taken from the organs of the senses. He said: **The senses composed of simple elements,** etc. That is, the organs of the senses which are ascribed to the dominant elements on account of their composition and nature, are three only, namely, the organ which is composed of air, namely, the organ of hearing, as was explained earlier, and the organ which is composed of water, the organ of vision, and third is what comes about from both, namely, the organ of smell. He said in regard to this sense that it comes from one of those two, namely, either water or air, because animals which are in water smell through water {329}, just as the animals which are in air smell

---

305. Arabic fragments correspond to Book 2, 129.66–71: ومن البين ان كل ما يتأدى عن طريق اللحم فهو اما ملموس أو مذاق وكل ما يتأدى بالهواء او الماء أو بكليهما فهو اما صوت (*Long Commentary* Fragments [1985], 41). In this last list of senses in the Arabic, touch is not mentioned. I read the printed text, فأما كل احساس احساس احساس, as a typographical error for فأما كل احساس.

306. I read *aut non est aut communis est,* following manuscript A, instead of *aut est communis.* The corresponding Greek has τὸ δὲ πῦρ ἢ οὐθενὸς ἢ κοινὸν πάντων, "while fire is found either in none or in all." Aristotle, *De Anima* (1984). The alternate translation is quite different: ثم لا تصير النار حاسة لشيء واحد ، بل تكون شائعة بينهما (ibid. [1954]); "Then fire does not come to sense one thing, but rather it is common to both."

through air. Next he said: **Fire, however,** etc. That is, fire, however, either has no sense ascribed to it in this way or it is ascribed in a common way. For it appears that no sense can carry out its action when it is cooled. This is weakly indicated by this word, **or,** which notes repetition. He said this because its relation to something aside from fire is just as the relation of something to matter and its relation to fire is as the relation of something to its form. Next he said: **Earth either does not belong to** one, etc. That is, earth either is not ascribed to one of the organs of those senses, since it does not seem to serve sensibles in some way, or if it is ascribed, it is ascribed to flesh, because that medium or that organ needs constitution and fortification; hence, earth is dominant in it. Next he said: **It remains,** therefore, etc. That is, it remains, therefore, that there is no sixth sense apart from water and air, since there is no body apart from those two bodies, because it is impossible to find an organ of sense made of fire or of earth, but rather it is [only] possible that it be of water, of air, or of both. Since matters of the organs of senses are finite in number, it is necessary that the senses be so. If, therefore, there were a sixth sense, it would happen that there is a fifth element, for the senses which are composed of air or of water are those of the eye, the ear, or the nose. {330}

131. **These two are now in certain animals, in such a way that all the senses are discerned in these which neither are weak nor have injury. For the mole is seen to have eyes under the skin.** (425a8–11)

The senses ascribed to these two elements[307] are found only in certain animals, namely, those fully formed for the sake of better living, to the extent that, on account of the care of nature concerning this, it is necessary that all senses be discerned as existing in an animal of fully formed creation which has not suffered injury, and that from a fully formed animal, such as a human being, no sense be lacking. For the mole seems to have eyes under the skin, although it does not see.[308] [It is] as if he means by this that if there were a sixth sense, it would have to be found in a human being, which is the most fully formed of the animals, for it would be necessarily for better living. This is evident concerning the care of nature in giving senses to animals, to the extent that on account of this it gave to the mole eyes and covered them with skin, since it does not need them for the greater part of its operation, besides the fact that its matter cannot receive more; and if it could, perhaps it would be superfluous.

---

307. That is, air and water.

308. The *Middle Commentary* (2002), at 92.9–10, refers to another account: "Thus, we find that the mole, though not [a] seeing [animal] has two eyes under the skin—though some say, according to a non-Aristotelian report (فيما حكى غير أرسطو), that it sees the shadows of bodies."

132. **It is necessary, therefore, if there is no other body or [there is no] af-fection which is not of one of the bodies which are present with us, that no sense be lacking.** (425a11–13)

This is the third demonstration. The antecedent is missing. The syllogism is composed completely in this way: If there were a sixth sense, it is necessary that there be a sensible body different from all the sensible bodies which those five senses sense, and {331} that there be an affection and quality—which the sensing organ receives from sensibles, so that it will be qualified through it—different from those qualities and affections. But there is no sensible body different from those sensible bodies, nor an affection other than those affections, nor a quality. Therefore, there is no sense in addition to those five senses.

133. **Furthermore it is impossible that there be a sensory organ for the common [sensibles] which we sense unless [we sense] through each sense accidentally, for instance, [the common sensibles] motion, rest, shape, quan-tity, number, and unity. For all those are sensed through motion, for in-stance, quantity through motion, hence shape also, for shape is a certain quantity. Rest, however, [is sensed] through lack of motion, while number [is sensed] through the negation of continuity and through its properties, for each of the senses senses unity.**[309] (425a14–20)

Furthermore it is impossible for there to be a sensing organ different from the five senses, in such a way that its sensible object be one of the common sensibles, under which are the sensible objects proper to each of the five senses, unless the sensibles were common to each of the senses in an acciden-tal way. He said this because if they were to belong to them in an accidental way, it would happen that they would belong to some sense in an essential way, for what is found to belong to something in an accidental way ought to be found belonging to something else in an essential way. Next he said: **for instance, [the common sensibles] motion**, etc. That is, the common sensibles are not apprehended by the five senses in an accidental way, for instance, mo-tion, rest, shape, quantity, and number, {332} for all those are sensed by the five senses through some motion and affection. Because it is so it is necessary that it be in an essential way. Next he said: for instance, **quantity**, etc. That is, for instance, quantity, for the senses are naturally constituted to apprehend it through some affection and motion. It is similarly the case for shape, for shape

---

309. The Arabic Text may have been corrupt. I take Averroes as my guide to under-standing *unum* here. See his remarks in the Comment which follows. The Greek, how-ever, carried a different meaning: ἑκάστη γὰρ ἓν αἰσθάνεται αἴσθησις, "for each sense perceives one class of sensible objects." Aristotle, *De Anima* (1984). The alternate text is in accord with the Greek: وذلك أن كل حس إنما يحس بشيء واحد (ibid. [1954]).

is quantity with some quality. Next he said: Rest, however, [is sensed] through lack of motion, etc. That is, the apprehension of rest is through the apprehension of the privation of motion. For when it has apprehended motion in an essential way, it will apprehend its privation in an essential way, namely, rest. The apprehension of number and multitude by the senses is through apprehension of the privation of the continuous which is magnitude. It was already explained that the continuous is apprehended in an essential way; therefore its privation is also apprehended in an essential way.[310]

134. **It is therefore evident that it is impossible for there to be an organ of sense proper to one of those, for instance, motion. For it would be as we now sense sweet through sight. This was [so for us now] because we have a sense in which each [sensible] is [apprehended] and which is such that it knows these [sensibles] when they are both joined together. If it were not so, we would sense it only in an accidental way, for instance, the son of Socrates.[311] For we do not sense the son of Socrates, but rather what is white and it just happens that it was the son of Socrates. For common [sensibles], however, we have a sense which is common in a non-accidental way; therefore they do not have a proper sense. Unless this were so, we would not sense these at all, except such as we said {333} that we see the son of Socrates. A particular sense senses the sensibles of these [other senses] only in an accidental way. [This] is not [something] belonging to one of the senses [alone] since the senses are [perceptive] in regard to the same thing at the same time,[312] for instance, there is bile, for it is bitter and yellow. For**

310. Ivry (1995), 89–90, cites this text as an example of the dependence of the *Middle Commentary* (2002), at 92.17–93.2, on the *Long Commentary*, Book 2, 133 {331–332}. His 1995 translation of the passage differs only slightly from that of 2002, which is as follows: "Nor, again, is it possible for there to be some sense here other than the five senses whose object is one of the common sensibles, unless the perception of the common sensibles by each one of the senses is had incidentally. However, the common sensibles— motion, rest, magnitude, figure and number—are not perceived incidentally. The senses perceive them all, as affected, moved and the like, essentially. We perceive magnitude, for example, by a certain affection—as we do figure, which is a quality joined to magnitude. The senses' perception of rest, however, is due to the perception of the absence of motion, while their perception of number is due to the perception of the absence of continuity in the object."

311. Throughout this passage this Latin translation from the Arabic substitutes "Socrates" for the Greek text's "Cleon."

312. *Et sensus quidam non sentit sensibilia quorundam nisi accidentaliter. Et non est unius cum sensus fuerint insimul in eodem.* τὰ δ᾽ ἀλλήλων ἴδια κατὰ συμβεβηκὸς αἰσθάνονται αἱ αἰσθήσεις, οὐχ ᾗ αὐταί, ἀλλ᾽ ᾗ μία, ὅταν ἅμα γένηται ἡ αἴσθησις ἐπὶ τοῦ αὐτοῦ. "The senses perceive each other's special objects incidentally; not be-

the judgment that each is of the same [object] does not belong to one [of those senses]. For this reason error also occurs such that what is yellow is thought to be bile. (425a20–b4)

After it had been explained that the common sensibles are apprehended by the five senses in an essential way, it is evident that it is impossible for there to be a proper sense for one of those common sensibles, for instance, motion or quantity. For if it were so, then we would sense motion or what is like it from the common sensibles, not per se but through a medium, as we apprehend by sight that something is sweet through the mediation of color. Next he said: **This is because there is in us a sense**, etc. That is, such an apprehension occurs for us, namely, to judge through some sense regarding the sensible object of another sense, because it happens that those two senses have been joined in the act of apprehending those two sensible objects from the same thing in some [moment of] time. When later it happens that we apprehend through one of the two senses the other sensible object from the same thing, through that sense we will judge regarding the sensible object of the other in virtue of the precedent joining. For instance, we do not know by sight that something is sweet, unless it earlier happened for us in some [moment of] time that we apprehended by sight that honey is yellow and by taste that it is sweet. Since, therefore, in the second place we will sense it through vision alone to be yellow, immediately we will apprehend it to be sweet and honey. Next he said: **Unless this were so, we would not sense**, etc. That is, if it had not been conceded by us that if any of those {334} common sensibles had a proper sense, it would happen that to sense these things would be just as to sense through sight that something is sweet, then it would be necessary that to sense these things would be of the kind of sensing which is properly said [to be] **in an accidental way.** For instance, we sense by sight that this is the son of Socrates, because we would sense him to be white and because it happens that the son of Socrates is white. Next he said: Common things have **a common sense**, etc. That is, after it had been explained that if one of the common sensibles were to have a proper sense, then it would be sensed by us in an accidental way (just as we sense by sight that this is the son of Socrates, because he is white, or just as we

---

cause the percipient sense is this or that special sense, but because all form a unity: this incidental perception takes place whenever sense is directed at one and the same moment to two disparate qualities in one and the same object" (Aristotle, *De Anima* [1984]); وقد يدرك الحس بالعرض ما كان خاصاً لغيره من الحواس ، وليس ذلك على حال اجتماع من الحواس بل إنما يكون ذلك في الحس الواحد إذا اجتمع شيئان في شيء واحد (ibid. [1954]); "The sense may perceive incidentally what is proper to another one of the senses, but this is not a state of affairs joining the senses. Rather, this is only in regard to one sense, when it joins two things in one thing." The Text's Arabic version did not render ἢ αὐταί, ἀλλ .

judge something to be sweet because it is yellow, for these two are two modes in an accidental way). It was already explained that the common sensibles are apprehended in an essential way. Therefore, none of the common sensibles has a proper sense, but rather a common one. For if it were to have a proper sense, then it would be sensed either as we sense by sight that this is the son of Socrates because he is white, or as some sense senses a sensible proper to some other. That way is also accidental but it differs from the first way which is simply called accidental (and it is to apprehend by sight that this is the son of Socrates), although each was considered as accidental. They differ, namely, in this: because to apprehend by sight that something is sweet was because with sight there was joined in the same thing the power of one kind, namely, the sense of taste, with the power of sight. But to judge by sight that this is the son of Socrates happens because at some time a power other than a sensory power was joined with sight. For the power by which we apprehend that this is Socrates or the son of Socrates is superior to the power of sense. For this reason that way seems to be more accidental {335} than the second; hence he said simply that this one is accidental and not the second. Next he said: **It does not belong to one**, etc. That is, the judgment does not belong to one of those powers when two senses are joined in judging regarding the same thing that it is the same, but that judgment belongs to each sense, not to a sense different from them, as one might think. But if it were said of one in this way, it will be said in an accidental way. Next he said: **for instance, there is bile**, etc. That is, for instance, something is bile because it is bitter and yellow. For to judge that these two are of the same thing, namely, bile, does not belong to a power different from these two. And because the judgment regarding this thing being one belongs to two powers, rather than to one, error occurs in judging something which is not bile to be bile because [it is] yellow.

135. **One ought to investigate why we have more senses than one and not just one. Let us say, therefore: so that we do not fail to recognize the common things which follow, such as motion, quantity, and number. For if we were to have only sight alone, then it would be more proper that sight itself not fail to recognize what is white, to the extent that it would think all things are this [color].**[313] **For color and quantity are immediately consequent upon**

313. *Quoniam, si non haberemus nisi visum solum, tunc ipse visus esset magis dignus ut ignoraret album, adeo ut existimaret hoc esse omnia.* The corresponding Greek has εἰ γὰρ ἦν ἡ ὄψις μόνη, καὶ αὕτη λευκοῦ, ἐλάνθανεν ἂν μᾶλλον καὶ ἐδόκει ταὐτὸν εἶναι πάντα. "Had we no sense but sight, and that sense no object but white, they would have tended to escape our notice and everything would have merged for us into an indistinguishable identity." Aristotle, *De Anima* (1984). The alternate Arabic

one another. Now, however, because the common sensibles are from something else, it is made evident that any of them is distinct [from the proper sensibles]. (425b4–11)

He wants to give the reason why these common sensibles are not apprehended by one sense. He said: **One ought to investigate,** etc. That is, it should be asked why these common sensibles are apprehended by more senses than one {336} and not apprehended by one alone. Next he gave a response. He said: **Let us say, therefore: so that we do not fail to recognize,** etc. That is, so that we do not fail to recognize the dissimilarity of the common sensibles from proper sensibles. Next he said: **For, if we were to have [. . .] sight alone,** etc. That is, this is necessary because if we were to assert that sight alone apprehends those [common sensibles] and that it alone is in us in this intention, then it would happen for sight that it would not recognize and not distinguish white from something else, to the extent that it would consider color, quantity, and shape to be the same things. This would happen from the fact that color and quantity follow upon one another, namely, that color is found only on a surface, and a surface on a body. Next he said: **Now, however, because the common,** etc. That is, now, however, because we see that common [sensibles], such as quantity and magnitude, are apprehended through a sense different from sight. . . .[314] His account in this passage, therefore, should be understood in accord with this, not as his words sound in a superficial way, namely, what is said concerning why the senses are more than one. For the formal cause in this is evident, namely, the multitude of

---

translation has ولو كان الحس واحداً كالبصر ، والبصر مدرك البياض ، لذهب علينا ما خلف ذلك ، و [إن] كان في الأبيض الجميع (ibid. [1954]); "If sense were one such as sight, and sight perceives <only> white, then what is after that would escape us and everything would be in white." The question of the precise stage at which a corruption of the Text here might have occurred is difficult to determine. Averroes' Comment on this gives no indication of his being aware of a problem.

314. Crawford indicates that the Comment's text here suffers from omission. In the *Middle Commentary* (2002), at 94.1–8, Averroes' argument takes a different approach: "For the inquirer who asks why we perceive these common sensibles through more than one sense, [we say] that it is in order not to overlook the difference between common and particular sensibles. This is necessary, for, if we were to posit, for example, that sight alone is that which perceives these [common sensibles], the distinction between white, magnitude, and figure would be overlooked. This would happen because magnitude and color entail each other, that is, color is not perceived other than with magnitude. Now, however, since senses other than sight perceive magnitude and figure, it does not happen that these two (common sensibles) and the object of visible apprehension will be thought of as the same thing."

sensible things.[315] This was already said. The final cause should be investigated later at the end of this book.[316]

136. **Since, however, we sense that we hear and see, it is necessary that sensing that we see either is through sight or through something else. But that {337} will be [perceptive] of sight and of color, the subject [of sight]. Either the two [senses are perceptive] of one [object] or the same thing of itself. And also, if the sense by which we sense that we see is different, either this will be [so] into infinity, or the same will be [perceptive] of itself. It is necessary, therefore, that this happen in the first place.** (3.2, 425b12–17)

After he had completed the account of the five senses and had explained that there is no sixth sense, he began to explain that those five senses have a common power. He began first to express doubt in accord with his custom. He said: Because **we sense that we see**, etc. That is, because we see and we sense that we see, and we hear and we sense that we hear, and so forth for each of the senses, it is necessary that this come about through the power of sight or through another power. Next he said: **But that will be [perceptive] of sight and of color**, etc. That is, but if this, namely, to sense that we see, belongs to a sense different from sight, it will happen that this sense has a twofold apprehension. For it will apprehend that it apprehends sight and it will apprehend color, which sight apprehends. For it is impossible for it to apprehend that sight

---

315. Arabic fragments correspond to Book 2, 135.13–32: يعني للباحث ان يبحث لِمَ صرنا ندرك هذه المحسوسات المشتركة بأكثر من حاسة واحدة ⟨ولا ندركها كلها بحاسة واحدة⟩ فأجاب عن ذلك بقوله : فنقول انما كان ذلك لئلا يذهب علينا... يعني لكي لا يذهب علينا مغايرة المحسوسات المشتركة للمحسوسات الخاصية ثم قال :لأنه لو فرضنا ان البصر وحده هو الذي يدركها دون سائر الحواس ⟨.. ⟩ فقد يعرض للبصر ان يذهب عليه تمييز الأبيض من غيره فيظن ان الأبيض والمقدار والشكل هو معنى واحد وهذا يعرض له من قبل ان المقدار واللون يلزم كل واحد منهما صاحبه – أعني أنه انما يدرك الكون في مساحة والمساحة في جسم ما ⟨.. ⟩ ويريد بقوله : اما الآن فلما ⟨كنا نرى⟩ ان المشتركة ⟨أعني⟩ المقدار والعظم ، انما يدركها بحس غير البصر ⟨لم يعرض للبصر ان يظن انهما ومدركة شيء واحد وهكذا يجب ان نفهم⟩ هذا البحث الذي فحص عنه هنا لا كما يظهر من ظاهر ⟨كلامه⟩ أي : لِمَ صارت الحواس أكثر من حاسة واحدة ، لأن السبب ⟨سهل⟩ التصور وبين بنفسه ، وهو كثرة المحسوسات (*Long Commentary* Fragments [1985], 42). I understand the words preceding this in this edition to have been supplied by Ben Chehida. His text is missing the closing bracket < indicating the end of his interpolation from the Latin. الكون seems to be an error for اللون. The mention of "formal cause" at 135.31 is likely the result of a corruption in the translator's Arabic manuscript. The Arabic has, "The reason is easy to see and self-evident, namely, the multiplicity of sensibles." The opening words of this fragment are identical to what is found in the *Middle Commentary*: و للباحث ان يبحث لِمَ صرنا ندرك هذه المحسوسات المشتركة بأكثر من حاسة واحدة (*Middle Commentary* [2002], 94.1–2).

316. See *De Anima* 3.12–13, 434a22ff.

apprehends color unless it also apprehends color. Next he said: **Either the two [are] of** the same object **or the same thing of itself.** That is, one of the two will, therefore, follow from this. For, if we assert that there are two powers, it will happen that two senses are of the same intention, namely, a sense which senses it and a sense which senses that this sense senses it. For both sense that [intention]. Or we will assert that the same thing senses itself such that the agent is the patient, which is unthinkable. Next he said: **And also, if the sense** of sight, etc. That is, and if we assert that there are two powers, namely, that the sense which apprehends that we see is different from the one which sees, it will happen {338} also in the case of that sense what happens in the first. For it is necessary that it have a twofold apprehension, namely, the apprehension of its first subject which it senses and the apprehension that it apprehends it. If we also assert this of the two powers, there will happen in regard to a third what happens in the case of the second, and so forth into infinity, which is impossible. Hence, it is necessary for us to assert that it is the same power which apprehends both, namely, its first subject, and which apprehends that it apprehends. Since it is necessary to forestall an infinite regress, it is better to do this in the first instance and to assert that through the same power we apprehend color and we apprehend also that we apprehend it. For what will arise for us later should be dealt with earlier. He meant this when he said: It is necessary, **therefore**, to do **this** in the first place, or to assert that the same thing is affected by itself and apprehends itself.

137. **There is a question in regard to this and it is that if seeing is sensing through sight, and it sees color, and one does not see what has color except when one sees something, [then] it will happen that what sees in the first place also has color.** (425b17–20)

But that account also raises a question, namely, to assert that through the same power we apprehend color and we apprehend that we apprehend color. For if seeing is sensing through sight, and sight apprehends color, and one does not see that he sees color except when he sees something, it will happen that what sees in the first place, when it judges that it sees, also has color. {339} He meant by this that if it is necessary that everything able to be apprehended by sight be colored and sight apprehends the apprehension of color, it will therefore happen from this that the very apprehension is colored, which is unthinkable.[317]

138. **Let us say, therefore, that it is evident that to sense through sight is not one [in intention]. For we judge darkness and light through sight, when**

317. Arabic fragments correspond to Book 2, 137.13–16: ويريد بهذا القول انه ان كان كل مدرك للون بالبصر — وهو يدرك انه ادرك اللون — فقد يجب ان يكون الادراك نفسه ملوّنا ، وذلك أمر شنيع (Long Commentary Fragments [1985], 42).

not seeing, but not in the same way. **Even what sees is colored, as it were, for the sensing organ receives the sensible without matter, any [sense] whatever, any [sensible] whatever.**[318] **For this reason, when the sensibles are separated, the sensations and imaginings will be in the sensing organ. The action of the sensible and of the sense is the same; but in being they are not the same in them, for instance, sound which is in act, hearing which is in act. For it is possible that something has hearing and does not hear and that something have sound but does not always sound. But when what is in potency to hear does so and what is in potency to sound sounds, then hearing and sound will be simultaneous. Someone can say that the first of those is to hear and the second is to sound.** (425b20–426a1)

After he had given the questionable account, he began to resolve it. He said: **Let us say, therefore, that it is evident that to sense**, etc. That is, let us say, therefore, that it is evident that to sense through sight is not of the same intention such that it would follow from it that everything which can be apprehended {340} by sight is colored. Next he said: **For we judge darkness and light through sight**, etc. That is, what indicates this is that we judge by sight though not seeing something colored, when we judge darkness to be darkness and light to be light, although neither has color. But we do not judge darkness and light by sight in the same way, for we judge light in its own right and darkness because it is a privation of light. When he had given this way of resolution, he gave the second resolution for the question, saying that sight ought to be colored if the power of vision apprehends sight. He said: **Even what sees is colored, as it were**, etc. That is, we can also concede that sight is colored, for what sees, when it apprehends color, is made colored, as it were, in some way. The reason for this is that the sensing organ receives the sensible and is assimilated to it. So the organ of sight receives the color which the body outside the soul receives. But they differ in that the reception on the part of the sensing organ is not material, while the reception of the body outside the soul is material. Next he said: **any [sense] whatever, any [sensible] whatever.** That is, for the sensing organ receives the sensible immaterially, whichever of the senses, whichever of the sensibles. Because the senses receive sensibles in some way, they are also said of these in some way. Next he said: **For this reason, when the sensibles are separated**, etc. That is, because the senses receive the sensibles without the matter, sensations and imaginations arise in the organs of sense rather than the sensible colors, flavors, or the other sensible qualities which exist in matter outside the soul. Next he said: **The action of the sensible and of the sense**, etc. That is, the action of the sensible outside the soul in mov-

---

318. *Quidlibet quodlibet.* This added phrase has nothing corresponding in the Greek text of Aristotle or in the alternate translation.

ing the sensing organ, and {341} the action of the sense which is in the sensing organ, namely, the quality by which the sensing organ is qualified in moving also the power of sight, is the same action, although the mode of sensible being outside the soul differs from the mode of its being in the sensing organ. For instance, [consider] sound, which is in act outside the soul in such a way that it moves the organ of hearing just as hearing which is in act moves the power of hearing. Likewise the disposition of color in moving what sees is just as the disposition of quality which accrues in what sees from color in moving the power of vision. Next he said: **For it is possible for something to have hearing,** etc. That is, this was so because it is possible for something to have hearing in potency as it has sound in potency and that it may have sound in act as it has hearing in act. When it has hearing in act, it will have an apprehension of what hears in act, that is, apprehension that it hears. He said: **For it is possible** to say **something has hearing and [. . .] that something has sound** although it **does not always sound**, on account of the fact that they are such as this in potency. . . .[319]

139. **If action, affection, and motion are in what is affected, it is necessary that sound and hearing which are in act be in what is in potency. For the action of the agent and of the mover are in the patient. For this reason it is not necessary that what causes motion be moved. And the action of what sounds either is sound or is to sound and the action of what hears is either hearing or to hear, for hearing has two modes and sound has two modes.** (426a2–8)

After he had asserted that the action of what senses and of the sensible object is the same, although they differ in being, he began to explain this from the general things {342} mentioned earlier. He said: **If action [. . .] and motion,** etc. That is, if it is necessary that every action which proceeds from an agent and every motion which proceeds from a mover be found only in the thing which is affected and moved, while the senses are affected by sensibles and sensibles act upon them, [then] it is necessary that the action of the sensible be in what senses that which is sensible in potency. Thus sound and hearing which are in act are in what is sounding in potency, namely, what is struck, and [in] what is hearing in potency, namely, the hearing sense. Next he said: For this reason **it is not necessary that what causes motion be moved.** That is, because motion is in the patient and not in the agent, it is not necessary for every agent to be a patient, as was explained in the general accounts.[320] He

319. Crawford at {341} indicates that the Comment is incomplete in its Latin version here.

320. *Physics* 3.3, 202a12–22. Also see 3.1, 201a25–28 and 8.5.

brought up all this to explain that the senses move the powers as the sensibles which are outside the soul move the senses. Next he said: for **sound has two modes**, etc. That is, it was necessary that it be so for sound as for hearing, namely, that they move in the same way and that the action come about in the recipient, not in the agent, on account of the fact that each is found in two modes, a mode in potency and a mode in act.

140. **That same account is [true] for the other senses and for the other sensibles. For just as action and affection are in the patient, not in the agent, so too the actions of the senses and sensibles are in what senses. But in some cases they have names, such as "to sound" and "to hear," while in others one of them has no name. For the action of seeing is called sight, while the action of color does not have a name in the Greek language.**[321] (426a8–14)

That same account which we gave in regard to sound and hearing, namely, that their action is in the patient, is [true] for the other senses. {343} Next he repeated the proposition from which he began this explanation. He said: **For just as action and affection**, etc. That is, the reason for this is that as action and affection are in the patient, not in the agent, so too the actions of the senses and sensibles are in what primarily senses, since the sensibles are active powers, while the senses [are] agents and patients, and what primarily senses[322] is only passive. Because this is obscure, namely, that sensibles are active powers and the senses are patient [powers], on account of their [way of] being named (for most sensibles lack names insofar as they are agents and the names of most of them are passive instead of expressing active powers), he said: **But in some cases they have names**, etc. That is, but in regard to some senses names are given both for the action of the sensible itself and for the affection of the very thing which senses, for instance, **to sound and to hear**, for to sound is an action of sound, while to hear is an affection of the sense of hearing. In some cases one of them lacks a name, for instance, in sight, for the affection of sight has a name and it is "to see" (although it is the form of name indicating action); but the action of its sensible (which is color) lacks a name in the Greek language. I say that in Arabic actions of positive dispositions of the senses reaching them from sensibles into the first sensitive powers do not seem to have names in any idiom, since this is not known by the common folk, for they are not apprehended by sense nor [grasped] at first consideration.

---

321. *In lingua Greca*. These words are additions to the Greek and not found in the alternate translation. These words are also found at *Middle Commentary* (2002), 108.

322. That is, the sense organ. See {313–314}.

141. **Because the action of the sensible and of what senses is the same but they differ in being, it is necessary that the hearing {344} which is said in this way and the sound be corrupted at the same time and be preserved at the same time, and similarly for flavor, taste and the rest. But in these things which are said to be in potency it is not necessary.** (426a15–19)

The action of the sensible is the same as the action of what senses, namely, that the positive disposition which reaches from [the sensible] to what senses and the positive disposition by which the sensible acts on what senses are the same in subject, although they differ in being and form. Hence it is necessary that the corruption and the preservation of the two positive dispositions be at the same time, namely, the positive disposition through which the sensible is moving in act after it was in potency and the positive disposition through which what senses is what senses in act after it was in potency. Next he said: **the hearing which is said in this way and the sound**. That is, this follows in regard to sound which is said according to this mode, i.e., sound in act. It happens in the same way in regard to flavor which is in act and in regard to taste which is in act and in regard to all the senses. But in the sensible which is in potency and in what senses which is in potency, it does not follow, namely, that when one of them is corrupted, the other also is corrupted, or when one is, that the other is [too].

142. **But the ancient natural scientists did not speak soundly in regard to this, since they thought that nothing is white or black without sight and [that there is] no flavor without taste. For this is true in one way and in another {345} way not true. For, because the sense and the sensible are said in two ways, in potency and in act, what was said follows in regard to the latter but not in regard to the former. But these spoke in an unqualified way about what is not spoken about in an unqualified way.** (426a20–26)

But the ancient natural scientists did not speak correctly in regard to this intention. For they said that there is no color without sight nor flavor without taste. They said this in an absolute way, that is, they held that the sensible and what senses are related in an unqualified way, and if one exists, so does the other, and [if] one be corrupted, so is the other. Next he said: **For this is true in one way**, etc. That is, what the ancients said is true in one way and in another not true. Sometimes the sense and the sensible are said to be in potency and sometimes in act. But the account of the ancients follows in regard to their being in act, while in regard to their being in potency it does not follow, namely, that their being and corruption is always at the same time. But the error of the ancients was in that they spoke in an absolute way in regard to what is indeterminate.

143. If, therefore, harmony is sound and sound[323] and hearing are the same, as it were, and harmony is ratio, it is also necessary that hearing be a certain ratio. For this reason anything[324] is corrupted when hearing is intense, namely, high or low. In a similar way taste is corrupted in regard to flavors, sight in regard to colors by intense light {346} and darkness, and in smell by strong smell, both sweet and bitter, because sense is a certain ratio. On account of this, when sour, sweet, and salty are placed with what is like, while being pure and unmixed, they will then be pleasant.[325] Generally things that are mixed are more fit to be harmonious than high and low. In the case of touch [the pleasant is what is such that] it is possible that it become warm and be cooled. The sense is a similar ratio. And when [the sensibles] are intense, they will be harmful and corruptive.[326] (426a27–b8)

After he had asserted that a sense which is in act is in a way relative, he began to explain this and to give from this the causes for many accidents in sense. He said: **If, therefore, harmony is sound**, etc. That is, therefore, harmonious pitch in hearing—that is, what is mixed in a pleasant mixture—is sound and sound in act is hearing in act; and the harmony found in pitch is only a moderate ratio between extremes, namely, between deep and high sound which are said in reference to hearing. [If that is so,] it is necessary that the moderate [sound] existing between them (this is harmony) be itself hearing, since the being of hearing in act is found only in this ratio which is moderation.

323. *Sonus, et sonus*: ἡ φωνὴ ... ἡ ... φωνή, "voice ... the voice." Aristotle, *De Anima* (1984). Both the alternate translation in ibid. (1954), and the *Middle Commentary* (2002), at 97.8, have forms of صوت, "voice."

324. *Quidilibet* is a typographical error for *quidlibet*.

325. *Quando fuerint posita cum simili*: ἄγηται εἰς τὸν λόγον, "when e.g. acid or sweet or salt, being pure and unmixed, *are brought into the proper ratio*" (Aristotle, *De Anima* [1984]), my emphasis; من أجل ذلك كانت المحسوسة لذيذة عند الحس ، إذا دنت اليها (ibid. [1954]), my emphasis; ‹بعد أن كانت نقية› وليست مخالطة لغيرها: كالحامض ، والحلو والمالح "On account of this what is sensed is pleasant to sense, *when it draws near to it*, <when it is pure> and is unmixed with anything else, like the sour, the sweet, and the salty." The angle-bracketed phrase is added by the editor. Thus, it appears that the Greek phrase (indicated here by overbar and italics) was corrupt or confused in both Arabic translations.

326. *Et sensus est similis proportio; et cum fuerint intensa, nocebunt et corrumpent*: ἡ δ' αἴσθησις ὁ λόγος· ὑπερβάλλοντα δὲ λύει ἢ φθείρει; "the sense and the ratio are identical; while excess is painful or destructive" (Aristotle, *De Anima* [1984]); وأما الحس فهو المعنى ، ومتى أفرطت هذه أفسدت به وأفسدته (ibid. [1954]). The *Middle Commentary* (2002), at 109, has والسبب في ذلك كله أنه من الحس الطبيعي إنما وجوده في النسب المعتدلة; "The reason for all this is that the existence of a natural sense consists of an equitable ratio."

Because what moderates and what is moderated are relative and the being of hearing in act is natural in moderated sound, it happens that hearing and what can be heard will be in the category of relation. He said that it is necessary that hearing be a certain ratio and he did not say ratio without qualification, because it is thought that this ratio, although it is in the category of relation, is nevertheless {347} an active ratio; and ratios, insofar as they are ratios, are not active, but [they are active] insofar as they are qualities. The senses, therefore, are considered in [the category of] relation in one way and in [that of] quality in another way. And so it will be understood. Next he said: **For this reason anything is corrupted**, etc. That is, on account of what we said it happens that any one of the senses is corrupted when that ratio is changed in an intense way going over to the other of the extremes, for instance, the corruption of hearing with sound intensely high or deep, the corruption of taste with intense flavor, the corruption of sight with intense light and intense darkness, and the corruption of smell with intense smells. The reason for this is that the being of the natural sense is in a moderate ratio. When that ratio is corrupted, the sense will be corrupted, since that ratio is the form of sense. [It is] just as health is in the moderate ratio between the four qualities and when that ratio is corrupted, health will be corrupted, since the form of health is in this moderate ratio. Next he said: **On account of this, when sour**, etc. That is, because sense is a certain intention and a certain ratio, for that reason sour, sweet, and salty added to their like, not mixed with something else, will be pleasant, for when they come together with similar things, while pure, they will be pleasant; for then they will be more separate from matter. Next he said: **Generally things that are mixed**, etc. That is, generally things mixed from the contraries which are in any of the senses are more fit to be a ratio than the contraries themselves, for instance, sound which is between high and deep {348} is more fit to be a ratio than the high and the deep. It is likewise for touch with hot and cold, wet and dry, although a body which touches can be made warm and be cooled, contrary to the other senses, as we already said earlier. Nevertheless, what is moderate is more fit to be a ratio than the extremes.

144. **Each of the senses is of the sensible thing subject to it and it exists in what senses it insofar as it is what senses and it judges the differences of the sensible subject to it, namely, sight [judges] white and black, taste sweet and bitter, and so forth for the other [senses].** (426b8–12)

After he had begun to investigate whether the power by which we sense that we sense is the same as the power of the senses which is proper to each sense or different, he gave initially an account from which it follows that it is one and later on another from which it follows that it is many. Then next [he gave] an account concluding that it is one and a solution from which he went on to explain that the sense and the sensible are one in act, not different (on account of which it would happen that what judges of the sense itself would be different from what judges of the sensible itself). When he had done this, he returned afterwards to that same investigation. He said: **Each of the senses**, etc. That is, it is self-evident that each of the senses judges its proper subject which belongs to it insofar as it is that thing which senses and judges besides the proper differences which are in that proper subject. For instance, [consider] that sight judges {349} color, which is the subject proper to it insofar as it is sight, and it judges the contrary differences existing in it, for instance, white, black, and the intermediaries, and likewise hearing judges sound, which is its subject, and deep, soft, and the intermediaries, which are the differences of sound.

145. **But because we also judge white and sweet and each of the sensibles by comparing them to one another, in virtue of what, therefore, do we sense these things to be different? Indeed, it is necessary that this be through sense, for they are sensibles.** (426b12–15)

Since the senses apprehend the contrary differences which are in the subjects proper to each sense, in virtue of what power, therefore, do we judge that those are different, when we have compared them to one another? It is indeed apparent that there follows from this account what [followed] from the first. [This] is that the power by which sight judges white to be different from sweet is different from the power of sight, just as the power by which it judges that it sees seems to be different from the power of vision. For the difference between the sensibles is able to be sensed.

146. **Let us say, therefore, that it is evident that flesh is not the ultimate thing which senses. For it would happen, when it would touch, that it would judge. But it is impossible that what judges judge sweet to be different from white through two different things,[327] but rather it is necessary that both belong to the same [thing] through two organs. Unless this were so, {350} it would be possible, when I would sense this and you that, that I would understand them to be different things. But it is necessary that one thing say this to be different from that and sweet different from white. What says [this], therefore, is the same. Hence it is necessary that, as we say, we act[328] and sense in this way. However, that it is impossible to judge different things through different [things] is evident. That this does not occur**

327. That is, by two different senses.

328. *Agamus.* The corresponding Greek is νοεῖ, "thinks." Aristotle, *De Anima* (1984). The manuscript of the alternate Arabic translation has يفسر (explain), which Badawi corrects to يفكر (think). See ibid. (1954). Note that in the Latin Comment Averroes quotes the Text precisely as *agamus* and yet explains it as discussing sensing and think-

at two different times will be explained. For just as the same thing says good
is different from evil, so too when it says something is different, in that
same instant it also says it in reference to the other. [This is] not in an accidental way, as I say now there is something different, not that there is
something different now, but I speak out in this way in an instant and [I
say in this way] that it is in an instant. By what will it therefore be? It will
not be divisible and [it will be] in indivisible time.[329] (426b15–29)

Let us say, therefore, that it is evident from what I say that the ultimate
thing which senses in touch is not in flesh, nor in the case of sight in the eye,
and so forth for the others. For if the ultimate thing which senses were in the
eye, or in the case of taste in the tongue, then it would be necessary to judge
by two different [things] when we judge sweet to be different from white. For
what apprehends what is sweet according to this position is altogether different from what apprehends color. For that is in the eye alone and this in flesh
alone, or what is similar to it.[330] But flesh in regard to touch is not as the eye in

---

ing. See below {351}. In Arabic manuscripts confusion between forms of فعل (to act) and
عقل (to understand) is not uncommon. It appears here that the original translation
from Greek was likely correct as يعقل, which became corrupted to يفعل in the transmission of Averroes' Text and Comment. Averroes himself read the Text in accord with
the Greek, as his Comment indicates. Thus, *agamus* reflects a corruption in the Latin
translator's Arabic manuscript of Averroes' Commentary, not the understanding of
Averroes. Cf. Book 2, n. 129.

329. *Et non accidentaliter, sicut dico nunc esse aliud non quia nunc est aliud, sed
dico sic instans et quod est instans. A quo igitur erit? Erit non divisibile, et in tem-
pore indivisibili.* καὶ θάτερον, οὐ κατὰ συμβεβηκὸς τὸ ὅτε (λέγω δ', οἷον νῦν λέγω
ὅτι ἕτερον, οὐ μέντοι ὅτι νῦν ἕτερον), ἀλλ' οὕτω λέγει, καὶ νῦν καὶ ὅτι νῦν · ἅμα
ἄρα. ὥστε ἀχώριστον καὶ ἐν ἀχωρίστῳ χρόνῳ. "And the other to be different is not
accidental to the assertion (as it is for instance when I now assert a difference but do
not assert that there is now a difference); it asserts thus—both now and that the objects
are different now; the objects therefore must be present at one and the same moment.
Both the discriminating power and the time of its exercise must be one and undivided."
Aristotle, *De Anima* (1984). Aside from the phrase *A quo igitur erit?*, a corruption or misunderstanding of the Arabic rendering ἅμα ἄρα, "the objects therefore must be present at one and the same moment," this is a literal rendering of the text of Aristotle and
difficult because of that. The Greek expresses a distinction between the time at which
an assertion is made and the time at which the state of affairs described in the assertion
is true.

330. Ivry (1995), 90–91, cites this text as an example of the dependence of the *Middle Commentary* (2002), at 98.11–18, on the *Long Commentary*, Book 2 {350}. In the *Middle
Commentary* (2002) he has: "We say that it is evident in what I say that the ultimate sense
organ for the sense of touch, for example, is not in the flesh; nor [is it] in the eye for the

regard to sight. Next he explained that this is impossible. He said: **but it is
necessary that both be on the part of the same [thing]**, etc. That is, but it is
necessary that they be apprehended by the same thing but {351} through two
organs, and unless this were so, it will not be able to judge that this is different
from that. For if it were possible to judge these two to be different through two
different powers, each of which individually apprehends one of those two,
then it would be necessary that when I would sense that this is sweet and you
that it is white, and I did not sense what you sensed nor you what I [sensed],
that I apprehend my sensible to be different from yours, although I do not sense
yours. [It would also be necessary that] you apprehend yours to be different
from mine, although you in no way apprehend mine. This is clearly impossible.
Next he said: **But it is necessary that one thing say this to be different from
that and sweet different from white**, etc. That is, but just as it is necessary that
the same person say this to be different from that, so too it is necessary that
the power by which one judges sweet to be different from white be the same
power. For it is so in this with regard to individuals as with regard to the sensory parts, since they are also several in number. He meant this when he said:
Hence it is necessary that, as we say, we act[331] **and sense**. That is, hence it is
necessary that as the one who says this to be different from that is the same
person, so too that which senses and understands this to be different from that
is the same power. Next he said: **However, that it is impossible**, etc. That is, it
is therefore evident from this account that we do not judge sensibles to be different through different powers. Next he said: **That this**, etc. That is, that this
apprehension, besides {352} the fact that it is of one power, ought also to be in
the same instant, is evident since, just as one person says good to be different
from evil, so too when he says in regard to one of two that it is different in
some instant, it is evident that, in the instant in which he says that one of them
is different, in that same [instant] he says in regard to the other that it is different, since otherness is a certain relation, and relative things exist at the same
time in act. Next he said: and [this is] **not in an accidental way**, etc. That is,
and I do not understand by **instant** this instant which is said in an accidental
way in regard to what is divisible, as the instant in regard to which we say for
an extrinsic reason to be a different instant, since it is apprehended for an intrinsic reason to be different. (For the instant of which it is said that it is dif-

---

sense of sight, and so forth. Were the ultimate sense organ for sight, for example, to be
in the eye and [were] that for taste [to be] in the tongue, then our judgment that sweet
is different from white would require two separate faculties; for, that [faculty] which
apprehends sweet in this fashion is different from that which apprehends white, since
the latter is in the eye and the former in the tongue."

331. See n. 328.

ferent is different from the instant in which it is apprehended that it is different. He meant this when he said: **not because** the instant **is different**, that is,
the instant about which I said that it is different is not the [same] instant in
which it is apprehended that it is different.) But we say this instant to be different and that now it is different; and that instant is different from the instant
of apprehension. Next he said: **By what will it**, etc. That is, by what, therefore,
will this judgment be? I say: it will be by a power indivisible and one, and in
a time indivisible and one.

147. **But it is impossible for the same thing to be moved by contrary motions at the same time inasmuch as it is indivisible and in indivisible time.**[332]
**For if something is sweet, {353} it will move the sense or intellect with some
sort of motion, while bitter [will move it] in a contrary way, but white in a
different way. Is it, therefore, possible for what judges them to be at the
same time indivisible in number and divisible in being, in such a way that
in one way, that is, by way of division, it senses divisible things and in
another way it senses the indivisible, since it is divisible according to being
and indivisible according to place and number?** (426b29–427a5)

After he had explained that the same power ought to be the ultimate thing
which senses[333] in regard to all senses, he began to ask about the mode in
which it is able to be the same thing and to judge contraries at the same time.
He said: **But it is impossible for the same thing to be moved**, etc. That is, but
it is impossible to assert that the same thing receives contraries at the same
instant, insofar as it is the same and indivisible. Next he said: **For, if something
is sweet**, etc. That is, for instance, that if this is sweet, it will move what primarily senses with some kind of motion, and when it is bitter, it will move it
in a contrary way, and likewise for white and black. When, therefore, the sense
judges this to be different from that (for this is sweet while that is bitter), a
power same and indivisible will then be affected by contraries at the same
time insofar as it is one and indivisible, which is impossible. Next he said: **Is
it, therefore, possible** that **what judges**, etc. That is, is it, therefore, possible
that this power judging contraries at the same time be same in subject and

332. The *Middle Commentary* (2002), at 99.9, has the following corresponding to this
passage: "That apprehension of this sort, with its single faculty, has to occur in a single
moment is evident. Just as one of us will say at a single moment that the good is different from the bad, so one will say at a certain moment that one of two things is different;
and in that moment he will be saying of the other that it [too] is different, since difference is a relation between two things, and two actual correlatives exist simultaneously.
This is not the sort of moment which, being divisible, is spoken of metaphorically; but
rather it is predicated as indivisible, having a truly indivisible moment."

333. *Ultimum sentiens*. That is, the common sense.

indivisible, but divisible through intentions which it receives, so that by this the question is resolved in this way? For that power, insofar as it is divisible, apprehends things numbered and divisible, and insofar as it is the same [power] it judges {354} these things by a single judgment. Next he said: for **it is divisible according to being and indivisible according to place and number**. That is, perhaps what judges different things and contraries is divisible according to being and form, but indivisible according to subject and according to matter, as we say about the apple that it is indivisible in subject and divisible according to different kinds of being in it, namely, color, smell, and flavor.

148. **Let us say, therefore, that this is impossible. For the same indivisible thing is two contraries in potency, not, however, in being, but rather it is divisible in act, and it is impossible for it to be white and black at the same time. Hence it is necessary that it also not receive their forms if sensing and understanding are such.** (427a5–9)

After he had asserted that way of solving the question mentioned earlier, he returned now to recounting that this is not sufficient for the solution. He said: **Let us say, therefore, that this is impossible**, etc. That is, let us therefore say that this is impossible, namely, that this power be unique in subject and several according to beings and forms. For it is not possible that the same thing be indivisible in subject and also receptive of contraries at the same time except in potency, not in act and being. For instance, [consider] that the same body may be said to be hot and cold at the same time in potency, but not in act, except insofar as it is divisible,[334] namely, because a certain part of it is hot and a certain part is cold. He meant this {355} when he said: **but rather it is divisible in act,** etc. After he had explained this, he said: **Hence it is necessary that it also not receive their forms,** etc. That is, hence it is necessary that this power not receive the contrary forms of sensibles, if that same power, namely, the sensitive [power], is such as this, namely, unique in subject and several in being. He said: **and understanding** because understanding in this intention is like sensing, namely, because in each there is a receiving and judging power which judges contraries at the same time, as we will explain in regard to the rational power. He intends by all these things to explain that this power is not the same insofar as it is in potency, as is prime matter, but is unique in concept, in being, and in act, and many according to organs, as we will explain afterwards.

334. Lyons (in Themistius, *De Anima Paraphrase* [1973], 150, note) notes the likely influence of ibid. (1899), 86.12–16; (1973), 150.4–8; and (1996), 108–109, on Averroes' thought here.

149. **But what is called by some a single point is divisible insofar as it is two.**[335] **Insofar as it is indivisible, what judges is one and insofar as it is divisible, it uses the same point twice. Therefore, insofar as it uses an end point as two endpoints, it judges two which are different. This, therefore, will be through the divisible; and insofar as it is one, through one.**[336] **In this way, therefore, we will determine the principle by which we say that an animal is sentient.** (427a9–16)

After he had related that it is impossible that this potency be one in subject and many in powers, he began to give the way according to which it is one and the way according {356} to which it is many. Because this is difficult to say and it is easier to explain by example, he brought forth an account as an example. He said: **But what**, as it were, etc. That is, but that power is one and many as a point which is the center of a circle when many lines are drawn out from it from the center to the circumference.[337] He meant this when he said **a single point**; this is a point which is contained by one line. Next he said: **is divisible**

335. *Sed illud quod dicitur a quibusdam punctus unicus secundum quod est duo est divisible.* ἀλλ᾿ ὥσπερ ἦν καλοῦσί τινες στιγμήν, ἦ μία καὶ δύο, ταύτῃ <καὶ ἀδιαίρετος> καὶ διαιρετή. "Just as what is called a point is, as being at once one and two, properly said to be divisible." (Aristotle, *De Anima* [1984]); فكما أن النقطة التى سماها أقوام نقطة إنما هي نقطة إذا كانت واحدة أو إذا كانت اثنتين ، فهي مجزأة من هذه الجهة (ibid. [1954]). In lieu of Crawford's *punctus unius* I instead suggest and translate *punctus unicus*. The corresponding Greek has στιγμήν, "a point" (ibid. [1984]), and the alternate Arabic translation rightly renders this as نقطة, not نقطة واحدة (ibid. [1954]). This Text seems to have suffered two corruptions at two differing stages. As Averroes' Comment makes clear, this Arabic translation was faulty as he read it with واحدة (*unicus*) or some similar form of that word misplaced with نقطة, an apparent error in the transmission of this translation. A second error seems to have taken place in the transmission of the Latin text, with *unicus* being replaced by *unius* early in that tradition.

336. The Greek ἅμα, "in a single moment of time," occurs here three times, none of which is reflected in this Text. The alternate Arabic translation reflects this term twice with معًا. See Aristotle, *De Anima* (1954). The Greek is translated as follows in ibid. (1984). "Just as what is called a point is, as being at once one and two, properly said to be divisible, so here, that which discriminates is *qua* undivided one, and active in a single moment of time, while *qua* divisible it twice over uses the same dot at one and the same time. So far then as it takes the limit as two, it discriminates two separate objects with what in a sense is separated; while so far as it takes it as one, it does so with what is one and occupies in its activity a single moment of time."

337. As Lyons notes in Themistius, *De Anima Paraphrase* (1973), 150, note, this sentence has its origin in Alexander, *De Anima* (1887), 63.8–13; (1979), 76. Averroes' proximate source was likely Themistius, *De Anima Paraphrase* (1899), 86.18ff.; (1973), 150.11ff.; (1996), 109.

insofar as it is two. That is, therefore, insofar as that power is two and several in virtue of the senses which are united with it, just as the point is two and several in virtue of the ends of line going out from it, [the power] is divisible in regard to its being affected by different sensible things.[338] Next he said: therefore, **insofar as it is indivisible, what judges is one.** That is, insofar as that power is something indivisible, namely, insofar as it is the end of the motions of the senses from sensible things, just as the point is something indivisible insofar as it is the end of lines coming from the circumference to it, it is able to judge different things which are united with it from the senses. After he had explained the way in which it can be understood that this power is indivisible and the way in which it can be understood that it is divisible, he began to distinguish what it does insofar as it is divisible and what it does insofar as it is indivisible. He said: therefore **insofar as it is divisible, it uses,** etc. That is, therefore, insofar as that power is divisible through sense, it operates through that one thing which is in regard to it as a point for two different operations at the same time. Insofar {357} as it uses things which are in regard to it as end points of lines, namely, the senses inasmuch as they have this similarity, it judges different things by different judgments. And insofar as it is one [power], it judges different things by a single judgment. It is as if it is held that it is better to say that the power of what primarily senses is said to be one in form and many with respect to the organs united with it, through which there pass on to it the motions of sensibles to the extent that they are united with it, than to say that it is one in subject and many according to the forms which will be delineated in it. For that being is more deserving of it insofar as it is what judges, while the other insofar as it is what receives. But, nevertheless, since we do not assert there that this intention is the same according to form, we will not be able to find anything through which it will judge different things to be different. For judgment is more deservingly ascribed to that potency insofar as it is act than insofar as it is potency, just as its passive motion from the senses is more deservingly ascribed to it insofar as it is a receiving subject than insofar as it is agent. Therefore, in its case it seems to be what receives according to the senses and what acts according to judgment, for to receive something is different from judging it, and these two ought to be found in something in two different ways. For this reason we see that this power judges the intentions which it properly receives and their privations. It is similarly the case for the rational power, but they differ in that this power

338. Arabic fragments correspond to Book 2, 149.21–25: وهو يريد من طريق ان هذه
القوة اثنين وأكثر بعدد الحواس التي تتصل بها كما ان هذه اثنين او أكثر بعدد أطراف الخطوط
الخارجة منها هي من هذه الجهة منقسمة للقبول والتأتي المحسوسات المختلفة (Long Commentary Fragments [1985], 42).

is of material intentions while the latter is of intentions unmixed with matter,[339] as will be explained later on.[340] {358}

150. **Because they determined the soul properly by these two differences, namely, to be moved in place and to understand, judge, and sense, while holding that understanding is in some way just as bodily sensing[341] (for the soul judges and knows something in these two ways), the ancients also said that understanding is the same as sensing. So does Empedocles when he said that judgment in human beings receives according to what is present [to them] and he said in another place that on account of this understanding in it always changes.[342] And this is the same thing which Homer meant when he said that it is so for the intellect.** (3.3, 427a17–26)

339. Arabic fragments correspond to Book 2, 149.54–66: فان الحكم أحرى أن ينسب الى هذه القوة من جهة ما هي فعل من ان ينسب اليها من جهة ما هي قوة. كما ان تحريكها عن الحواس أحرى ان ينسب أليها من حيث ما هي قابل وموضوع ⟨من ان ينسب اليها من جهة ما هي فعل⟩. فكأنها عنده قابلة من جهة الحواس ، ففعله من جهة الحكم والقضاء بان قبول الشيء غير القضاء والحكم عليه. وينبغي ان يؤخذ هذان الأمران للشيء من جهتين ولذلك ما نرى ان هذه القوة تحكم على المعاني المختصة التي تقبلها وعلى أعدامها كالحال في القوة الناطقة ، لكن الفرق بينهما ان هذه القوة معنى هيولاني وتلك معنى غير هيولاني ولا مختلطة بهيولى (*Long Commentary* Fragments [1985], 42).

340. Book 3, Comment 4.

341. *Existimando quod intelligere est quasi sentire corporale quoquo modo.* δοκεῖ δὲ καὶ τὸ νοεῖν καὶ τὸ φρονεῖν ὥσπερ αἰσθάνεσθαί τι εἶναι. "Thinking and understanding are regarded as akin to a form of perceiving" (Aristotle, *De Anima* [1984]); وقد يظن أن الإدراك بالفهم يشبه الإدراك بالحس (ibid. [1954]); "It may appear that apprehension by understanding is similar to apprehension by sensation." Apparently both Arabic translations were faulty: the first seems not to reflect καὶ τὸ φρονεῖν and adds (not unreasonably) *corporale*, while the alternate translation only fails to reflect καὶ τὸ φρονεῖν.

342. *Ut Empedocles cum dixit quod consilium in hominibus recipit secundum presens, et dixit in alio loco quod propter hoc transmutatur intellectus in eo semper.* ὥσπερ καὶ Ἐμπεδοκλῆς εἴρηκε "πρὸς παρεὸν γὰρ μῆτις ἀέξεται ἀνθρώποισιν" καὶ ἐν ἄλλοις "ὅθεν σφίσιν αἰεὶ καὶ τὸ φρονεῖν ἀλλοῖα παρίσταται. "E.g. Empedocles says 'For 'tis in respect of what is present that man's wit is increased,' and again 'Whence it befalls them from time to time to think diverse thoughts.'" Aristotle, *De Anima* (1984). The alternate Arabic translation omits this and merely states that "Empedocles and the poet Homer were among them," i.e., among the ancients: منهم أنبادقلس وأوميرش الشاعر (ibid. *Anima* [1954]). The translators rendering the Greek into Arabic seem to have found these quotations from Empedocles in more archaic Greek particularly difficult. The *Middle Commentary* (2002), at 101.11–13, is more faithful to the text of Aristotle: "Empedocles, for example, said in one place that man's intellect judges and distinguishes only things present to sense." The word *recipit* is likely the Latin translator's mistranslation of the Arabic يقبل, which is found as يقبل بحسب الحضر in Themistius, *De Anima*

The ancients agree in defining the soul properly through these two differences, namely, through local motion and through knowledge and apprehension, which seem to be understanding and sensing. Next he said: **while holding that understanding**, etc. That is, they considered that understanding is a kind of sensing, which is either a body or bodily, for the soul in these two judges and knows things. Because the ancients thought that understanding and sensing are of the same power and potency, for that reason it is necessary for us to investigate this. Next he said: **So does Empedocles**, etc. That is, so Empedocles said that intellect in human beings judges the sensible thing which is present. In another place he said that sense is the same as intellect and on account of this the intellect is always changed in regard to these [present sensible things] just as the sense is changed.[343] He means by change {359} the error which happens to each power, or forgetfulness, and other accidents in which they are thought to share. Homer meant this when he said that sense is similar to intellect.

151. **All those consider that understanding is bodily, just as sensing, and that sensing and understanding are from like to like as we determined earlier, although they ought besides to speak of error as well. For this is more proper to animals and the soul delays over it for a long time. For this reason it is necessary for it to be the case, as some say, that all the things which pass through the mind be true or [that] error be touching what is unlike, for this is the contrary and like is known through its like. It is considered that error in regard to contraries is the same.**[344] (427a26–b6)

After he had explained that after the account concerning the power of sense it is necessary to investigate the difference between this power and the power of the intellect, he said that it was considered that intellect is bodily as is sense. This is because many of the ancients believed that sensing and understanding are the same. Next he related the reason leading them to say this and explained how inadequate they are in regard to this. He said: therefore, **all those consider**, etc. That is, those people, therefore, considered that both understanding and sensing are body because they believed {360} that understanding and sensing come about through like, and because these two powers apprehend body, it is necessary that they be bodily, as we earlier determined concerning this with

---

Paraphrase (1973), 152.14, "is in accord with what is present," rendering the Greek πρὸς παρεὸν . . . αέξεται (ibid. [1899], 87.22); "according to what is present" (ibid. [1996], 110).

343. 1.2, 404b7ff.

344. The corresponding Greek has, "But it seems that error as well as knowledge in respect to contraries is one and the same." Omitted here is the Greek, "as well as knowledge," καὶ ἡ ἐπιστήμη. The alternate Arabic translation has والعلم والغلط شيئان مضادان (Aristotle, *De Anima* [1954]); "Knowledge and error are two opposite things."

reference to the opinion of the ancients. Next he said: **although they ought to speak**, etc. That is, although it was necessary for them to mention the cause of error from this perspective, for error is found more among animals, and the soul for the greater part of time is found ignorant and erroneous rather than knowing. Next he said: **For this reason it is necessary**, etc. That is, on account of the fact that they give that cause in regard to knowledge, it happens for them either to concede what the Sophists say, namely, that all things which pass through the mind, that is, all things imagined, are true or to say that the true is the soul touching what is like, since it is body, and error is [the soul] touching what is unlike, for unlike is a contrary and error is a contrary as well.[345] What he said is evident, namely, that if the soul apprehends things through things existing in it, as they say, if they say that [the soul] is similar to all things because they are all in it, it happens for them that there is no error at all. Or they may say that it is composed of one of two contraries existing in things and thus it will find truth when it apprehends the like contrary and will err when it apprehends the unlike contrary. Next he gave the impossible [consequence] which follows from this. He said: **It is considered that error in contraries is the same**. That is, but it happens for this position that there is error in regard to the proper contrary from any of the contrary things. But it is evident that error can occur in regard to each contrary indifferently and that it is not proper to a single contrary alone. {361}

152. **Let us say, therefore, that sensing is not understanding. This is evident. For one exists in all animals and one is found only in a few animals. Nor is understanding, in which the true and the not true exist as contraries to these, the same as sensing.**[346] **For the sensing of proper objects is always**

345. Averroes seems to have in mind the teaching of Protagoras. At *Metaphysics* 4.5, 1009a7ff. Protagoras is mentioned at the beginning of this chapter, while at 1009b10–16 Aristotle writes, "And this is why Democritus, at any rate, says that either there is no truth or to us at least it is not evident. And in general it is because these thinkers suppose knowledge to be sensation, and this to be a physical alteration, that they say that what appears to our senses must be true; for it is for these reasons that Empedocles and Democritus and, one may almost say, all the others have fallen victims to opinions of this sort." Aristotle, *Metaphysics* (1984).

346. *Neque intelligere, in quo existunt verum et non verum contraria istis, est idem cum sentire.* Omissions here leave this text corrupt and unclear with the referent of *istis,* "to these," indeterminate. The corresponding Greek has ἀλλ οὐδὲ τὸ νοεῖν, ἐν ᾧ ἐστὶ τὸ ὀρθῶς καὶ τὸ μὴ ὀρθῶς, <u>τὸ μὲν ὀρθῶς φρόνησις καὶ ἐπιστήμη καὶ δόξα ἀληθής, τὸ δὲ μὴ ὀρθῶς τἀναντία τούτων</u>—οὐδὲ τοῦτό ἐστι ταὐτὸ τῷ αἰσθάνεσθαι. "Further, thinking is also distinct from perceiving—I mean that in which we find rightness and wrongness—*rightness in understanding, knowledge, true opinion, wrongness* in their opposites." Aristotle, *De Anima* (1984); my emphasis indicating the missing text. In light

true and exists in all animals. But discerning can be false and is not in any animal unless it has opinion.[347] (427b6–14)

This account can be a response to the word **because**,[348] from which he began [this discussion] above, since it requires a response. It is as if he says: because the ancients defined the soul through motion and apprehension—it was considered that apprehension by intellect and sense are the same since each is a [form of] knowledge—and also many of the ancients believed this on account of the fact that they held that only like knows its like. Because they said this, let us say that sensing is not understanding by intellect. It can be understood in such a way that the response is weak and that account will be the starting point. It is as if he says: since it was already explained that it is necessary that there be investigation into this intention, let us say that sensing is not understanding. Next he said: **This is evident**, etc. That is, that understanding is different from sensation is self-evident. For sensation exists in all animals, while understanding is in few, namely, in human beings. He said **few** on account of the fact that one considers that several animals share in this power with human beings. Because this was not evident in this passage, he accepts what was conceded, and it is that we cannot say that all {362} animals have understanding. Since these two powers are different in subject, it is necessary that they be different in being, for things which differ in subject differ in being. Next he said: **Nor is understanding, in which the true and the not true are**, etc. That is, nor are things understood in which there is [division into] what is true for the most part and what is not true for the most part, insofar as they

---

of the Greek, *istis*, "to these," apparently refers to the missing terms, understanding, knowledge, and true opinion. The alternate Arabic translation has وليس الإدراك بالعقل (دون الإدراك إذا صح أو لم يصحّ إدراكاً واحداً ، وذلك أن صحة الإدراك بالعقل فَهْمٌ وعلم وثبت صادق ، والإدراك به على غير صحة خلاف لهذا كله)، وليس من هذه شيء مشاكل للإدراك بالحس (ibid. [1954]); "Nor is intellectual apprehension (الإدراك بالعقل) <in other animals> (<for they are> without <this sort of> apprehension since true and not true are in virtue of one apprehension, for the soundness of intellectual apprehension is understanding, knowledge, and true opinion, while apprehension which is not true is contrary to all this) and among these there is nothing similar to sensory apprehension." The *Middle Commentary* (2002), at 102.9–11, is more succinct: "He said: We say it is apparent that sensation is not the intellect and comprehension, for [the faculty of] sense is found in all animals, whereas it is known that the intellect is found only in a few animals, not in all."

347. *Distinguere . . . non est in aliquo animali nisi existimet*. καὶ οὐδενὶ ὑπάρχει ᾧ μὴ καὶ λόγος; "and thought is found only where there is discourse of reason" (Aristotle, *De Anima* [1984]); ولا يكون في من لا نطق له (ibid. [1954]); "and it is not in one who does not have reason."

348. This is found at the beginning of Book 2, Text 150 {358}.

are contraries, the same as the contraries which are [found] in the case of sensation, namely, in one of these there is the true for the most part and in the other error for the most part. For sensation always indicates the true in proper things and the false in universals, while understanding, on the contrary, indicates the true in universals and the false in proper things.[349] Furthermore, in regard to proper things the truth of sensation is more firm than that of understanding in regard to universals. For this reason he said **always** when he said: **For the sensing of** proper things **is always true**; and he said later: **But discerning can be false**.

153. **Imagination, however, is different from sensation and different from discernment. This does not occur without sensation nor does judgment occur without it. That, however, it is not the same as understanding and judging is evident.[350] For that affection[351] is with us whenever we wish, for we can put [images] before our eyes, just as things placed in storage, and [we can] fashion forms. Formation of opinion, however, is not [something solely] up to us, for it is necessary that it be false or true.[352]** (427b14–21)

After he had explained that discernment is only in what has rationality, he began to explain that the discernment which {363} is reputed to be reason in certain animals is only a discernment which comes about from imagination and that imagination is neither sensation nor understanding. He said: **Imagination, however, is different from sensation**, etc. That is, discerning is found only in what has reason, for imagining is different from sensing and from

349. Particular things are proper to sense, while universals are proper to thought. Hence, each power is a sound witness to its proper objects and an unreliable witness to objects not proper. *Middle Commentary* (2002), 102.11–15, is clearer: "Moreover, universals and particulars are contrary things; and we find that the veracity of the intellect is more involved with one of these contraries (namely, the universals) and its mistakenness more involved with the other contary (namely, particulars), while the situation with the sense is the contrary—that is, its veracity is more involved with particulars and its mistakenness more involved with universals." As Ivry notes at *Middle Commentary* (2002), 197, n. 38, Averroes seems to be drawing on Themistius here. See Themistius, *De Anima Paraphrase* (1899), 88.21–23; (1973), 154.5–9; (1996), 111.

350. *Quoniam autem non est cum intelligere et consiliari idem manifestum est.* ὅτι δ᾽ οὐκ ἔστιν ἡ αὐτὴ [νόησις] καὶ ὑπόληψις, φανερόν. "That this activity is not the same kind of thinking as judgement is obvious." Aristotle, *De Anima* (1984).

351. That is, imagination.

352. Imagination's ability to form images from past sensory experience is something fully in our power and within us and is without external reference and consequent truth value. The formation of opinions, however, is in our power but not absolutely and in its entirety since it has assertive reference to things external and so has truth value.

discerning by intellect and [imagining] does not occur without sensing, and without [imagining] no judging occurs. It is as if he indicated here the distinctiveness of those three powers according to the prior and posterior in nature. For if there is sensation, it does not follow that there is imagination, but if there is imagination, there is sensation. Similarly, if there is understanding, there is imagination and not the converse. Next he said: **That, however, it is not the same as** understanding **and** judgment, etc. That account is evident. Next he said: **For that affection is with us**, etc. That is, for imagination is voluntary for us. For when we wish to imagine things sensed previously and placed in the preserving power, we can do so. He meant this when he said: **we can put [images]**, etc. That is, through this power we can also fashion imaginary forms, individual instances of which we have never sensed. Next he said: **Formation of an opinion, however,** etc. That is, formation of an opinion, however, is not [fully] voluntary. He meant this when he said: **for it is necessary that** it be true or false. That is, for it necessarily follows for us that formation of an opinion is true or false and it is not so in the case of imagination. That is one of the arguments from which it is apparent that imagining is different from understanding. {364}

154. **Furthermore, when we form an opinion that something is very fearful, we are immediately affected. [It is] similarly [so], if we form an opinion of something inspiring courage. Through the imagination, however, our disposition will be just as our disposition if we were seeing things in the forms of things fearful or inspiring of courage. The differences of judgment itself**[353] **are knowledge, opinion and understanding and what are contrary to those. Let the account concerning their differences be elsewhere.** (427b21–26)

What he said is evident. There is another argument that imagination is different from judgment and opinion. For when we form the opinion that something fearful is going to occur, we are in some way affected by some affection, but not by the [same] affection as if that fearful object were present. Similarly when we form the opinion that something inspiring courage is going to occur, immediately we are affected, but not with the sort of affection as there would be if that source of inspiration were actually existing. When, however, we have imagined that fearful thing, immediately we are affected as if it were present. He means here by **judgment** assent. The place in which he promised to speak of those differences seems to me to be the book *Sense and Sensibilia*. For there he speaks about particular things belonging to those powers and in regard to all their last accidents.

353. That is, the distinct kinds of judgment.

155. Because understanding is different from sensing and the opinion is held that understanding is a type of imagining and a type of judging, we should first come to a determination concerning {365} imagination, then next we will speak of the other intention. Let us say, therefore, that if the imagination which occurs[354] is what is called imagining in a way which is not metaphorical, it is one of those powers or a disposition through which we indicate assent and say what is true or false. And among those are sensation, formation of opinion, knowledge, and understanding. (427b27–428a5)

After he had completed the account of sensation, he began afterward to speak of the imaginative power. He said: **Because understanding**, etc. That is, because it is evident, or nearly so, that understanding is different from sensing, but it is not so evident that understanding is different from imagination (for it is held that of the actions of intellect, one is imagining, another believing, and that there is no difference between imagination and understanding). Hence, we should make some determinations first concerning the power of imagination, then later we will speak about the rational power. Next he said: **Let us say, therefore, that if the imagination**, etc. That is, let us therefore say that if there is an action which comes about in us which is called imagination in a way which is not metaphorical, as sensation is frequently called false, it is necessary that it be either one of those apprehensive discerning powers, namely, either sensation or formation of opinion or knowledge or understanding, or a power different from those and a disposition different from those dispositions through which we ascertain beings, that is, we select them out. It is one of the things through which we ought to state the true or the false. Next he began to explain that it is not {366} one of those powers. He means by **understanding**, as it seems to me, the primary propositions and by **knowledge** what arises from them.

156. That, however, it is not sensation was explained from those things, if sensation is either a potency or an act, for instance, vision or sight, and sometimes something is imagined which is neither, for instance, what is imagined in sleep. Furthermore, sensation is always of the present, while imagination is not. If it were the same thing in act, then it would be possible for imagination to belong to all beasts and reptiles,[355] which is not held to be the case, for instance, for ants, bees, and worms. Furthermore, that is

354. *Dicamus igitur quod, si ymaginatio est que fit que dicitur ymaginari non secundum similitudinem.* The Greek ἡμῖν, "for us," may have been lost at some stage in the tradition of the text. This phrase is found in the *Middle Commentary* (2002), at 103.13, as فينا.

355. *Et reptilibus* is an addition to the Greek. It is also found in the *Middle Commentary* (2002), at 104.7.

always true, while imagination is false for the most part. Moreover, when we know in reality[356] **that this sensible thing is a human being, we do not say that we imagine this to be a human being, for we say this only when it is not clearly a human being**[357] **and then it will be either true or false. And from these things which we said earlier it is the case that people imagine images when their eyes are closed.** (428a5–16)

That, however, imagination is not sensation will be explained from the things which we will say. One of them is that sensation is in two modes, namely, either in potency (for instance, vision when it is not active) or in act (for instance, sight). There is a sort of imagination {367} which is not sensation in act or in potency, namely, the imagination which comes about in sleep. For it is evident that the imagination which is in sleep, insofar as it is in act, is not sensation in potency, and insofar as that act belongs to it without the presence of the sensible things, [imagination] is also not sensation in act. Next he said: **Furthermore, sensation is always of the present,** etc. This is the second argument and it is that sensation always occurs in the presence of a sensible object, while imagination does not, but rather [imagination can occur] in absence [of sensation]. Next he said: **And if it were the same thing in act,** etc. This is the third argument. For the opinion is held that not every animal imagines and that there are animals which are moved toward sensibles only in the presence of them in act, such as worms and flies. Bees and ants, however, necessarily imagine, bees because of their expertise, ants because of their disposition. But he does not trouble himself over the example.[358] Next he said: **Furthermore, that is always true,** etc. This is a different argument and it is that the senses are always true, that is, for the most part, while imagination is false for the most part. Next he said: **Moreover, when we know in fact,** etc. This is the fifth argument and it is self-evident. For we do not say, when we sense something to be such in fact, that we imagine it, but [we do say so] when the sense does not truly apprehend it to be such. If sensation were the same as imagination, it would be necessary that where sensation is spoken of, there too imagination

356. *In rei veritate*: ἀκριβῶς, "precisely." Aristotle, *De Anima* (1984).

357. *Quando non manifeste fuerit homo* is an interpretive rendering of μὴ ἐναργῶς αἰσθανώμεθα, "when there is some failure of accuracy in its exercise." Aristotle, *De Anima* (1984).

358. Note that Averroes corrects Aristotle here. Cf. Averroes' remarks at {159}. It may also be worth noting that some of the Greek manuscripts omit mention of bees at 428a11. The *Middle Commentary* (2002), 104, mentions animals and reptiles as well as "the worm and fly" (104.7–8) but not bees. As Ivry notes (198, n. 7), the *Short Commentary* mentions flies, worms, and crustaceans. *Short Commentary on the De Anima* (1985), 83.3; (1987), 173; (1950), 59.14–15.

would be spoken of. Next he said: **And from these things which we said earlier,** etc. That is, and there is another argument, one close to the earlier ones, namely, that frequently people imagine a form when their eyes are closed. {368}

157. **It also is not one of those which are always true, such as knowledge and understanding,**[359] **for imagination is false. It remains, therefore, to consider whether it is opinion, since opinion is sometimes true and sometimes false. But belief**[360] **follows upon opinion,**[361] **for it is impossible for someone who holds something not to believe what he holds. And no beast and reptile**[362] **has belief, while imagination is present in most of them. Belief therefore follows upon all opinion, while satisfaction**[363] **follows upon assent, and rationality**[364] **upon satisfaction. And of the reptiles**[365] **and beasts, some have imagination but not reason.**[366] (428a16–24)

After he had refuted the notion that the imagination is sensation, he began to refute the notion that it is knowledge, understanding, or opinion. He said:

359. *Intellectus*. The corresponding Greek is νοῦς, which in this context denotes the intellectual power which discerns first principles and cannot err. In this sense, "thought" can never be false or incorrect, although it can fail to exist as thought. See 430a26ff.

360. *Fides*: πίστις. From this point through the end of Book 2 *fides* generally has the meaning of "belief." But elsewhere it has the meaning of judgment and is rendered "assent." See {364}, where Averroes writes of Aristotle, "He means here by judgment (*consilium*) assent (*fidem*)."

361. *Existimationem*: δόξῃ. In what follows, for consistency I continue to translate *existimatio* as "opinion," though this is at times problematic.

362. *Et reptile* added to the Greek.

363. *Sufficientia*. قانع is found in the corresponding text of Averroes' *Middle Commentary* (2002), at 104.18, and is rendered "powers of persuasion" by Ivry. This Arabic form of the root قنع has the different basic senses of "to be convinced" and "to be content." Apparently the Latin translator chose incorrectly to use the latter instead of the former. The corresponding Greek is τὸ πεπεῖσθαι, "conviction." Aristotle, *De Anima* (1984). The corresponding text in the *Middle Commentary* has "As everyone with an opinion assents to it, and every assenting person has powers of persuasion, and everyone with powers of persuasion reasons, it follows that everyone with an opinion reasons." 104.18–105.1.

364. *Rationabilitas*: λόγος.

365. *Et reptilium* is an addition to what is found in the Greek.

366. *Omnem igitur existimationem . . . rationem autem non*. The corresponding Greek text at 428a22–24 is marked for excision by Ross (following Biehl). See Aristotle, *De Anima* (1956). It is translated, "Further, every opinion is accompanied by belief, belief by conviction, and conviction by discourse of reason, while there are some of the brutes in which we find imagination, without discourse of reason." Ibid. (1984). This text was preserved by both of Averroes' Arabic translations. See ibid. (1954).

It also is not one **of those**, etc. That is, and if imagination were knowledge or understanding, it would always be true, that is, it would indicate what is true. But this is not so. Therefore, it is not knowledge or understanding. Next he said: **It remains, therefore,** etc. That is, it remains, therefore, to consider whether it is opinion, since each[367] is said to be truthful sometimes and false sometimes, and this causes people to hold that they are the same power, according to two affirmatives in the second figure.[368] Next he said: **But belief follows upon opinion**, etc. That is, but belief always follows upon opinion, so, if imagination were opinion, {369} it would happen that everything which imagines would have belief. But many [animals] imagine, but nevertheless do not have belief. For none of the beasts have belief, although several of them imagine. Next he said: **Assent, therefore, follows upon all opinion,** etc. That is, and because everything which holds opinions is something which believes, and everything which believes is self-sufficient,[369] and everything which is self-sufficient has reason, it is necessary that everything which holds opinions have reason. And if imagination were opinion, then everything which imagines would have reason. But many of the beasts and reptiles seem to have imagination but no reason at all. Therefore, imagination is not opinion.

158. **It is also evident that it is impossible for imagination to be opinion with sensation[370] or a composite of opinion and sensation, from those things and from the fact that it is evident that opinion is not of something different from that of which there is sensation also, namely, if the composite which comes to be from opinion of something as white and from sensation of it is imagination. For it is impossible for it to be from the opinion of good and**

367. That is, opinion and imagination.

368. That is, some people fallaciously hold the view that imagination and opinion are identical on the basis of the following argument: Opinion is sometimes true, sometimes false. Imagination is sometimes true, sometimes false. Therefore imagination is opinion.

369. *Sibi sufficit.* See Book 2, n. 363.

370. The Text here omits οὐδὲ δι᾿ αἰσθήσεως; "It is clear then that imagination cannot, again, be opinion *plus* sensation, *or opinion mediated by sensation,* or a blend of opinion and sensation." Aristotle, *De Anima* (1984); my emphasis to indicate missing text. Averroes' Comment evidences no knowledge of the omission, although the alternate translation does render the Greek accurately as بحس ولا. Ibid. (1954). The *Middle Commentary* (2002), at 105.3–4, also gives no indication of awareness of the omission on the part of Averroes: "Again, it is clear that imagination is neither opinion connected to sensation nor a faculty compounded of opinion and sensation, since we can have an opinion about something without having a sensation of it at the moment of the opinion."

from the sensation of white. Rather, imagination is[371] **the opinion of what is sensed in a way which is not accidental.** (428a24–b2)

After he had explained that it is impossible for imagination to be opinion, sensation, knowledge, or understanding, and generally any of the powers of reason, he began to explain also that it is not a composite of opinion and sensation, as some of the ancients said.[372] He said: **It is also evident** {370} **that it is impossible for imagination**, etc. That is, it is also evident from the previous accounts in which we explained that imagination is not one of those powers that imagination is not opinion joined with sensation or a power composed of opinion and sensation. For if it were composed of them, it would happen that the properties of those powers from which it is composed would be truly said of it in some way. For in the case of what is composed from certain things it is necessary that there exist in it in some way the things which exist in the components. From this it is [necessarily] evident also that opinion would truly be only of that of which there is sensation, but they ought to be of the same intention,[373] namely, if the composition which comes to be from the opinion of something as white and from the sensation of it, as some said, were imagination. He indicates that Plato held the opinion, as I figure, that imagination is such that opinion and sensation are simultaneously composed in the same thing for us.[374] Next he said: **For it is impossible for it to be**, etc. That is, for

---

371. *Sed imaginatio est*: τὸ οὖν φαίνεσθαι ἔσται, "to imagine is therefore (on this view)." Aristotle, *De Anima* (1984). In the Greek context it is clear that this is a consequence which follows but is not what is in fact the case.

372. Plato, *Timaeus*, 52A-B.

373. Arabic fragments correspond to Book 2, 158.16–27: ومن البين أيضا ان التخيل ليس هو ظنا مقترنا بحس ولا قوة مركبة من ظن وحس فيما قيل ⟨من قبل⟩ من ان التخيل ليس هو واحدا من هذه القوى لأنه لو كان مركبا منها لزم ⟨..⟩ التي تركب منها بنحو متوسط ⟨..⟩ يجب على جهة ما ان يوجد فيه جميع ما في الأشياء المركبة من قبل انه من البين ان الظن كان يجب الا يكون ⟨صادقا الا على⟩ الذي الحس له أي : بل يجب ⟨أن يكون⟩ لمعنى ,بنحو متوسط واحد بعينه (*Long Commentary* Fragments [1985], 42–43). It is not clear how توسط "in a middle way," fits into this passage, perhaps due to the omission which follows. Much of the opening lines of this text is found in the *Middle Commentary*: ومن البين أيضا ان التخيل ليس هو ظنا مقترنا بحس ولا قوة مركبة من ظن وحس من قبل أنا نظن بالشيء ;ولا نحسه فى وقت الظن. وبالجملة فبما قيل من أن التخيل ليس هو واحدا من هذه القوى "Again, it is clear that imagination is neither opinion connected to sensation nor a faculty compounded of opinion and sensation, since we can have opinion about something without having a sensation of it at the moment of the opinion. In general, inasmuch as it has been said that imagination is not one of these faculties, . . ." *Middle Commentary* (2002), 105.3–5.

374. As Lyons notes at Themistius, *De Anima Paraphrase* (1973), 159, Averroes is here drawing on Themistius. See ibid. (1899), 90.28–32; (1973), 159.1–5; (1996), 113–114.

opinion is of something as good and sensation of something white and it is impossible for imagination to be something composed from the opinion of the fact that the same thing is white and good. For opinion and sensation, according to this way, will not be of the same thing except accidentally. Imagination, however, in their view is opinion and sensation of the same thing in a way which is not accidental. It is necessary that it be so, since if imagination is of the same thing (and this is evident) and it is composed of opinion and sensation, it is necessary that opinion and sensation be of the same thing essentially.[375]

159. **We also imagine false things and we have true opinion besides in regard to them, for instance {371} we imagine the size of the sun to be a foot, while we believe it to be greater than the earth. It happens, therefore, either that a person rejects the opinion which he used to hold, and this is while the state of affairs remains the same, without [his] awareness[376] and sufficiency[377] to the contrary, or, if he remains firm in regard to [this opinion], this same thing will necessarily be true and false. But it is not made false except when the thing is changed without it having been perceived. (428b2–9)**

The indication that opinion and sensation are not of the same apprehensible thing is that frequently they contradict one another in regard to the same thing. For we sense false things and yet we have true opinion in regard to them. For instance, we sense in a visible way that the size of the sun is a foot and yet we hold the true opinion that the sun is greater than the earth. Next he said: It

375. The *Middle Commentary* (2002), at 105.6–18, is clearer here. "Moreover, if imagination were [both] opinion and sensation together, then opinion and sensation would belong to the same thing, essentially. This is not possible, however, since there can be an opinion that this white object [for example] is good, while the sensation is only that it is white or some other sensible thing. This [dual judgement], however, would be necessary since imagination belongs to one thing; and, if opinion and sensation belonged to the same thing, then the opinion [obtained] through a sensible object (qua sensible) that it is good would not be held in an incidental way, like our having the opinion that a white object which we perceive is good or evil."

Arabic fragments correspond to Book 2, 158.38–41: فلو كان التخيل هو لشيء واحد على ما هو الظاهر من أمره – وكان مركبا من الظن والحس ⟨معا⟩ لكان الظن والحس هما لشيء واحد بالذات. (*Long Commentary* Fragments [1985], 43)

376. *Sine vigilia*: μὴ ἐπιλαθόμενον, "and the observer has *neither forgotten* nor lost belief in the true opinion which he had" (Aristotle, *De Anima* [1984]); my emphasis to indicate the relevant words); إذا ذهب علم الشيء عليه جملة (ibid. [1954]); "when knowledge of the thing on his part slips away completely."

377. See Book 2, n. 363.

happens, therefore, either that a person rejects, etc. That is, it happens, therefore, if opinion and sensation in such things are of the same apprehensible object, either (1) that a person rejects the true opinion in regard to those things, although the opinion is preserved. [That opinion is] not changed from one disposition into another on account of change on the part of the thing which is the object of opinion nor on account of the fact that the person having the opinion also changed because of some illness or awareness or argument which has led to a conclusion to the contrary. Rather [the opinion] changed per se, since sensation and opinion are, as it were, the same, because they are of the same thing. Or (2) I say, it is such that he rejects it in such a way that he persists in it {372} by believing two contraries simultaneously, and the thing will be in itself both true and false at the same time. Next he said: **But it is not made false except when the thing is changed**. That is, it is impossible for true opinion to turn about and become false per se; rather, it becomes false only when the thing is changed in itself without it being the case that this is perceived. Since it is impossible for the same thing to be true and false and it is impossible for what is true to be changed of itself without a change on the part of the thing, it is therefore impossible that opinion and sensation be of the same thing.

160. **Imagination, therefore, is not one of those nor composed from them, but just as one thing is moved through the motion of another, and imagination is thought to be a motion, and it is impossible for it to be without sensation, but [it is] in regard to these things which are sensed and in these which have sensation, [so] too [then] does motion come to be by the action of sensation.**[378] (428b9–14)

After he had refuted [the notion that] imagination is one of those powers or a composite of them, he began to show its substance and being. He said: **Imagination, therefore**, etc. That is, it was explained, therefore, from this account that imagination is not one of those powers or a composite of them, but rather the substance of that power is what I mention [here]. For there are certain things

---

378. This long Latin sentence reflects only part of a long and complex Greek sentence which was broken into several sentences in the Arabic translation. "But since when one thing has been set in motion another thing may be moved by it, *and imagination is held to be a movement and to be impossible without sensation, i.e. to occur in beings that are percipient and to have for its content what can be perceived, and since movement may be produced by actual sensation* and that movement is necessarily similar in character to the sensation itself, this movement cannot exist apart from sensation or in creatures that do not perceive, and its possessor does and undergoes many things in virtue of it, and it is true and false." Aristotle, *De Anima* (1984); my emphasis to indicate the lines translated in this Text.

which are moved by others and move others and imagination seems to be a power which is movable and affected by something else.[379] It is impossible for it to be without sensation, but it is in reference to sensible things and [present] in animals having fully formed [powers of] sensation, and it is possible for motion to come about from sensation which is in act. Hence, it is then necessary that imagination in act be nothing other than the actuality of that power through sensible intentions {373} existing in sensation in the way in which the senses are perfected through sensibles which are outside the soul. [It is also necessary] that the first actuality of that part of the soul be the power which is naturally constituted to assimilate itself to sensations which are in the common sense itself.[380] But Aristotle set forth the antecedent in this account and was silent about the consequent, because it is evident and because later he will explain it in a more complete way.[381] For this reason he sets that aside in this passage.

161. It is necessary that [the motion of the imagination] be similar to sensation (for it is impossible for that motion to be without sensation or that it

379. *Virtus mobilis et passiva ab alio.* Or perhaps the sense requires "a power [both] able to cause motion and able to be affected by another." See the following Text and Comment.

380. Arabic fragments correspond to Book 2, 160.10–24: انه قد تبين من هذا القول انه ليس التخيل واحدا من هذه القوى ولا مركبا من أكثر من واحد منها ، لكن جوهر هذه القوة هو ما أقوله : وكذلك فان كان التخيل قوة متحركة عن شيء ⟨ومحركة غيرها⟩ فان التخيل يظهر من أمره انه ليس يمكن أن يوجد دون حس بل انما يكون في الأشياء المحسوسة وفي الحيوانات التي لها الحس الكامل موجود وكان يمكن ان تحدث في النفس الحركة عن الحس الذي بالفعل ، فقد يجب ان يكون التخيل ليس هو شيئا غير قوة واستكمالها بمعاني ⟨المحسوسات⟩ الموجودة في الحس ⟨على جهة ما تستكمل هذه⟩ الحواس بالمحسوسات التي من خارج النفس وان يكون الاستكمال الأول لهذا الجزء من النفس ⟨عن طريق⟩ القوة التي من شأنها تتشبه بالاحساسات التي في الحاسة المشتركة (*Long Commentary* Fragments [1985], 43). The Latin omits في النفس at 160.17: "and it is possible for motion to come about *in the soul* from sensation which is in act;" omitted text emphasized. Portions of this text are also found in the *Middle Commentary*: فقد تبين من هذا القول انه ليس التخيل واحدا ;من هذه القوى ولا مركبا من أكثر من واحد منها ، لكن جوهر هذه القوة ما أقوله "It has thus been explained by this statement that imagination is not one of these faculties, nor is it compounded of more than one of them; rather, the essence of this faculty is what I shall say it is." *Middle Commentary* (2002), 106.5–6. فقد يجب ان يكون التخيل ليس هو شيئا غير قوة واستكمالها بالمعاني الموجودة في الحس المشترك على جهة ما تستكمل هذه القوة بالمحسوسات التي خارج النفس; "Thus, imagination must be nothing other than a faculty perfected by the intentions found in the common sense, in the same way that that faculty [that is, common sense] is perfected by sensible objects outside the soul." Ibid., 106.11–14.

381. See the Text and Comment which follow immediately below.

be in something lacking sensation) and that what has it be something that affects and is affected by many things. [The motion] will be true and false. This happens on account of what I will report. Sensation of proper objects is true and scarcely does falsity occur in it. Next afterward [there is] sensation of the thing which those follow and in this place there can be falsity, for instance, that this is white, for in this case it is not incorrect. However, that what is white is this or that [can] be false.[382] Next the third [kind of] sensation is the sensation of common things consequent upon the things which follow the proper [sensibles], and they are these in which the existence of the proper [sensibles] is located (I mean motion and quantity), and they are the things which accrue to sensibles. In regard to those properly speaking there is error. Therefore, sensation and motion which come to be from act differ from sensation and they differ from those three modes of sensation.[383] The first, therefore, when the sensation is present, will be true; the other[384] is false whether it is present or absent, and chiefly when the sen-

382. *Deinde post sensus rei quam sequuntur ista; et in hoc loco potest falsari; v.g. hoc esse album; in hoc enim non falsat; quoniam autem album est hoc aut aliud falsatur.* δεύτερον δὲ τοῦ συμβεβηκέναι ταῦτα <ἃ συμβέβηκε τοῖς αἰσθητοῖς>· καὶ ἐνταῦθα ἤδη ἐνδέχεται διαψεύδεσθαι· ὅτι μὲν γὰρ λευκόν, οὐ ψεύδεται, εἰ δὲ τοῦτο τὸ λευκὸν ἢ ἄλλο τι, ψεύδεται. "Next comes perception that what is incidental to the objects of perception *is* incidental to them: in this case certainly we may be deceived; for while the perception that there is white before us cannot be false, the perception that what is white is this or that may be false" (Aristotle, *De Anima* [1984]); وإنما يجوز أن يغلط فيكذب إذا عَرَض له عارض: وليس يغلط في أن الأبيض أبيض ، ويغلط في أن كان هذا أبيض أم الآخر ، فهذا ضربٌ ثانٍ مِن الخطأ (ibid. [1954]); "It is possible for error to occur and for one to be wrong when something occurs for it: there is no error regarding the fact that the white thing is white, while there is error regarding the fact that this or that is white. This is a second sort of error." The Latin Text here reflects τοῦ συμβεβηκέναι ταῦτα, "of the fact that these are attributed" (my translation) with awkward literalness, the sense of which may have been clear in Arabic but is hardly so in the Latin. Also note that if *sequuntur* is used to render the verb وَلِيَ, then the Arabic might have had a sense close to that of the Greek: "sensation of the thing which those accompany."

383. *Sensus igitur et motus qui fiunt ab actu differunt a sensu, et differunt ab istis tribus modis sensus.* ἡ δὲ κίνησις ἡ ὑπὸ τῆς ἐνεργείας τῆς αἰσθήσεως γινομένη διοίσει, ἡ ἀπὸ τούτων τῶν τριῶν αἰσθήσεων. "The motion which is due to the activity of sense in these three modes of its exercise will differ," Aristotle, *De Anima* (1984). وبين حركة فعل الثلاثة الحواس فرق (ibid. [1954]); "The motion of the activity belonging to the three sensations differs (for each of the three)." The Latin fails to render the Greek accurately here.

384. *Alius:* αἱ δ ἕτεραι. The Greek here is plural, referring to the other two "modes of exercise," while the Latin is singular. The sense of the text requires the plural here, and Averroes' Comment understands the Text in this way.

sible {374} is at a distance. If, therefore, what we reported is not otherwise than we said, and what was reported is imagination, then imagination is a motion from sensation which is in act. (428b14–429a2)

If imagination is a motion from sensation in act, that motion which is imagination must be similar to sensation in these things which occur for sensation and it must be impossible for that motion to exist outside of sensation and outside of animals. [It must also be the case] that those animals which have this power by it affect [many things] and are affected by many things and [that imagination] be true and false, as is the case for sensation. Next he said: **This happens**, etc. That is, it happens that true and false occur in the imagination since it is a motion from sensation which is in act, on the basis of what I will report about what happens in the case of sensation. For there is a kind of sensation which is true for the most part and [this] is the sensation of proper [sensibles], for instance: this is white or black. Another kind is false for the most part and this is in two ways, namely, sensation of accidental sensibles, for instance, that this white [person] is Socrates or Plato, and sensation of common sensibles, for instance, of quantity and motion, for error occurs in those two types of sensibles. Since this is so, there must happen for imagination regarding this what happens for sensation, and more. First, because the motion which comes about in imagination from sensation which is in act differs from the motion which comes about in sensation from sensible things because of the absence of sensibles, and on account of this falsity occurs in imagination. Second, because the motions of those three kinds of sensation in reference to the imaginative power differ from one another: the imagination which is of proper sensibles is true in every way, when sensation {375} apprehends them first; but the imagination which is of the other modes of sensibles is false, although it apprehends them, since sensation errs in regard to them. Next he said: **Therefore, sensation and motion which come to be from act differ from sensation**, etc. That is, as it seems to me, therefore the apprehension and the motion which arise from actual sensation and which are both imagination, differ from actual sensation in what concerns truth in the sensation as well. He meant by this that sensation is true but when the sensible vanishes, its remaining signs are perhaps changed because of this in the common sense and this will be a cause of error for the imaginative power even though the sensation was true. Then he said: **and they differ from those three modes**, etc. That is, and that motion which comes from the three modes of sensation in act, namely, the one which comes to be in the imaginative power, is different from those three modes of sensation. Motion, therefore, which comes to be from sensation which [in turn] comes to be from the first proper sensibles, will be true when the sensation is present, that is, when the sensation of them in act precedes imagination. But for the two other motions which come to be from the two other modes of sensation in act, which comes to be from two different kinds of sensibles, it is false, although the sensation is present and it has sensed those things before imagination, and chiefly when the time of the sensible apprehension is distant from the sensation.

If imagination is a motion from sensation in act, imagination must be similar to sensation in all its dispositions and it must be possible to trace the causes of all the things appearing in it to sensation. And if it is similar to sensation in all its dispositions, [imagination] must be a motion from sensation in act. It does appear that it is similar [to sensation]. It already appeared also from this account that we can trace the causes of all the things appearing in [imagination] {376} insofar as it is motion from sensation and that it is impossible to trace them to another power. Then, because all this is necessary, he brought together all that he said and set forth the conclusion which he intended. He said: **If, therefore, what we reported**, etc.[385] That is, if, therefore, what we have reported concerning this part of the soul seems to be [the case] and if all the things which occur in [imagination] occur in it only insofar as it is a motion from sensation which is in act only [and] not through another power of the soul, then imagination is a motion of sensation which is in act. (But if we assert it to be a different power among the apprehensive powers of the soul or composed of more than one of them, the impossible will happen, as was explained from this account. However, what we reported is what is truly called imagination.) You also ought to know that imagination seems to be a motion from sensation in act[386] in one of two ways. One of them is that since it has been asserted that it is a mode which it is possible to mention as being only one of the previously mentioned modes, namely, such that it is knowledge, understanding, opinion, sensation, or a composite of these, or a motion caused by sensation, and from all these the impossible occurs except from the position that it is a motion from sensation (for from this nothing impossible happens), then imagination must be a motion from sensation in act.[387] The second

---

385. Arabic fragments correspond to Book 2, 161.83–84: فان كان ما وصفنا (*Long Commentary* Fragments [1985], 43). Cf. *Long Commentary* Fragments (2005), 89.

386. Arabic fragments correspond to Book 2, 161.93–94: وقد يجب ان ⟨يكون⟩ التخييل حركة عن الحس الذي بالفعل (*Long Commentary* Fragments [1985], 43). This phrasing is repeated several times throughout Book 2, Comment 161.

387. Arabic fragments correspond to Book 2, 161.95–102: وهو يريد انه اذا وضع الأنحاء التي تقدمت وهي أن تكون اما علما أو عقلا أو ظنا أو حسا أو مركبة منها ، او حركة حادثة عن الحس وفي سائر الأقسام – ⟨التي⟩ يعرض لمن أنزلها محال ⟨سوى انها هنا⟩ حركة عن الحس ⟨فانه⟩ ليس يعرض عنها محال. فلقد يجب ضرورة أن يكون التخيل هو حركة عن الحس الذي بالفعل (*Long Commentary* Fragments [1985], 43). يريد انه اذا وضع أن ليس هاهنا إلا الأنحاء التي / تقدمت وهي أن تكون إما علما أو عقلـ⟨ا⟩ أو ظنـ⟨ا⟩ أو حسـ⟨ا⟩ أو مركبـ⟨ا⟩

way is that since it has been asserted that [imagination] is with the sensible and in the sensible and similar to it in all its dispositions, we will then be able to trace the causes of all the things which appear in it in this way. Hence it is necessary that it be a motion from sensation in act. Aristotle brought both together and concluded that it is necessary that the substance of the imagination be that substance. We ought to understand in this way the account of Aristotle in this passage. {377}

162. Because sight properly is sensation, the name was derived for [imagination] from light,[388] for it is impossible to see without light. And because sensations are firmly fixed in it and it is of the same mode, for this reason an animal does many things by it, some of which are because they do not have[389] intellect, such as beasts, and some because perhaps intellect in it is muddled by some accident,[390] illness or sleep, such as [happens to] human beings. This, therefore, is the end of our account concerning imagination, what it is and why. (429a2–9)

Because sight properly is what is called sensation first of all, since it is the most noble of the senses and [since it] is actualized by light, for this reason the

---

منها او حركة / حادثة عن الحس وكان سائر الأقسام يعرض من إنزالها محال وكونه حركة عن الحس ليس / يعرض عنه محال. فقد يجب ضرورة أن يكون التخيل هو حركة عن الحس بالفعل (*Long Commentary* Fragments [2005], 89–90); "He means to say that if one asserts that there are no other modes than those set forth earlier, and which are that it [the imagination] is either knowledge or intellect or opinion or sense, or composed of these [things], or a movement which arises from the sense, and that there results an impossibility from asserting the other alternatives, while from the fact that it is a movement of the sense there does not result any impossibility, then it must necessarily be that imagination is a movement of the sense in act." My translation of the French of Sirat and Geoffroy.

388. The corresponding Greek has ἐπεὶ δ' ἡ ὄψις μάλιστα αἴσθησίς ἐστι, καὶ τὸ ὄνομα ἀπὸ τοῦ φάους εἴληφεν: "As sight is the most highly developed sense, the name φαντασία (imagination) has been formed from φάος (light)" (Aristotle, *De Anima* [1984]). Averroes' alternate translation is closer to the Greek, although the editor has to add وإذا كان البصر حسا ⟨بالمعنى الأكمال⟩ ، (*proprie*) for the Greek μάλιστα. ⟨بالمعنى الأكمال⟩ يسمى التوهم باليونانية باسم مشتق من الضوء (Aristotle, *De Anima* [1954]); "If sight is sense in the most perfect meaning, then imagination in Greek is derived from the word light." The *Middle Commentary* (2002) at 107.15–17 is clear: "And, since the sense of sight is the most noble of the senses and needs light to be perfected, this faculty [namely, imagination] was called in the Greek language by a name derived from the word for light."

389. *Non habent*: The Latin Text shifts from singular to plural and then back to singular in this discussion of animals.

390. *Ab aliquo accidente*: πάθει, "by feeling." Aristotle, *De Anima* (1984).

name of that power is derived from the name of light in the Greek language. Next he began to report the usefulness of that power in animals, namely, the final cause. He said: **Because sensations are firmly fixed in** it, etc. That is, because sensations are firmly fixed in it and in the absence of sensibles they remain in the imagining animal in the way they were when the sensibles were present, for this reason the animal is moved. [It is moved] by those sensations in virtue of this power in the absence of sensibles by many motions in reference to sensibles and non-sensibles, in seeking what is useful and avoiding what is harmful, to the extent that it was moved through the sensation by the sensibles, in such a way that the animal does not lack the usefulness present in the sensibles during their absence, but that power remains such as it was when the sensibles were present. And generally the usefulness of the senses in the presence of sensibles {378} was given for this power in the absence of sensibles, in such a way that the animal in virtue of this have the most excellent being by having health. Next he said: **some of which [are] because they do not have intellect**, etc. That is, some animals act in virtue of this power because they do not have intellect and they have that power in place of intellect for attaining health. And some act through it when the intellect has been muddled by illness or something else, and they are the animals having intellect, such as human beings, for then for these it occupies the place of intellect. This, then, is the account concerning imagination, what it is and why, and these two [accounts] are naturally desired. {379}

Book 3

1. **Concerning the part of the soul in virtue of which the soul knows and understands[1] [and] whether or not it differs [from other parts of the soul] with respect to spatial magnitude, or rather [only] in intention[2], we should investigate what its difference[3] is and how conceptualizing takes place.[4]** (3. 4, 429a10–13)[5]

    1. *Cognoscit et intelligit*: γινώσκει . . . καὶ φρονεῖ, "knows and thinks." Smith and Barnes (Aristotle, *De Anima* [1984]) omit "thinks" by typographical error. الذي به تدرك النفس و تَعقِل (ibid. [1954]); "by which the soul perceives and understands."

    2. *Utrum est differens aut non differens in magnitudine, sed in intentione*: εἴτε χωριστοῦ ὄντος εἴτε καὶ μὴ χωριστοῦ κατὰ μέγεθος ἀλλὰ κατὰ λόγον; "whether this is separable from the others in definition only, or spatially as well" (Aristotle, *De Anima* [1984]); أمفارق هو كمفارقة الجسم الجسم؟ أو إنما مفارقته بالمعنى وليس هو بمفارق البتة؟ (ibid. [1954]); "Is it separate as one body is separate from another? Or is its separation in intention only while it is not in fact separate?" The paraphrasing *Middle Commentary* (2002), 108.6–7, has إن كان مفارقا لسائر قوى النفس بالموضع من البدن وبالمعنى; "whether it is separate from the rest of the faculties of the soul in location and intention."

    3. That is, what is its differentiating characteristic.

    4. *Formare per intellectum*: γίνεται τὸ νοεῖν. This phrase corresponds to the Arabic التصور بالعقل, literally "representation by intellect," which Ivry rightly renders as "conceptualization" in the *Middle Commentary* (2002), at 108.10. It first appears in the present work at {6}, where it is rendered by the phrase *ymaginatio per intellectum*, a phrase which also occurs frequently in the Latin of the *Long Commentary on the Metaphysics*, corresponding to the Arabic التصور بالعقل. See Book 1, n. 14. At {220} in the present work, Averroes discusses the human rational ability for intellectual understanding whenever wished and contrasts it with sense perception, which requires an extrinsic object. This ability is characterized by Averroes as *formare* in the Latin, which I also render as "to conceptualize." At {454}, Book 3, Text 21, *formare . . . res indivisibles* corresponds to the Greek Ἡ μὲν οὖν τῶν ἀδιαιρέτων νόησις (430a26). In the Comment at Book 3, 21, {455}, this is paraphrased as *comprehendere autem res simplices non compositas erit per intellecta que non falsantur neque veridicantur, que dicitur informatio*. "That is, apprehending simple incomposite things will be through intelligibles which are neither false nor true, which is called *conceptualization*." Hence, I render both *formare* and *formare per intellectum* by forms of "to conceptualize." Both *formatio* and *informatio* are rendered as "conceptualization."

    5. Averroes gives no explanation of why he begins the third book of his *Long Commentary* after the completion of Aristotle's Book 3, chapter 3, on the imagination, rather than at the traditional beginning of Aristotle's third book (424b22). The division may have been in the Text itself. Gutas (1988), 61, n. 3, mentions that the *De Anima* used by Avicenna began its final book at this point also. The reason for such a division is obvi-

After he had completed the account of what the imaginative power is and why it exists, he began to investigate the rational [power] and to seek how it differs from the other apprehensive powers, namely, from the power of sense and [the power] of imagination. The difference lies in both the first and the final actuality as well as in proper action and affection, since it is necessary that the diverse powers differ in these two respects. Hence, it is evident that they will necessarily differ in the category of action, if they are active, or in the category of affection, if they are passive, or in both if both. Because his intention is just this, he first began to show that the existence of that power is self-evident, namely, that it differs from the other powers of the soul, since it is in virtue of this power that human beings differ from other animals, as has been said in many places. What is in doubt—whether it differs from the other powers in subject as well as in intention, or only in intention[6]—need not be known

---

ous: Aristotle's discussion of the rational power begins here, as Averroes says at the beginning of his first Comment. Averroes' *Middle Commentary*, however, observed the traditional divisions of Aristotle's book. See *Middle Commentary* (2002), 90, and Book 2, n. 301, above. For a general discussion of the Arabic versions of the *De Anima*, see Elamrani-Jamal (2003) and Puig (2007). Also see the introduction, pp. lxxvi–lxxix.

6. Arabic fragments correspond to Book 3, 1.19–25: بهذه القوة أعني كونها مباينة لسائر ⟨قوى⟩ النفس هو شيء معروف بنفسه إذ كان بهذه القوة ⟨يتميز⟩ الانسان من سائر الحيوان *. واما الشك فيه هل هي ⟨. . .⟩ قوى او تفارق بالموضوع ⟨. . .⟩ كما هي مباينة بالمعنى أم هي مباينة بالمعنى فقط (*Long Commentary* Fragments [1985], 43); "By this power, I mean its being distinct from the rest [of the powers] of the soul, this is something self-evident since by this power human beings are distinguished from the rest of the animals. What is in doubt regarding it is whether it <. . .> power or separate in subject <. . .> as well as being distinct in notion or it is distinct in notion alone." At* the Arabic fragment has nothing corresponding to the Latin *ut dictum est in multis locis*, "as has been said in many places." Sirat and Geoffroy (*Long Commentary* Fragments [2005]) find considerably more text in the fragments. See the note which follows.

Averroes here has in mind 413b13–16. See his discussion at Book 1, Text and Comment 19 {157–158}, where he explains the issue: "That those powers in certain animals are the same in subject and different in definition is not difficult. In regard to certain others, however, it is difficult and involves difficulty. Likewise, whether every one {158} of those principles is in the soul or not, in regard to certain [ones] is clear and in regard to certain others obscure." For Averroes the issue of the rational power and intellect is complex since the subject of knowledge is twofold, the individual person's theoretical intellect and the separate material intellect. The power is in two subjects, one as a power existing in an individual corporeal subject, the other as a power existing in an incorporeal and immaterial subject. While Aristotle's distinction between an organ of sense and the sense κατὰ λόγον or λόγῳ might allow for this to be characterized as a logical or notional distinction, Averroes' understanding of the relationship of the theoretical intellect and the material intellect leaves this as an issue which he rightly characterized as "difficult."

beforehand {380} in the course of this investigation, though perhaps from this investigation how it exists will be explained. And he said: **Concerning the part of the soul**,[7] etc. That is, [consider] the part of the soul by which we apprehend

"{بــ}ـالاستكمال الأول أو بالاستكمال الأخير والفعل الذي يخصه / {والانف}ـعرا)ال 7.
لأن القوى المفارقة تفارق في هذين المعنيين / {فلما تفار ق}ـت بهذين المعين فظاهر أن
التف)ا)رق يكون في / {كيفية الـ}ـفعل إن كانت من القوى الفاعلة أو في كيفية الـ /
{انفعال إن} كانت من القوى المنفعلة أو في الأمرين جميعا / {ولما كان} الوجود بالشيء
قبل الماهية ابتدأ أولا بتعريف / {أن الو}جود بهذه القوة أعني كونها مباينة لسائر / {قوى
النـ}ـفس هو شيء معروف بنفسه إذ كان بهذه القوة / {يتميز} الإنسان من سائر الحيوان وأما
الشك فيه هل هي مفا) رق / {عن سائر} قوى النفس بالموضع كما هي مباينة بالمعنى /
أو هي مباينة بالمعنى فقط فتقديم معرفة ذلك غير / {ضرور}ي في هذا الفحص بل لعل من
(Long Com- هذا الفحص يبين كيف الأمر / {في ذ}لك فابتدأ فقال فأما الجزء من النفس
mentary Fragments [2005], 93–94). "by the first perfection or by the last perfection, and the action which is proper to it and the affection, because the distinct powers are distiguished by these two criteria. And, given that it [the rational faculty] is distinguished by these two criteria, then it is clear that the difference will consist in the quality of the action if it is among the active faculties, or in the quality of affection if it is among the passive qualities (sic), or by the two things at once. And given that the existence, in the thing, precedes the quiddity, he [Aristotle] begins first by making it known that the existence of this faculty, I mean the fact that it is distinct from other faculties, is something self-evident, because it is by this faculty that man is distinguished from the other animals. As for the question on this subject: is it distinct from the other faculties of the soul in place as it is distinct from it in notion, or is it distinct from it only in notion, this knowledge does not have to precede necessarily in this inquiry. On the contrary, it is perhaps by this inquiry that how the thing is will be revealed. This is why he [Aristotle] begins by saying, 'Concerning the part of the soul, etc.'" Because of complicated textual matters and conjectural interpretations regarding matters such as the proper intended placement of the marginal manuscript notes which make up the fragments, I provide an English translation of the French of Sirat and Geoffroy. In some cases, however, I provide my own English version of the Arabic, as in the present case.

I prefer to render the Arabic somewhat differently: "by the first actuality or by the last actuality, and the activity which is proper to it and the affection, because the distinct powers are distiguished by these two criteria. And given that it [the rational faculty] is distinguished by these two criteria, then it is clear that the difference is in the quality of the activity if it is among the active powers, or in the quality of affection if it is among the passive powers, or by the two at once. And given that the existence, in the thing, precedes the quiddity, he [Aristotle] begins first by making it known that the existence of this power, I mean the fact that it is distinct from other powers, is something self-evident, because it is by this power that human beings are distinguished from the other animals. As for the question in regard to this about whether it is distinct from the other powers of the soul in place just as it is distinct from it in notion, or is it distinct from it only in notion, this knowledge does not necessarily have to take precedence in this inquiry. Rather, it is perhaps by this inquiry that how the thing is in reference to that with the [sort of] apprehension which is called knowing and understanding, since it is evident that it differs from the other powers. It does no harm in this investigation we are undertaking for us not to know from the start whether it differs from the other powers of the soul in subject and intention (as Plato and others used to say that the subject of that power in the body is other than the subject of the other powers)[8] or does not differ from the others in subject but only in intention. [Hence] we now must investigate the difference by which that power differs from the others. Next he said: **and how conceptualizing takes place**. That is, we should investigate whether it is an action or a reception before [investigating] how conceptualizing takes place. For from our perspective knowing the actions of the soul is prior to knowing its substance. It seems that by *to know* he meant here theoretical knowledge and by *to understand* practical knowledge,[9] since [practical] understanding is common to all but knowing is not.[10]

---

will become evident. This is why he begins by saying, 'Concerning the part of the soul, etc.'" Note that Sirat and Geoffroy render قوة *quwah* as "faculty," while I prefer "power."

This corresponds to Book 3, 1.12–28.

8. Averroes is here using Themistius, *De Anima Paraphrase* (1899), 93.32–94.5; (1996), 117. This text is corrupt in Arabic, but see Arabic in ibid. (1973), 163.5–8. Arabic fragments correspond to Book 3, 1.32–34: ‹. . .› ان موضوع هذه القوة من البدن ‹. .› كما يذهب أفلاطون غير موضوع سائر القوى (*Long Commentary* Fragments [1985], 43). Sirat and Geoffroy conjecture ‹إلى› at ‹. . .› (*Long Commentary* Fragments [2005], 99). Cf. *Middle Commentary* (2002), 108.5–9, where the text of Themistius was not used.

9. Arabic fragments correspond to Book 3, 1.39–44: وفحص هل التصور بالعقل فعل أو انفعالا وقبول ‹. .› اسم «المعرفة» يقع على المعرفة النظرية و «الفهم» على العملية (*Long Commentary* Fragments [1985], 43). "And he investigated whether conceptualizing by intellect is an action or an affection and reception <. . .> the term 'knowledge' stands for theoretical knowledge and 'understanding' for practical [knowledge]." فعل العقل أشد تقدما من علم / [من] جوهره والفحص هل الـ/ تصور بالعقل فعل أو / انفعال أو قبول (*Long Commentary* Fragments [2005], 100). Sirat and Geoffroy indicate that these correspond to Book 3, 1.40–41 and 1.39–40. اسم المعرفة تقع على الـ/معرفة النظرية و الفهم على / ‹الـ›عملية إذ كان الفهم مشتركا {للجميع وأما المعرفة فلا} (ibid., 98). "The term *ma'rifa* is applied to theoretical knowledge and the term *fahm* to practical [knowledge], because this latter is common [to all, contrary to the first]." My translation of the French. I prefer to render the Arabic as follows: "The term *ma'rifah* is applied to theoretical knowledge and the term *fahm* to practical [knowledge], because *fahm* is common [to all, while *ma'rifah* is not]." This corresponds to Book 3, 1.42–45. Note that the Latin translator rendered الفهم with *intelligere*, which usually renders a form of عقل.

10. Cf. *Epistle 1 On Conjunction* in Geoffroy and Steel (2001), 218 and 220. With "practical knowledge" I render *cognitionem operativam*. It is not immediately obvious how

2. Let us then say that if conceptualizing is just the same as sensing,[11] then either [the soul] is affected in some way by the intelligible, or something else similar to this [occurs]. (429a13–15)

After he had recounted that the starting point of the investigation concerning the substance of this power is to investigate the genus of this activity of conceptualizing—knowing the genus precedes knowing the difference—he began first to express doubt {381} as to whether conceptualizing is one of the passive powers, as is sensation, or one of the active powers. If it is one of the passive powers, whether it is passive because it is material in some way and mixed with the body, i.e., it is a power in a body, just as sensation is passive, or is not at all passive because it is neither material nor mixed with the body at all,[12] but [rather] has only [the characteristic of] receptivity from the intention

---

Averroes got this interpretation of knowing (*cognitio* and *cognoscere,* in each case المعرفة for γινώσκει) as indicating theoretical knowledge (المعرفة النظرية) and understanding (*intelligere, intellectus,* الفهم for φρονεῖ) as indicating practical knowledge. The text of Aristotle as Averroes had it does not make this distinction evident. The ultimate source seems to be Themistius, who explains these activities as θεωρίαν καὶ πρᾶξιν, "contemplation and action." Themistius, *De Anima Paraphrase* (1899), 93.32–33; (1996), 117. The Arabic version of Themistius edited by Lyons is corrupt here, but cf. Arabic in ibid. (1973), 163.5–8. At Book 3, Text 49 (433a14) *intellectus operativus* corresponds to the Greek ὁ πρακτικός (νοῦς), the practical mind, which is distinguished from theoretical mind by its end, since practical mind concerns action while theoretical mind is concerned with knowing for its own sake. That is, intellect in the sense of practical intellect is something common to all healthy human beings who partake in normal human goal-oriented actions, but the grasp of theoretical knowledge is not common to all human beings. The term "intellect" is equivocal for Averroes, having four or more senses. See {452}.

11. See n. 14 for a corresponding Arabic fragment.

12. Arabic fragments correspond to Book 3, 2.4–14: فنقول : لما ابتدأ بالقول ان مبدأ الفحص عن جوهر هذه النفس هو الفحص اولا عن جنس التصور بالعقل ، ولما كانت معرفة جنس الشيء تتقدم المعرفة بفصله ابتدأ يشكك ⟨في⟩ معرفة جنس التصور هل هو من القوى المنفعلة كالحال في الحس أو من القوى الفاعلة ، وإن كان من القوى المنفعلة هل هو من القوى المنفعلة كالحال في الحس أو من القوى الفاعلة ، وان كان من القوى المنفعلة هل هو منفعل من قبل انه هيولاني بجهة ما ومخالط للجسم أي انه قوة في جسم بمنزلة الحس أم غير منفعل لأنه غير ⟨هيولاني ولا⟩ مخالط للجسم أصلا (*Long Commentary* Fragments [1985], 44). Note that while the Arabic has جوهر هذه النفس, "substance of this soul," the Latin has "substance of this power." Sirat and Geoffroy read القوة, faculty or power. See below. The second occurrence of كالحال في الحس أو من القوى الفاعلة is a mistake in the Ben Chehida edition and should be deleted, as evident in the text provided by Sirat and Geoffroy: فنقول : لما ابتدأ ان مبدأ قوة ناطقة الفحص عن جوهر هذه القوة / هو الفحص اولا عن جنس التصور بالعقل وكانت معرفة جنس الـ / شيء يتقدم المعرفة بفصله ابتدأ أولا يشكك معرفة / جنس التصور هل هو من القوى المنفعلة كالحال في الحس أو من القوى الفاعلة وإن كان من القوى المنفعلة / هل هو منفعل من / قبل انه

of affection.[13] And he said: **Let us then say that if conceptualizing,** etc. That is, let us then say that if we assert that conceptualizing is just the same as sensing, namely, one of the passive powers, to the extent that the first intellective power receives the intelligibles and apprehends them just as the sensing power receives sensibles and apprehends them, then one of the following alternatives is necessary. Either some change and affection occurs to it from the intelligible

---

قوة في جسم / أو غير منفعل / أصلا لأنه غير مخالط / لجسم أصلا (*Long Commentary* Fragments [2005],101–102); "Intellective faculty: 'We say. . . .' Having begun [by saying] that the principle of inquiry concerning this faculty is the inquiry, in the first place, about the genus [to which it belongs] as a thing preceding the knowledge of its difference, he begins first by asking about the subject of the knowledge of the genus of representation: is it among the affective faculties, as sense, or the active faculties? And if it is among the affective faculties, is it affective insofar as it is a faculty of the body? Or [on the contrary] is it in no way affective, insofar as it is not in any way mixed with the body?" My translation of the French.

I prefer to render the Arabic as follows: "Rational faculty: 'We say. . . .' Having begun [with the understanding] that the starting point of inquiry concerning this power is the inquiry first about the genus of intellectual conceptualizing—for knowledge of the genus of a thing precedes knowledge of its species—he begins first by asking about the knowledge of the genus of conceptualizing: is it among the passive powers, as is the case for sense, or among the active powers? And if it is among the passive powers, is it passive insofar as it is a power in a body? Or is it not passive, insofar as it is not in any way mixed with a body?"

Sirat and Geoffroy understand this to correspond to Book 3, 2.4–10 and 2.11–14. They also find another fragment to correspond to Book 3, 2.10–12: لأنه هيولاني ومخالط / للأجسام أي هي قوة في / جسم (ibid., 103); "because it is material and mixed with bodies, that is to say, it is a power in a body."

13. That is, of the various characteristics manifested by what has the intention or nature of affection, this intellect has only that of receptivity. إلا القبول فقط (*Long Commentary* Fragments [2005], 107); "if this is receptivity alone." This corresponds to Book 3, 2.14–15. As Sirat and Geoffroy also indicate on 106, the *Long Commentary*'s Book 3, 2.8–15, is quite similar to what is found in the *Middle Commentary*: فنقول إنه إن كان التصور بالعقل موجودا في القوى المنفعلة بمنزلة الإحساس على ما هو الظاهر من أمره فإما أن يكون انفعاله عن المعقول على نحو انفعال الحواس عن المحسوسات وإما أن يكون أبعد من الانفعال الحقيقي من انفعال الحواس فيكون ليس يوجد فيه شيء من معنى الانفعال الذي في الحواس. "We say that, if conceptualization exists among the passive faculties comparable to sensation, as appears to be its nature, then either its being affected by an intelligible object resembles the passivity whereby the senses are affected by sensible objects, or it is more remote than that true passivity of the senses, such that nothing of the intention of passivity which is in the senses will be found in it." *Middle Commentary* (2002), 108.10–14. Sirat and Geoffroy then add إلا القبول فقط, "except receptivity alone," to the end of this passage. *Long Commentary* Fragments (2005), 98.

thing, a change similar to the change which occurs to the sense from the sensed object, because the actuality of the sense is a power in the body. Or there occurs no change similar to the change of the senses and to the affection of these by the sensed object, because the first actuality of the intellect is not a power in a body; rather, this does not come about for it at all. He meant this when he said: **or something else similar to this.** That is, or it does not undergo affection equivalent to the affection of the sense, namely, there does not come about for it a change similar to the change which comes about for the sense, but it is only likened to sense in regard to receptivity, because it is not a power in a body.[14]

3. It, therefore, must not be something affected, but it does receive the form and is in potency just as that, [while] not [being] that. Its disposition will be according to an analogy: as what senses is in relation to the sensibles, so is the intellect in relation to the intelligibles. (429a15–18) {382}

After he had set forth that first it is necessary to investigate whether this activity of conceptualizing is passive or active, he began to set forth what he

---

14. Arabic fragments correspond to Book 3, 2.18–32: الحواس حتى تكون القوة العاقلة الأولى تقبل المعقولات وتدركها كما تقبل القوة الحساسة المحسوسات وتدركها ، فقد وجب على هذه القوة أحد أمرين : أما ان ‹يلحقها تغير› وانفعال عن المعقول مثل انفعال الحاس وتغيره عند هذه المحسوسات من قبل ان ‹الاستكمال الذي› للحس قوة في جسم. وأما ان لا يلحقها تغير وانفعال كالحواس عن المحسوس من قبل الاستكمال الأول للعقل ليس قوة في جسم . . . الحس الا الحواس (*Long Commentary* Fragments [1985], 44). في القبول فقط من قبل أنّه ليس قوة في جسم حتى يكون القوة العاقلة الأولى تعقل المعقولات وتدركها / [كما يدرك] {كما تقبل} القوة الحساسة المحسوسات وتدركها فقد يجب فى هذه القوة أحد أمرين إما أن / {يلحقها} تغير وانفعا‹ل›‹ل› عن المعقول مثل انفعا‹ل›‹ل› الحواس وتغيرها عند قبول المحسوس من قبل /{أن الا} ستكم‹را›‹ل› للحس قوة في جسم وإما ألا يلحقها تغير وانفعال كالحواس عن المحسوس من قبل / {أن الا} ستكم‹را›‹ل› الأول للعقل ليس قوة في جسم بل ‹يفعل› فعلا مخالفا له فما نسبة شب‹ـ›‹ـ›ـه‹ـ›هما› ؟؟؟ / {. . .} لا يشب‹ـ›ـه المحسوس إلا في القبول فقط من قبل أنه ليس قوة في يجب جسم فنقول إنه (*Long Commentary* Fragments [2005], 104–105); ". . . the senses so that the first intellective faculty understands and apprehends the intelligibles, in the same way that the sensitive faculty receives and apprehends sensibles. However, there must come about for this faculty one of two things: either that they bring about a change and an affection on the part of the intelligible, similar to the affection of the senses and their change when they receive the sensible; or they do not bring about change and affection similar to that by which the senses [are affected] on the part of the sensible, from the fact that the first perfection of the intellect is not a faculty in a body; but on the contrary, it accomplishes an action opposed to it [the body], of the sort that the relation of resemblance [between the two (?) . . . and that the intellective faculty is not like] the sense except from the perspective of reception, since it is not a faculty in a body. Let us say, then, that it must, etc." My translation of the French. This corresponds to Book 3, 2.18–27 and 31–32. Note that Ben Chehida reads تقبل (receives) in agreement with the Latin (*recipiat*), while Sirat and Geoffroy read تعقل (understands) at the beginning of the passage.

wants to explain, namely, that it is that of a passive power in some way and [yet] that it is not changeable because it is neither a body nor a power in a body.[15] He said: **It, therefore, must not be something affected**, etc. That is, when there has been a thorough investigation of this, it will be apparent that this part of the soul by which conceptualizing comes about must be a power not changeable by the form which it apprehends. Rather, it has of the intention of affection only this alone: it receives the form which it apprehends.[16] [This is] because it is in potency what it apprehends, as [is] what senses, not because it is a determinate particular[17] in act, or a body, or a power of a body, as is what senses. He meant this when he said: **and is in potency just as that, [while] not [being] that.** That is, it is in potency, as is the sense, [but] not because that power is a determinate particular, a body or a power in a body. Next he said: Its being **will be according to** the example of sense **as what senses is in relation to the sensibles.** It can be understood in this way: it must be among the passive

15. Sirat and Geoffroy print a fragment which they identify as related to the Latin at Book 3, 3.9–11, 4.56–57, 4.60–61, 2.1–2, and 2. 17. { . . . }مـ{ـن القوى المنفعلة بجهة ما وبجهة م وبجهة ما من الفاعلة وأنه غير متغير / {من قبل} أنه ليس هو قوة في جسم وبعد يقول إنها من القوى / {الفاعـ}ـلة لأنها يخلق المعقولات ‹بـ›أن يجردها من المواد / {ويصرح بـ} ـأن كلاهما غير كائن ولا فاسد ويبين أولا أن فصل الانفعال والقبول موجود فيها / { . . . الـ} تصور بالعقل وبعد يقال ثم فصل الفعل موجود فيها / { . . . الـ}تصور بالعقل بمنزلة الإحساس) (*Long Commentary* Fragments [2005], 109–110); ". . . among the passive faculties under a certain aspect, and under another, those active, and that it is not subject to change, from the fact that it is not a faculty in a body. And next he says that it is among the active faculties because it created the intelligibles in abstracting them from matters. And he explains that neither one nor the other of these are generable or corruptible. It is explicated first that the difference 'passivity and reception' exists in it. And next he says: then the difference 'action' exists in it. To conceive by intellect is similar to the sense." My translation of the French.

16. Sirat and Geoffroy find a similar text in the fragments, though the correspondence is not literal. لأنـ‹ه› عند القبول لا ينفعل أصلا / من الصورة التي تذكرها / وبهذا المعنى فقط هو / مِن القوى المنفعلة أعني القبول / فقط (*Long Commentary* Fragments [2005], 111); "because at the time of the reception, it absolutely does not undergo affection under the effect of the form which it apprehends, and it is according to this meaning only that it is among the affective faculties, I mean to say the reception alone." My translation of the French.

17. *Aliquid hoc*. See Book 1, n. 25, and the introduction, pp. lviii–lxi. What is a "this," الشخص المشار إليه, *aliquid hoc*, is a particular which is a member of a species containing more than one member and which derives its particularity from the contraction of the form to matter in a composite. As such, what is received by a determinate particular or a "this" is particularized by reception into it. This notion is central to Averroes' arguments asserting the necessity of the single, shared material intellect in which understood intentions are not particularized. See {387–388}.

powers in such a way that the relation of sense to the sensibles is as the relation of the intellect to the intelligibles. In accord with this there will be a transposition in the order of the account and then it ought to be read in this way:
Its disposition must then be according to [this] analogy: as sense is in relation
to the sensibles, so is intellect in relation to the intelligibles. [It must be] that it is
not something passive with an affection as with the affection belonging to the
senses, but rather it receives the form and is just as that in potency, [while] not
[being] that. It can be understood [as follows]. Its disposition will be thus: as
what senses is in relation to the sensibles, so is the intellect in relation to the
intelligibles, i.e., to assert that it is not {383} something passive does not contradict the view that its relation to the intelligible is as the relation of what
senses to the sensed. But perhaps in conceding it to have this relation, it will
be necessary that it not be changeable. The fact that it is self-evident or nearly
so that the intellect has this relation, together with the fact that it is the starting point for knowing that it is not something passive or changeable, compelled us to give this exposition.[18]

**4. Therefore, if [the intellect] understands all things, it must not be mixed,
as Anaxagoras said, as it appears, namely, so that it may know.[19] For if
[something] appeared in it, the foreign element appearing in it would be an
impediment because it is different. (429a18–20)**

After he had asserted that the recipient material intellect ought to be of the
genus of passive powers and furthermore[20] that it is not changed in the reception because it is neither a body nor a power in a body, he gave a demonstration
of this. He said: It is **therefore** necessary, **if it understands**, etc. That is, it is
therefore necessary, if it apprehends all things existing outside the soul, that
before [its] apprehension [of things] it be named for this reason to be in the

---

18. That is, his understanding of the relevant epistemological and metaphysical
principles required Averroes to give this account.

19. Arabic fragments correspond to Book 3, 4.1–3: قال أرسطو : قد يجب ان هو يعقل
الأشياء كلها ان يكون غير مخالط كما قال أنكساغورش كيما يعقل ‹ . › لقبول الصور
المعقولة (*Long Commentary* Fragments [1985], 44). The fragments omit "as it appears" and
add an interpretive comment: "by receiving the understood forms." I follow the suggestion of Janssens and read *appareat* with the manuscripts instead of Crawford's conjecture
of *imperet*, following the Greek. Janssens (1998), 722, remarks that the Arabic original
may have been *zahara*, which has the primary sense of "to appear" but a secondary sense
of "to have power over." The latter fits the sense of the Greek, but the former is in accord
with the Latin manuscripts. His reasoning may be supported by Averroes' comment "so
that it may apprehend" (*ut comprehendat*). That is, it is likely Averroes read the Arabic
correctly in accord with the Greek while the Latin translator did not.

20. Cf. Janssens (1998), 722.

genus of passive, not active, powers and that it not be mixed with bodies, namely, [that it be] neither a body nor a natural or animate power in a body, as Anaxagoras said. Next he said: **so that it may know**, etc. That is, it is necessary that it be unmixed so that it may apprehend and receive all things. For if it is mixed, then it will be either a body or a power in a body, and if it is {384} either of these, it will have its own form and this form will impede its reception of another foreign form. He meant this when he said: **If [something] appeared in it**, etc. That is, for if it has its own form, then that form will impede its receiving other extraneous forms because they are other than it.

Now we must consider these propositions by which Aristotle makes these two claims about the intellect, namely, that it is in the genus of passive powers and that it is unchangeable because it is neither a body nor a power in a body. For these two claims are the starting points of all the things which are said about the intellect.[21] And as Plato says, the greatest discussion ought to be in the beginning;[22] for the smallest error in the beginning is cause of the greatest error in the end, as Aristotle says.[23]

Let us therefore say that the fact that conceptualizing is in some way concerned with receptive powers, as is the case for the power of sense, is evident from the following. Passive powers are able to be moved by that in reference to which they are ascribed; active [powers], however, move that in reference to which they are ascribed.[24] A thing moves [something else] only inasmuch as it is in act and it is moved inasmuch as it is in potency, insofar as the forms of things are in act outside the soul. Hence, it is necessary that they move the rational soul inasmuch as it apprehends them, just as, in the case of sensibles, insofar as they are beings in act, they necessarily move the senses and the senses are moved by them. For this reason the rational soul needs to consider the intentions which are in the imaginative power, just as sense needs to view sensibles. But since it seems that the forms of external things move this power in such a way that the mind abstracts them from matters and makes them first to be intelligibles {385} in act after they were intelligibles in potency, on the

---

21. Arabic fragments correspond to Book 3, 4.25–31: وقد يجب ان ننظر في هذه المقدمات التي بين بها أرسطو هذين الشيئين من أمر العقل أعني أنه داخل في جنس القوى المنفعلة ⟨وانه⟩ غير متغير من قبل انه ليس بجسم ولا قوة في جسم فان هذين المعنيين من أمر العقل هما ⟨. . .⟩ المبدآن (*Long Commentary* Fragments [1985], 44).

22. Cf. *Nicomachean Ethics* 1.2, 1095a31–32. There Aristotle may be referring to *Republic*, 511A–C or to the oral teachings of Plato.

23. *De Caelo* 1.5, 271b12–14.

24. That is, the actualization of passive powers lies in their being moved by something external to which the actualization is to be ascribed, while the actualization of active powers lies in their moving themselves in such a way that the actualization is ascribed to the active powers themselves.

basis of this it seems that this soul is active, not passive. Therefore, inasmuch as the intelligibles move it, it is passive, and inasmuch as they are moved by it, it is active. For this reason Aristotle will say later that it is necessary to assert that these two differences are in the rational soul, namely, the power of activity and the power of affection.[25] And he says plainly that each part of it is neither generable nor corruptible, as will be evident later.[26] But here he began to make known the substance of this passive power, since this is necessary in the doctrine. On the basis of this, then, it is declared that this difference, namely, of affection and reception, exists in the rational power.[27]

However, that the substance receiving these forms must be neither a body nor a power in a body is evident from the propositions which Aristotle uses in this discussion. One of these is that this substance receives all material forms, something known concerning this intellect. The second is that everything receiving something else must be devoid of the nature of the thing received[28] and its substance must not be the same in species as the substance of the thing received. For if the recipient were of the nature of the thing received, then the thing would receive itself and then the mover would be the moved. Thus, it is necessary that the sense receiving color lack color and that receiving sound lack sound. This proposition is necessary and indubitable. From these two [propositions] it follows that this substance which is called the material intellect has none of those material forms in its nature. Because the material forms are either a body or forms in a body, it is evident that this substance which is called the material intellect {386} is neither a body nor a form in a body; it is, therefore, altogether unmixed with matter.[29] You ought to know that what he set forth is necessarily so, because that is a substance and what is a recipient of the forms

---

25. 3.5, 430a13–14 {436}.

26. "It was necessary that the agent intelligence be separate, unmixed and impassible, insofar as it is what makes all forms intelligible. If, therefore, it were mixed, it would not make all forms, just as it was necessary that the material intellect, insofar as it is what receives all forms, also be separate and unmixed. For if it were not separate, it would have this singular form and then necessarily one of two alternatives would come about, either it would receive itself and then the mover in it would be moved, or it would not receive all the species of forms" {441}.

27. See n. 14 for a corresponding Arabic fragment.

28. Arabic fragments correspond to Book 3, 4.63–68: ⟨و⟩ لا جسم ولا قوة في جسم
هذا بيّن بنفسه ⟨. . .⟩ انها تقبل جميع الصور الهيولانية . . . ⟨وذلك ان كل⟩ قابل لشيء من
الأشياء يجب أن يكون ⟨عاريا⟩ من الطبيعة ذلك الشيء الذي يَقبله (*Long Commentary*
Fragments [1985], 44).

29. Arabic fragments correspond to Book 3, 4.73–80: وهذه لا شك فيها فيلزم من هاتين
المقولتين ان هذا الجوهر الذي يسمى عقلا هيولانيا ليس في طبيعته واحد من الصور الهيولانية
المشار اليها الا ⟨ان⟩ الصور الهيولانية هي أما جسم وامّا صورة في جسم فظاهركنهها

of material things or material [forms] does not have a material form in itself, namely, [it is not] a [substance] composed of matter and form. Neither is it again one of the material forms, for material forms are not separable. Nor is it again one of the simple first forms, for those are separable, but [the material intellect] does not . . . receive forms unless they are diverse [from its own nature],[30] and inasmuch as they are intelligibles in potency, not in act. [The material intellect] is, therefore, a being which is other than form and matter and the composite of these.[31] But whether this substance has its own form other in being from material forms has not yet been explained from this discussion. For the proposition saying that the recipient ought to be devoid of the nature of the thing received is understood of the nature of the species of that thing received, not of the nature of its genus, especially its remote [genus] and especially for what is said by equivocation. For this reason we said that in the sense of touch there is found a mean between the contraries which it apprehends; for contraries are other than the means in species. Since such is the disposition of the material intellect, namely, that it is one of the beings,[32] that it is a separate potency, and it does not have a material form, it is evident that it is not passive (since passive things, namely, changeable things, are as material forms) and that it is simple, as Aristotle says,[33] and separable. In this way Aristotle understood the nature of the material intellect; and later we will speak about his doubts.[34] {387}

5. So it will have no nature except this, namely, what is possible. Therefore that part of the soul which is called the intellect (and I call the intellect that

---

ان هذا الجوهر الذي يسمى العقل الهيولاني ليس هو جسم ولا قوة في جسم فهو غير مخالط للهيولي ضرورة ولا قوة (*Long Commentary* Fragments [1985], 44). Note that the Arabic has ولا قوة في جسم, "nor a power in a body," while the Latin has *neque forma in corpore*, "nor a form in a body," at Book 3, 4.79.

30. Crawford marks this passage as corrupt. An alternative to my conjectural rendering of this corrupt passage might be to understand the passage as asserting that for the forms to be received in the material intellect they must be separable from matter by the power of intellect. Janssens (1998), 722, conjectures the omission of *habet in se naturam materialem, quae non* by homeoteleuton and provides another reading of this entire section. If his conjectured text is correct, my translation would read "but [the material intellect] does not *have in itself a material nature which* receives forms only if they are diverse [from its own nature], and inasmuch as they are intelligibles in potency, not in act."

31. "One should hold that it is a fourth kind of being" {409}.

32. This sort of phrasing is used by al-Fârâbî in his *Letter on the Intellect*. See ibid., أحد موجودات العالم, 17.9–18.1 :(1983). It follows Aristotle's lead in passages such as in the next Text, *De Anima*, 429a24, τῶν ὄντων.

33. See 405a13–19 {40}.

34. See {399ff}.

part by which we discern and cogitate[35]**) is not one of the beings in act before it understands.** (429a21–24)

After he had explained that the material intellect does not have some form characteristic of material things, he began to define it in the following way. He said it has no nature according to this except the nature of the possibility for receiving intelligible material forms. And he said: **And so it** has **no nature**, etc. That is, then that part of the soul which is called the material intellect has no nature and being by which it is constituted inasmuch as it is material except the nature of possibility, since it is devoid of all material and intelligible forms.

Next he said: **and I call the intellect**, etc. That is, and I mean here by **intellect** the power of the soul which is truly called intellect, not the power which is called intellect in the broad sense in Greek, namely, the imaginative power, but the power by which we discern theoretical things and cogitate concerning things which will come about by our action.[36] Next he said: **it is not one of the beings in act before it understands.** That is, the definition of the material intellect, therefore, is that which is in potency all the intentions of universal material forms and is not any of the beings in act before it understands any of them.

Since that is the definition of the material intellect, it is evident that according to him it differs from prime matter in this respect: it is in potency all the intentions {388} of the universal material forms, while prime matter is in potency all those sensible forms [and is] not something which knows or apprehends [things]. The reason why that nature is something which discerns and knows while prime matter neither knows nor discerns, is because prime matter receives diverse forms, namely, individual and particular forms, while this [nature][37] receives universal forms. From this it is apparent that this nature is not a determinate particular nor a body nor a power in a body. For if it were so, then it would receive forms inasmuch as they are diverse and particular;

---

35. *Per quod distinguimus et cogitamus*: ᾧ διανοεῖται καὶ ὑπολαμβάνει ἡ ψυχή. The Latin here lacks the Greek subject and substitutes for "the soul" the first person plural, "we." The fault may lie in the Greek textual tradition since Averroes' alternate translation also lacks this mention of soul: فلا محالة أن عقل النفس المسمى عقلاً (وهو الذى يتفكر به فيرى الرأى أيّه) ليس بموجود في شيء من الأشياء بالفعل قبل أن يدرك الشيء بفهمه (Aristotle, *De Anima* [1954]); "So it must be the case that the intellect of the soul called intellect (which is that by which it cogitates so that opinion may be formed regarding anything) is not an existent in act in any of the things before it grasps the thing with its comprehension."

36. Cf. Themistius, *De Anima Paraphrase* (1899), 89.26–29, 94.27–29; (1996), 112, 118. The corresponding Arabic text is corrupt.

37. The material intellect.

and if it were so, then the forms existing in it would be intelligibles in potency; and thus it would not discern the nature of the forms inasmuch as they are forms, as is the disposition in the case of individual forms, be they spiritual or corporeal. For this reason, if that nature which is called intellect receives forms, it must receive forms by a mode of reception other than that by which those matters receive the forms whose contraction by matter is the determination of prime matter in them. For this reason it is not necessary that it be of the genus of those matters in which the form is included,[38] nor that it be prime matter itself. Since if this were so, then the reception in these would be of the same genus; for the diversity of the received nature causes the diversity of the nature of the recipient. This, therefore, moved Aristotle to set forth this nature, which is other than the nature of matter, other than the nature of form, and other than the nature of the composite. {389}

This same consideration brought Theophrastus, Themistius, and several commentators to hold the opinion that the material intellect is a substance which is neither generable nor corruptible.[39] For everything which is generable and corruptible is a determinate particular; but it has already been demonstrated that [the material intellect] is not a determinate particular nor a body nor a form in a body.[40] This brought them to hold the opinion, as well, that this is the opinion of Aristotle. For that intention, namely, that this intellect is such, is quite apparent to those who regard the demonstration of Aristotle and his words, with reference to the demonstration as we have explained [it] and with reference to [his] words because he said that it is unaffected and he said that it is separable and simple. For these three words are used with regard to it by Aristotle and it is not right—rather it is highly unlikely—for him to use any of

38. That is, it is not a composite form which necessarily has matter included in its definition.

39. Cf. *Short Commentary on the De Anima* (1950), 83–84; (1985), 121–122; (1987), 206–207. Avicenna is grouped with these because he holds for the incorruptibility of the material intellect, but Averroes also characterizes him as contradicting himself because he holds that the material intellect comes into being by generation of the individual and then is eternal. On Theophrastus as available to Averroes, see Gutas (1999b). On Averroes and the Greek Commentators, see the introduction pp. lxxix–lxxxix.

Arabic fragments correspond to Book 3, 5.53–59: اختلاف طبيعة القابلين ، فهذا هو الذي حرّك أرسطو الى ادخال هذه الطبيعة التي هي غير طبيعة الهيولي وغير طبيعة الصورة وغير طبيعة المجموع منها. وهذه هي البراهين التي قادته الى ذلك ولهذا قال انه جوهر غير كائن ولا فاسد (*Long Commentary* Fragments [1985], 44). The fragment does not specify "Theophrastus, Themistius, and several commentators" as does the Latin, but rather has "These are the demonstrations which force him [Aristotle] to this. On account of this he said that it is a substance neither generated nor corruptible."

40. {387–388}.

these [words] in a demonstrative doctrine about something generable and corruptible.

But they later saw Aristotle say that if there is an intellect in potency, there must also be an intellect in act, namely, an agent (it is this which draws out what is in potency from potency into act), and the intellect [must] be drawn out from potency into act (this is what the agent intellect places into the material intellect as artistry places forms pertaining to artistry in the matter of the artisan). Since they saw this later, they held the opinion that this third intellect which the agent intellect places into the recipient material intellect (this is the theoretical intellect) must be eternal. For since the recipient was eternal and the agent eternal, then the product must necessarily be eternal. Because[41] they held this opinion, it happens in reality that {390} it is neither the agent intellect nor the product, since agent and product are understood only with reference to generation in time.[42] Or it may be said that this "agent" and this "product" are said only by analogy and that the theoretical intellect is nothing but the actuality of the material intellect in virtue of the agent intellect such that the theoretical [intellect] is something composed of the material intellect and the intellect which is in act.[43] What seems to be the case, that the agent intellect sometimes understands when it is united to us and sometimes does not un-

41. *Et quia.* The sense requires "while." Perhaps وَكَكَن corrupted into وَلَأَن or was read as such by the translator.

42. "If the world were by itself eternal and existent (not insofar as it is moved, for each movement is composed of parts which are produced), then, indeed, the world would not have an agent at all. But if the meaning of 'eternal' is that it is in everlasting production and that this production has neither beginning nor end, certainly the term 'production' is more truly applied to him who brings about an everlasting production than to him who procures a limited production. In this way the world is God's product and the name 'production' is even more suitable for it than the word 'eternity,' and the philosophers only call the world eternal to safeguard themselves against the word 'product' in the sense of 'a thing produced after a state of non-existence, from something, and in time.'" *Incoherence of the Incoherence* (1930), 162; (1969), 96–97.

43. *Intellectu qui est in actu.* This phrase is used to denote an intellect or power of intellect which is in a state of actuality. As such, it can denote the agent intellect or the acquired intellect. Here I take it to refer to the agent intellect. The phrase *intellectus qui est in actu* occurs only in Book 3, where it is found nine times, here and at {394}, {410}, {430}, {476}, {479}, {483}, and twice at {484}. In its sole appearance in the *De Anima* Text, at Book 3, Text 36 {479}, it corresponds to the Greek ὁ νοῦς . . . ὁ κατ᾽ ἐνέργειαν. At {394} it appears in a quotation of the text of Alexander's *De Intellectu*. At {484–485} Averroes identifies "the intellect which is in act" with the acquired intellect. See the introduction pp. xix–xx, n. 10, and p. xxiv, n. 20; and Book 2, n. 440, regarding the use of *intelligentia agens* and *intellectus agens* to denote the agent intellect. The doctrine Averroes is expounding in the present sentence sounds much like his own doctrine in the *Middle Commentary*.

derstand, results for it because of the mixture, namely, on account of its mixture with the material intellect. From this consideration alone Aristotle was forced to assert [the existence of] the material intellect, not because the theoretical intelligibles are generated and made [to exist].[44]

They confirmed this by the fact that Aristotle insisted that the agent intellect exists for us in the soul, since we seem to strip forms from matter first and then to understand them. To strip them is nothing but to make them intelligibles in act after they were [intelligibles] in potency, to the extent that apprehending them is nothing but receiving them. They saw that this activity of creating and generating intelligibles is due to our will and is able to be augmented in us in accord with the augmentation of the intellect which is in us, namely, the theoretical intellect. And it was already explained that the intellect which creates and generates intelligibles and things understood is the agent intelligence. For this reason they said that the intellect in a positive disposition is that intellect, though sometimes weakness afflicts it and sometimes an addition [accrues to it] because of the mixture. This, therefore, moved Theophrastus, {391} Themistius, and others to hold this opinion about the theoretical intellect and to say that this was the opinion of Aristotle.

The questions on this are not few. The first is that this position contradicts what Aristotle asserted, namely, that the relation of what is understood in act to the material intellect is like the relation of what is sensed to what senses. This contradicts truth in itself. For if conceptualization were eternal, then it would be necessary for what is conceptualized to be eternal. Hence, it would be necessary for the sensible forms to be intelligibles in act outside the soul and not [be] material at all.[45] But this is contrary to what is found regarding those forms.

See the introduction, pp. xxxv–xlii. Cf. the interpretation of de Libera at *Long Commentary, Book 3* (1998), 193, n. 85.

44. In this context the meaning seems to be that the interaction of the material intellect and the agent intellect is not such that the material intellect by which we know is always in constant reception of intelligibles of material things by way of the "light" of the agent intellect. (At {441} Averroes asserts for himself that the agent intellect understands nothing of things of this material world. For him it is always in act of its own nature and so, in a different sense, always understanding.) Hence, since the material intellect is not always receiving the intelligibles of material things, the cause of the lack of receptivity is not the agent intellect but must have to do with the nature of the material intellect or its reception. The fact of intermittent intellectual receiving indicates that there are two intellects, not the fact that theoretical intelligibles are generated in us. Cf. {450–451}. The reason for the inability of the material intellect to function at all times would be simply because it depends not on the agent intellect alone but also on the internal and external senses to provide intelligibles in potency.

45. Cf. *De Anima* 3.4, 429b27ff., and Book 3, Text and Comment 13 at {427–428}.

Aristotle even says plainly in this book that the relation of that rational discerning power to the intentions of the imagined forms is just as the relation of the senses to the things sensed. For this reason the soul understands nothing without the imagination, just as the senses sense nothing without the presence of the sensible. Therefore, if the intentions which the intellect apprehends from the imagined forms were eternal, then the intentions in the imaginative powers would be eternal. And if those were eternal, then the sensations would be eternal, for the sensations are related to this power just as the intentions which can be imagined are related to the rational power. And if the sensations were eternal, then the things sensed would be eternal or the sensations would be intentions other than the intentions of things existing outside the soul in matter. For it is impossible to assert these same intentions to be sometimes eternal and sometimes corruptible, unless it were possible that a corruptible nature be changed and converted into an eternal one. {392} For this reason it is necessary, if those intentions which are in the soul are of generable and corruptible things, that those [intentions] be generable and corruptible. On this there was lengthy discussion elsewhere.[46]

This, therefore, is one of the impossible things which seem to contradict this opinion, namely, this [opinion of Themistius, Theophrastus, and others] which we asserted: that the material intellect is a power which has not come into being. For it is thought impossible to imagine how intelligibles will have come into being while that [power][47] will not have come into being. For when the agent is eternal and the patient is eternal, the product must be eternal. Also, if we assert that the product is generated (this is the intellect which is in a positive disposition), how can we say in reference to this that it generates and creates the intelligibles?

The second question is much more difficult.[48] It is this: if the material intellect is the first actuality of a human being, as it is explained concerning the definition of the soul, and the theoretical intellect is the final actuality, but a human being is generable and corruptible and [yet also] one in number in virtue of his final actuality by the intellect, then it is necessary that he be so in virtue of his own first actuality. That is, [it must be the case] that I be other than you in virtue of the first actuality in reference to intelligibles and you be

46. Averroes discussed this issue at Book 1, Comment 13 {19}. A lengthy discussion is found below in Book 3, Comment 36 {483–486}.

47. The material intellect.

48. What is at issue here is whether each person has his or her own material intellect from the start as a rational animal.

Janssens (1998), 723, is likely correct in suggesting one read *impossibilia contingentia* (understanding *sunt* to be supressed) with manuscripts B and C instead of Crawford's conjectural *contingunt impossibilia*. This does not affect my English translation.

other than I. If not, you would exist in virtue of the being belonging to me and
I would exist in virtue of the being belonging to you. Universally a human
being would be a being before having existed, and so a human being would
not be generable and corruptible inasmuch as he is a human being, but if he
were [generable and corruptible], he would be [so] inasmuch as [he is] an animal. For it is thought that just as it is necessary that the final actuality be of
this sort if the first actuality will have been a determinate particular and nu-
merable the way individuals are, {393} so too it is necessary for the contrary,
namely, that the first actuality be of this sort if the final actuality is numbered
in virtue of the numbering of individual human beings.[49]

Many other impossible things result from this position. For if the first actuality were the same for all human beings and [were] not numbered the way
these [individuals] are, then it would happen that when I acquire some intelligible, you too would also acquire that same thing, and when I forget some
intelligible, you [would] also.

Many other impossible things also result from this position. For it is thought
there is no difference between either position insofar as something impossible
results, namely, from the fact that we assert that the final [actuality] and the first
actuality are of the same sort, namely, [that they are] not numbered the way
individuals are. Since we seek to avoid all those impossibilities, we consequently
assert that the first actuality is this [particular] intention, namely, [the intention]
of an individual human being both generable and corruptible in matter and
numbered the way individuals are. [Yet] it was already explained from the
demonstration of Aristotle mentioned earlier that [the intellect] is not a determinate particular nor a body nor a power in a body.[50] How, then, can we escape
from this error, or what sort of way is there to solve this question?

Alexander,[51] however, bases his position on this last account and says that

49. De Libera is certainly right to call attention to this text. As it stands in the Latin,
it does not make a strong contribution to the argument but merely states that if the first
human actuality is individual for each human being, so too the final actuality of knowing is individual for each. But if the final actuality of knowing is individual for each,
then the first actuality would be individual for each. This is how I have translated the
Latin. I understand Averroes to start here by giving the first of two problematic explanations in relation to individuals. Then he contrasts this with the equally problematic
account which would hold that both the first and the final actuality do not belong to
human begins as individuals. For his interpretation, de Libera understands *huiusmodi*,
"of this sort," to refer ahead to "of the same sort, namely [they are] not numbered the
way individuals are." See *Long Commentary, Book 3* (1998), 62–63 and 196–199.

50. {387–388}.

51. Regarding the understanding of Alexander put forth here by Averroes, see the
introduction, pp. lxxxi–lxxxiii.

it belongs more to Natural Philosophy, namely, [to] the account which concludes that the material intellect {394} is a generated power such that we understand regarding it the opinion which is held also in regard to the other powers of the soul, that dispositions[52] come to be in the body per se from mixture and compounding. He says this is not unthinkable, namely, that from a mixture of elements there comes to be such a noble and marvelous thing, though it is far from the substance of the elements because of the great extent of the mixture. He testifies regarding this that it is possible in light of the fact that it appears that the composition which first occurred in elements—the composition of the four simple qualities—even while that composition is small, is the cause of the greatest diversity, inasmuch as one is fire and another is air. Since this is so, it is not implausible that through the multiplicity of composition which is in a human being and in animals, so many diverse powers are made there from the substances of the elements.

He propounded this plainly and in a general way in the beginning of his book *On the Soul*,[53] and he enjoined that when considering the soul in the first place one ought to know beforehand the wonders of the composition of the body of a human being. He said also in the treatise which he authored, *On the Intellect According to the Opinion of Aristotle*, that the material intellect is a power made from the compound. These are his words:

"Since, therefore, from this body, when it is mixed in a certain mixture, something will be generated from the whole mixture such that it is fit for being an instrument of that intellect which is in this mixed thing, since it exists in all the body, and that instrument is also a body, then it will be called the intellect in potency. It is a power made from a mixture which occurred in bodies, [a power] disposed to receive the intellect which is in act."[54] {395}

---

52. The Latin Averroes' *praeparatio* renders اﺳﺘﻌﺪاد and corresponds to Alexander's ἐπιτηδειότης, "suitability, fitness." See n. 54 and 55 below. Hence, it is a disposition for the reception of forms.

53. Alexander, *De Anima* (1887), 15.26ff.; (1979), 21ff.

54. ὅταν μὲν οὖν ἐκ τοῦ σώματος τοῦ κραθέντος πῦρ γένηται ἤ τι τοιοῦτον ἐκ τῆς μίξεως, ὡς καὶ ὄργανον δύνασθαι τῷ νῷ τούτῳ παρασχεῖν, ὅς ἐστιν ἐν τῷ μίγματι τούτῳ (διότι ἐστὶν ἐν παντὶ σώματι, σῶμα δὲ καὶ τοῦτο), τοῦτο τὸ ὄργανον δυνάμει νοῦς λέγεται ἐπιτήδειός τις δύναμις ἐπὶ τῇ τοιᾷδε κράσει τῶν σωμάτων γινομένη πρὸς τὸ δέξασθαι τὸν ἐνεργείᾳ νοῦν (Alexander, *De Intellectu* [1887], 112.11–16). "When, from the body that was blended, there comes to be fire or something of this sort as the result of the mixture, which is able to provide an instrument for this intellect, which is in this mixture—for it is in every body, and this too is a body—then this instrument is said to be intellect potentially, supervening on this sort of blending of bodies as a suitable potentiality for receiving the intellect that is in actuality" (ibid. [2004], 39–40; [1990], 55–56). Regarding the Arabic version, which is available in two editions, Davidson re-

This opinion regarding the substance of the material intellect is extraordinarily distant from the words and demonstration of Aristotle. [It is distant] from his words where he says that the material intellect is separable, that it does not have a corporeal instrument, and that it is simple and impassible, that is, unable to be affected, and where he praises Anaxagoras because he said that it is not mixed with the body. And [it is distant] from demonstration as it is known on the basis of what we have written.

Alexander expounded the demonstration of Aristotle by which he concluded that the material intellect is not passive nor a determinate particular nor a body nor a power in a body, in such a way that [Aristotle] meant that disposition, not the subject of that disposition. For this reason he says in his book *On the Soul* that the material intellect is more likened to the disposition which is in the tablet unwritten upon than to the tablet which has been disposed [with writing]. He says that this disposition can be said truly not to be a determinate particular nor a body nor a power in a body, and that it is not passive.[55]

---

marks that "neither edition of the Arabic is wholly adequate. I have translated from my own ad hoc eclectic text, which I base on both editions and their apparatuses, with corrections here and there from the Greek." Davidson (1992), 7, n. 2. For the Arabic text, see Alexander, *De Intellectu* (1971), 40.3–7. The text is corrupt in the faulty Jarullah manuscript used as base by Finnegan (1956), 181–199; see esp. 195. Also see Geoffroy (2002). Note that although the Latin might allow "intelligible" for *intellectum* here, it is more reasonable to translate *intellectum* as "intellect," which happens to be in accord with the thought of Alexander as we have it in the Greek and in the extant Arabic: لقبول العقل الذى بالفعل (Alexander, *De Intellectu* [1971], 40.7, and [1956], 195).

55. ἐπιτηδειότης τις ἄρα μόνον ἐστὶν ὁ ὑλικὸς νοῦς πρὸς τὴν τῶν εἰδῶν ὑποδοχὴν ἐοικὼς πινακίδι ἀγράφῳ, μᾶλλον δὲ τῷ τῆς πινακίδος ἀγράφῳ, ἀλλ᾿ οὐ τῇ πινακίδι αὐτῇ. αὐτὸ γὰρ τὸ γραμματεῖον ἤδη τι τῶν ὄντων ἐστίν. διὸ ἡ μὲν ψυχὴ καὶ τὸ ταύτην ἔχον εἴη μᾶλλον ‹ἂν› κατὰ τὸ γραμματεῖον, τὸ δὲ ἄγραφον ἐν αὐτῇ ὁ νοῦς ὁ ὑλικὸς λεγόμενος, ἢ ἐπιτηδειότης ἡ πρὸς τὸ ἐγγραφῆναι. ὡς οὖν ἐπὶ τοῦ γραμματείου τὸ μὲν γραμματεῖον πάσχοι ‹ἂν› ἀντιγραφόμενον, ἐν ᾧ ἡ πρὸς τὸ γραφῆναι ἐπιτηδειότης, ἡ μέντοι ἐπιτηδειότης αὐτὴ οὐδὲν πάσχει εἰς ἐνέργειαν ἀγομένη (οὐδὲ γάρ ἐστί τι ὑποκείμενον), οὕτως οὐδ᾿ ἂν ὁ νοῦς πάσχοι τι, μηδέν γε ὢν τῶν ἐνεργείᾳ (Alexander, *De Anima* [1887], 84.24–85.5), "We must say, then, that the material intellect is only a kind of propensity suitable for the reception of intelligible forms; it is like a tablet on which nothing has been written, or (to express this better) more like the blank condition of the tablet than the tablet itself, since the writing surface is an existent. Hence the soul, or the subject to which it belongs, might more properly be compared to the writing surface, and the intellect called material likened to the unmarked condition of the page or its suitability for being written on. Using these terms, we can state the analogy thus: As the surface of a tablet in which there inheres a disposition for being written on would be affected if it were inscribed, but the disposition itself would undergo no change by being actualized, since it is not the subject [of the writing]; so the intellect is

But there is nothing to what Alexander said. For this is truly said of every disposition, namely, that it is neither a body nor this [particular] form in a body. Why, then, of [all] the other [sorts of] dispositions did Aristotle select this for the disposition which is in the intellect, if he did not intend to show us the substance of the thing disposed but rather the substance of the disposition? But it is impossible to say that the disposition is a substance, while we say that the subject of that disposition is neither a body nor a power in a body. What Aristotle's demonstration reaches is an intention different from this one according to which it is said that the disposition is neither a body nor a power in a body.

This is evident from the demonstration of Aristotle. {396} For the proposition saying that everything which receives something must not have anything of the nature of the thing received existing in it in act is evident from the fact that the substance and nature of the thing disposed is able to have this aforementioned thing inasmuch as it is disposed . For the disposition is not the recipient but rather the being of the disposition on the part of the recipient is as [the being] of a proper accident. For this reason, when there is a reception, there will not be a disposition [any more] and the recipient will remain [in existence]. This is evident and thought by all the commentators from the demonstration of Aristotle.

For there are four different ways in which something can be said to be neither a body nor a power in a body. The first is as the subject of intelligibles, and this is the material intellect, the nature of whose being has been demonstrated. The second is the disposition itself existing in matters, and this is close to the way in which it is said that privation without qualification is neither a body nor a power in a body. The third is prime matter, the being of which has also been demonstrated. The fourth is the separate forms, the being of which has also been demonstrated. All these are diverse.

This led Alexander to this far-fetched and obviously erroneous explanation, namely, to evade and take refuge from the questions mentioned above.[56] We also see that Alexander is bolstered by the fact that the first actuality of the intellect ought to be a generated power on the basis of general accounts said in regard to the definition of the soul, namely, because it is the first actuality of a natural organic body. He says that this definition is true of all the parts of the soul with the same intention. And he gives the reason for this: since to say that all the parts of the soul are forms is [to speak] univocally, or nearly so, and because it is impossible for form, inasmuch as it is the end of a thing having

---

not a subject which is acted upon because it is none of the things which actually exist." (ibid. [1979], 109–110).

56. I follow the suggestion of Janssens (1998), 723, and read *scilicet evadere et fugere* with manuscripts A and C.

{397} a form, to be separate, then since the first actualities of the soul are forms, they must not be separate. By this he refuted [the position] that there is a separate actuality in the first actualities of the soul, as it is said of the sailor and the ship, or generally that there will be some part which is called an actuality with an intention different from the intention with which it is said elsewhere.[57] What he supposes is evident concerning general accounts in regard to the soul [is something] Aristotle himself clearly said is not evident in regard to all the parts of the soul. For to say *form* and *first actuality* is to speak equivocally about the rational soul and about the other parts of the soul.

Abû Bakr,[58] however, in the literal understanding of his discussion, seems to intend for the material intellect to be the imaginative power inasmuch as it is disposed so that the intentions which are in it may be intelligibles in act and [so] that there is no other power [which is] the subject for intelligibles other than that power. Abû Bakr, however, seems to intend this in order to avoid the impossible results [reached] by Alexander, namely, that the subject receiving the intelligible forms is a body made from the elements or a power in a body. Since, if it were so, then it would happen either that the being of the forms in the soul would be the being they have outside the soul, and so the soul will not be apprehending [them] or [it would happen] that the intellect would have a corporeal instrument, if the subject for the intelligibles were a power in a body, as is the case for the senses.

57. Averroes remarks at {405} that Alexander has taken the notion that the soul is the first actuality of the natural organic body and applied it to the material intellect. That is, insofar as the material intellect is a first actuality for knowing awaiting actualization by the agent intellect, then it too must be an actuality of parts or powers of a body. Yet the first actualities here are not of the same sort since one is the life of a material body while the other is the receptivity of an immaterial intellect. See the introduction, p. lxxxii.

58. Abubacher: Abû Bakr Muḥammad Ibn Bâjjah. As noted above, in Book 2 and throughout Book 3 with the exception of the two occurences in this paragraph, the translator has Avempache for Ibn Bâjjah. Referring to the present account, Davidson writes, "Either by reading out the implications of that statement and similar statements of that sort in Ibn Bâjjah or by drawing on sources no longer extant or still undiscovered—as, for example, Ibn Bâjjah's *De anima*, the published text of which breaks off tantalizingly in the middle of the discussion of the intellect—Averroes reports that Ibn Bâjjah construed the material intellect as a disposition located in the imaginative faculty of the soul." Davidson (1992), 261. For what we have of this work, see Ibn Bâjjah, *Book on the Soul* (1960), (1961). For discussion of the position of Ibn Bâjjah, see the introduction, pp. xxv–xxvii and lxxxix–xciii. Albert the Great apparently understood Abubacher in this paragraph to refer to the physician Abû Bakr Muḥammad Ibn Zakarîyah al-Râzî (d. 925), known in Latin as Rhazes. See Albertus Magnus, *De Anima* (1968), III, tr. 1, c. 6, 184B–185B. III. For more texts with this identification by Albert, see Bach (1881), 122–129.

A more unthinkable aspect of the opinion of Alexander is that he said that the first dispositions for the intelligibles and for the other later actualities of the soul are things produced from the mixture, not powers produced by an external mover as is well known of the opinion of Aristotle and all the Peripatetics.[59] For that opinion regarding the apprehensive powers of the soul, {398} if it is as we have understood it, is false. For from the substance and the nature of the elements there cannot come to be an apprehensive discerning power. For if it were possible that there come to be such powers from their nature and without an external mover, then it would be possible for the final actuality, which is the intelligibles, to be something produced from the substance of their elements, as color and taste come to be. This opinion is similar to the opinion of those who deny agent causes and those who allow only material causes: these are those who speak of chance.[60] Alexander has greater nobility than to believe this, but the questions which were posed to him regarding the material intellect forced him to this [position].

Let us then return to our [own discussion] and say that perhaps these are the questions that led Ibn Bâjjah to say this regarding the material intellect. But it is evident that what occurs to him is impossible. For the imagined intentions are what move the intellect, not what are moved. For it is explained that they are such that their relation to the discerning rational power is just as the relation of what is sensed to what senses, not as of what senses to the positive disposition which is sensation. If it were what receives the intelligibles, then the thing would receive itself and the mover would be the moved.[61] [But] it was already explained that it is impossible that the material intellect have a form

---

59. Averroes has in mind Aristotle's famous mention of τὸν νοῦν . . . θύραθεν, reason or intellect which enters human beings from outside, at *Generation of Animals* 2.2, 736b27.

60. Cf. Aristotle, *Physics* 2.4, 196b5–6, where Aristotle says, "Others there are who believe that chance is a cause, but that it is inscrutable to human intelligence, as being a divine thing and full of mystery." When Averroes comments on this text of the *Physics*, he may have in mind the Occasionalist view that things do not of themselves have causal natures but depend on God for their existence at every moment. There he remarks that the quiddity of a thing could not be known and that this would be a divine matter (*res divina*). *Long Commentary on the Physics* (1962), 66rA-B. This is in accord with his critique of Occasionalism found in his *Explanation of the Sorts of Proofs in the Doctrines of Religion* (1998), 166; (1947), 291–292; (2001), 83–84.

61. That is, the imagination would be both what gives rise to intelligibles by providing intentions of material things (mover) and what receives intelligibles (moved) if the receptive material intellect is to be identified with the imagination. As indicated in the introduction, pp. xxv–xxvii, Averroes adopted the view of Ibn Bâjjah in his *Short Commentary on the De Anima*.

in act, since its substance and nature is to receive forms inasmuch as they are forms. {399}

All the things which can be said regarding the nature of the material intellect seem to be impossible, except what Aristotle said, to whom also no few questions occur. One concerns the fact that the theoretical intelligibles are eternal. The second is the most formidable of them, namely, that the final actuality of a human being is numbered the way individual human beings are and the first actuality is one in number for all [human beings].[62] The third is the question of Theophrastus, namely, that it is necessary to assert that this intellect has no form and it is necessary to assert also that it is a being; and if not, there would be neither a reception nor a disposition. For the disposition and reception result from the fact that they are not found in a subject. Since it is a being and does not have the nature of a form, then it remains that it has the nature of prime matter, which is altogether unthinkable, for prime matter is neither apprehensive nor discerning. How can this be said regarding something the being of which is such that it is separate?[63]

Since there are all those things [which can be raised regarding the material intellect], for this reason it seemed [best] to me to write what seemed to me to be the case on this topic. If what appears to me is not complete, it will be a start for a complete account. So I ask my brothers seeing this exposition to write down their doubts and perhaps in that way what is true regarding this will be found out, if I have not yet found [it]. If I have found [it], as I suppose, then it will be clarified through those questions. For truth, as Aristotle says, is fitting and gives testimony to itself in every way.[64]

The question addressing how the theoretical intelligibles will be generable and corruptible while their agent and {400} recipient will be eternal and [that of] what the need is for setting forth an agent [intellect] and a recipient intellect if there is not something generated there, this question would not occur if there were not another thing here which is the cause that the theoretical intel-

---

62. The issue here is that all human beings are from birth rational in definition by species, yet they reach their full actuality of intellect only individually.

63. These issues are raised by Theophrastus in a long text quoted by Themistius. See Themistius, *De Anima Paraphrase* (1899), 107.30–108.7; (1973), 195–196; (1996), 133. The Arabic of the account of Theophrastus is translated by Dimitri Gutas in Huby (1999), 120.

64. Aristotle, *Prior Analytics* 1.32, 47a5–6: δεῖ γὰρ πᾶν τό ἀληθὲς αὐτὸ ἑαυτῷ ὁμολογούμενον εἶναι πάντῃ. "For everything that is true must in every respect agree with itself." (ibid. [1984]). لأنه يجب أن يكون الحق شاهد لنفسه ومتفقا من كل جهة (ibid. [1948]). Cf. Averroes' *Faṣl al-Maqâl* in *Decisive Treatise* (1959), 13: فان الحق لا يضاد الحق ، بل يوافقه ويشهد له; "Truth does not contradict truth but rather is consistent with it and bears witness to it." My translation. For a discussion of this, see Taylor (2000b).

ligibles are generated. Now, however, because those intelligibles are constituted through two things, one generated and the other not generated, what was said regarding this follows naturally. Conceptualizing, as Aristotle says, is just as apprehending by sense. But apprehending by sense is something which is actualized through two subjects, one the subject in virtue of which the sense is[65] true (this is the thing sensed outside the soul) and the other the subject in virtue of which the sense is an existing form (this is the first actuality of the sense organ). Hence, the intelligibles in act must also have two subjects, one the subject in virtue of which they are true, namely, the forms which are true images, and the other that in virtue of which the intelligibles are among the beings in the world, and this latter is the material intellect. For there is no difference regarding this between sense and intellect except that the subject of the sense in virtue of which it is true is outside the soul and the subject of the intellect in virtue of which it is true is inside the soul. This was said by Aristotle regarding this intellect, as will be seen later.[66]

This intellect's subject, which is its mover in some way, is what Ibn Bâjjah held to be the recipient, because he found it sometimes to be intellect in potency and sometimes to be intellect in act—that is, the disposition of a recipient subject—and he thought the converse [as well].[67] {401} That proportionality is found to be more exact between the subject of vision which moves [vision] and the subject of the intellect which moves [intellect]. For just as the subject of vision moving [vision], which is color, moves it only when color is made to exist in act through the presence of light after it was in potency, so too the imagined intentions move the material intellect only when the intelligibles are made to exist in act after they were in potency. For this reason Aristotle had to posit the agent intellect, as will be seen later.[68] It is this which draws out these intentions from potency into act. Therefore, just as color which is in potency is not the first actuality of the color which is the apprehended intention but rather the subject actualized through that color is vision, so too the subject

65. Crawford lists no variants for *fit* ("comes to be"). The sense of the argument which follows indicates the likelihood that this was originally *sit* ("is"). For my translation I read this as *sit*.

66. See {409–412}. On this topic see the insightful remarks of Michael Blaustein (1984), 63ff. Also see Blaustein (1986). The notion of the intelligibles being true in virtue of a subject external to the soul is discussed in the *Short Commentary on the De Anima* (1985), 116–117 and (1987), 203–204; and the notion of the subject by which the intelligibles exist as such is mentioned at (1985), 125 and (1987), 210. Ibn Bâjjah is inspiration for this. See Ibn Bâjjah, *Treatise on the Conjoining of the Intellect with Man* (1942), 15–16; Spanish, 33–35; (1968), 163–164; (1981), 188.

67. The text is problematic here and far from clear. See Janssens (1998), 724.

68. 430a10ff. Book 3, Text and Comment 17 {436ff}.

actualized through the thing understood is not the imagined intentions which are intelligibles in potency, but rather the material intellect, which is actualized through the intelligibles. And so it is + that the relation of [the material intellect] to [the intelligibles] + is as the relation of the intention of color to the power of vision.[69]

Since all those things are as we recounted, it happens that those intelligibles which are in act, namely, the theoretical [intelligibles], are generable and corruptible only in virtue of the subject in virtue of which they are true, not in virtue of the subject in virtue of which they are one of the beings, namely, the material intellect.[70]

The second question, how the material intellect is one in number in all individual human beings, neither generable nor corruptible, and the intelligibles [are] existing in it in act (this is the theoretical intellect), [yet it is also] enumerated in virtue of the numbering of individual human beings, generable {402} and corruptible through generation and corruption of individuals, this question is very difficult and has the greatest ambiguity.

For if we hold that this material intellect is enumerated through the numbering of individual human beings, it will happen that it is a determinate particular or a body or a power in a body. When it is a determinate particular, it will be an intention intelligible in potency. But an intention intelligible in potency is the subject moving the recipient intellect, not the subject moved. Therefore, if the recipient subject is held to be a determinate particular, it will happen that the thing receives itself, as we said,[71] which is impossible.

Also, if we concede that it receives itself, it would happen that it would receive itself insofar as it is different. Thus, the power of the intellect will be the same as the power of sense, or there will be no difference between the being of a form outside the soul and [the being of one] in the soul.[72] For this indi-

69. Crawford marks this passage as corrupt. What one would expect here is rather that the relation of the material intellect to the intelligibles is as the relation of the power of vision to the intention of color.

70. That is, here intelligibles exist as intelligibles in act only in the material intellect. If it were not for intellect, the intentions would remain at the level of intelligibles in potency, that is, at the level of imagination or at the level of forms in things, both of which are corruptible particulars.

71. {385}, {398}.

72. That is, intellect's power for receiving forms will be just as sense's power for receiving forms—namely, that an intention different in being is received in the sense as the actuality of the sense from the sensed object. If such were not the case and the being of the form in the sensed object were the same as the being in the soul, then they would not differ in being at all. Clearly this latter cannot be so. But neither can it be the case that intellect receives the forms just as sense does, since sense receives them in

vidual matter receives the forms only as these [determinate particular forms] and individual [forms]. This is one of the things which attest that Aristotle holds this intellect not to be an individual intention.[73]

If we hold that it is not enumerated through the numbering of individuals, it will happen that its relation to all the individuals existing in their final actuality in generation is the same. Hence, if any of those individuals acquired some intelligible, then that intelligible must be acquired by all of them. Consider whether the conjoining of those individuals is owing to the conjoining of the material intellect with them. Now, the conjoining of a human being with a sensible intention is owing to the conjoining of the first actuality {403} of sense with one who is receptive of the sensible intention. But the conjoining of the material intellect with all human beings existing in act in their final actuality at some time ought to be the same conjoining; for there is nothing to cause difference in the relation of conjoining between these two conjoinings. If this is so, I say, then when you have acquired some intelligible, it is necessary that I also would acquire that intelligible, which is impossible.

It makes no difference whether you hold that the final actuality generated in any individual is made the subject for that intellect, namely, [the actuality] in virtue of which the material intellect is united [to individuals] and [hold that] it is from this [actuality] as a form separable from its subject with which it is conjoined, if there is such a thing, or whether you hold that this actuality is one of the powers of the soul or [one] of the powers of the body, [still] the same impossible consequences result.

For this reason one should hold the opinion that if there are some living things whose first actuality is a substance separate from its subjects, as is thought concerning the celestial bodies,[74] it is impossible that there be found

---

their determinate particularity and individuality while intellect receives forms as intelligibles in act, which allows for the aspect of universality which makes science possible.

73. That is, the material intellect cannot be a determinate particular as an individual being because it would then have to receive things as particular individuals receive them—that is, in accord with its own individuality and not in accord with the universality which knowledge requires. In that case, they would become intelligibles in potency, not in act. This understanding is central to Averroes' teaching that there cannot be a plurality of material intellects—that is, that it is not possible for each human being to have his or her own material or possible intellect as Avicenna held.

74. "And generally, since it is clear that the activity of this body is eternal, it is also clear concerning the nature of its form that it does not subsist in a subject, and that its subject is simple, not composed of matter and form, for if the latter were the case, the celestial body would be generated and corruptible." *De Substantia Orbis* (1986), 72. As Geoffroy makes clear, analogy with the celestial bodies and souls is central to Averroes'

more than one individual from one species of these. For, if among these, namely, from the same species, we find more than one individual, for instance, with regard to a body moved by the same mover, then the being of these [others] would be useless and superfluous, since the motion of these [bodies] would be owing to an intention which is the same in number.[75] For example, for there to be more than one ship in number for one sailor at the same time is useless; and similarly for there to be more than one tool in number of the [very] same kind of tools for one artisan is useless.[76]

This is the intention of what was said in the first book of *On the Heavens and the World*,[77] namely, that if there were another world, there would be another celestial body. If there were another celestial body, then it would have a mover different {404} in number from the mover of this celestial body. And if this were so, then the mover of the celestial body would be material and numbered in virtue of the numbering of the celestial bodies, namely, because it is impossible that a mover singular in number belong to two bodies different in number. For this reason the artisan does not use more than one instrument since only a unique activity results from it. Generally it is thought that the impossible things which result for this position result for our position because the intellect which is in a positive disposition is one in number.[78] Ibn Bâjjah already listed most of these in his short work, which he called *The Conjoining of the Intellect with Human Beings*.[79] Since this is so, how then is there a way to solve this difficult question?

Let us say, then, that it is evident that a human being is intelligent in act only

---

mature doctrine of the material intellect. See Geoffroy and Steel (2001), 48–51, 68–69; 261. Also see the introduction, pp. xlivff.

75. The argument here is that a plurality of celestial souls of the same species causing the one movement of a single celestial body would be superfluous since only one soul is required. For Averroes the distinct celestial movements are indicative of distinct intentions in distinct celestial souls which receive those intentions from contemplation of distinct separate intellects. Regarding the celestial bodies, souls, and intellects, see Endress (1995) and Twetten (1995).

See n. 78 below.

76. That is, it is useless for the artisan to have multiple copies of the same tool at hand since he can use only one when in the very actuality of exercising his skills.

77. *De Caelo* 1.8–9. He probably has specifically in mind the discussion at 1.8, 277b8–13, though the argument here goes well beyond that text. See his comments on this text in his *Long Commentary on the De Caelo* (2003), 164–165 where he discusses conceptualization on the part of the movers of the heavens.

78. That is, if the same applies analogically to Averroes' doctrine of the intellect, then the intellect in a positive disposition would be one, not many.

79. Ibn Bâjjah, *Treatise on the Conjoining of the Intellect with Man* (1942), 14–16; Spanish, 31–35; (1968), 161–164; (1981), 186–189.

owing to the conjoining of the intelligible with him in act. It is also evident that matter and form are united to one another in such a way that the composite of these is a singular thing, and [this is likewise so] to the greatest extent [in the case of] the material intellect and the intention which is intelligible in act. For what is composed from these is not some third thing different from these as it is for other things composed of matter and form. Therefore, it is impossible for there to be a conjoining of the intelligible with human beings except through the conjoining of each of those two parts with [human beings], namely, of the part which is related to one as matter and of the part which is related to another as form.[80]

Since it was explained among the doubts mentioned earlier that it is impossible for the intelligible to be united with each human being and be numbered in virtue of the numbering of these by way of the part which belongs to it as matter, namely, the material intellect, {405} then it remains that the conjoining of intelligibles with us human beings is through the conjoining of the intelligible intention with us (these are the imagined intentions), namely, of the part which is related to it in us in some way as form. For this reason the statement that a boy is intelligent in potency can be understood in two ways, one because the imagined forms which are in him are intelligible in potency, the second because the material intellect which is naturally constituted to receive the intelligible of that imagined form is receptive in potency and conjoined with us in potency.[81]

It has therefore been explained that the first actuality of the intellect differs from the first actualities of the other powers of the soul and that this word "actuality" is said of these in an equivocal way, contrary to what Alexander thought.[82] For this reason Aristotle said in regard to the definition of the soul that it is the first actuality of a natural organized body, because it was not yet evident whether the body is actualized through all the powers in the same way or [whether] there is some [power] among these in virtue of which the body is not actualized, and if [that other power] is actualized, it will be in another way.

However, the disposition for intelligibles which is in the imaginative power is similar to the dispositions which are in the other powers of the soul, namely, [similar] to the first actualities of the other powers, inasmuch as each of these

80. That is, the material intellect and the agent intellect. Note that I remove Crawford's insertion of *scilicet intellecto*.

81. That is, the boy is intelligent in potency in virtue of (a) the imagined intentions in him which are intelligible in potency, and (b) the material intellect that is in potency with respect to those imagined intentions which are able to become intelligible in act when they come to exist in the material intellect.

82. Cf. {396–397}.

two [sorts of] dispositions is generated through the generation of an individual, corrupted through its corruption, and generally numbered through its numbering. They differ in this: one is a disposition in a mover insofar as it is a mover, namely, the disposition which is in the intentions {406} imagined;[83] the other is a disposition in the recipient and is a disposition which is in the first actualities of the other parts of the soul.[84]

Owing to this similarity between these two dispositions, Ibn Bâjjah thought that there is no disposition for the thing coming to be understood except the disposition existing in the imagined intentions. But these two dispositions differ as [much as] the earth from the heavens. For one is the disposition in the mover insofar as it is a mover and the other is a disposition in the moved insofar as it is moved and receptive.

For this reason one should hold the opinion, which already was apparent to us from the account of Aristotle, that in the soul there are two parts belonging to the intellect, one is the recipient whose being is explained here, the other is the agent which is what makes the intentions which are in the imaginative power to be movers of the material intellect in act after they were movers in potency, as will be apparent later from the account of Aristotle.[85] [Also from Aristotle it is apparent] that these two parts are neither generable nor corruptible and that the agent is related to the recipient as form to matter, as will be explained afterwards.[86]

For this reason Themistius held the opinion that we are the agent intellect and that the theoretical intellect is nothing else but just the conjoining of the agent intellect with the material intellect.[87] It is not as he thought. Rather, one

83. "The imaginative form is the first mover in man." Ibn Bâjjah, *Treatise on the Conjoining of the Intellect with Man* (1942), 12; Spanish, 29; (1968), 159; (1981), 185.

84. The intentions imagined there constitute an active predisposition insofar as they are intelligible in potency, while in other parts of the soul there are first actualities which are predispositions for receptivity.

85. {438–439}.

86. {409ff}.

87. Themistius, *De Anima Paraphrase* 100.16–21; (1973), 182.1–7; (1996), 124–125. "We, then, are either the potential intellect or the actual [intellect]. So if, in the case of everything that is combined from what is potential and actual, something (*to tode*) and what it is to be something (*to tôide einai*) are distinct, then the I (*to egô*) and what it is to be me (*to emoi einai*) will also be distinct, and while I am the intellect combined from the potential and the actual [intellects], what it is to be me comes from the actual [intellect]. Thus while the intellect combined from the potential and the actual [intellects] is writing what I am [now] discursively thinking about and composing, it is writing not *qua* potential but *qua* actual [intellect], for the activity from the [potential intellect] is channelled to it." Todd also translated this text in ibid. (1990), 93–94. Note that Todd changed

should hold the opinion that there are three parts of the intellect in the soul, one is the receptive intellect, the second is that which makes [things], and the third is the product [of these]. Two of these three are eternal, namely, the agent and the recipient; the third is generable and corruptible in one way, eternal in another way.[88]

On the basis of this account we have held the opinion that the material intellect is one for all human beings and also {407} on the basis of this we have held the opinion that the human species is eternal, as was explained in other places.[89] The material intellect must not be devoid of the natural principles common to the whole human species, namely, the primary propositions and singular conceptions common to all [human beings]. For these intelligibles are unique according to the recipient and many according to the intention received.[90]

---

his mind regarding the referent of αὐτῷ in τὸ γὰρ ἐνεργεῖ ἐκεῖθεν αὐτῷ ἐποχετεύεται. In the 1990 translation Todd understood the referent to be the actual intellect, while in the 1996 translation he understood the referent to be the potential intellect. This revision seems to be correct since Themistius is speaking of the activity of the composite human being, which, while traced to the actual intellect, is existing in the composite only via the actual intellect's actualization in the potential intellect.

88. The agent intellect and the material intellect are eternal. The theoretical intellect is eternal insofar as the theoretical intelligibles are in the material intellect and generable and corruptible insofar as the theoretical intelligibles are in human individual knowers for Averroes.

89. Averroes may be referring to *Epistle 1 On Conjunction*, where he speaks of the possibility of the material intellect being "a substance one in number for all human beings in itself, but many by accident, which is not the case for material forms." Geoffroy and Steel (2001), 210. Also see *Long Commentary on the Metaphysics* (1952), 1487–1490; (1962), 302I–303D; (1984), 103–105. In his *Commentary on the De Intellectu of Alexander*, Averroes sets forth his doctrine that العقل الهيولاني هو قوة واحدة مشتركة للنفوس الشخصية ("the material intellect is one power shared by individual souls") and that the theoretical intelligibles are في ذاته غير كائنة ولا فاسدة ("in its essence ungenerable and incorruptible"). *Commentary on the De Intellectu of Alexander* (2001), 29. On Averroes' position in this work also see Davidson (1992), 293–295. Davidson suggests as relevant *Incoherence of the Incoherence* (1930), 180; (1969), 108.

90. For Averroes here the intelligibles are described as the same but received individually into differing individuals. The common conceptions and first principles of understanding here seem to be the first principles of demonstration—that is, such as that a thing cannot both be and not be at the same time in the same respect—attained via sense perception. Averroes' understanding of these seems to follow the accounts of al-Fârâbî and Avicenna, who hold that these are communicated to all human beings by the separate agent intellect. This terminology and this understanding of primary or first intelligibles are dependent on the thought of al-Fârâbî. In *The Perfect State*, al-Fârâbî speaks of first intelligibles and the voluntary intelligibles which can be brought about

Therefore, according to the way by which they are unique, they are necessarily eternal, since being does not desert the subject received, namely, the mover which is the intention of the imagined forms,[91] and for this there is no impediment on the part of the recipient. Therefore, generation and corruption belong to these only owing to the multiplicity accruing to them, not owing to the way by which they are unique. For this reason, since in relation to some individual, one of the first intelligibles is corrupted through the corruption of its subject insofar as it is united with us and true, it is necessary that this intelligible not be without qualification corruptible but [rather be] corruptible in relation to any given individual. In this way we can say that the theoretical intellect is one in all [human beings].

Since consideration is given to those intelligibles insofar as they are simply beings, not with reference to some individual, and insofar as they are not sometimes understood and sometimes not, but rather always [understood], they are truly said to be eternal. It is as if that being is intermediate for them between being which perishes and being which persists.[92] For according to the multiplicity and diminution accruing to them from final actuality [in indi-

---

later. "The presence of the first intelligibles in man is his first perfection, but these intelligibles are supplied to him only in order to be used by him to reach his ultimate perfection, i.e. felicity." Al-Fârâbî, *Principles of the Opinions of the People of the Virtuous City* (1985), 204–205. See Druart (1997a). The same sort of description of the primary propositions is given by Avicenna at Ibn Sînâ, *Kitâb al-Nafs* (1959), 49; (1972), 96–97. Also see Averroes' *Short Commentary on the De Anima* (1950), 79.15–16; (1985), 115.13–14; (1987), 202, where he writes of المعقولات التي لا ندري متى حصلت ، ولا كيف حصلت, "the intelligibles which are such that we do not know when they arose nor how they arose." Later, at {496–497}, Averroes distinguishes between these first principles of the understanding, which he calls natural intelligibles, and voluntary intelligibles. Also see {506}.

91. The words *cum esse non fugiat a subiecto recepto, scilicet motore, qui est intentio formarum ymaginatarum* ("since being does not desert the subject received, namely, the mover which is the intention of the imagined forms") are far from clear. What it is precisely to which "the subject received" corresponds is problematic. Averroes has already established the necessity of the material intellect's eternal existence and set forth his view that the human species is eternal. His point may be that the subject into which the intentions are received as intelligible in act always exists as knower and so the mover, "the intention of the imagined forms," must always exist. He draws the consequences of this in the following paragraphs, where he asserts that human beings will always exist to provide intentions for the material intellect.

92. Cf. Averroes' *Commentary on the De Intellectu of Alexander* (2001), 29–30, where he writes that وجودها كأنه وجود متوسط بين الوجود الشخصى والوجود الذى هو صورة مفارقة باطلاق; "their existence is as an existence intermediate between individual existence and the existence which is a separate form absolutely."

vidual human beings] they are generable and corruptible, while insofar as they are unique in number [in the material intellect] they are eternal.

This will be the case if it is not asserted that the disposition in regard to the final actuality in human beings is just as the disposition in regard to {408} the intelligibles common to all [human beings], namely, that worldly being is not devoid of such individual being.[93] For that this is impossible is not evident. Rather, one saying this can have a reason sufficient and able to quiet the soul. For since it is the case that wisdom exists in some way proper to human beings, just as it is the case that [various] kinds of arts exist in ways proper to human beings, it is thought that it is impossible that the whole habitable world shun philosophy, just as one should hold the opinion that it is impossible for [the whole habitable world] to shun the natural arts. For if some part of [the habitable world], for example, the northern quarter of the earth, were to be devoid of them, namely, the arts, the other quarters will not be devoid of them, because it was explained that habitation[94] is possible in the southern as in the northern quarters. Perhaps, then, philosophy is found in the greater part of the subject[95] in every era, as a human being is found [to come about] from a human being and a horse from a horse.[96] The theoretical intellect, therefore, is neither generable nor corruptible in this way. And generally it is for the agent intellect creating the intelligibles just as [it is] for the discerning recipient intellect. For insofar as the agent intellect never rests from generating and creating without

93. Intelligibles are able to be present in members of the human species, though they exist independent of any perishable individual and are unchanging. As is evident in what follows, Averroes is here asserting that there will always exist at every time one or more individual human beings supplying intentions which are intelligibles in potency for the material intellect. The same teaching is found in *Epistle 1 On Conjunction*, where he asserts that it is not necessary that each and every human being have intellectual knowledge but only that it be manifested in the species. See Geoffroy and Steel (2001), 218.

94. That is, human habitation and the consequent presence of the natural arts can be found in the southern part as well as in the northern.

95. As de Libera notes in his preface to *Long Commentary* Fragments (2005), at 11, n. 2, it is evident that the Latin translator read the Arabic موضع as *maudu'* (subject, *subiecti*) instead of *maudi'* (place). Hence, the sense in the Arabic is that philosophy is found in most places. In this de Libera is following the remarks of Janssens (1998), 721.

96. That is, philosophy exists in every age as a human activity. Even if it seems to be hardly evident in some societies and eras, still it is an endeavor which is generated and passed on inevitably by individual human beings, just as humans generate humans and horses horses. This is because of the eternal nature of intellectual activity in the material intellect.

qualification, even if some subject is removed from this, namely, from generation, so it is concerning the discerning intellect.[97]

Aristotle indicates this in the beginning of this book when he says: **And
conceptualizing**[98] **and contemplating are diverse, such that something else
undergoes corruption internally, but it in itself does not suffer corruption.**[99]
He means by **something else** human imagined forms. He means by **conceptualizing** {409} the reception which is always [existent] in the material intellect.
Concerning this he intended to raise doubts in this passage and in that other,
when he said: **We do not remember because that is not passive; the passive
intellect, however, is corruptible and without this it understands nothing.**[100]
He means by **the passive intellect** the imaginative power, as he will later explain.[101] And generally that notion appeared from extrinsic considerations,
namely, that soul—the theoretical intellect—is immortal.

97. That is, strictly speaking, the agent intellect is distinct and continues to carry out
its activity. And similarly, the material intellect is a being in its own right and distinct
from transient individuals: it does not cease to exist when one or another individual
perishes.

98. *Formare per intellectum*: At Book 1, Text 66 {88}, the corresponding term is instead
intelligere. The corresponding Greek there is καὶ τὸ νοεῖν δὴ καὶ τὸ θεωρεῖν (408b24).

99. **To understand and to contemplate are distinguished when something else
inside undergoes corruption, but it is in itself {89} affected by nothing.** Book 1, Text
66 {88–89} (408b24–25). Note that "it," *ipsum*, is neuter nominative and must refer to the
activity of intellect. Crawford lists no variants for this difficult reading. See Book 1,
n. 252, regarding the mistranslation of this text.

100. Note the difference between the Latin here and the Latin at Book 3, Text 20.
Here we have: *Et non sumus memores, quia iste est non passivus; intellectus autem
passivus est corruptibilis, et absque hoc nichil intelligit.* Later we read: *Et non re-
memoramur, quia iste est non passibilis, et intellectus passibilis est corruptibilis,
et sine hoc nichil intelligitur.* "We do not remember, because that is not passible, while
the passible intellect is corruptible, and without this nothing is understood." Book 3,
Text 20 {443} (430a24–25). This difference is likely due to the understanding of the
translator, which is more subtle in the later text.

101. Aristotle's remarks at Book 3, Text 20 (430a24–25), that "the passible intellect is
corruptible and without this nothing is understood" {443} are interpreted by Averroes
as referring to "the forms of the imagination insofar as the cogitative power proper to
human beings acts upon them." {449} This power is "a kind of reason," *aliqua ratio* {449},
thanks only to its connection to the material intellect. But it is a kind of reason which
is bound up with the body for Averroes, a "particular material power," *virtus particularis
materialis* {476}. Thomas Aquinas follows Averroes in calling this "cogitative power"
(*vis cogitativa*) "the passive intellect" (*intellectus passivus*) and "particular reason" (*ratio
particularis*) and describes this bodily power as "what gathers particular intentions"

Hence, Plato said that the universals are neither generable nor corruptible and that they exist outside the mind. The account is true in this way [which was just explained] and false with respect to the intent of his words. This latter is the sense which Aristotle worked to refute in the *Metaphysics*.[102] Generally that intention in reference to the soul is the part which is true in the probable propositions which attribute to soul both kinds of being, namely, mortal and non-mortal. For it is impossible for probable things to be completely false.[103] The ancients recounted this and all the religious laws alike reflect it.

The third question (how the material intellect is a being and [yet] is not one of the material forms nor even prime matter) is resolved in this way. One should hold that it is a fourth kind of being. For just as sensible being is divided into form and matter, so too intelligible being must be divided into things similar to these two, namely, into something similar to form and into something similar to matter. This is [something] necessarily present in every separate intelligence which understands something else.[104] And if not, then there would be no multiplicity {410} in separate forms.[105] It was already explained in First Philosophy that there is no form free of potency without qualification except the First Form, which understands nothing outside itself.[106] Its being is its quiddity. Other

---

(*quae est collativa intentionum particularium*). Thomas Aquinas, *Quaestiones disputatae de anima* (1996), q. 13 resp., 118.266–267.

102. *Metaphysics* 1.9, 990a32ff.

103. Cf. *Epistle 1 On Conjunction* in Geoffroy and Steel (2001), 214, 270. In his n. 63, Geoffroy cites Aristotle, *Metaphysics* 8, 1047b3–5, and Averroes' Commentary on that passage indicating the meaning that what is possible must necessarily be realized at some time. His reference is to *Long Commentary on the Metaphysics* (1952), 1139–1140.

104. That is, this division of what is analogous to form and what is analogous to matter, or of act and potency, must be present in any separate intellect which is capable of knowing anything outside itself. For insofar as it is an intelligence with itself as its object, it need have no potency. But insofar as it is in potency for knowing something other than its own essence or nature, it must have a certain materiality or potency for receiving form which contains essentially a reference to something outside the nature of that particular intelligence, namely, God. The exception among the separate substances or intelligences is God, who, in thinking the highest being, thinks nothing outside himself.

105. That is, there will not be a plurality of separate forms or intellects.

106. The "separate forms" to which he refers here are the separate intelligences. The "First Form" is God for Averroes. Averroes holds that the separate substances or intelligences are distinguished from one another in virtue of their potency for knowledge, a certain equivocal "materiality" found in each which is sufficient to allow their distinction from one another and to make reasonable the assertion that there is a multiplicity of separate substances. This doctrine is also found in the *Incoherence of the Incoherence*. "The difference between the First's understanding of Itself and the understanding of

forms, however, are in some way different in quiddity and being.[107] If it were not for this genus of beings which we have come to know in the science of the soul, we could not understand multiplicity in separate things, to the extent that unless we know here the nature of the intellect, we could not know that the separate moving powers ought to be intellects.[108]

This was unknown to many modern [thinkers] to the extent that they denied what Aristotle says, in the Eleventh Book of First Philosophy, that the separate forms moving the bodies must be in accord with the number of celestial bodies.[109] To this extent knowledge of the soul is necessary for knowledge of First Philosophy. That receptive intellect must understand the intellect which is in act. For while it understands material forms, it is even more befitting that it

---

themselves which the rest of the intellects have is that the First Intellect understands Itself as existing through Itself, not as what is related to a cause, while the rest of the intellects understand themselves as being related to their cause so that plurality enters into these in this way. For it is not necessary that they all be in one grade of simplicity since they are not in a single grade in regard to the First Principle and none of them exists simply in the sense in which the First is simple, because the First is considered to exist by Itself, while they are in related existence." *Incoherence of the Incoherence* (1930), 204; (1969), 122. My translation. Cf. *Long Commentary on the Metaphysics* (1952), 1696–1697; (1962), c. 51, 335H; (1984), 192–193, where Averroes follows Aristotle in stressing that what requires something other than itself is less than the most excellent of all entities. In his *Short Commentary on the De Anima* in the context of his summary of the views of Ibn Bâjjah he writes that "The First Intellect is the most simple of all the intellects and neither is It caused at all nor does It conceptualize (ولايتصور) anything external to Its own essence." *Short Commentary on the De Anima* (1950), 93; (1985), omitted; (1987), 218–219, My translation.

107. *Essentia eius est quiditas eius; alie autem forme diversantur in quiditate et essentia quoquo modo.* With the First Form (الصورة الاولى) as its probable antecedent, this is in all likelihood ووجودها فهو ماهيتها. Cf. {422}, where Averroes is concerned to assert the simplicity of *all* immaterial substances and there states that "in simple beings the quiddity and being are the same." As indicated in n. 128 below, in the corresponding passage of the *Middle Commentary* (2002), 113.17, Averroes asserts that إنّ الأشياء البسيطة الوجود والماهية فيها هو شيء واحد بعينه; "the existence and essence of simple things are one and the same."

108. In this, then, lies the reason why the study of the soul is more worthy and more noble than other studies and why it should precede others: we understand the nature of intellect first through understanding the nature of intellect in ourselves, and only when something of that understanding has been achieved can there be any understanding of intellect in higher beings. See Book 1, Text 1 (402a1–4) {3}, with n. 11 there also, and the introduction, pp. liff.

109. *Metaphysics* 12. 8, 1073a26–38. Book 11 in Averroes corresponds to Book 12 because Book 11 of the *Metaphysics* was not available to Averroes.

understand immaterial forms. What it understands of separate forms, for example, of the agent intelligence, does not impede it from understanding material forms.

The proposition saying that the recipient ought to have in act nothing of what it receives is not said without qualification but conditionally. [This is] because it is not necessary that the recipient be nothing at all in act but rather that it not be in act something of what it receives, as we said earlier.[110] Rather, you ought to know that the relation of the agent intellect to that intellect is [the same as] the relation of light to the transparent [medium], and the relation of the material forms {411} to [the material intellect] is [the same as] the relation of color to the transparent [medium]. For just as light is the actuality of the transparent [medium], so the agent intellect is the actuality of the material [intellect]. Just as the transparent [medium] is not moved by color and does not receive it except when there is light, so too that intellect does not receive the intelligibles which are here except insofar as it is actualized through that [agent] intellect and illuminated by it. Just as light makes color in potency to be in act in such a way that it can move the transparent [medium], so the agent intellect makes the intentions in potency to be intelligible in act in such a way that the material intellect receives them. This, then, is how the material intellect and the agent [intellect] should be understood.

When the material intellect is united with us[111] insofar as it is actualized through the agent intellect, we then are united with the agent intellect. This disposition is called acquisition and the acquired intellect,[112] as we will see later.[113] That way in which we posited the being of the material intellect solves all the questions resulting from our holding that the intellect is one and many. For if the thing understood in me and in you were one in every way, it would happen that when I would know some intelligible, you would also know it, and many other impossible things [would also follow]. If we assert it to be many, then it would happen that the thing understood in me and in you would be one in species and two in individual [number]. In this way the thing understood will have a thing understood and so it proceeds into infinity.[114] Thus, it

110. {385–386}.

111. I read *copulatus nobiscum* with manuscripts A and C, following Janssens (1998), 724.

112. *Adeptio et intellectus adeptus.*

113. See {445}, but especially the extended discussion of the thought of Alexander of Aphrodisias on this at {482–485}.

114. That is, if there is a unity in species but the object in the intellect is different in each individual, then an infinite regress would arise insofar as the object understood in any one mind would have a higher unity which yet again when understood would be grasped differently by different individuals, and so forth. It is better, then, to say

will be impossible for a student to learn from a teacher unless the knowledge which is in the teacher is a power generating and creating the knowledge which is in the student, in the way in which one fire generates another {412} fire similar to it in species, which is impossible. That what is known is the same in the teacher and the student in this way caused Plato to believe that learning is recollection. Since, then, we asserted that the intelligible thing which is in me and in you is many in subject insofar as it is true, namely, the forms of the imagination, and one in the subject in virtue of which it is an existing intellect (namely, the material [intellect]), those questions are completely resolved.

The way Ibn Bâjjah thought to solve the questions arising from the fact that the intellect is one or many, namely, the way which he gave in his treatise entitled *The Conjoining of the Intellect with Human Beings,* is not a way fit for resolving that question. For the intellect which he demonstrated in that treatise to be one, when he worked to resolve that question, is different from the intellect which he demonstrates there also to be many, since the intellect which he demonstrated to be one is the agent intellect inasmuch as it is necessarily a form of the theoretical intellect. But the intellect which he demonstrated to be many is the theoretical intellect itself. This name, however, namely, "intellect," is said equivocally of the theoretical and the agent [intellects].[115]

For this reason, if that which is understood concerning this word "intellect" in two opposed accounts—namely, concluding that the intellect is many and concluding that the intellect is one—is an intention which is not equivocal, then what he gave later in regard to this—that the agent intellect is one and the theoretical is many—does not resolve this question. If {413} what is understood in these two opposite accounts concerning this word intellect is an equivocal intention, then the problem will be sophistical, not subject to argument. For this reason we should believe that the questions which that man raised in that treatise are resolved only in this way, if those problems are not sophistical but subject to argument. In this way the question regarding what he was uncertain about concerning the material intellect—whether it is external or united—is resolved. Since this has been explained, let us return to the exposition of Aristotle's account.

6. For this reason it must not be mixed with the body. For if it were mixed with the body, then it would be in some disposition, either hot or cold, or it

---

that each individual mind grasps the same intelligible thing. This argument is from Themistius, *De Anima Paraphrase* (1899), 104.2–14; (1973), 189.2–15; (1996), 129. But another source is Ibn Bâjjah, *Treatise on the Conjoining of the Intellect with Man* (1942), section 8; 14–15; Spanish, 32–33; (1968), 162–163; (1981), 187.

115. Ibn Bâjjah, *Treatise on the Conjoining of the Intellect with Man* (1942), 13–14; Spanish, 30–32; (1968), 162; (1981), 187.

would have some instrument[116] as does sense. Yet[117] it is not so. Those, therefore, saying the soul is the place of forms did speak rightly. But [it is] not the whole [soul] but rather the part which understands, and the forms [are] not in actuality, but rather in potency. (429a24–29)

This is another demonstration that the material intellect is not a determinate particular nor a body nor a power in a body. He said: **For this reason it was necessary**, etc. That is, because its nature is what we have recounted, it was right and necessary that it not be mixed with the body, that is, that there is no power in it in virtue of which it is mixed with the body, as was explained.[118] Next he gave {414} a second reason for this. He said: For **if it were** mixed, etc. That is, for if it were a power in a body, then it would be a disposition and a bodily quality. And if it were to have quality, then that quality either would be ascribed to what is hot or what is cold (namely, to the compound in what is a compound), or it would be a quality existing in a compound only added to the compound, as it is for the sensitive soul and for things similar to it, and thus it would have a bodily instrument.[119] Next he said: But **it is not so**. That is, but [the material intellect] does not have the quality ascribed to what is hot and what is cold nor does it have an instrument. Therefore it is not mixed with the body. You ought to consider in regard to the consequence and the refutation whether they require demonstration or not. Let us say then: but that the consequent of what follows upon the antecedent is true is evident from what was mentioned earlier. For it was explained that every power in a composite body either is ascribed to primary qualities, namely, to the form of the compound, or it will be a power existing in the compounding form, and thus it will necessarily be an organic soul. But the refutation is evident also from what was mentioned earlier, for it was explained that there is no instrument different from the instruments of the five senses (where it was explained that there is no sixth sense).[120] Generally, if intellect were a living power in a body, then either it would be a sixth sense or something consequent upon a sixth sense, namely, something whose relation to a sixth sense is as the relation of imagina-

116. *Instrumentum*: ὄργανόν, "organ."

117. Janssens (1998), 724, notes that *modo* corresponds to the Greek νῦν, "now."

118. See {387–388}.

119. That is, if it is a bodily quality, then this predisposition which arises from the compound of bodily parts would be either a quality such as hot or cold, which are accidental qualities attributed to a subject, or a quality which arises from the compound as something additional to the blend. For example, the sensible soul is something over and above the compound of bodily parts. If the material intellect were either of these alternatives, it would be a bodily instrument.

120. See {325ff}.

tion to the common sense.[121] That the material intellect is not a power ascribed to the compound is evident {415} from what was mentioned earlier, for since the sensitive soul is not a power ascribed to the compound, how much more is this so for the intellect!

If [the material intellectual power] were ascribed to the compound, then, as Aristotle says, the being of the form of the stone in the soul would be the same as its being outside the soul,[122] and so the stone would be something which apprehends, and many other impossible things would follow for this position. Some people were uncertain about what was said (namely, that the intellect does not have an instrument) because it was said that the imaginative power is in the anterior of the brain, the cogitative power in the middle, and the power of memory in the posterior. This was not only said by physicians but is said in *Sense and Sensibilia*.[123] But Galen and other physicians[124] reasoned regarding this that those powers are in those places by virtue of an argument of concomitance, which is an argument which causes one to hold an opinion, not a true argument.

But it was already explained in *Sense and Sensibilia* that such is the order of those powers in the brain through a demonstration giving the being and the cause.[125] But that does not contradict what was said here. For the cogitative power according to Aristotle is an individual discerning power, namely, because it discerns something only in an individual way, not in a universal way. For it was explained there that the cogitative power is only a power which discerns the intention of a sensible thing from its imagined image. That power is one which is such that its relation to those two intentions, namely, to the image of the thing and to the intention of its image, is just as the relation of the common sense to the intentions of the five senses.[126] The cogitative power, therefore, is of the genus of powers existing in bodies. Aristotle explicitly said

121. The common sense and the imagination use the same instrument but are different actualities or powers. Cf. *Sense and Sensibilia* 7, 449a14–19.

122. That is, the activity of thought (composing receptive potency with received form) attributed to the material intellect would also have to be attributed to things.

123. Cf. *Short Commentary on the Parva Naturalia* (1949), 57–59; (1961), 26–27; (1972), 42–43. The reference may be to the discussion at *De Memoria* 1, 449b29ff.

124. Reference not found.

125. That is, there have been demonstrations of the fact and of the reason for the fact.

126. The common sense unites what is received from the five senses and also has its own operation related to the common sensibles. Cf. *Sense and Sensibilia* 7, 449a14–19. Similarly, the cogitative power unites the reports of imagination in the image and performs its own operation of discernment, by which it grasps the denuded individual intention and places it in memory.

this in that book, when he placed the individual discerning powers in four orders. In the first he placed {416} the common sense, next the imaginative power, next the cogitative power, and after that the power of memory. He set forth the power of memory as the more spiritual, then the cogitative, then the imaginative, and after that the sensible. Although, therefore, a human being properly has a cogitative power, nevertheless this does not make it that this power is rational and discerning, for [the rational power] discerns universal intentions, not individual ones. This was explicitly said by Aristotle in that book.[127] If, therefore, the discerning rational power were a power in a body, it would happen that it would be one of those four powers, and so it would have a bodily organ. Or it would be an individual discerning power different from those four. But it was already explained there that this is impossible. Because Galen thought that this cogitative power is rational and material, the argument of concomitance made him err in regard to this. For because the rational power belongs to human beings and the cogitative belongs to them, it was thought on account of the conversion of the universal affirmative that the cogitative power is the rational power.[128] One of those who erred in regard to this is Abu al-Faraj in his *Commentary on [Aristotle's] Sense and Sensibilia*.[129] Next he said: **Those, therefore, saying the soul is the place of forms did speak rightly.** That is, since it was explained that it is not mixed with some body, then those describing the soul as the place of forms spoke correctly, although in making known its substance they did not accept more than that similarity and congruity which there is between it and a place. Next he said: **But [it is] not the whole [soul] but rather the part which understands.** {417} That is, but that similarity ought not to be taken in understanding all the parts of the soul, but only in regard to the rational soul, for the other parts of the soul are forms in matter, while the rational part is not. Next he said: And **the forms [are] not in** actuality, **but rather in potency.** That is, but place is different from the soul which discerns and understands insofar as a place is none of these things which exist in it, while the rational material soul is the forms existing in it, not in act,

127. Aristotle is by no means as explicit about this in the *Parva Naturalia* as Averroes indicates here. But Averroes discusses just this in detail in his *Short Commentary on the Parva Naturalia* in the section on Aristotle on dreams. See *Short Commentary on the Parva Naturalia* (1949), 109–113; (1961), 46–48; (1972), 79–82.

128. This is the fallacy of false cause, which involves the second figure syllogism with two affirmative premises, leading to a conclusion which is not necessary or, as Averroes puts it, yields an opinion, not a true argument. It is a version of *post hoc ergo propter hoc*. Cf. {513} and Book 3, n. 301.

129. Abelfarag Babilonensis. Abu al-Faraj Ibn al-Tayyib's *Commentary on Sense and Sensibilia* is not extant. Peters (1968), 46, remarks that it is mentioned by Hajji Khalifah and cited by a disciple of Avicenna. See the introduction, p. xcvi.

but in potency. He did this lest someone understand from this description that the genus taken in this is the true genus, not a rhetorical one. But human beings are forced in regard to such things which are understood only by analogy to make them known through such rhetorical genera.

7. But the fact that the impassibility in sensing and in conceptualizing[130] is not similar is evident in the sense.[131] For the sense cannot sense after a strong sensible object, for instance, after loud sounds, after bright colors, or after strong scents. But when the intellect has understood something highly intelligible, then it will understand what is below that first object not less well but rather better. For what senses is not outside the body, while [the intellect] is separate. (429a29–b5)

After he had explained that the material intellect is not mixed with matter, he began to make it known that this fits the appearances. For this is a neces-sary condition for necessary demonstrations, namely, that things apparent to sense do not differ from what is seen through reason. And he said: **But the fact that the impassibility,** etc. That is, but the fact that the privation of change {418} existing in sense is not similar to the privation of change existing in in-tellect, as had been demonstrated by reason, this is [something] also evident from the appearances. For the privation of change in intellect ought to be pure and the privation of change in sense is not so, since sense is a material power. Next he said: **For the sense cannot sense,** etc. That is, the indication of this is that sense is unable to sense its sensibles coming to it when it has sensed something strong and has immediately retreated from it to a different sensi-ble, for instance, when the sense of hearing has retreated from a loud sound, sight from bright color, or smell from a strong scent. The reason for this is the affection and change which occurs for what senses from the strong sensible object. And the reason for this change is that it is a power in a body. After he had demonstrated what is seen regarding the change in the sense, he began to make it known that the contrary is the case for the intellect. And he said: But when **the intellect has understood something highly,** etc. That is, but when the intellect has understood something highly intelligible, then it will understand more easily something which is not highly intelligible. Hence, it follows that it is not affected nor is it changed by something highly intelligi-ble. After he had demonstrated that these are different in this regard, he gave

130. *Privatio passionis in sentiente et in formatione per intellectum*: ἡ ἀπάθεια τοῦ αἰσθητικοῦ καὶ τοῦ νοητικοῦ, "the impassibility of the sensitive faculty and that of the faculty of thought." Aristotle, *De Anima* (1984).

131. The Greek is more specific in mentioning that this is evident in consideration of what senses (the sense organ) and the sense itself: ἐπὶ τῶν αἰσθητηρίων καὶ τῆς αἰσθήσεως.

the reason. He said: **For what senses is not outside the body, while [the intel-
lect] is separate.** That is, the reason for this is what was explained earlier,
namely, that what senses is not outside the body, while the intellect is separate.
We can set out this account as a third demonstration per se, but {419} one less
powerful. For when we have said that if the intellect is changed essentially,
not accidentally and through the mediation of something else (for this was
conceded in the case of the intellect), it is necessary that the change occur for
it in the course of its proper activity (which is to understand), just as it is in the
case of sense. And if it is not changed per se and essentially, it must not be a
power in a body at all. For every receptive power in some body ought to be
changed insofar as it is receptive.

For this reason one must not object to this argument on the basis of the fact
that some change occurs in the intellect due to the change belonging to the
powers of the imagination, and especially [due to a change occurring in] the
cogitative power. For fatigue is thought to happen to the intellect in this way
but it is so only accidentally. For the cogitative power is of the genus of sensible powers. But the imaginative, cogitative, and memorative powers are only
in place of the sensible power, and for this reason there is no need for them
except in the absence of the sensible [power]. They all cooperate to present an
image of the sensible thing, so that the separate rational power[132] may behold
it and extract the universal intention and after that receive it, that is, apprehend it. And perhaps, as we said, he presented this account to verify the earlier demonstrations.

8. **And when it has in this way been any of these, namely, as knowledge
is said in act (and this will occur when he has been able to understand in
virtue of himself), then he will also be in potency in a certain way, but not
in the same way by which he was previously [in potency], before he had
knowledge or discovered [something]. He is then able to understand in
virtue of himself.[133]** (429b5–9) {420}

132. That is, the material intellect in cooperation with the agent intellect.

133. Although it is almost certainly not what Averroes himself read in his Arabic
manuscript of the *De Anima*, I translate the Latin as edited by Crawford here and in the
quotation of this text on {420}. However, Averroes' Comment shows he understood this
text to concern self-knowledge and that he read an Arabic text with the same meaning
as what we find in the alternate Arabic translation: ويمكنه في ذلك الوقت أن يعقل نفسه
(Aristotle, *De Anima* [1954]); "and in this moment he would be able to know himself."
Manuscript A omits *per* here and so is in accord with the generally accepted Greek version. *Per se* would be in accord with the Greek text published by Ross, who follows
Bywater in emending δὲ αὐτὸν to δι' αὐτοῦ. See Aristotle, *De Anima* (1961), 292, and
also see Owens (1976), who argues for the traditional interpretation found in the Greek
manuscript tradition.

When each of the intelligibles is in it in such a way that it is said in regard to the knower that he is a knower in act, that is, when the intelligibles have been in him as beings in act (this occurs for the intellect when it has been able to understand in virtue of itself, not when it has understood in virtue of something else). What he stated is the difference between proximate active powers and remote ones, for those proximate to act are those which act in virtue of themselves and do not need something drawing them out from potency into act, while remote ones need [something else]. For this reason he said that when the intellect has been in this disposition, then it will be a potency in a way, that is, then this word potency will be said of it not truly but by analogy. Next he said: **And he** has been able **to understand in virtue of himself.** That is, when the intellect has been in this disposition, then it will understand itself insofar as it is nothing else but the forms of the things, inasmuch as it draws them out from matter. It is as if it understands itself in an accidental way, as Alexander says,[134] that is, insofar as it happens to the intelligibles of things that they have been it, that is, its essence. This is contrary to the disposition in separate forms, for since their intelligible is not different from them in terms of the intention in virtue of which they are intelligibles belonging to that intellect, for this reason they understand themselves essentially and not accidentally. This is found more perfectly in the First Knower, who understands nothing outside Himself. We can expound that passage in accord with what al-Fârâbî says in his treatise *On the Intellect and the Intelligible.*[135] This is that when the intellect has been in act, it will be one of the beings and it will be able to understand itself through an intention which it will abstract from itself, insofar as it abstracts the intentions of things which are outside the soul. Thus the intelligible will have intelligibles. We will later investigate whether or not this is possible.[136] {421}

9. **And since magnitude is one thing and the being of a magnitude another and water is one thing and the being of water another, and so for many other cases (but not for all, for in certain cases the being of flesh is the same as the flesh), [the soul] must ascertain [these] in virtue of two [distinct powers] or in virtue of a different disposition [of a single power]. For there is no flesh without matter, but, as is the case for snubness, it is a determinate particular and in a determinate particular.**[137] (429b10–14)

134. Alexander, *De Anima* (1887), 109.4–23, esp. 109.17; (1979), 141–142.

135. Al-Fârâbî, *Letter on the Intellect* (1983), 19.1ff.; (1973), 216ff.; (1974), 99ff.

136. {434ff}.

137. *Aliquid hoc et in aliquo hoc:* τόδε ἐν τῷδε, "a *this* in a *this*" (Aristotle, *De Anima* [1984]); شيء في شيء (ibid. [1954]); "a thing in a thing." تلك الماهية هي في ذلك الشخص "a thing in a thing." المشار إليه, "a particular essence is in a given individual" (*Middle Commentary* [2002]), 113.22. Cf. Book 1, n. 24, and the introduction, p. lvi.

After he had completed the demonstration making known the substance of
the material intellect and had given the difference between it and the substance
of a material sentient being, he also began to give the difference between the
intellect in act and the imagination in act. For it is thought that the imagination
itself is the intellect, and especially when we say that its relation to the intellect
is as the relation of the sensible to the sense, namely, because it moves it, and
it is thought that the mover and the moved ought to be of the same species.
And he began to say: **And since magnitude is one thing**, etc. That is, and since
this individual is one thing and the intention in virtue of which this individual
is a being, namely, its quiddity and form, is another thing. For instance, this
water is one thing and the intention, that is, the form in virtue of which this
water is a being, is different from the water. Next he said: **and so for many
other cases**. That is, and this occurs in a similar way in many things, namely,
in all things composed of matter and form. He said **but not for all** to make an
exception of separate things and generally simple incomposite things. Next he
said: **for in certain cases the being of flesh is the same as the flesh**. That is,
the reason why these two intentions are not found in all beings is {422} that in
simple beings the quiddity and being are the same, so that, for instance, the
being of flesh is the same as flesh, because [what is analogous to] the intention
of flesh in these [simple beings] is not in matter.[138] After he had introduced the
antecedent in this account, he gave the consequent. He said: **[the soul] must
ascertain [these]**, etc. That is, after it had been explained that sensible beings
are divided into a twofold being, namely, into this singular and its form, the
ascertaining power, that is, the apprehending [power], must apprehend these
things either in virtue of two powers or in virtue of one but [one operating] in
two different dispositions. It will, however, be with two powers when it has

---

138. *Quiditas et essentia in entibus simplicibus est idem.* The same is found in the corresponding passage of the *Middle Commentary* (2002), 113.17: فإن الأشياء البسيطة الوجود
والماهية فيها هو شيء واحد بعينه, "for the existence and essence of simple things are one
and the same." Since the simple entities are the immaterial and separate intellects, the
meaning must be that if they were able to be said to have some essential nature—for
example, X—then in them the being of X and X would be the same. This is because they
are not forms in subjects but rather just simple forms. Averroes seems compelled to
state it this way because he is closely following a faulty translation of Aristotle's text,
but the meaning is clear enough. There is no distinction of being or essence from subject such that these simple beings would be composite. Rather, in these the actual being
of the simple entity is identical to its essence. Nevertheless, it should be noted that at
{410} he asserts that "It was already explained in First Philosophy that there is no form
free of potency without qualification except the First Form, which understands nothing
outside itself. Its being is its quiddity. Other forms, however, are in some way different
in quiddity and being." Cf. Book 3, nn. 106 and 107.

apprehended each of those per se, namely, the form alone and the individual alone; but it will be in virtue of one power and a different disposition when it has apprehended the divergence which there is between these two intentions. For what apprehends the divergence between the two, as was explained, must be one in one way and many in another way. That is the disposition of the intellect in apprehending the divergence which there is between the form and the individual, for it apprehends the form per se and it apprehends the individual through the mediation of sense. It therefore apprehends the divergence between these in virtue of a disposition which is diverse, just as the common sense apprehends the divergence between the sensibles in virtue of a diverse disposition, namely, that of a particular sense. But because the intellect does not apprehend those forms except with their matters, for this reason it apprehends them through a disposition which is diverse.[139] And after he had revealed that the soul must apprehend these two intentions in virtue of a diverse power and apprehend the divergence of these through a single {423} power but according to a diverse disposition, he gave the reason why the soul needs a diverse disposition to apprehend those two intentions. He said: **For there is no flesh without matter.** That is, the reason why the form is not apprehended by the intellect except with matter—the consideration which makes it apprehend it by a different disposition—is that the forms do not exist without matter. For the form of flesh is never denuded of matter, but [rather] it is always understood with matter,[140] as snubness with nose, since snubness is a determinate particular in a determinate particular. So too it is regarding sensible forms, namely, that they are a determinate particular in a determinate particular.

10. **[The soul], therefore, ascertains hot and cold through what senses. And the things which are in flesh are likened to those which belong to that. It ascertains what the being of flesh is in virtue of something else, or according to the disposition of a spiral line, as long as it lasts.**[141] (429b14–18)

139. That is, while intellect must apprehend them as intelligibles without matters, its apprehension of them with their natural matters takes place by way of its use of sense. Judgments, then, which concern the specific or generic classification of individuals, will require intellect and the particular powers in a body.

140. That is, the intellectual consideration of a material form necessarily requires that reference to matter be contained in the understanding of that form, since matter is contained in the definition of the thing insofar as it is the definition of a physical entity.

141. The corresponding Greek has τῷ μὲν οὖν αἰσθητικῷ τὸ θερμὸν καὶ τὸ ψυχρὸν κρίνει, καὶ ὧν λόγος τις ἡ σάρξ· ἄλλῳ δέ, ἤτοι χωριστῷ ὡς ἡ κεκλασμένη ἔχει πρὸς αὑτὴν ὅταν ἐκταθῇ, τὸ σαρκὶ εἶναι κρίνει. "Now it is by means of the sensitive faculty that we discriminate the hot and the cold, i.e. the factors which combined in a certain ratio constitute flesh: the essential character of flesh is apprehended by something dif-

Since it is necessary that diverse things be ascertained in virtue of diverse powers (in virtue of what senses and the like the soul ascertains hot and cold and the like), then analogously it is necessary that the thing existing in flesh in virtue of which flesh is what it is, not that in virtue of which it is hot or cold,[142] be like the power apprehending it and it must ascertain [this] in virtue of another power. And he said: **are likened to those which belong to that**, because the relation which is of an intention to an intention, {424} namely, of an individual [intention] to a universal [intention], is just as the relation of a power apprehending one of these to the power apprehending the other. Since the two intentions must be diverse, the powers must be diverse. The understanding power, therefore, is not the imaginative power, since it was already explained that what is apprehended on the part of the imaginative power and the sensible power is the same thing. Next he said: **It ascertains what the being of flesh is in virtue of something else, or according to the disposition of a spiral line**, etc. That is, it must ascertain the form in virtue of another power. And this will be from this power either in virtue of a disposition similar to a straight line, since it will have understood the first form existing in this single thing, or according to the disposition similar to a spiral line, when it has been turned about, in seeking to understand also the quiddity of that form, then the quiddity of that quiddity, until it reaches the simple quiddity in that thing. For instance, initially it understands the quiddity of flesh, then it seeks to understand the quiddity of that quiddity, then the quiddity of that quiddity. This will go on until it finds the quiddity in the quiddity and it will not cease until it reaches the simple form. He meant this when he said: **as long as it lasts**, that is, the understanding of

---

ferent either wholly separate from the sensitive faculty or related to it as a bent line to the same line when it has been straightened out." Aristotle, *De Anima* (1984). The alternate translation has فبالحس يقضى على الحار والبارد ، وبموضع النطق يقال ما جزء اللحم ويقضى على الغيرية : إما كشىء مفارق وإما كخط أعوج عند نفسه إذا مر هكذا قضاؤه على ما كان لجزء اللحم (ibid. [1954]); "By sense it judges the hot and the cold and by way of reason what is called the flesh part. It judges distinction: either as something separate or as a line bent upon itself when it has thus reached its term in accord with what belongs to the part of the flesh." Averroes seems not to be fully aware of the corrupt status of the text of Aristotle. Rather, he devises an interpretation (perhaps inspired by Ibn Bâjjah) in which he understands the notion of intellect being likened to a spiral line to represent what seems almost a Platonic view of dialectic (*Republic* 6, 511b–d) with intellect moving from quiddities through quiddities to quiddities until it finally reaches a simple form itself. See {424}. In his *Middle Commentary*, there is nothing corresponding to this text of Aristotle. Note, however, that Averroes seems to have had some awareness that there may have been faults in the manuscript of Aristotle's Text here and in the one which follows. See his remarks at the end of the next Comment at {426}.

142. That is, in virtue of its form, not in virtue of its subject.

the intelligible will go on in a similar way in regard to flesh as long as it will be possible in regard to flesh that its quiddity have a quiddity.[143]

11. **And also in the case of things existing in mathematics, the straight is like snubness, for it has continuous quantity. According to being,[144] however, the being of the straight is different from this.[145] If, therefore, {425} [the soul] ascertains[146] [the being of something], it then does so in virtue of something else and because its disposition is different. And generally the disposition of things which are in the intellect is the same as [that of] things separate from matter.** (429b18–22)

This understanding on the part of the intellect is found not only in regard to material things, but also in regard to mathematical things. For because the straight is in what is continuous, just as snubness is in a nose, insofar as the intellect understands snubness in composition with a nose, so too it is necessary that it understand the quiddity of the straight in composition with what is continuous. He said: **And also in the case of things,** etc. That is, and the being of the straight and its like from among mathematical things is similar to the being of snubness in a nose, for the straight is in what is continuous just as snubness is in a nose. Next he said: **According to being, however,[147]** the being in the straight is different from the quiddity of the continuous, although one of them is found only in the other. Next he said: **If, therefore,** etc. That is, when, therefore, we have asserted that in mathematics there are also two things of which one is in the other, then the soul does not ascertain these except through another power, or through the same [power] but nevertheless through a disposition which is diverse, since it understands these only with the thing, although it does not understand them with sensible matter. For it should be known that the disposition possessed by the intellect which [disposition] is diverse in it when it apprehends the first sensible forms of things, [this disposition] belongs to it in virtue of the senses. And the disposition which is diverse in it in virtue of the apprehension of the quiddity and form belongs to it as a disposition diverse in itself, not in virtue of the senses. For this reason Aristotle likens it to a spiral line in this disposition, while Plato [likens it] to a circular line,[148] and by this disposition he understands the forms

143. Cf. Averroes' discussion of Ibn Bâjjah on {491–492}.

144. *Secundum autem esse*: τὸ δὲ τί ἦν εἶναι.

145. The Greek text here has: "its constitutive essence is different, if we may distinguish between straightness and what is straight: let us take it to be two-ness." Aristotle, *De Anima* (1984).

146. *Experimentatur*: κρίνει.

147. Although Crawford does not italicize this, I read it as a quotation of the Text since these are the exact words used in the Text.

of mathematical things, since he does not allow a sensible magnitude to be involved in the understanding of these. {426} Next he said: **And generally the disposition of things**, etc. That is, as it seems to me, and generally the disposition of things which the intellect apprehends is found in [the intellect] in the way in which they are in themselves in reference to proximity and distance by separation from matter. Those, therefore, which are remote from matter are able to be separated by the intellect without matter, although they may have being only in matter, as it is in the case of mathematics. And those of them which are proximate to matter will not be able [to be separated]. When, then, he said **as [that of] things separate from matter**, he means according to the mode of being in things separate from matter in the order in which they exist with respect to separation, if that account is complete in the manuscript.

12. **And someone will doubt that the intellect is simple and impassible and that it is impossible for it to have something in common with something else, as Anaxagoras said. How, therefore, is it understood that conceptualizing is an affection? For because there is something common to both, it is thought that one of them acts and the other is affected.** (429b22–26)

After he had given the difference between understanding and imagining, he returned to express uncertainty concerning the passible intellect. He said: **And someone may be uncertain**, etc. That is, and one is uncertain regarding what was said, that the material intellect is simple and impassible, because it is not thought that it has anything in common with a material thing, as Anaxagoras said, and as was explained earlier.[149] The question, however, is how it is understood that conceptualizing is an affection, that is, [is] of the genus of passive powers, {427} and has nothing in common with the thing by which it is affected. For it is thought that one acts and the other is affected in virtue of something common to the agent and to the patient. For unless there were matter, there would be no affection. And when we will have asserted the intellect not to be matter nor to be in matter, how then will we understand [this] when we also hold that understanding is an affection, not an activity? We are therefore between two considerations: either we do not assert that understanding is in the category of affection or we assert that the material intellect has something in common with the body, to the extent that the form of the imagination which moves it is common to the body.

13. **And also is it in itself intelligible? For either intellect will belong to the other things (if it is not an intelligible in another way, but what is**

148. *Timaeus* 37Bff.
149. See Book 1, Comment 31 at {40}.

conceptualized is one in its form) or there will be in it a mixture from something which has made it intelligible, as is the case for other things.[150] (429b26–29)

That is the second uncertainty about the material intellect, whether it is intelligible in itself, not in virtue of a nature existing in it, to the extent that the intellect and the intelligible in it will be the same in every way, as is the disposition in the case of separate things, or is the intelligible of it different from it in some way. And he said: **And also is it in itself**, etc. That is, and also is it that which is the intelligible of it. For it must be one of these two alternatives: either the other things which are outside the soul have intellect (if the intellect is the intelligible of it in every way and is not a different way in the case of understanding things, but understanding is the same in regard to all {428} things), or it is not intelligible per se, but in virtue of the intention in what made it intelligible, as is the disposition in things which are outside the soul. He was silent, as it seems, about what follows from this position, namely, that the intellect in itself is not something which has understanding.[151] The short account of the uncertainty, as it seems, is the following: for either it will be an intelligible just as the other separate intelligible things, and so the things which are outside the soul will have understanding, or it will be intelligible as are the other things which are outside the soul, and thus it will in itself not be something which understands or apprehends.[152]

14. **Let us say, therefore, that affection, as was seen earlier, is a general notion and that the intellect is somehow the intelligibles in potency, but not in actuality, until it understands. And what happens in the case of the intel-**

---

150. The corresponding Greek is clearer: "For if thought is thinkable *per se* and what is thinkable is in kind one and the same, then either thought will belong to everything, or it will contain some element common to it with all other realities which makes them all thinkable." Aristotle, *De Anima* (1984).

151. That is, the intellect will have understanding only when it has received the intelligible, not as an intelligible in its own right. If so, it differs from other separate intellects in this regard.

152. Other separate intelligible things, scil. the self-thinking separate intellects, have intellectual understanding of themselves as intelligibles in act. The material intellect has as its function the grasping of intelligibles in act which derive from the world. If, then, the material intellect in the same way thinks things which are intelligibles in act and thinks things of the world, then the things of the world must be intelligibles in act essentially. If they are so essentially, then they are also intellects in act essentially and thereby have understanding. If, on the other hand, the material intellect is intelligible as are things outside the soul in the world, it would be an intelligible in potency, not in act, and so would not have understanding.

lect ought to follow such a pattern, namely, as the tablet is disposed for drawing, [but is] not at all drawn upon in act. (429b29–430a2)

After he had presented these two questions concerning the material intellect, he began to resolve them, and first [he resolves] the first, saying: How is it that we understand that the material intellect is something simple and unmixed with anything, when we hold the opinion that understanding is an affection, and [yet] it was already explained in the general accounts that things which act and are affected have a subject in common?[153] And he said: **Let us say, therefore, that affection**, etc. That is, and that question is resolved by means of the knowledge that the term affection, which we used earlier in regard to the question, is more general than something said in regard to material things because [this latter] is [something which is] passive. Next he expounded {429} what this term affection signifies in the case of the intellect. He said: **that the intellect is somehow the intelligibles in potency**, etc. That is, that general intention of affection in the case of the intellect is nothing but that something is in potency in the intellect, not in act until it understands. And also to say that it is in potency is [to speak] in a manner different from those [ways] according to which it is said that material things are in potency. This is what we said earlier, that it should be understood here that these terms, namely, *potency, reception*, and *actuality*, are said equivocally of these in relation to material things. For the diversity of that intention, namely, [of the intention] of the reception which is in the intellect, from the reception which is in material things is a thing to which reason leads. Hence, one should not hold the opinion that prime matter is the cause of reception considered without qualification, but [that it is] the cause of the changeable reception which involves the reception belonging to a singular thing. The cause of reception considered without qualification is that nature. And in this way it was possible for heavenly bodies to receive the separate forms and understand them, and it was possible for separate intelligences to be actualized per se with respect to one another. And if not, it would not be possible to understand there [among the heavenly bodies] any thing receptive or able to be received. Hence we see that what is free of this nature [of receptivity] is the first thing which has understanding.[154]

153. That is, the actuality of the agent as agent and the actuality of the patient as patient take place in the same subject—namely, in the patient. The patient, then, is the common subject for an actualization which is one in being but two in description. This is the topic of discussion in *Physics* 3.3, 202a12–29.

154. What is completely free of such potency is the first thinking entity—namely, God. See below {520}, where God is described as pure actuality, *pura actio*. In his *Long Commentary on the Metaphysics*, Averroes also characterizes the First as pure actuality: فانه فعل محض. *Long Commentary on the Metaphysics* (1952), 1599; (1984), 151. This char-

By asserting that nature [to be such as this], the following question is resolved: How is plurality understood and how are the separate forms understood to be many, with the intellect being the same as the intelligible in these? After he had made known the way of affection in the case of the intellect and that it is said equivocally in regard to the intellect and in regard to material things, he began to give an example from sensible things in virtue of which that intention is understood in regard to the material intellect. Although it is not true [for the separate intellects in precisely the same way], nevertheless it provides a way {430} for understanding. This manner of teaching is more necessary in regard to such things, although it is rhetorical. And he said: **And what happens in the case of the intellect**, etc. That is, and it should be understood that what we said concerning this general intention, namely, [concerning] the affection which is in the intellect, which[155] is just reception without a change, just as the reception of the drawing on the tablet. For just as the tablet is not affected by the drawing and there occurs no change to it by this but there is only found in it of the intention of the affection that it is actualized by the drawing after [the tablet] was drawn upon in potency, so too is there this disposition in the case of the material intellect. This example which he provided is very similar to the disposition of the intellect which is in potency with the intellect which is in act. For just as the tablet has no drawing in act nor in potency proximate to act, so too in the material intellect there is none of the intelligible forms which it receives, neither in act nor in potency proximate to act. And I call here *potency proximate to act* a disposition intermediate between a remote potency and a final actuality. This is so that there is in it no intention which is intelligible in potency. This is proper to the intellect alone. For the first actuality of a sensory power is something in act with respect to a remote potency and is something in potency[156] with respect to a final actuality. For this reason Aristotle likened the first actuality of sense

---

acterization of the First is not reflected in the Latin translation of the text of Aristotle in the *Long Commentary on the Metaphysics*. See the 1574 text (1962), v. 8, 319G, for the corresponding Latin. However, in this printing, v. 8, 321 C–D, in his Comment we find *illud quod movet primum motum, cum sit non motum, quia est actus purus sine aliqua potentia*, which corresponds to *Long Commentary on the Metaphysics* (1952), 1610: ان الذى يحرك; المتحرك الأول اذ هو غير متحرك من قبل انه فعل محض ليس فيه قوة اصلا, "that which moves the first moved while being unmoved because it is pure actuality completely free from any potentiality" (ibid. [1984], 156).

155. I follow Janssens (1998), 725, in reading *quae* with all the manuscripts rather than Crawford's conjecture of *quod*.

156. Arabic fragments correspond to Book 3, 14.58–65: وهذا المثال شبيه المناسبة جدا لحال العقل الذي بالقوة مع العقل الذي بالفعل ووجه الشبه انه كما ان اللوح ليس فيه من الكتابة شيء موجود لا بالفعل ولا بالقوة القريبة من الفعل كذلك العقل الهيولاني ليس فيه شيء من الصورة المعقولة التي لا بالفعل ولا بالقوة القريبة من الفعل وذلك لأن لا يكون

to the geometer when he is not using geometry. For we know certainly that we have a sensible power existing in act, although then we are sensing nothing. The manner of similarity of that example to what was said by Aristotle in regard to the material intellect has been explained.[157]

To say, however, that the material intellect is similar to the disposition which is in the tablet, not to the tablet insofar as it is what is disposed, as Alexander expounded {431} this account,[158] is false. For the disposition is a certain privation and has no nature of its own except owing to the nature of the subject and for this reason it was possible for the dispositions to be different in each being. Oh, Alexander, you figured that Aristotle intends to demonstrate to us the nature of the disposition alone, not the nature of what is disposed (the nature of that disposition is not proper to it, if it has been possible [to know it] without knowing the nature disposed), but [with regard to] the nature of the disposition considered without qualification, in what sort of thing would it be? But I am ashamed of this account and of this fantastic exposition. For if Aristotle meant to demonstrate the nature of the disposition which is in the intellect through all the aforementioned accounts in regard to the material intellect, either he must mean to demonstrate through them the nature of the disposition considered without qualification or the nature of the proper disposition. It is impossible, however, that the nature of the disposition proper to the intellect be demonstrated without the nature of the subject, since the disposition proper to each subject is consequent upon the actuality and form it has from it. But knowing the nature of the disposed subject must necessarily be through knowledge of the nature of the disposition. And if he meant by these accounts to demonstrate the nature of the disposition considered without qualification, then that is not something proper to the intellect and all this is confusion. For every disposition, insofar as it is a disposition, is truly said to be nothing in act [apart] from these things which it receives and [to be] something which is impassible, and it is truly said to be neither a body nor a power in a body.

How, therefore, can we expound that what Aristotle intended to demonstrate

---

فيه معنى هو بالقوة معقول وهذا شيء يخص العقل وحده لا كالحس فان الاستكمال الأولي
هو شيء ما بالفعل بالاضافة الى قوة بعيدة وشيء ما بالقوة (*Long Commentary* Fragments [1985], 45). The Arabic text omits Book 3, Comment 14.65–67: "And I call . . . and a final actuality." It appears that the Latin translator's Arabic text was faulty with لا كالحس, "unlike sense." The Arabic differs slightly: "This is proper to the intellect alone, unlike sense. For the first actuality is something in act with respect to a remote potency and is something in potency. . . ." Also note that there is nothing in the Arabic corresponding to the Latin *quas recipit*, "which it receives," at Book 3, Comment 14.64.

157. Cf. {135–136}.
158. See {395ff}.

to us here concerning the nature of the material intellect [is] what is common to all recipients, namely, [all those things] in which there is a disposition for receiving {432} any kind of form, and [that he did] not [intend] to demonstrate the nature of what is disposed through knowledge of the nature of the disposition proper to it? Unless the material intellect were only a disposition, without some subject, which is impossible, for the disposition indicates a disposed subject. Hence Aristotle, when he found the disposition which is in the intellect to be diverse from the others, judged in a precise way that the nature which is a subject for it differs from the other disposed natures. What is proper to that subject of disposition is that there is in it none of the intentions intelligible in potency or in act. Hence it was necessary that it not be a body nor a form in a body. And since it is not a body nor a power in a body, it will also not be the forms of the imagination, for those are powers in bodies and they are intentions intelligible in potency.[159] Since the subject of that disposition is neither a form of the imagination nor a mixture of elements, as Alexander intended, nor can we say that some disposition is stripped from a subject, we rightly see that Theophrastus, Themistius, Nicolaus,[160] and others among the ancient Peripatetics hold faster to the demonstration of Aristotle and preserve his words to a greater degree. For since they attend to the accounts and words of Aristotle, none could bring these to bear upon the disposition itself alone nor upon the thing subject to the disposition [as] if we had asserted it to be a power in a body, while saying that it is simple, separate, impassible, and unmixed with the body. If that were not the opinion of Aristotle, it would be necessary that it be held that it is the true opinion. But on account of what I say, no one ought to doubt that this is the opinion of Aristotle. {433} For all those who hold this opinion believe only on account of what Aristotle said. For this is so difficult that if Aristotle's account of this were not found, then it would be very difficult to come upon it, or perhaps impossible, unless someone such as Aristotle were found. For I believe that this man was a model in nature and the exemplar which nature found for showing the final human perfection in the material realm.[161] Perhaps the opinion ascribed to Alexander was contrived by him

159. This is precisely Averroes' own position in the *Short Commentary on the De Anima*. See the introduction, pp. xxiii–xxviii.

160. This is presumably a reference to "On the Philosophy of Aristotle," by Nicolaus of Damascus (d. ca. 25 CE), a work translated into Syriac in the ninth century. For detailed discussion of the text, its tradition in Arabic and Syriac, and its use by Averroes, see Nicolaus of Damascus in the primary sources.

161. Cf. Endress (2005), 251. This often-cited passage is frequently understood out of context. Note that while praising Aristotle himself as an extraordinary work of nature for his high intellectual achievement, Averroes in the previous lines states that it is not mere authority that governs this judgment but rather intellectual excellence: "If that

alone and in his time it was unthinkable and rejected by everyone. For this reason we see Themistius dismissing it altogether and avoiding it just as we guard against unthinkable things. This is contrary to what happens for modern [thinkers], for no one is knowing and perfect in their eyes unless he is an Alexandrian.[162] The reason for this is the notoriety of that man and because he is believed[163] to be one of the good commentators. Although al-Fârâbî, while he was the greatest among them, followed Alexander in this intention, he also added to this opinion something unthinkable. For in his *Commentary on the Nicomachean Ethics*[164] he seems to deny that there is conjoining with the separate intelligences. He says that this is the opinion of Alexander and that it should not be held that the human end is anything but theoretical perfection.[165] Ibn Bâjjah, however, expounded his own account and said that his opinion is the opinion of all the Peripatetics, namely, that conjoining is possible and that it is the end [for human beings]. Perhaps this is one of the reasons why we see that the customs and habits of most of those devoting themselves to philosophy in this time are corrupt. This has other causes not unknown to those giving themselves over to study of practical philosophy.[166] {434}

15. It too is intelligible, just as the intelligibles. For the conceptualizing and that which is conceptualized in these things which are without matter

---

were not the opinion of Aristotle, it would be necessary that it be held that it is the true opinion." Still, in his *Middle Commentary on the Prior Analytics* Averroes writes, "How wonderful is this man and how different is his nature from human natures generally. It is as though divine art (*sinâ'ah*) brought him forth so as to inform us, humans, that ultimate perfection is possible in the human species perceptibly and demonstrably. Such [a person] is not human, that is why the ancients used to call him divine." Translated in Fakhry (2001), 41, from Ibn Rushd, *Middle Commentary on the Prior Analytics* (1982), 213. 20–24.

162. That is, a follower of Alexander.

163. Janssens (1998), 725, suggests *credimus* ("we believe [him]") in lieu of *creditur* following manuscripts A, C, D, and G.

164. See the introduction, pp. lxx and lxxxvii.

165. That is, al-Fârâbî is reported to have moved late in life to the view that human perfection consists in the perfection of human intellects by knowledge, not in reaching a state of conjoining with separate intellects. See Davidson (1992), 71. This teaching has obvious eschatological consequences. Regarding al-Fârâbî's lost *Commentary on the Nicomachean Ethics*, see the introduction, p. xlv, n. 84, and p. lxxxvii, n. 162.

166. Averroes could be complaining that too much concern by contemporary philosophical thinkers has been given over to theoretical study and the perfection of the intellect to the neglect of the proper character formation which must precede true intellectual excellence. His target may be a familiar one: Avicenna. Regarding Avicenna, see Gutas (1988). Regarding the views of al-Fârâbî, see Druart (1997a).

are the same. For theoretical knowledge and what is known are the same in this way. (430a2–5)

He was uncertain about the material intellect as to whether what is intelligible in it is the intellect itself or something else in some way. If the intellect in it is the very thing intelligible, it must be intelligible per se, not through an intention in it; and if it were in some way something else, it must be intelligible through an intention in it. He began to explain that it is intelligible through an intention in it, just as other things intelligible, but it differs from these in that this intention is in itself the intellect in act, while in the case of other things it is the intellect in potency. He said: **It too is** intelligible, **just as the intelligibles.**[167] That is, it is intelligible through an intention in it just as other intelligible things. Next he gave a demonstration of this. He said: **For the conceptualizing,** etc. That is, it is necessary that it be an intelligible through an intention in it, because the conceptualizing and that which is conceptualized are the same in immaterial things. And if that intellect were an intellect per se, it would follow that theoretical knowledge and what is known would be the same, which is impossible [in this case].[168]

16. **We must investigate why it is not always understanding. In the case of what has matter, however, any of the intelligibles is only in potency. These, therefore, will not have intellect (for in relation to those intellect is only as a potency belonging to those when they have been separated from matter), while [intellect does belong] to that, since it is intelligible.** (430a5–9) {435}

It is necessary to investigate why it does not always understand in such a way that its intelligibles are the intellect in itself. The reason for this is that with respect to those intelligibles which do not have matter, their intelligible is the intellect in itself and it is always understanding. But for those things which have matter, each of the intelligibles is in it in potency and for this reason material intelligible things do not understand. He meant this when he said: these, **therefore**, do **not** have **intellect.** That is, for this reason material intelligibles do not have intellect. What is missing from the account is understood through its opposite and through this word, **while**, which indicates division. It is as if he says:

167. The difference between the Lemma's *intelligibilis* and the Comment's *intellectum* here is likely indicative of the difficulty the Latin translator had in rendering soundly the Arabic *maʿqûl*. The alternate translation has [*sic*] وهو أيضا معقول مثل سائر المعقولة (Aristotle, *De Anima* [1954]), "It too is intelligible just as the rest of the intelligibles," substituting the plural المعقولات for the singular المعقولة.

168. That is, in the case of the separate immaterial intellects, intellect and its intelligible are per se the same, while in the case of the material intellect this cannot be so because it knows things of the world by way of intentions of those things in it.

the reason for this is because the intelligible of what does not have matter exists always and in act, while the intelligible of what has matter is in potency.

Next he said: **These, therefore,** do **not have intellect**, etc. That is, those intelligibles, then, on account of this, namely, because they are intelligible in potency, do not have intellect. For intellect is not ascribed in reference to them but in reference to the form of those as separate from matter. For this reason those forms in relation to these [material things] will not be intelligible in act, that is, will not be apprehended by these [material things] nor will they be [actually] understanding in virtue of these [material things]. In relation to what separates them from their matters they will be intelligible in act and in virtue of these [intellect] will be understanding and in virtue of that same intention those will not be understanding. This is the conclusion of the account resolving the question mentioned earlier. For that account forced us to one of two alternatives: on the one hand, if intellect were identical with the intelligible in the material intellect, [then it would be the case] that other things which are outside the soul would have understanding; on the other hand, if [the intellect] is different [from the intelligible in the material intellect, then it would be the case] that it is intelligible in virtue of an intention in it, [and] hence it will require [another] intellect in order to be thought, and this proceeds in infinite regress.[169] {436}

The resolution of this question, therefore, lies in the fact that the intention in virtue of which the material intellect comes to be intellect in act exists such that it is intelligible in act. But the intention in virtue of which the things which are outside the soul are beings is such that they are intelligible in potency, and if they were [intelligible] in act, then they would [themselves] have understanding.

17. **And because, just as in nature there is something in every genus which is matter (and this is what is all those things in potency) and something else which is a cause and agent (and this is that on account of which it brings about anything, as the disposition of artistry to matter), these differences must exist in the soul.** (3.5, 430a10–14)

After he had explained the nature of the intellect which is in potency and [the nature of the intellect] which is in act and had given the difference between it and the power of the imagination, he began to explain that it is necessary for there to be a third kind of intellect, namely, the agent intelli-

169. That is, if the objects thought (the things outside the soul) are identical with thought, then each would be thinking. And if they are not identical but rather are different, then the only way thought can be thought is in virtue of another higher intellect. But an infinite regress is generated if in that intellect what is thought and what thinks are different.

gence[170] which makes the intellect which is in potency to be intellect in act. And he said that the assertion that the agent intelligence is in this genus of beings is just as the disposition [found] in all natural beings. Just as it is necessary in any genus of natural and generable things that there be three things from the nature of that genus and ascribed to it, namely, the agent, the patient, and the product, so ought it to be in the case of the intellect. And he said: **And because, just as in nature**, etc. That is, and because this is just as it is the case in natural things. That is to say, and because the consideration of the soul is a consideration of what is natural, because the soul is one of the natural beings, while it is common to natural beings that they have {437} matter in any genus (namely, what is in potency all the things which are in that genus), and [that they have something else] which is a cause and agent (this is that on account of which everything which is of that genus is generated, as the artistry is to the matter), then it is necessary that there be these three differences in the soul.

18. **It is necessary, therefore, that in [the soul] there be the intellect which is intellect insofar as it is made everything, and the intellect which is intellect insofar as it makes it understand everything, and the intellect insofar as it understands everything, as a positive disposition, which is like light.[171] For light in a way also makes colors which are in potency to be colors in act.** (430a14–17)

170. Note that Averroes' understanding here seems to be influenced by the faulty Text 18, which follows below. As indicated in the introduction, pp. xix–xx, n. 10, the terms *intelligentia* and *intellectus* translate one Arabic word, العقل, so any distinction is from the mind of the Latin translator. See the introduction, n. 209; Book 2, n. 138; and Book 3, n. 43.

171. This account of three intellects is absent from the Greek text of Aristotle and absent from Averroes' alternate translation. It is also not mentioned by Averroes in the corresponding passage in his *Middle Commentary*. See *Middle Commentary* (2002), 116. The Greek text has καὶ ἔστιν ὁ μὲν τοιοῦτος νοῦς τῷ πάντα γίνεσθαι, ὁ δὲ τῷ πάντα ποιεῖν, ὡς ἕξις τις, οἷον τὸ φῶς. "And in fact thought, as we have described it, is what it is by virtue of becoming all things, while there is another which is what it is by virtue of making all things: this is a sort of positive state like light." Aristotle, *De Anima* (1984). The Hebrew (ibid. [1994]) corresponds well with the Greek and thereby reveals that Averroes' primary translation is faulty here. The text seems to have suffered two corruptions, something verified by consultation of the Hebrew translation, which is from the same tradition as the Arabic translation. First, consider "**and the intellect insofar as it understands everything, as a positive disposition, which is like light**," for the Latin *et intellectus secundum quod intelligit omne, quasi habitus, qui est quasi lux*. The Latin *intelligit* likely renders the Arabic يعقل, a corruption of يفعل, "makes," corresponding to the Greek ποιεῖν, "making." Second, what was perhaps a marginal gloss on the originally sound version of this text may have been moved from the margin into the text—namely, the phrase, "**and the intellect which is intellect insofar as it makes**

Since those three differences must be found in the part of the soul which is called intellect, it is necessary that there be in it a part which is called intellect insofar as it is made everything by way of likeness and reception. There must also be in it a second part which is called intellect insofar as it makes that intellect which is in potency to understand everything in act. For the reason why it makes the intellect which is in potency to understand all things in act is nothing other than that it is in act; for this fact, that it is in act, is the cause that it understands all things in act. And there must also be in it a third part which is called intellect insofar as it makes every intelligible in potency to be an intelligible in act. He said: **It is necessary, therefore**, etc. He means by that the material intellect. This, therefore, is his description mentioned earlier.[172] Next he said: **and . . . the intellect insofar as it makes it understand everything.** He means {438} by that what comes to be, which is in a positive disposition. This [latter] pronoun can be understood to refer to the material intellect, as we said, and can be understood to refer to the human being who is the one understanding. It is necessary to add in the account: insofar as it makes it understand everything in its own right and when it wishes.[173] For this is the definition of a positive disposition, namely, that what has a positive disposition understands in virtue of it what is proper to itself in its own right and when it wishes, without it being the case that it needs something external in this. Next he said: **and the intellect insofar as it understands**, etc. He means by that the agent intelligence. When he said this: **it understands everything, as** a certain **positive disposition**, he means that it makes everything intelligible in potency to be intelligible in act after it was in potency, as a positive disposition and form. Next he said: **like light**, etc. Now he gives the way on the basis of which it was necessary to assert the agent intelligence to be in the soul. For we cannot say that the relation of the agent intellect in the soul to the generated intelligible is just as the relation of the artistry to the art's product in every way. For art imposes the form on the whole matter without it being the case that there was something of the intention of the form existing in the matter before the artistry has made it. It is not so in the case of the intellect, for if it were so in the case of the intellect, then a human being would not need sense or imagination for apprehending intelligibles. Rather, the intelligibles would enter into the material intellect from the agent intellect, without the material intellect needing to behold sensible forms. And neither can we even say that the imagined intentions are solely what move the material intellect and draw it out from potency into act. For if it were so, then

---

it understand everything," **et intellectus qui est intellectus secundum quod facit ipsum intellegere omne.** See Taylor (1999a). Cf. Davidson (1992), 317, n. 10.

172. {387}.

173. Cf. {220ff}, {439–440}, {495–496}, {499}.

there would be no difference between the universal and the individual, and then the intellect would be of the genus of the imaginative power. Hence, in view of our having asserted that the relation of the imagined intentions {439} to the material intellect is just as the relation of the sensibles to the senses (as Aristotle will say later), it is necessary to suppose that there is another mover which makes [the intentions] move the material intellect in act, and this is nothing but to make [the intentions] intelligible in act by separating them from matter.

Because this intention, which forces the assertion of an agent intellect different from the material intellect and different from the forms of things which the material intellect apprehends, is similar to the intention on account of which sight needs light, in view of the fact that the agent and the recipient are different from light, he was content to make this way known by means of this example. It is as if he says: and the way which forced us to suppose the agent intellect is the same as the way on account of which sight needs light. For just as sight is not moved by colors except when they are in act, which is not realized unless light is present since it is what draws them from potency into act, so too the imagined intentions do not move the material intellect except when the intelligibles are in act, because it is not actualized by these unless something else is present, namely, the intellect in act.[174] It was necessary to ascribe these two activities to the soul in us, namely, to receive the intelligible and to make it, although the agent and the recipient are eternal substances, on account of the fact that these two activities are reduced to our will, namely, to abstract intelligibles and to understand them. For to abstract is nothing other than to make imagined intentions intelligible in act after they were [intelligible] in potency. But to understand is nothing other than to receive these intentions. For when we found the same thing, namely, the imagined intentions, is transferred in its being from one order into another,[175] we said that this must be

174. That is, the agent intellect.

175. *Idem transferri in suo esse de ordine in ordinem.* Averroes surely has in mind al-Fârâbî's explanation in his *Letter on the Intellect*: واذا حصلت معقولات بالفعل فليس وجودها من حيث هى معقولات بالفعل هو وجودها من حيث هى صور في مواد ووجودها فى نفسها ;ليس هو وجودها من حيث هى معقولات بالفعل "But when they become intelligibles in actuality, then their existence, insofar as they are intelligibles in actuality, is not the same as their existence insofar as they are forms in matters. And their existence in themselves [as forms in matters] is not the same as their existence insofar as they are intelligibles in actuality." Al-Fârâbî, *Letter on the Intellect* (1983), 16; (1973), 216; (1974), 98. A description of this transference of intelligibles from potency to act is given in al-Fârâbî's *The Perfect State*, where he writes, "Neither in the rational power nor in what nature gives (أعطى) is there something sufficient to become by itself an intellect in actuality. Rather, to become an intellect in actuality it needs something else to transfer it (ينقلها) from potentiality to actuality. However, it becomes an intellect in actuality

from an agent cause and a recipient cause. The recipient, however, is the material [intellect] and the agent is [the intellect] which brings [this] about.

We found that we act in virtue of these two powers of intellect {440} when we wish; and nothing acts except through its form; [so] for this reason it was necessary to ascribe to us these two powers of the intellect. The intellect which is responsible for abstracting and creating the intelligible necessarily precedes in us the intellect which is to receive it. Alexander says that it is more correct to describe the intellect which is in us through its agent power, not through the patient [power], since affection and reception are common to the intellect, the senses, and discerning powers, while activity is proper to [intellect]. It is better that the thing be described through its activity.[176] I say: this would be necessary in every way only if this name affection were said in a univocal way in regard to these, but in fact it is said only equivocally.

All the things said by Aristotle in regard to this are so that the universals have no being outside the soul, [for that sort of separate being] is what Plato intended. For if it were so, then there would be no need to assert the agent intellect.

19. **And that intellect is also separate, unmixed, and impassible, and in its substance it is activity. For the agent is always more noble than the patient**

---

when the intelligibles arise in it. The intelligibles which are in potentiality become intelligibles in actuality when they come to be understood by the intellect in actuality. But they need something else to transfer them from potentiality to make them come to be in actuality. The agent which transfers them from potentiality to actuality is a certain essence the substance of which is a certain intellect in actuality and separate from matter. For this intellect gives the material intellect which is in potentiality an intellect something like light." Al-Fârâbî, *Principles of the Opinions of the People of the Virtuous City* (1985), 198–200. Translation substantially modified. Cf. *The Political Regime*, where al-Fârâbî writes that the agent intellect "makes (يجعل) the things which are not in their essences intelligible to be intelligible." It raises (يرفعها) things which are not per se intelligibles to a rank of existence higher than they possess naturally so that they are intelligibles for the human intellect in act. In this way the agent intellect causes them to become intelligibles in act for the human rational power, assisting it to reach the rank of the agent intellect, which is the end of human beings in their perfection and happiness. Al-Fârâbî, *The Political Regime* (1964), 34–35.

176. Cf. Aristotle, *Physics* 2.1, 193b7–8. I am grateful to my Marquette University colleague Owen Goldin for help with this reference to Aristotle's *Physics*. Regarding Alexander, see Alexander, *De Intellectu* (1887), 111.8–15; (1990), 53–54; (2004), 35–36. At 112.4 he writes, ἴδιον γὰρ τοῦ νοῦ τὸ ποιητικόν. *"For being productive is peculiar to intellect*, and its thinking is being active, not being affected" ([2004], 38; [1990], 55). My emphasis. خاصة العقل انه فاعل ([1971], 39.12; [1956], 195.3); "It is characteristic of the intellect that it is active [or: agent]." I am also grateful to Victor Caston for his suggestions regarding the reference of this comment by Averroes.

and the principle more noble than the matter. And knowledge in act is the same as the thing [known]. (430a17–20)

After he had explained the second kind of being of the intellect, this is the agent [intellect], he began to make a comparison between it and the material [intellect]. He said: **And that intellect is also,** etc. That is, and that intellect is also separate, as is the material [intellect], and it is also impassible and unmixed, as that. After he had recounted these things which it has in common with the material intellect, he gave the disposition proper to the agent intellect. He said: **and in its substance it is activity,** that is, there is in it no potency {441} for something, as there is in the recipient intellect potency for receiving forms. For the agent intelligence understands nothing of the things which are here. It was necessary that the agent intelligence be separate, unmixed, and impassible, insofar as it is what makes all forms intelligible. If, therefore, it were mixed, it would not make all forms, just as it was necessary that the material intellect, insofar as it is what receives all forms, also be separate and unmixed. For if it were not separate, it would have this singular form and then necessarily one of two alternatives would come about: either it would receive itself and then the mover in it would be moved, or it would not receive all the species of forms. Likewise, if the agent intelligence were mixed with matter, then it would be necessary either that it understand and create itself or that it not create all forms. What, therefore, is the difference between these two demonstrations when they are considered in reference to these [two intellects]? For they are altogether similar. The marvel is how they all concede this demonstration to be true with reference to the agent intellect and then do not agree in regard to the demonstration in reference to the material intellect, although [the demonstrations] are also altogether similar, such that it is necessary to concede one when conceding the other. We can know that the material intellect ought to be unmixed from its judgment and apprehension. For because we judge in virtue of it things infinite in number in a universal proposition—and it is evident that the judging powers of the soul, namely, mixed individual [powers], judge only finite intentions—according to the conversion of the opposite the consequence is that what does not judge finite intentions necessarily is not a mixed power of the soul. And when we have joined to this that the material intellect judges things infinite and not acquired by sense and that it does not judge finite intentions, the consequence is that it is an unmixed power. {442} Ibn Bâjjah, however, seems to concede this proposition to be true in his *Letter of Farewell*,[177] namely, that the power in virtue of which we judge with a universal judgment is infinite. But he thought this power to be the agent intel-

---

177. Ibn Bâjjah, *Letter of Farewell* (1943), 36.11–12, Spanish, 80; (1968), 138.

lect, according to the evidence of his account there. Yet it is not so, for judgment and discernment in us are ascribed only to the material intellect. Avicenna certainly used this proposition, and it is true in its own right.[178] After he had made it known that the agent intellect is different from the material [intellect] in that the agent [intellect] is always pure activity while the material is both[179] on account of the things which are here, he then gave the final cause for this. He said: **For the agent is always more noble than the patient.** That is, the former is always activity in its substance, while the latter is found in each disposition. It was already explained that the relation of the agent intellect to the patient intellect[180] is just as the relation of the moving principle in some way to the moved matter. The agent, however, is more noble than the patient and the principle [more noble] than the matter. For this reason it should be held according to Aristotle that the last of the separate intellects[181] in the hierarchy is that material intellect. For its activity is less [immaterial] than the activity of those [other separate intellects], since its activity seems more to be affection rather than activity, not because there is something else in virtue of which that intellect differs from the agent intellect other than this intention alone.[182] For just as we know the plurality of separate intellects only through the diversity of their activities, so too we know the diversity of that material intellect from the agent intellect only in virtue of the diversity of their activities. And just as it happens for the agent intellect that sometimes it acts on things existing here and sometimes not, so too it happens for [the material intellect] that sometimes it judges things existing here and sometimes {443} it does not. But they differ only in that the judgment is something in the category of the actuality of the judge, while the activity is not in that way in the category of the perfection of the agent. Therefore consider this: there is a difference between these two intellects and unless there were, there would be no divergence between them. Oh, Alexander, if this term *material intellect* had signified for Aristotle only the disposition alone, how would he make the comparison between it and the agent intellect, namely, in giving these [characteristics] which they have in common and these in which they differ? Next he said: **And knowledge in act is** the same thing **as the thing [known].** He indicates, as I figure, something

178. See Ibn Sînâ, *Kitâb al-Nafs* (1959), 206ff.; (1968), 76ff. Averroes also discusses material intellect and universal judgments in his *Incoherence of the Incoherence* (1930), 579; (1969), 358, as noted in Davidson (1992), 254.

179. That is, it is both activity and passivity or actuality and potentiality.

180. That is, the material intellect.

181. Instead of *intellectus*, I read *intellectuum* with manuscript C, following Davidson (1992), 292, n. 151.

182. That is, they are intellect but differ by way of this intention of receptivity in knowing present in material intellect.

proper to the agent intellect in which it differs from the material [intellect], namely, that knowledge in act in the agent intelligence is the same as what is known, and it is not so in the material intellect, since its intelligible is the things which are not intellects in themselves. After he had made it known that its substance is its activity, he gave the reason for this. He said:

20. **And what is in potency is prior in time in an individual, while in general it is not [prior] even in time. Nor does it sometimes understand and sometimes not understand. And when it is separate, it is what it is alone and that alone is eternally immortal. We do not remember, because that is not passible,**[183] **while the passible intellect**[184] **is corruptible, and without this nothing is understood.** (430a20–25)

That section can be understood in three ways: (1) according to the opinion of Alexander, (2) according to the opinion {444} of Themistius and the other commentators, and (3) according to the opinion which we have reported (and this one is the more obvious according to the words).

(1) For it can be understood according to Alexander that [Aristotle] meant by "intellect in potency" the disposition existing in the human compound, because the potency and disposition which is in a human being for receiving the intelligible with respect to any given individual is prior in time to the agent intellect. The agent intellect, however, is prior without qualification. When he said: **Nor is it sometimes** understanding **and sometimes not**, he means the agent intellect. When he said: **And when it is** separate, **it is what it is alone**, not mortal, he means when that intellect has been united to us and in virtue of it we understand other beings insofar as it is form for us, then this alone of the intellect's parts is not mortal. Next he said: **We do not remember**, etc. This is a question concerning the agent intellect insofar as it is united to us and we understand in virtue of it. For someone can say that when we have thought in virtue of something eternal, it is necessary that we understand in virtue of that after death as before. He said in response that this intellect is united with us only in virtue of the mediation of the material intellect [which is] generable and corruptible in us; and when that intellect has been corrupted in us, we will also not remember. Perhaps, then, Alexander expounded this section in this way, although we have not seen his exposition on this passage.

(2) Themistius,[185] however, understands by "the intellect which is in potency"

183. *Non passibilis:* ἀπαθές.

184. *Passibilis:* ὁ δὲ παθητικὸς νοῦς.

185. The account which follows is based on Themistius, *De Anima Paraphrase* (1899), 98–99; (1973), 169–181; (1996), 122–124.

the separate material intellect, whose being was demonstrated. And he intends by the intellect {445} with which he made the comparison with this the agent intellect insofar as it is conjoined with the intellect which is in potency. This is in fact the theoretical intellect according to him. And when [Aristotle] said: **Nor does it sometimes understand and sometimes not,** he understands the agent intellect insofar as it is not in contact with the material intellect. When he said: **And when it is separate, it is only what it is,** not mortal, he means the agent intellect insofar as it is form for the material intellect, and this is the theoretical intellect according to him. That question will concern the agent intellect insofar as it is in contact with the material intellect (this is the theoretical intellect), namely, when he said: **We do not remember.** For he said that it is highly unusual that this doubt on the part of Aristotle would concern the intellect except insofar as the agent intellect is a form for us. For he says that for one asserting the agent intellect to be eternal and the theoretical intellect not to be eternal, this question, namely, why we do not remember after death what we understand in life, does not arise. It is as he said, for to pose that question about the agent intellect insofar as it is acquired, as Alexander said, is highly unlikely. For the knowledge existing in us in the state of acquisition is predicated equivocally in reference to the knowledge existing through nature and instruction. That question, therefore, as it appears, is only in reference to knowledge existing through nature. For it is impossible for that question to arise except in reference to eternal knowledge existing in us either through nature, as Themistius says, or through an intelligible acquired afterward.[186] Because this question in the view of Themistius concerns the theoretical intellect and the beginning of Aristotle's account concerns the agent intellect, for this reason he held that the theoretical intellect is the agent [intellect] according to Aristotle insofar as it is in contact with the material intellect. {446} He attests to all those things on the basis of what [Aristotle] said in the first treatise concerning the theoretical intellect. For there he posed the same question as here and he resolved it by the same solution. For he said in the beginning of that book: **The intellect, however, seems to be a substance** existing in reality and **not to be** corrupted. For **if it were corrupted, then this would rather be** with **the weariness of old age.**[187] Later on he provided the way on the basis of which

186. *In postremo.* That is, as coming about in us afterwards in time.

187. **Intellect, however, seems to be a substance which comes to be in a thing and is not subject to corruption. For if it were subject to corruption, it would be more appropriate for it to undergo corruption in the feebleness which accompanies old age.** (408b18–20), Book 1, Text 65 {87}. From consideration of the Latin Text it would appear that the translator did not bother to go back to find the text and to make this translation consistent with what he did earlier. But perhaps Averroes did not bother to coordinate the statements precisely.

it is possible for the intellect to be incorruptible but understanding in virtue of it to be corruptible, and he said: Conceptualizing **and contemplating** are diverse in such a way that **something else is corrupted inside, but in itself it has no** failing. Discernment **and love are not the being of that, but rather of that** to which this belongs, **insofar as** it belongs to it. **And for this reason**, when **that is corrupted, we will not remember nor will we love.**[188] Themistius, therefore, says that [Aristotle's] account in that treatise in which [Aristotle] said, **The intellect, however, seems to be a substance existing in reality and not to be corrupted**, is the same as that in which he said this: **And when it is separate, it is only what it is**, not mortal, eternal. And what he said here: **And we do not remember, because that is not passible**, while **the passible intellect is corruptible, and without this nothing is understood**, is the same as what he said there, namely: Conceptualizing **and contemplating are distinguished**, etc. He says this on account of the fact that he meant here by **passible intellect** the concupiscible part of the soul. For that part seems to have some [share in] reason, for it listens to what the rational soul considers.

(3) Since, however, we have seen the opinions of Alexander and Themistius to be impossible and have found the words of Aristotle evident according to our {447} exposition, we believe that this is Aristotle's opinion which we voiced and that it is true in its own right. That, however, his words are clear in this section will be explained as follows. For when he said: **And that intellect is also separate, unmixed, and impassible**, he speaks of the agent intellect, and we cannot say otherwise. This word, **also**, indicates another intellect to be impassible and unmixed. Likewise, it is evident that the comparison among these is between the agent intellect and the material intellect, insofar as the material intellect has something in common with the agent [intellect] in many of those dispositions. And in this Themistius agrees with us and Alexander differs.

When he said: **And what is in potency is prior in time** to **the individual**, it can be understood in the same way for the three opinions. For according to our opinion and [that] of Themistius, the intellect which is in potency is conjoined with us before the agent intellect.[189] And according to Alexander the

---

188. Book 1 {88–89}: **To understand and to contemplate (intelligere et considerare) are distinguished when something else inside undergoes corruption, but it is in itself affected by nothing. Discerning, loving, and hating are not the being of the [intellect] but rather of this [whole human being], namely, what has [them] insofar as it has [them]. Furthermore, for this reason, when this is corrupted, we will not remember or love others.** (408b24–25)

189. Cf. Themistius, *De Anima Paraphrase* (1899), 95.9–10; (1996), 119: "Now this potential intellect comes into existence even among infants."

intellect which is in potency will be prior in us in being or generation, not according to conjoining. When he said: **while in general it is not** [so] **even in time**, he speaks about the intellect which is in potency. For when it is taken without qualification, not with respect to the individual, then it will not be prior to the agent intellect in any kind of priority, but posterior to it in all ways. That account agrees with each opinion, namely, the one saying that the intellect which is in potency is generable or [the one saying it is] not generable.

When he said: **And it** is **not sometimes** understanding **and sometimes not** understanding, it is impossible for that account to be understood according to its literal meaning, neither according to Themistius nor according to Alexander. For this phrase, **it is,**[190] when {448} he said: **And it** is **not sometimes** understanding **and sometimes not** understanding, refers according to them to the agent intellect. But Themistius, as we said, holds that the agent intellect is the theoretical [intellect], insofar as it is in contact with the material intellect. Alexander, however, holds that the intellect which is in a positive disposition (this is the theoretical [intellect]) is different from the agent intellect. And it is necessary to believe this, for the artistry is different from the artistic product and the agent different from [its] act. But insofar as it appeared to us, that account is in accord with its literal meaning and that phrase **it is** will be related to the nearest referent, which is the material intellect when it has been taken without qualification, not with reference to an individual. For it does not occur for the intellect which is called material, according to what we have said, that sometimes it understands and sometimes it does not, except in regard to the forms of the imagination existing in each individual, not with regard to the species. For instance, it does not occur for it that sometimes it understands the intelligible of horse and sometimes it does not, except with regard to Socrates and Plato. But without qualification and with regard to the species, it always understands this universal, unless the human species be altogether defunct, which is impossible. According to this the account will be according to its literal meaning. And when he said: **while in general it is not** [so] **even in time**, etc., he meant that when the intellect which is in potency is not received in reference to some individual, but is taken without qualification and in regard to any given individual, then it will not be found sometimes understanding and sometimes not, but will be found always understanding. Just as when the agent intellect is not taken in reference to some individual, then it will not be found sometimes understanding and sometimes not understanding, but will be found always to understand when it is taken without qualification; for the mode in {449} the activity of the two intellects is the same. According to this, when he said: **And when it is separate, it is only what it is,**

---

190. The Arabic is likely هو, "it," without an expressed verb, something which made it difficult for the translator to render the text literally.

not mortal, he meant: and when it is separate in this way, in this way alone is it not mortal, not insofar as it is taken in reference to the individual. His account in which he said: **and we do not remember**, etc., will be in accord with his literal meaning. For contrary to this opinion there ultimately arises a question. For one asking will say: Since the common intelligibles are not generable or corruptible in this way, why do we not remember after death any of the knowledge had in this life? It will be said to resolve this: because remembrance comes about by virtue of possible apprehensive powers, namely, material [powers]. There are three powers, the being of which was explained in *Sense and Sensibilia*, namely, the imaginative, the cogitative, and the memorative. For those three powers are in human beings for presenting the form of a thing imagined when the sense is not present. For this reason it was said there that when those three powers assist each other, perhaps they will represent the individual nature of the thing insofar as it is in its being, even though we may not sense it.[191] He meant here by **possible intellect** the forms of the imagination insofar as the cogitative power proper to human beings acts upon them. For that power is a kind of reason[192] and its activity is nothing but the placing of the intention of the form imagined in its individuality[193] in memory or the discerning of it from [the individual] in conception[194] and imagination. And it is evident that the intellect which is called material receives the imagined intentions after this discernment. That passible intellect, therefore, is necessary for conceptualization. He, therefore, rightly said: **And we do not remember, because that is not passible, while the passible intellect is corruptible, and without this nothing** understands. That is, and {450} without the imaginative power and the cogitative [power] the intellect which is called material understands nothing. For these powers are, as it were, things which prepare artistry's matter for receiving the activity of artistry. This, therefore, is one exposition.

It can be expounded in another way, and it is this: when he said: **And it** is **not sometimes** understanding **and sometimes not** understanding, he meant: when it has not been taken insofar as it understands and is informed by generable and corruptible material forms, but has been taken without qualification and insofar as it understands separate forms freed from matter, then it will not be found sometimes understanding and sometimes not understanding, but it will be found in the same form. For instance, [it will be found] in the way in virtue of which it

191. Cf. *Short Commentary on the Parva Naturalia* (1949), 54ff.; (1961), 25ff.; (1972), 40ff.

192. Themistius mentions that imagination can be called intellect in a way at Themistius, *De Anima Paraphrase* (1899), 89.27–29 and 94.27–29; (1973), 157; (1996), 112 and 118. Cf. Book 3, n. 98.

193. Literally, with its individual.

194. *Formationem*. Conceptualization, properly so called, can take place only by intellect, so here Averroes is indicating the activity of imagination or cogitation together with the material intellect.

understands the agent intellect, whose relation to it is, as we said, like that of light to the transparent. For it should be held that when it was explained that this intellect which is in potency is eternal and that it is naturally constituted to be actualized through material forms, it is [even] more fitting that it be naturally constituted to be actualized through non-material forms which are intelligible in themselves. But in the beginning it is not conjoined with us in this way but rather later on when the generation of the intellect which is in a positive disposition is actualized, as we will explain later. According to this exposition, when he said: **And when it is separate, it is only what it is**, not mortal, he indicated the material intellect insofar as it is actualized through the agent intellect, when it has been united with us in this way, then it will be separated. Perhaps he indicated the material intellect in its first conjoining with us, namely, [in] the conjoining which is through nature. He specified it through this word only in indicating the corruption of the intellect which is in a positive disposition in the way it is corruptible. And generally, when someone will consider the material intellect with the agent intellect, {451} they will appear to be two in a way and one in another way. For they are two in virtue of the diversity of their activity, for the activity of the agent intellect is to generate while that of the former is to be informed. They are one, however, because the material intellect is actualized through the agent [intellect] and understands it. In this way we say that two powers appear in the intellect conjoined with us, of which one is active and the other of the genus of passive powers.[195] How well does Alexander liken that to fire! For fire is naturally constituted to transform every body through a power existing in it, but nevertheless in the course of this it is affected in a certain way by what it transforms and is assimilated to that in some way, that is, it acquires

195. Cf. Book 3, n. 44. I am in agreement with Davidson (1992), 292, 293, 332–333, that Averroes holds for the existence of two distinct intellects. Still, the account in the *Long Commentary on the Metaphysics* is sufficiently equivocal to leave some doubt for its readers. See *Long Commentary on the Metaphysics* (1952), 1489–1490; (1962), 302M–303D; (1984), 104–105. Cf. Themistius, *De Anima Paraphrase* (1899), 108.32–34; (1973), 198.2–4; (1996), 134: "and that another [intellect] is like a combination from the potential and actual [intellects], which they posit as separate from the body, imperishable, and uncreated. These intellects are natures that in different ways are one as well as two, for what [is combined] from matter and form is one." Also cf. *Long Commentary on the Metaphysics* (1952), 1489; (1962), 302M–303D; (1984), 104: "but most commentators think that the material intellect survives and that the separate active intellect is like the form in the material intellect, as happens in the compound of matter and form, and that it is that which creates the intelligibles in a way and receives them in another way. I mean it makes them as form and receives them as material intellect." In what follows this passage of the *Long Commentary on the Metaphysics* Averroes goes on to explain that highest human happiness would be attained when the material intellect is fully actualized by the agent intellect.

from it a form less fiery than the fiery form which causes the transforming. For this disposition is precisely similar to the disposition of the agent intellect with the passible [intellect] and with the intelligibles which it generates, for it makes these in one way and receives them in another way. And in accord with this will be the account in which he said: **And we do not remember**, etc. [This is] the solution of the question which made the ancient commentators believe the intellect which is in a positive disposition to be eternal and which made Alexander hold that the material intellect is generable and corruptible. In regard to this question it was said: How are the things understood by us not eternal, while the intellect is eternal and the recipient is eternal? It is as if he says in response that the reason for this is that the material intellect understands nothing without the passible intellect, although there is an agent and there is a recipient, just as there is no apprehending of color, although there is light and there is sight, unless there is some colored thing. Then, according to whichever of those expositions it may be said, the letter [of the text] will agree with the words of Aristotle and his demonstrations without any contradiction or departure from his literal account. For this reason it is not right to use in the doctrine concerning equivocal words {452} except for these which, although they are diverse, nevertheless agree in all the intentions regarding which they can be said. He shows that he meant here by **passible intellect** the human imaginative power because of what lies in the other translation in place of what he said: **because that is not passible, while the passible intellect is corruptible**. For he says in the other translation: "And what brought us to say that this intellect is not transformed or affected is that opinion[196] belongs to the passible intellect and that it is corruptible, and does not apprehend the intelligible and nothing understands without imagination."[197] This term **intellect**, therefore, is accordingly said in this book in four ways. For it is said of the material intellect, of the intellect which is in a positive disposition, of the agent intellect, and of the imaginative power.

You ought to know that there is no difference between the exposition of Themistius and the other ancient commentators and the opinion of Plato in regard to the fact that the intelligibles existing in us are eternal and that learn-

---

196. *Existimatio*: التوهّم. The translator should have rendered this as *ymaginatio*, "imagination," as he does at the end of this quotation. But perhaps his Arabic manuscript was faulty and had الوهم.

197. (والذى دعانا الآن ﴿إلى أن﴾ قلنا إن هذا العقل لا يستحيل ولا يألم أن التوهّم هو العقل الآلم ، وإنه يفسد﴾ وليس يدرك العقل ولا يفهم شيئًا بغير توهّم). (Aristotle, *De Anima* [1954], 75); "What led us to our having said that this intellect is not passible and not undergoing affection is that the opining faculty is the intellect undergoing affection. The intellect does not apprehend nor does it understand anything without the opining faculty." This is an addition to the text of Aristotle not found in the Greek. In spite of the use of التوهّم here, Averroes understands this to denote the imagination.

ing is recollection. But Plato says that those intelligibles sometimes are in us and sometimes are not, owing to the fact that the subject is sometimes prepared for receiving them and sometimes not. They exist in themselves in this way before we receive them as well as after; and thus they are outside the soul as well as in the soul. Themistius, however, says that this, namely, that they are sometimes united and sometimes not, occurs for them due to the nature of the recipient. For he holds that the agent intellect is not naturally constituted to be conjoined with us at first except insofar as it is in contact with the material intellect. And this declination occurs for it in this way, since the conjoining with the intentions of the imagination is in one way a reception, as it were, and in another way an activity, as it were. For this reason the intelligibles are in [the material intellect] in a disposition diverse from their being in the agent intellect. Assurance {453} in regard to understanding this opinion is [found in the fact] that the reason moving Aristotle to propose the existence of the material intellect is not because here there is a produced intelligible. Rather, the reason for this is either because when there were found the intelligibles which are in us according to dispositions not in accord with the simple intelligibles, then it was said that this intellect which is in us is composed of what is in act, namely, the agent intellect, and of what is in potency. Or [it is] because the conjoining of this according to this opinion is similar to generation and is, as it were, likened to agent and patient, namely, in its conjoining with intentions of imagination. According to this opinion, therefore, the agent, the patient, and the product will be the same and it was said from those three dispositions in virtue of the diversity which occurs for it. We, however, hold that nothing moves him to impose the agent intellect except that the theoretical intelligibles are generated in the way which we said.

Therefore consider this: there is difference among the three opinions, namely, that of Plato, that of Themistius, and our opinion. According to the exposition of Themistius in regard to those intelligibles there is need only to assert the material intellect alone, or the material intellect and the agent [intellect] by analogy, for where there is no true generation, there is no agent. We agree with Alexander in regard to the way of asserting the agent intellect and we differ from him in regard to the nature of the material intellect. We differ from Themistius in regard to the nature of the intellect which is in a positive disposition and in regard to the manner of asserting the agent intellect. We also agree with Alexander in a certain way in regard to the nature of the intellect which is in a positive disposition and in another way we differ. These, therefore, are the differences by which the opinions ascribed to Aristotle are divided. You ought to know that use and exercise[198] are the causes of what appears to be the case

198. Cf. Alexander, *De Anima* (1887), 83.1–3; (1979), 107.

concerning the potency of the agent intellect which is in {454} us for separating [things] and the material intellect for receiving [things]. They are, I say, causes on account of the positive disposition existing through use and exercise in the **passible** and corruptible intellect which Aristotle called **passible**, and [which] he said plainly is corruptible. If not, it would happen that the power which is in us making the intelligibles would be material and likewise the passible power. For this reason no one can reason on the basis of this that the material intellect is mixed with the body. For what one holding it to be mixed says in response to that account in regard to the agent intellect, we [ourselves also] say in response to this in regard to the material intellect. By that intellect which Aristotle called **passible** human beings are distinguished in terms of the four powers mentioned in *The Topics*[199] which al-Fârâbî listed in his *Sophistic Refutations*.[200] By that intellect a human being differs from the other animals. And if [it were] not [for this], then it would be necessary that the conjoining of the agent intellect and the recipient would be with animals in the same way.[201] Indeed, the practical intellect differs from the theoretical in virtue of the diversity of the disposition existing in this intellect. These things having been explained, let us return to our [account] and let us say:

21. **There will, however, be conceptualizing of indivisible things in the case of those things in which there is no falsity. However, in regard to things in which there is the true and the false that [conceptualizing] is then a composition in reference to intelligible things insofar as they are beings. As Empedocles said that many heads and necks are distributed . . . ultimately in virtue of the composition of friendship. So too do separate things exist in virtue of composition, for instance, say the incommensurate and the diameter.**[202] (3.6, 430a26–31) {455}

199. "The instruments whereby we are to become well supplied with deductions are four: one, the securing of propositons; second, the power to distinguish in how many ways an expression is used; third, the discovery of the differences of things; fourth, the investigation of likenesses." *Topics* 1.13, 105a22–25, *The Complete Works of Aristotle* (1984).

200. This work is not extant. See Peters (1968), 25, n. 10. This does not seem to arise in al-Fârâbî, *Book of Sophistic Refutations* (1986).

201. Cf. {502}.

202. "The thinking of indivisibles is found in those cases where falsehood is impossible: where the alternative of true or false applies, there we always find a sort of combining of objects of thought in a quasi-unity. As Empedocles said that 'where heads of many a creature sprouted without necks' they afterwards by Love's power were combined, so here too objects of thought which were separate are combined, e.g. 'incommensurate' and diagonal." Aristotle, *De Anima* (1984). The Arabic text used by Averroes does not render explicitly the Greek ἕν in the phrase ὥσπερ ἐν ὄντων, "in a quasi-unity." Averroes' alternate translation offers a quite different understanding: والتي فيها كذب

After he had completed making known the substance of the three intellects, namely, the material, what is in a positive disposition, and the agent, he began to consider the activities and properties of intellect. This is what remained [to be considered] concerning the knowledge of that power. Because the more well-known of the differences in virtue of which the activity of the intellect is divided are two activities, one called conceptualizing and the other assent, he began here to make known the difference between these two activities.[203] He said: **There will, however, be conceptualizing of indivisible things**, etc. That is, apprehending simple incomposite things will be through intelligibles which are neither false nor true, which is called conceptualization, while apprehending composite things by [intellect] will be by virtue of intelligibles in which there is falsity and truth. He was content with the first division without the second, since opposite is understood through its opposite. Next he said: **However, in regard to things in which there is** found **the true and the false**, etc. That is, intelligibles, however, in which truth and falsity are found involve in them a certain composition made by the material intellect and the intellect which first understands singulars.[204] If, therefore, this composition is [one] befitting the being, it will be true, but if not, it will be false.[205] And that activity of the intellect upon the intelligibles is similar to what Empedocles says concerning the activity of friendship upon beings. For just as Empedocles says that many heads had been separated from necks, then friendship brought them together and composed like with like, so too the intelligibles exist first as divided in the material intellect, for instance, say **the diameter of a square** and say **the incommensurate character of the sides**. For the intellect understands those singulars first; then it composes them, namely, what is commensurate or incommensurate. If, therefore, it has composed according to being, it will be true, if not, false. {456}

22. **And if they are past or future things, then it understands time together with this and composes it. For falsity is always in composition, since when you say what is white is not white, you have already composed white with not-white, as if speaking of a white thing. And it is possible to say all these are [cases of] division. But not only is this true and false, namely, that So-**

وصدق ولها تركيب معان كأنها قائمة فى نفسه ؛ (ibid. [1954]); "In the case of things in which there is falsehood and truth and which involve the composition of intentions, it is as if they are *subsistent per se.*"

203. These are تصور, "conceptualizing," and تصديق, "assenting." Cf. *Middle Commentary* (2002), 117.14–17.

204. By "singulars" he seems to mean singular concepts. See his remarks at the end of this comment.

205. That is, it is true if it is in accord with the being of things in the world and false if not.

crates[206] is white, but additionally that he was or will be [white]. **What makes this and its like one is intellect.** (430a31–b6)

If those singular intelligibles are among things which are naturally constituted to exist either in past time or in future time, then the intellect understands together with these things the time in which they exist. Afterwards it will compose [time] with these and will judge that those things were or will be, just as it judges that the diameter is incommensurate with the side [in the case of a triangle]. Because he reported first that truth and falsity are found in composition, he began to explain that falsity is in the composition and not found in any of the activities of intellect. He said: **For falsity is always in the composition.** The reason for this is that to say in regard to a white thing that it is not white is a composition similar to saying in regard to a white thing that it is white, although that is false and this true. Since it appears that affirmation is more fitting than composition and negation than division, he said: **And it is possible to say** in regard to all these that they are [cases of] division. That is, and just as we can say negation and affirmation are composition, so too we can say that each is division, although affirmation seems more deserving of this name, {457} **composition**, and negation of this name, **division**. For in affirmation the predicate is composed with the subject, while in negation first the intellect divides the predicate from the subject and later composes them. After he had explained that truth and falsity occur in the composition of things with one another, he also explained that this same thing occurs when it composes them with time. He said: **But not only is** that **true and false**, etc. That is, both truth and falsity do not occur only in composition in the case of propositions in which the predicate is a name, but [also] in these things in which the predicate is a verb, for instance, **Socrates was** or **will be**. Next he said: **What makes this**, etc. That is, what makes these singular intelligibles one through composition after they were many is the material intellect. For [the material intellect] discerns singular intelligibles and composes similar things and divides different things. For the power apprehending simple and composite things must be the same, since the relationship of that power to the intentions of imagined forms ought to be just as the relation of the common sense to different sensibles, not as it appears from the words of Ibn Bâjjah in the beginning of his account of the rational power, namely, that the composing power ought to be different from the imaginative.[207]

206. The Greek uses Cleon instead of Socrates.

207. فالقوة التي بها تدرك الأشخاص هي القوة المتخيلة على ما تبين قبل هذا. وأما الكليات فهي لقوة أخرى (Ibn Bâjjah, *Book on the Soul* [1960], 148–149); "As shown before, the faculty by which the particulars are perceived is the imaginative faculty. But the universals belong to another faculty." (ibid. [1961], 120). That faculty to which he refers is القوة المفكرة

23. And because the indivisible is of two modes, either in potency or in act, nothing prevents it from being the case that when [the intellect] has understood length, it understands the indivisible (and that is actually indivisible) and [does so] in indivisible time. For time according to this mode is divisible and indivisible [as is the case] in regard to length. For no one can say that he understands each {458} measure to be something, since it does not exist, to the extent that it is divided, except in potency. When, however, [intellect] has thought each of those two per se, then it will divide time also and then there will be, as it were, two lengths, brought together, however, in the time which encompasses them. (430b6–14)

After he had explained that the activity of the intellect is indivisible in relation to indivisible things, he began here to explain in what way [intellect] happens to understand divisible things having quantity with indivisible intellection and in indivisible time, and in what way it happens to understand these in a divisible way and in divisible time, as is the disposition in understanding a plurality of things. He said: **And because the indivisible is**, etc. That is, and because indivisible is said in two ways, in potency and in act, it is possible to say that the intellect understands things from among divisible things in potency and indivisible things in act (as length and the implicit time which is in these is indivisible in act), and that this comes about by indivisible intellection and in indivisible time, to the extent that it understands indivisible things in each way. For it necessarily understands the indivisible intention in an indivisible way, whether that intention will have been divisible in some way or in no way [at all]. When he said: **it understands the indivisible**, etc., he means: it understands the indivisible intention—and that intelligible is indivisible— and in indivisible time. Next he said: **For time according to that mode is divisible and indivisible.** That is, for time is also found to be divisible in one way and indivisible in another way, just as in the case of length. And when he explained that the intellect understands magnitude and time and generally everything which is indivisible in act and {459} divisible in potency, through an indivisible intellection and in indivisible time, he also explained that it is impossible for someone to say that understanding such things comes about through a divisible intellection and in divisible time. He said: **No one can say**, etc. That is, no one, therefore, can say that when the intellect understands a line, it does not immediately understand it, but first one part and then another. For those two parts are not two in act in the line until the line is divided, but rather they are only two in potency. And when he said **each measure**, he meant

---

([1960], 148), "the cogitative power," as I render it in the present translation, or "the thinking faculty" ([1961], 119).

each part of the line. [It is] as if he says: no one, therefore, can say that when the intellect understands a line, first it understands each part per se, then the whole. For those two parts do not exist in act until the line is divided, but rather they are two in potency. Next he said: **When, however, it will have understood each**, etc. That is, but it happens to understand each part of the length per se when it divides the length; then it understands that length just as it understands two lengths. He understood this when he said: **and** then there are, as it were, two lengths. Next he said: **brought together, however,** etc. That is, when, however, it understands these things which have been brought together, that is, the parts, and [understands them] as one length, it understands these in the same indivisible time and in the same instant in which they at once exist, not in two diverse instants. He meant this when he said (as it seems to me): **in the time which encompasses them.**

24. **But what is not indivisible in quantity but in form it understands in indivisible time and through an indivisible [aspect] of the soul, and [it does so] accidentally. But those two are divisible, namely, that in virtue of which it understands and the time in which it understands, because they are [themselves] {460} indivisible.**[208] **For even in these two there is something indivisible, but it is more fitting that it not be separable. It is what makes time to be one and length to be one. This is in a similar mode in everything continuous, both in time and in length.** (430b14–20)

After he had explained the way in which the intellect understands what is indivisible in quantity (this is what is indivisible in act and divisible in potency), he began also to explain the way in which it understands what is indivisible in form (this is what is indivisible in act and in potency, except accidentally). He said: **But what is not indivisible,** etc. That is, but what is indivisible in form and quality, not quantity (since indivisible is said in these two ways), is apprehended by the intellect in indivisible time and by an indivisible intellection. Next he said: **But [it does so] accidentally,** etc. That account is shortened and transposed, and it ought to be read in this way: but those two are divisible not essentially, but accidentally, namely, the time in which it under-

208. The Arabic text is faulty here, as Averroes is well aware. See {460}. The corresponding Greek has κατὰ συμβεβηκὸς δέ, καὶ οὐχ ᾗ ἐκεῖνα διαιρετὰ ὃ νοεῖ καὶ ἐν ᾧ χρόνῳ, ἀλλ' ᾗ ἀδιαίρετα· ἔνεστι γὰρ κἂν τούτοις τι ἀδιαίρετον. "But that which thought thinks of and the time in which it thinks are in this case divisible only incidentally and not as such. For in them too there is something indivisible." Aristotle, *De Anima* (1984). The alternate translation paraphrases the text: ﻻ كتلك ، ﻭ» بالعرض يتجزأ (ibid. [1954]); "<and> is divisible accidentally, not like these parts by which the intellect perceives, for in them is what is indivisible."

stands and the thing which is thought or by which it understands. Next he provided the reason for the fact that they are divisible accidentally. He said: **because they are [themselves] indivisible**, etc., that is, because the time in which it understands and the thing which it understands are indivisible in their own right, but they are nevertheless in divisible things, namely, the instant in which it understands and the form which it understands. For an instant is indivisible and is in time which is divisible; and the form is also indivisible and is in a magnitude which is divisible. Next he said: **For even in these [. . .] there is something indivisible**, that is, [indivisible] in magnitude and in time. Next he said: **but it is more fitting that it not be separable.** That is, but {461} what is indivisible in time and in magnitude is not separable from these, and for this reason it was divisible accidentally. Next he said: **It is what makes time to be one**, etc. That is, this indivisible [nature] existing in those things makes length to be one and time to be one. If not, then here neither one length nor one time would be understood, if this nature were not in them. This nature, therefore, is the cause for those things being one while they are also divisible. And because they are in those things, for this reason they happen to be divisible accidentally. That this nature is existent in those material things is the reason that understanding was one in time. This is the sum of what he intended in this section. Next he said: **This is in a similar mode in everything continuous**, etc. That is, that nature exists in a similar mode, namely, in time and length and in other species, inseparable from that in which it exists. For if it were separate, then division would not occur accidentally.

25. **The point, however, and every difference and what is indivisible in this way, are understood as an accident.**[209] **And so too for other things, for instance, how it knows blackness and what is black,**[210] **for it knows it through the contrary, as it were. And what knows in potency ought to be one in its own right.**[211] **If, therefore, there is something among things in which there**

209. For the Latin *quasi accidens*, the Greek has ὥσπερ ἡ στέρησις. "Points and similar instances of things that divide, themselves being indivisible, are realized in consciousness *in the same manner as privations.*" Aristotle, *De Anima* (1984); emphasis added. The alternate Arabic renders this sufficiently with العدم (ibid. [1954]); "privation." Averroes' remarks about an omission in the manuscript seem to refer to an omission of the Arabic corresponding to ἡ στέρησις. The Latin *accidens* may reflect العرض for العدم.

210. The Greek has οἷον πῶς τὸ κακὸν γνωρίζει ἢ τὸ μέλαν. "e.g. how evil or black is cognized." Aristotle, *De Anima* (1984). The alternate translation has كيف يعرف العقل السواد والأسود؟ (ibid. [1954]); "How does the intellect know the black or the dark?"

211. The corresponding Greek has δεῖ δὲ δυνάμει εἶναι τὸ γνωρίζον καὶ ἐνεῖναι ἐν αὐτῷ. "That which cognizes must be its objects potentially, and they must be in it." Aristotle, *De Anima* (1984). This part of the paraphrasing alternate translation reflects

is no contrariety, that understands itself alone and is in act [and] separate. (430b20–26)

After he had explained how the intellect understands things indivisible in act and divisible in potency, namely, magnitudes, and how also it understands things essentially indivisible [and] divisible accidentally, namely, qualities and forms, he began here to explain also how it understands indivisible things neither essentially nor {462} accidentally nor in potency nor in act, for instance, the point, the instant, and unity. He said: **The point, however,** etc. That is, to understand the point, however, and its like among the things which are said to be indivisible, and generally every privative difference, is accidental, namely, insofar as it happens to lack a thing [of which it is] deprived. For the point is understood only insofar as there occurs for it a privation of the divisibility existing in magnitude. Likewise with respect to the instant and the rest. Next he said: And in this way **it knows blackness and what is black;** for **it knows through the contrary, as it were.** A blank space falls in the manuscript in this way, namely, between the phrase **in [this] way** and **it knows.** The account is complete per se, but if something is lacking, perhaps it is this: and in this way the intellect or sight knows blackness or what is black.[212] Generally all privations are known only through contraries, namely, through the knowledge of a positive disposition and through knowledge of the lack of a positive disposition. Here he meant by blackness the privation of whiteness. For just as it is concerning the senses in regard to those things, so too is it concerning the intellect. For just as it was said there that sight apprehends darkness through apprehension of the lack of light, so too the intellect apprehends privation through apprehension of the lack of form. Next he said: **And what knows in potency ought to be one in its own right.** That is, the intellect knowing the positive disposition and its privation must be the same power in itself, just as

---

ويجب أن تكون المعرفة بحد قوة ، وإن أشياء لم يكن فيها ضدٌّ :the Greek ibid.) [1954]).

212. This comment may be one of an Arabic copyist or the Latin translator referring to "And in this way *it knows*." But it may be something reflected from consideration of the alternate translation quoted in n. 210.

The following account seems to be the result of Averroes' reading Themistius, *De Anima Paraphrase* (1899), 111.18–23; (1973), 203.7–12, "For to the intellect, as much as to sense-perception, there are some objects of thought that [occur] in respect of a [direct] encounter (*kat'epibolên*) where [the intellect] also grasps their nature, others that [occur] in respect of privation and abstraction. For just as for sense-perception white and light [occur] in respect of a [direct] encounter, and black and darkness in respect of privation (and for hearing sound in respect of a [direct] encounter, silence in respect of privation), so too for the intellect good depends on a [direct] encounter, bad on privation." Ibid. (1996), 137.

what knows darkness and light is the same power of sight. [It is necessary] that this knowing power apprehend privation by apprehending in itself being in potency, since it is in potency when it apprehends each in itself, namely, being in potency and being in act. And that is the disposition of the material intellect. Can we say, therefore, {463} that such a thing is the disposition alone and nothing else, as Alexander said? Next he said: **If, therefore, there is something among things**, etc. That is, if, therefore, there is some intellect in which there is no potency contrary to the act existing in it, that is, if there is some intellect which is not found sometimes understanding in potency and sometimes understanding in act, then that intellect will not understand privation at all. Rather, it will understand nothing outside itself. This is one of these things by which this intellect is distinguished from the agent intellect, namely, that in this intellect each is found, while in the agent [intellect] only act [is found], not potency. For this reason Aristotle rightly called that intellect material, not because it is mixed and has matter, as Alexander held.

26. **Both stating something of something, such as affirmation, and every composite [statement], is true or false. Not every sort of understanding is true, but [only] that which states the quiddity of the thing, not what [just] states something of something. But just as proper activities are true, while whether a white thing is a human being is not always true,[213] so likewise is the disposition of what is separate from matter.** (430b26–31)

To predicate something of something by intellect, such as affirmation and negation, is a composition by the activity of intellect. Every composed [predication] is true or false. In the material intellect, therefore, truth and falsity are always found mixed together. This is proper to this intellect.

Next he began to explain that this is not proper to all the activities of that intellect, but only to the activity which is called {464} assent, not intellective conceptualization. He said: **Not every sort of understanding**, etc. That is, truth and falsity are not found mixed together in every activity of that intellect, but [rather] the activity which is conceptualization is always true, not the activity which involves predicating something of something. Next he began to recount that what occurs for intellect is similar to what occurs for sense and that there is the same reason for this. He said: **But just as proper activities,**

213. The corresponding Greek ἀλλ᾽ ὥσπερ τὸ ὁρᾶν τοῦ ἰδίου ἀληθές, εἰ δ ἄνθρωπος τὸ λευκὸν ἢ μή, οὐκ ἀληθὲς ἀεί. "But, just as while the seeing of the special object of sight can never be in error, seeing whether the white object is a man or not may be mistaken." Aristotle, *De Anima* (1984). Apparently τὸ ὁρᾶν, "the seeing," was omitted from this text of Aristotle at some stage in the transmission or translation. Again, it is curious that Averroes did not consult his alternate translation, which renders the Greek adequately.

etc. That is, but the reason for this is the same as the reason in the case of sense. Activities proper to sight, namely, apprehending color, are true for the most part, while sensing the white thing to be Socrates or Plato is not always true but rather frequently falsity occurs in that case. This will likewise be [the case for] the disposition of intellect, namely, that it is always true in its proper activity. For assent occurs for it only because its intelligible is material, that is, composite. When he said: **so too is the disposition of what is separate from matter**, he meant: so too is the disposition of the material intellect which is separate from matter in regard to its activities of apprehension, namely, because it is correct in regard to things proper to it, namely, in conceptualization, and false in regard to things which are not proper. This can be understood in this way: so too is the disposition of intellects whose intelligible is separate from matter, in that they are always correct, since in them no activity which is accidental is found because their intelligible is separate from matter.[214]

27. **Knowledge which is in act is the thing itself. And what is in potency is prior in time to the individual, but universally not even in time.** {465} **For everything which is generated is generated by what is in act.** (3.7, 431a1–4)

Knowledge which is in act is the known object itself. Knowledge which is in potency is for the individual prior in time to knowledge which is in act. But universally and without qualification knowledge which is in potency is not prior to knowledge which is in act, since knowledge which goes out from potency into act is generated and everything generated is generated by what belongs in act to the species of that generated thing. Hence, it is necessary that knowledge which is in act be prior in every way to knowledge which is in potency. Perhaps he meant here by this account to indicate the reason why the apprehension belonging to the separate intellects is conceptualization only and truth in these is never mixed with falsity. It is the case that knowledge belonging to these [separate intellects] is the known object itself in every way, contrary to the disposition in regard to things known by the material intellect.

28. **We see the sensible make the sense to be in act after it was in potency and [to do so] without suffering an alteration. For this reason [sensation] is a different kind of motion. For motion is the activity of what is imperfect, while activity without qualification is a different [kind of] motion and is the activity of what is perfected. It seems, therefore, that to sense is similar to something being said only in words and to something being understood**

214. Note that, perhaps due to his faulty text, Averroes transforms Aristotle's epistemological generalization into a metaphysical account of the material intellect and any other separate intellect which apprehends an intelligible separate from matter.

by intellect. If, therefore, it is pleasant or unpleasant, as an affirmation or negation of it, it will be pursued or avoided. (431a4–10)

What he wants here to provide concerning the disposition of that power, namely, of the rational power, is more on account of its similarity to sense, {466} for these things in which they are similar are more evident in the case of sense than in the case of intellect. First he began to compare these things in the thing which is called motion and affection in them. He said: **We see** the sensible **make**, etc. That is, we see the sensible make what senses to be in act after it was in potency, not in such a way that what senses, at going out from potency into act, is transformed or altered as material things going out from potency into act are transformed. For this reason it should be held that there is a kind of motion and affection different from the kind which is in movable things. For this reason what was said in regard to the intellect, namely, that there is a going out from potency into act without change and without alteration, is not unthinkable. Next he said: **For motion is the activity of what is imperfect,** etc. That is, the reason why change and alteration occur for that motion but not for the other is because that motion, for which change occurs, is an activity not perfected and a process toward something complete, while the other is a perfect activity or rather something complete. It is as if he meant that since it is so, the fact that understanding is an imperfect activity happens for it on account of matter, not insofar as it is an activity. Since this happens for the activity, it is necessary that there be some activity free from this accident. For what happens to something accidentally must not belong to it insofar as it is what it is, and if it will not have belonged to it insofar as it is what it is, then it is necessarily separate from it. What he brought up here is, as it were, the solution of the greatest of all the questions arising in reference to this opinion. For someone can say: How can we imagine reception in a substance unmixed with matter when it was explained that the reason for reception is matter? It is as if he indicated {467} the solution in saying that matter is not the reason for the reception without qualification, but the reason for the changeable reception, namely, of the reception on the part of this individual being. Hence it is necessary that what does not receive by way of an individual reception not be material in any way.[215] In this way there remains no room for the question. When he had explained the kind of similarity between sense and intellect in this kind of affection and motion, namely, that in each there is perfect activity, he began to make known the similarity between sensing and understanding. He said: **therefore to sense is similar to something** being said **only in words and to something being understood by intellect.** That is, sensing, which is per se a perfect activity and without time, and without it being the case that an in-

---

215. Cf. {441}.

complete activity precedes it, is similar to understanding an intelligible intention when that intention is expressed by another, namely, because a perfect
activity comes about from this, without it being the case that an incomplete
activity precedes it. It is as if he meant by this to explain the reason why the
intellect understands without time. Next he said: **If, therefore, it is pleasant**,
etc. That is, if, therefore, that which is apprehended is pleasant or unpleasant
to the sense, it will be just as the intellect affirms this to be this or denies [it by
asserting] that this is not this. Then either it will be pursued or fled in virtue
of an intellectual apprehension, just as a thing will be pursued or fled in virtue
of a sensible apprehension.

29. **Feeling pleasure or feeling pain are activities with respect to a sensible
mean concerning good or bad insofar as they are such. This is to desire and
to avoid, which exist in act. What desires and what avoids do not differ** {468}
from one another nor from what senses, but the being differs. (431a10–14)

Feeling pain and feeling pleasure on the part of the soul is an activity belonging to it through the mediation of the sensitive power. Its motion in this
way concerns the good or bad insofar as the bad is painful and the good
pleasant, not insofar as the good is good and the bad bad, just as is the disposition in the intellect's seeking or avoiding. Next he said: **This is to desire and
to avoid, which exist in act.** That is, this is to desire and avoid a present thing
insofar as it is present and individual, namely, sensible desire. For this is
proper to sensible desire, namely, that it be moved only with the presence of
the object sensible in act, contrary to intellectual desire. Next he said: **What
desires and what avoids** are not diverse, etc. That is, the part of the soul which
pursues and flees is the same part, not two diverse ones, neither in the case of
intellect nor in the case of sense, but it is the same part in subject and diverse
ones in activity. He meant this when he said: but the being differs. He means
by this the concupiscible soul.

30. **In the sensitive soul**[216] **are found images according to the modes of the
senses. When we say in regard to something that it is bad or good not**[217] **ac-**

216. The corresponding Greek has τῇ δὲ διανοητικῇ ψυχῇ: "the thinking soul."
Aristotle, *De Anima* (1984). In his Comment Averroes prefers the alternate translation,
which is closer to the Greek: عند النفس الناطقة (ibid. [1954]); "in the rational [or: reason-
ing] soul."

217. *Non* occurs here without any corresponding negation in the Greek: "(and when
it asserts or denies them to be good or bad it avoids or pursues them)." Aristotle, *De
Anima* (1984). This problem does not occur in the alternate translation, which itself is
less than a clear rendering of the Greek. Averroes' Comment shows no awareness of
the problem.

cording to affirmation and negation, then we either pursue or avoid [it]. For this reason the soul understands nothing without imagination. (431a14–17)

In the sensitive soul, that is, in the common sense, images are found the modes of which are according to the modes of the senses {469} and the sensibles such that the relation of those images to the material intellect is just as the relation of sensibles to the senses. This is found in a more evident way in the other translation. For it says: "In the rational soul, however, the image is, as it were, the sensible things."[218] Next he said: **When we say in regard to** a thing, etc. That is, when the rational soul discerns an image and judges it to be good or bad not insofar as it is known to be such or not such alone (this is the difference proper to the theoretical intellect), then the concupiscible soul either will pursue that, if the rational soul has judged its image to be good, or will avoid [it], if [it has judged its image to be] bad. This is similar to what happens for sense with what is painful and what is pleasant. Next he said: **For this reason the soul understands nothing without imagination.** That is, because the relation of the images to the material intellect is just as the relation of the sensibles to sense, for this reason it was necessary that the material intellect not understand any sensible without imagination. In this he says expressly that universal intelligibles are gathered with images and corrupted with their corruption. He also expressly says that the relation of the intelligibles to images is just as the relation of color to the colored body, not as the relation of color to the sense of sight as Ibn Bâjjah thought.[219] But the intelligibles are the intentions of forms of the imagination separated from matter. For this reason they necessarily need in this [sort of] being to have matter different from the matter which they used to have in the forms of the imagination. This is self-evident to those who give it consideration. If the imagined intentions were receptive of intelligibles, then the thing would receive itself and the mover would be the moved. Aristotle's explanation that it is necessary that there be in the material intellect none of the intentions existing in act or there [not] have been {470} an intention intelligible in act or in potency, is sufficient to refute the opinion. But what made that man err, and us too for a long time, is that modern thinkers set aside the books of Aristotle and consider the books of the commentators, and chiefly in the case of the soul, in their believing that this book is impossible to understand. This is on account of Avicenna, who followed Aristotle only in dialectics,

---

218. *Apud autem animam rationabilem ymago est quasi res sensibiles*: وأما عند النـفـس الـناطقة فالتخييلى بمنزلة الأشياء المحسوسة (Aristotle, *De Anima* [1954]); "In the rational soul image forming is in place of the sensible things." التـخـييـلـى is Badawi's correction of the manuscript's التخييل, but in this note I translate the Arabic manuscript reading.

219. This is likely a reference to a discussion in the account of the rational soul in Ibn Bâjjah, *Book on the Soul* (1960), (1961), which is incomplete in manuscript.

but in other things he erred, and chiefly in the case of metaphysics. This is because he began, as it were, from his own perspective.

31. **[This is] just as air is what makes the organ of sight to be of such a disposition, and this [follows] from something else; and [it is] similarly so in the case of hearing. For what is last in this is one and the same thing and one and the same mean, while in being it is many. It had already been said earlier what it is in virtue of which we judge that sweet differs from hot or cold. Let us speak, therefore, as follows. For just as it is the same in being, so is it in definition.**[220] (431a17–22)

After he had explained the similarity between intellect and sense in reference to the need for a subject from which they receive the intentions which they apprehend, he began now to explain that the relation of that material intellect to the images numbered according to the species of sensibles is just as the relation of the common sense to diverse sensibles. He said: **[This is] just as air**, etc. That is, it was explained that air moves the organ of sight and is moved by another, and likewise the organ of hearing is moved by air, and air by another, until the motion passes {471} in all sensibles to one final [point] which is in relation to those motions as a point which is the center of a circle with lines going out from the circumference. It is likewise concerning the material intellect with the intelligible intentions of images. Next he said: **For** what is ultimate **is one . . . and the mean is one.** That is, for the last of the sensible motions is one and of these what is, as it were, the center of a circle is also one (this is the common sense). Next he said: **it was already said earlier**, etc. That is, it was said earlier generally what that is in virtue of which we judge the diversity of diverse sensibles, for instance, the diversity of sweet from hot and of color from sound. Therefore in that way by which there followed there that such be the case in regard to sense, it is necessary that it be [likewise so] here in apprehending things of diverse images by intellect. He meant this when he said: **For just as it is** one **in being, so is it in definition.** That is, for it was shown by the aforementioned account that just as what judges diverse being in reference to sense ought to be one, so too what judges the images of diverse things ought to be one. It can be understood in this way: just as in the being of diverse things there is one intention which makes what apprehends these to be one—this is the relation which the comprehensive power takes up when it makes a comparison between two different things—so too in diverse images there is one intention which makes what judges these to be one. It can be understood in this way: that

---

220. ἔστι γὰρ ἕν τι, οὕτω δὲ ὡς ὁ ὅρος. "That with which it does so is a sort of unity, but in the way a boundary is" is the rather interpretive translation in Aristotle, *De Anima* (1984).

is, the reason for this, namely, for the similarity between intellect and sense in regard to this, is that just as in this singular being there is one which is a being according to sense, so too in the imagined object there is one according to intellect {472} which is what is imagined. When there will have been many things according to what is imagined, many things will be in the imagination. This is more in agreement with the account which follows.

32. **This is found in proportional numbers and its disposition in them is just as their disposition with respect to one another. For there is no difference between a shape and a quality in the consideration of things unequal in genus or of contrary things, for instance, of white and black. The disposition, therefore, of A (white) toward B (black), and of C to D, is just as the disposition of those to one another, as it is found in contrary things. If, therefore, C and D, existing in the same thing, are found only in virtue of A and B, they are the same in this. If A will have been sweet, for instance, and B white, for instance, then the intellect will be understanding, as it were. For it understands the forms through the first imaginings.** (431a22–b2)

This evident consequence is found in these according to their proportionality in number. The disposition of the part of the soul which judges in the case of each being, namely, the sensible and the imaginable, is just as the disposition of each being with respect to one another. Next he said: **For there is no difference**, etc. That is, it makes no difference whether the judgment will have been about contrary things or diverse things. For shape and quality in the consideration ought to be one and the same with the sensitive and rational power in things diverse in genus and contraries. When he had explained that there is no difference in the consideration of those two kinds in the case of the sensitive and rational power, he gave a demonstration of this from the proportionality {473} and equality which they have in number, namely, the images of things with their individuals. He said: **The disposition, therefore, of A (white)**, etc. That is, there is, therefore, A (white) and B (black), and C (an image of white) and D (an image of black); the proportion, therefore, A to B will be just white to black, and the proportion of C to D [will be] as the image of white to the image of black. He meant this when he said, as it seems to me: the disposition **of C to D, is just as the disposition of those to one another, as it is found in** two contraries, that is, as it is found in two contraries from true images. When he had explained that they ought to have such a proportionality, drawing the consequence he gave the conclusion. He said: **If, therefore, C and D**, etc. That is, since the proportion of A to B is as C to D, and A and B are apprehended by the same power, therefore C and D ought to be apprehended by the same power. He leaves that conclusion out of his account. Next he gave what follows upon that. He said: **If, therefore, C and D**, etc. That is, if C and D are apprehended by the same power because

A and B are of the same power, then the two powers in this intention and in this way are the same and they do not differ at all, although they do differ in their natures. In virtue of the analogy between the rational power and the sensitive power many of the ancients thought, according to what Aristotle reported in the second treatise, that the two powers are the same. When he had explained that the disposition of these in apprehending contrary things is the same, he also explained that it is so in apprehending things different in genus. He said: **if A will have been sweet, for instance**, etc. That is, if we put in place of the contraries two things different in genus, for instance, sweet and white, {474} then the intellect will also apprehend these in a way similar to the apprehension of these by sense. For then it will understand the forms of these with the mediation of their first images, that is, true [images], just as sense apprehends the intentions of these through the presence of sensible individuals themselves.

33. It is so concerning what is pursued and what is avoided according to this determined pattern in these things. Sometimes it is moved without the use of sense, when it is existing in the imagination, as when it is imagined that a fire is lit in the towers of cities. For it is commonly thought that the moving thing is fire and it is a signal for the soldier.[221] For one cogitates,[222] as it were, that one sees a thing in virtue of the ways of the imagination, and cogitation of it in reference to future things is according to things present. (431b3–8)

It is so for the intellect with respect to what is pursued and what is avoided as it is with respect to apprehension. For just as it apprehends things by me-

---

221. οἶον αἰσθανόμενος τὸν φρυκτὸν ὅτι πῦρ, τῇ κοινῇ γνωρίζει, ὁρῶν κινούμενον, ὅτι πολέμιος. "E.g. perceiving by sense that the beacon is fire, it recognizes in virtue of the general faculty of sense that it signifies an enemy, because it sees it moving." Aristotle, *De Anima* (1984). The Latin *principium preliatori*, "signal for the soldier," corresponds to منذرة بالحرب (ibid. [1954]); "a signal for war" or "a battlefield signal" in the alternate translation. The sense of *principium* here in the Latin seems to be that of a signal or a first event which initiates action.

222. Note that *cogitat* corresponds to λογίζεται and *cogitatio . . . est* to βουλεύεται at 431b7–8. This Text omits rendering the Greek ἐν τῇ ψυχῇ and ἢ νοήμασιν, which I emphasize in the following translation. Aristotle, *De Anima* (1984) renders this sentence as follows: "But sometimes by means of the images *or thoughts which are within the soul*, just as if it were seeing, it calculates and deliberates what is to come by reference to what is present." The alternate translation, which is less literal and appears also to omit ἐν τῇ ψυχῆ, renders this as the protasis in a sentence which has as its apotasis the initial sentence of the Text which follows. فأما إذا صار إلى التفكر والارتياء فيما يأتى وفيما حضر. . . . (ibid. [1954]); "When it comes to cogitate and give consideration to what it is going to do and what is presently the case. . . ."

diating forms of images and sense apprehends in virtue of the presence of sensible things, so too intellect is moved by things to pursue or avoid when the forms of their images are present, just as sense pursues or avoids in the presence of its sensible [object]. Next he said: **Sometimes it is moved without the use of sense**, etc. That is, for this reason a human being is moved toward something, although he does not sense it, when he imagines it, just as the soldier is moved when he imagines fire to be lit in the towers, although the fire {475} has not yet been lit. Next he said: **For it is commonly thought that the thing moving is fire and it is a signal for the soldier.** That is, when the soldier will internally imagine the fire in the towers, immediately he will cogitate about putting that fire out and the opposed soldier [will immediately cogitate] about kindling it. They have a common cogitation, namely, in that the fire is the end set forth and sought on their parts, but in two different ways. What he said can be understood: **For it is commonly thought**, etc., that is, for the common proposition from which we can know all the things which follow is the first consequence of the existence of the fire in the towers. For this reason he said: **it is a signal**, in virtue of experiences of the soldier, that is, a signal for consideration. Next he said: **For one cogitates, as it were**, as one who is seeing. That is, for the signal, for his cogitation in regard to things will be in presenting the kinds of images of possible imaginings as existing in regard to that thing concerning which it cogitates, to the extent that it is as if he were to see that concerning which he cogitates. Next he said: **and cogitation of it in reference to future things**, etc. That is, the reason for this is because a human being puts the starting point of his consideration of possible things in present things which he sees. For this reason it is possible for a human being to cogitate in regard to some thing to the extent that he will find from this some individual thing which he will not have sensed before, but he will have sensed its like, not the very same thing. He indicates in virtue of this how there can be found through cogitation a true image of which the individual [instance] never had been sensed by someone cogitating. For he had already asserted that true images are numbered according to individual sensibles. It is as if he is explaining that this kind of imagining is found by cogitating on the basis of imaginings which are individual sensibles. {476} For, as was explained in *Sense and Sensibilia*, when the cogitative power draws aid for itself from the informative and the memorative [powers],[223] it is naturally constituted to present on the basis of the images of things something which it never sensed, in the same

223. See *On Memory* 1, 449b31–450a25. Also see *Short Commentary on the Parva Naturalia* (1949), 53ff.; (1961), 24ff.; (1972), 39ff. The three powers are those of cogitation, memory, and imagination. I translate the Latin *informativa* as "informative," but in the mind of Averroes it clearly refers to the power of the imagination.

disposition according to which it would exist if it had sensed it, by means of
assent and conceptualization. Then the intellect will judge those images with
a universal judgment. The intention of cogitation[224] is nothing but this, namely,
that the cogitative power presents a thing absent from sense as if it were a
sensed thing. For this reason things able to be apprehended by human beings
are divided into these two, namely, into the apprehensible which has as its
principle sense and the apprehensible which has as its principle cogitation. We
have already said that the cogitative power is neither the material intellect nor
the intellect which is in act,[225] but it is a particular material power. This is evident
from the things said in *Sense and Sensibilia*.[226] It is necessary to know this, since
the custom is to ascribe the cogitative power to the intellect. It should not be
the case that someone says that the cogitative power composes the singular
intelligibles. It was already explained that the material intellect composes them.
For cogitation is only for discerning individual instances among those intelligibles and to present them in act as if they were present in sensation. For this
reason when they are present in sensation, then cogitation will cease and the
activity of intellect in regard to them will remain. On the basis of this it will be
explained that the activity of intellect is different from the activity of the cogitative power, which Aristotle called the passible intellect and which he said is
generable and corruptible. This is evident concerning this [power], since it has
a determinate organ, namely, the middle chamber of the brain. A human being
is not generable and corruptible except in virtue of this power and without this
power and the imaginative power {477} the material intellect understands nothing. For this reason, as Aristotle says, we do not remember after death, not
because the intellect is generable and corruptible, as one can believe.

34. **When you have judged that something pleasant is here or there, then
something unpleasant will be either avoided or pursued, and so universally
in regard to actions. For falsity and truth are not involved in operation.
They both are in the same genus as also is the case in regard to what is good
and in regard to what is evil, but there is a difference because it is said
absolutely and in a limited way.[227]** (431b8–12)

224. That is, this is the meaning of cogitation in the present context. The cogitative
power is used both in apprehension and, as here, in the practical process of seeking out
individuals of a certain kind.

225. That is, the agent intellect.

226. See *On Memory* 449b31–450a25. Also see *Short Commentary on the Parva Naturalia* (1949), 55–56; (1961), 25; (1972), 41.

227. "That too which involves no action, i.e. that which is true or false, is in the same
province with what is good or bad: yet they differ in this, that the one is absolute and
the other relative to someone." Aristotle, *De Anima* (1984). The Greek ἥ seems perhaps

When you have judged by sense that something pleasant is here or there, then something unpleasant before the intellect will be either fled if the intellect has thought that this is evil or pursued if it has thought that this is good. It happens universally in this way for the intellect [working together] with sense in regard to all actions, namely, either to contradict this by seeing that something unpleasant is good and by seeking that which sense fled, or to be in agreement with sense by seeing that something pleasant is good. Next he said: **For falsity and truth are not involved in operation. They are . . . in the same genus.** A blank space was here in the manuscript. It could be: **For falsity and truth are**, etc., that is, for falsity and truth existing in the theoretical intellect are different from falsity and truth existing in the practical intellect.[228] Next he said: **They both are in the same genus as also is the case in regard to what is good and in regard to what is evil.** It can be understood that these two are in the same genus because each is a [sort of] knowledge and because truth is in the genus of what is good and falsity in the genus of what is evil. What he said, {478} **in regard to what is good and what is evil**, can be understood such that it is an exposition of what he said: **They are . . . in the same genus.** It is as if he says: they are in the same genus, that is, in regard to what is good and what is evil. When he had explained that both are united under [the notion of] the good and the evil, he explained what distinguishes them. He said: **but there is a difference**, etc. That is, but nevertheless they are distinct, because truth is in the theoretical intellect as absolutely good and falsity is in it as evil without qualification. Truth in the practical intellect is what is good[229] in a certain respect and conditionally (he meant this when he said: **and particular**), while falsity is what is evil with respect to that end which should be found

---

to have been lost, with the result that the Arabic translator understood the sentence as we have it above. It is not clear why Averroes apparently refrained from consulting the alternate translation, which renders the Greek accurately.

228. There are some Arabic fragments which correspond rather generally albeit unclearly to Book 3, 34.18–20: قول عوضه فأما الصدق والكذب فانهما يوجدان ‹في العقل النظري› في جنس آخر. . . غير الجنس العملي (*Long Commentary* Fragments [1985], 45). "a repetitive statement, for the true and the false both exist in the theoretical intellect in another kind . . . not the practical kind."

229. Some Arabic fragments correspond generally to Book 3, 34.28–33: جنس واحد لأن الصدق يقع تحت جنس الخير والكذب تحت جنس الشر. ثم قال : «لكنهما يفترقان» أي أن الصدق في العقل النظري خير مطلق والكذب فيه شر على الاطلاق فاطلاق الخير في العملي خير (*Long Commentary* Fragments [1985], 45); "one genus because the true falls under the genus of the good and the false falls under the genus of the evil. Then he said: **but they are distinguished**, that is, the true in the theoretical intellect is unconditioned good and the false in it is evil without qualification. So the unqualified nature of the good in the practical [intellect] is good."

[existing]. It can be understood in virtue of what he said: **and particular**, that is, in virtue of an end, namely, they are distinct because one is good without qualification and the other is good with respect to a given end. The closest intention is [to be found] in those two.

35. **It also knows things which are said by way of negation,**[230] **insofar as snub-nosed qua snub-nosed is indivisible. But in the case of what is concave, if the intellect has understood, then it will understand the intention of concavity denuded of flesh. But mathematical intentions are not [the same as] singular things in this way.** (431b12–16)

He means by **things which are said by way of negation** mathematical things. He means by negation separation from matter. He means that when the intellect understands things in separation from matter, it does not do this {479} because they in themselves are not in matter, as some have thought. But what it does, namely, that it understands these things as not in matter although they are in matter, is as if it were understanding snub-nose, insofar as it is snub-nose, separate from matter. But it is impossible for snub-nose insofar as it is snub-nose to be separate from matter. It is possible, however, for its genus, which is concavity, to be distinct from matter. He indicates by this that this possibility in reference to the separation of those by the intellect is consequent upon their natures and quiddities, not because it happens that they are not in matter. Next he said: And **mathematical intentions**, etc. That is, the mode of being of mathematical intentions outside the soul is not [the same] as the mode according to which they exist in the soul. That account can be read in this way: the intellect can also know mathematical things by some kind of definition, for understanding differs according to the diversity of the nature of the thought object. For instance, snub-nose, insofar as it is snub-nose, is not divided [into distinct parts] when it is thought; but insofar as it is concavity, then if the intellect understands it to be a singular per se, it will not understand the intention of concavity except as denuded of flesh. The example which he brings up supplies what is missing from the account.

36. **As a separate thing is thought when [the intellect] understands those things (for what is in act universally is the intellect which is in act), our cogitation later will concern whether or not it can understand any of the separate things while it is separate from magnitude.**[231] (431b16–19) {480}

230. *Res que dicuntur negative* corresponds to the Greek τὰ δὲ ἐν ἀφαιρέσει λεγόμενα, "The so-called abstract objects" (Aristotle, *De Anima* [1984]); وإدراك العقل الاشياء ([1984]); المعراة من الهيولى (ibid. [1954]); "the intellect's apprehending things stripped of matter."
231. This Text is far from the Greek: οὕτω τὰ μαθηματικά, οὐ κεχωρισμένα <ὄντα>, ὡς κεχωρισμένα νοεῖ, ὅταν νοῇ <ᾗ> ἐκεῖνα. ὅλως δὲ ὁ νοῦς ἐστιν ὁ κατ᾽ ἐνέργειαν

The intellect becomes the thing which the intellect separates when it separates and understands it, since it is necessary universally in regard to the intellect that what is intelligible in act be intellect in act. Hence, we must investigate and cogitate later on whether that intellect which is in us can understand something which is in itself intellect and separate from matter, just as it understands what makes it intellect in act after it was intellect in potency. He said: **while it is separate from magnitude**. It occurred this way in this manuscript. If it is correct, it should be understood this way, that is to say, we ought to cogitate later on whether it is possible for the intellect which is in us to understand things separate from matter insofar as they are separate from magnitude, without relation to something else. In place of that account there appeared in the other text the following: "Later on we will investigate whether or not the intellect, when existing in the body, not as separate from it, is able to apprehend any of those things which are separate from bodies."[232] This question is different from the one mentioned earlier. For that is a question on the part of one who allows that the intellect which is in potency understands

---

τὰ πράγματα. ἆρα δ᾿ ἐνδέχεται τῶν κεχωρισμένων τι νοεῖν ὄντα αὐτὸν μὴ κεχωρισμένον μεγέθους, ἢ οὔ, σκεπτέον ὕστερον. "It is thus that the mind when it is thinking the objects of mathematics thinks them as separate though they are not separate. In every case the mind which is actively thinking is the objects which it thinks. Whether it is possible for it while not existing separate from spatial conditions to think anything that is separate, or not, we must consider later." Aristotle, *De Anima* (1984). The alternate Arabic translation is less than completely accurate and literal but much better than Averroes' primary translation, which misses the point of this famous passage: وكذلك الأشياء المعلومية ليست بمفارقة الهيولى إلا بالتوهم. – وفى الجملة العقل يدرك الأشياء إدراك فعل. وسننظر أخيراً إن كان يمكن العقل ، وهو في الجسم ، إدراك شيء من مفارقات الأجساد ، أو ليس يمكنه ذلك. (ibid. [1954]); "Likewise the things known are not separate from matter except by imagination. And in general the intellect apprehends the things with an active apprehension. Later on we will investigate whether or not intellect is able to apprehend any of the things separate from bodies while it is in the body." Regarding this text, also see the following note.

232. *Et cecidit in alia scriptura loco istius sermonis sic: Et in postremo perscrutabimur utrum intellectus, essendo in corpore, non separatus ab eo, possit comprehendere aliquod eorum que separantur a corporibus, aut non.* وسننظر أخيراً إن كان يمكن العقل ، وهو في الجسم ، إدراك شيء من مفارقات الأجساد ، أو ليس يمكنه ذلك (Aristotle, *De Anima* [1954]). The Latin *non separatus ab eo,* "not as separated from it," is not reflected in the extant Arabic and yet seems to correspond precisely to the Greek of Aristotle: αὐτὸν μὴ κεχωρισμένον. Nevertheless, Dimitri Gutas, who has undertaken the task of preparing a new edition of the Arabic text of Averroes' alternate translation, has suggested to me that <غير مفارق له> was perhaps added from a marginal gloss and merely explains *essendo in corpore,* وهو في الجسم, which is a paraphrastic rendering of the Greek. This view is supported by the Text at *De Anima* 429a12. See Book 3, n. 3 {379}.

forms which are without qualification separate from matter, not insofar as the intellect is united with us. On this understanding there will be an investigation into the question of whether [intellect] can understand forms insofar as it is united with us, not whether it can understand forms at all. This understanding was mentioned by Themistius in his book on the soul,[233] and the first question, which [Aristotle] meant for later, was omitted.

It is necessary, therefore, first to investigate whether or not it is possible for the material intellect to understand separate things {481} and, if it does understand them, whether or not it is possible for it to understand them insofar as it is united with us. For this reason it is possible that in the copy from which we took this account the word "not" dropped out, so that it should be read this way: **our cogitation later on will concern whether . . . it can understand any of the separate things while it is** not separate from magnitude, that is, insofar as it is in contact with magnitude and united with us, in such a way that we ourselves understand the intellect which it understands. This investigation which he intends is extremely difficult and ambiguous and we must investigate this insofar as we are able.

Let us say, therefore: it seems to me that he who asserts that the material intellect is generable and corruptible can find no natural way by which we can be conjoined with the separate intellects. For the intellect ought to be intelligible in all ways, and chiefly in the case of things freed from matter. If it were therefore possible for a generable and corruptible substance to understand separate forms and be made to be the same as these, then it would be possible for a possible nature to become a necessary one, as al-Fârâbî said in [his] *Commentary on the Nicomachean Ethics*.[234] This follows necessarily according to the principles accepted by the wise.

[Such would be the case,] unless someone says that the intention which Alexander meant, namely, concerning the existence of the acquired intellect, is not a newly created conceptualization in the material intellect which did not exist before. But, rather, [this intellect] is united with us by a uniting to the extent that [this intellect] is form for us in virtue of which we understand other beings, as appears from the account of Alexander. Still, it is not apparent from this how that conjoining is possible. For if we assert {482} that the conjoining came to exist after [previously] not existing, as is necessary, it follows that at that time at which it is asserted to exist, there is a change in the recipient or in the received object or in both. Since it is impossible for it to be in the received

233. See Themistius, *De Anima Paraphrase* (1899), 114.31–33; (1973), 209.13–16; (1996), 141.

234. Regarding this lost Commentary, see n. 163 and the introduction, p. lxx and lxxxvi–lxxxix and the notes there.

object, it remains that it is in the recipient. And since there is a change existing in the recipient after it did not exist, there will necessarily be there a newly created reception and a recipient substance newly created after it did not exist. When, therefore, we assert a newly created reception, the aforementioned question will arise. If we do not assert a reception proper to us, there will be no difference between its conjoining with us and its conjoining with all beings and between its conjoining with us at one time and at another time, unless we assert its conjoining with us to be in a way different from that of reception. What then is that way?

Owing to the obscure character of that way according to Alexander, we see he is uncertain in regard to this. Sometimes, therefore, he says that what understands a separate intellect is not the material intellect nor the intellect which is in a positive disposition, and these are his words in his book on the soul.[235] The intellect, then, which understands this is the one which is not corrupted, not the intellect which is a material subject. For the material intellect is corrupted in virtue of the corruption of the soul, because it is one power belonging to the soul; and when that intellect is corrupted, its power and its actuality will be corrupted. Next, after he had explained that it is necessary for the intellect which is in us and which understands the separate forms to be neither generable nor corruptible, he recounted that this intellect is the acquired intellect according to the account of Aristotle, and he said: "The intellect, therefore, which is not corrupted is that intellect which is in us as separate, {483} which Aristotle calls acquired because it is in us from outside, not a power which is in the soul nor a disposition in virtue of which we understand different things and also understand that intellect."[236]

If, therefore, by the acquired intellect in virtue of which we understand separate intelligences he meant the agent intelligence, then the account concerning the way of conjoining of that intellect with us still remains [to be given]. If he meant a separate intellect different from the agent intellect, as appears from the opinion of al-Fârâbî in his *Letter on the Intellect*,[237] and also

235. Cf. Alexander, *De Anima* (1887), 87.24–88.16; (1979), 114–115.

236. ὁ οὖν νοούμενος ἄφθαρτος ἐν ἡμῖν νοῦς οὗτός ἐστιν, <ὅτι χωριστός τε ἐν ἡμῖν καὶ ἄφθαρτος νοῦς, ὃν καὶ θύραθεν᾽ Ἀριστοτέλης λέγει, νοῦς ὁ ἔξωθεν γινόμενος ἐν ἡμῖν,> ἀλλ᾽ οὐχ ἡ δύναμις τῆς ἐν ἡμῖν ψυχῆς, οὐδὲ ἡ ἕξις, καθ᾽ ἣν ἔξιν ὁ δυνάμει νοῦς τά τε ἄλλα καὶ τοῦτον νοεῖ. Alexander, *De Anima* (1887), 90.23–91.4; (1979), 119.

237. Al-Fârâbî, *Letter on the Intellect* (1983), 20.1–22.8. "When the intellect in actuality thinks the intelligibles which are forms in it, insofar as they are intelligibles in actuality, then the intellect of which it was first said that it is the intellect in actuality, becomes now the acquired intellect (العقل المستفاد)." Ibid. (1983), 20.1–4; (1973), 217; (1974), 99–100. "However, these forms [i.e., separate forms which never existed in matter] can only be per-

insofar as we are able to understand from what is evident of that account, then the question in regard to the way of conjoining of that intellect with us is also the same as the question in regard to the way of the conjoining of the agent intellect on the view of one holding that the agent intellect is the same as the acquired intellect. This is more evident from the account of Alexander. He, therefore, said this in his *Book on the Soul*[238] in regard to the way of the conjoining of the intellect which is in act with us.

But what he said in a treatise which he composed, entitled *On the Intellect According to the Account of Aristotle*, seems to contradict what he said in his book on the soul. These are his words: "When the intellect which is in potency is complete and fulfilled, then it will understand the agent intellect. For just as the potency for walking which a human being has at birth becomes actual in time when that in virtue of which walking comes about is actualized, so too when the intellect is actualized, it will understand these things which are intrinsically intelligible and it will make sensibles into intelligibles, because it is the agent."[239] What is evident from that account {484} contradicts his account in the *Book On the Soul*, namely, that the intellect which is in potency does not understand the intellect which is in act.

But when one considers all the accounts by that man and brings them to-

---

fectly thought after all intelligibles or most of them have become thought in actuality, and the acquired intellect has come into being." Ibid. (1983), 21.8–22.1; (1973), 217; (1974), 100.

238. Alexander, *De Anima* (1887), 90.19ff.; (1979), 119ff.

239. *Et hec sunt verba eius: Et intellectus qui est in potentia, cum fuerit completus et augmentatus, tunc intelliget agentem; quoniam, quemadmodum potentia ambulandi quam homo habet in nativitate venit ad actum post tempus quando perficitur illud per quod fit ambulatio, ita intellectus, cum fuerit perfectus, intelliget ea que sunt per suam naturam intellecta, et faciet sensata esse intellecta, quia est agens.* τοῦτο δὴ καὶ αὐτὸ ὁ δυνάμει νοῦς τελειούμενος καὶ αὐξόμενος νοεῖ. ὥσπερ γὰρ ἡ περιπατητικὴ δύναμις, ἣν ἔχει ὁ ἄνθρωπος εὐθὺς τῷ γενέσθαι, εἰς ἐνέργειαν ἄγεται προϊόντος τοῦ χρόνου τελειουμένου αὐτοῦ οὐ κατὰ πάθος τι, τὸν αὐτὸν τρόπον καὶ ὁ νοῦς τελειωθεὶς τά τε φύσει νοητὰ νοεῖ καὶ τὰ αἰσθητὰ δὲ νοητὰ αὐτῷ ποιεῖ, ἅτε ὢν ποιητικός (Alexander, *De Intellectu* [1887], 110.30–111.2). "This then [is what] the potential intellect, when it is being perfected and has developed, thinks. For just as the power of walking, which a human being has as soon as he comes to be, is led to actuality, as time advances, by being perfected itself and not by being affected in some way, in the same way the [potential] intellect too when it has been perfected both thinks the things that are intelligible by nature and makes sensible things intelligible to itself, as being productive" (ibid. [2004], 34–35; [1990], 53). والعقل أيضا الذي بالقوة إذا تمّ وَمَّا عقل هذا ، لأنه كما أن قوّة المشى التي تكون للإنسان مع ولادته تصير إلى الفعل إذا أمعن به الزمان وكمل الشيء الذي به يكون المشى ، كذلك العقل إذا استكمل عقل الأشياء التي هي بطبيعتها معقولة ، وجعل الأشياء المحسوسة معقولة لأنه فاعل (ibid. [1971], 38.1–4; cf. [1956], 191.10–192.1).

gether, one will see that he holds that when the intellect which is in potency is actualized, then the agent intelligence will be united with us [and it is] in virtue of this that we understand separate things and in virtue of this that we make sensible things intelligible in act, insofar as it becomes form in us. It is as if he means by this account that when the intellect which is in potency is actualized and perfected, then that intellect [i.e., the agent intellect] will be united with [the material intellect] and the form will come to be in [the material intellect]. Then we will understand other things in virtue of that [agent intellect]. [This is] not in such a way that the material intellect understands [the agent intellect] and on account of that understanding there comes to exist a conjoining with that intellect [i.e., the agent intellect], but rather the conjoining of that intellect [i.e., the agent intellect] with us is the cause of the fact that [the material intellect] understands [the agent intellect] and we understand other separate things through [the agent intellect].[240]

You are able to know that this is the opinion of that man in virtue of what he said in that treatise: "Since what is intrinsically intelligible, which is intellect in act, is the cause of the material intellect's separating and conceptualizing any of the material forms by ascending in the presence of that form, then it is said that it is the acquired agent [intellect]. It is not part of the soul nor a power of the soul, but rather it comes to exist in us from outside when we have thought in virtue of it."[241] It is evident, therefore, that he understands in virtue of this

240. I have supplied the referents of pronouns in accord with my understanding of this passage. Without those referents supplied, the passage is pervasively ambiguous. The sense of the passage is that the material intellect's thinking is consequent upon conjunction with the agent intellect and not causative of the conjunction. Then in virtue of this conjunction, we are able to think separate things through the material intellect and through our conjunction with the material intellect. Averroes is stressing that understanding the agent intellect means nothing more than the actualization of intelligibles in act in the material intellect. Separate immaterial substances such as the agent intellect are not direct objects of our knowing. But when the material intellect is receptive of the intellectually transformative "light" of the agent intellect, it is appropriate to say that it is in a sense understanding the consequences of the activity of the agent intellect and thereby understanding the agent intellect. It is in our will and power—that is, in the ability of our imaginative or cogitative power taken broadly—to provide the images needed to bring about knowledge in the material intellect and thereby in ourselves. Note that the Arabic العقل can be rendered *intellectus* or *intelligentia*. Perhaps the translator's use of *intelligentia* here is to emphasize that the agent intellect is separate in existence.

241. *Et potes scire quod ista est opinio istius hominis per hoc quod dixit in illo tractatu: Illud igitur intellectum per suam naturam, quod est intellectus in actu, cum fuerit causa intellectus materialis in abstrahendo et in formando unamquanque formarum materialium ascendendo apud illam formam, tunc dicetur quod est adeptus agens; et non est pars anime neque virtus anime, set fit in nobis extrinseco quando nos intellexerimus per ipsum.* τοῦτο δὴ τὸ νοητόν

account that when the intellect which is in act has become formal cause of the material intellect in its proper action (this is through the ascension of the material intellect {485} in the presence of that form), then it will be called the acquired intellect. This is because in that disposition we will be understanding in virtue of it since it is form for us, for then it will be the final form for us.

What, therefore, supports that opinion is that the agent intellect is first a cause bringing to actuality the material intellect and the intellect which is in a positive disposition. For this reason it is not united with us and we do [not] understand separate things from the start in virtue of it. When, therefore, the material intellect has been actualized, then the agent will become the form of the material [intellect]²⁴² and will be united with us and we will understand other separate things in virtue of it. [This does] not [occur] in such a way that the intellect which is in a positive disposition understands this intellect, since the intellect which is in a positive disposition is generable and corruptible, while that one is not generable or corruptible.

But on this account the aforementioned question occurs, namely, that what now is form for the intellect which is in a positive disposition after it did not previously exist arises from some newly created disposition in the intellect which is in a positive disposition. This [newly created disposition] is the reason why that intellect is form for the intellect which is in a positive disposition after it previously was not. If that disposition is not a reception in the intellect which is in a positive disposition in reference to the agent intellect, what then is that disposition? For if there is a reception, it will happen that something generated receives something eternal and is made like it, and in this way what is generated will become eternal, which is impossible.

For this reason we see later that since al-Fârâbî believed the opinion of Al-

τε τῇ αὐτοῦ φύσει καὶ κατ᾽ ἐνέργειαν νοῦς, αἴτιον γινόμενον τῷ ὑλικῷ νῷ τοῦ κατὰ τὴν πρὸς τὸ τοιοῦτο εἶδος ἀναφορὰν χωρίζειν τε καὶ μιμεῖσθαι καὶ νοεῖν καὶ τῶν ἐνύλων εἰδῶν ἕκαστον καὶ ποιεῖν νοητὸν αὐτό, θύραθέν ἐστι λεγόμενος νοῦς ὁ ποιητικός οὐκ ὢν μόριον καὶ δύναμίς τις τῆς ἡμετέρας ψυχῆς, ἀλλ᾽ ἔξωθεν γιγόμενος ἐν ἡμῖν, ὅταν αὐτὸν νοῶμεν (Alexander, *De Intellectu* [1887], 108.19–24). "This thing that is both intelligible in its own nature and intellect in actuality comes to be the cause of the material intellect's, by reference to such a form, separating and imitating and thinking each of the enmattered forms as well, and making it intelligible. It is the intellect said to be 'from without,' the productive [intellect], not being a part or power of our soul, but coming to be in us from outside, whenever we think of it" (ibid. [2004], 29–30; فهذا المعقول بطبيعته ،الذي هو عقل بالفعل ، إذا صار علة للعقل الهيولاني. (49 ,[1990] للانتزاع والتقبل والتصور لكل واحد من الصور الهيولانيات ، وكل معقول بترقيه نحو تلك الصورة قيل فيه إنه العقل المستفاد الفاعل ، وليس هو جزءًا ولا قوة للنفس منا ، ولكنه يحدث فينا من خارج إذا كمل عقلنا به (ibid. [1971], 34.19–22; [1956], 186.2–6).
242. Cf. {445}, {486}.

exander to be true in regard to the generation of the material intellect, it was necessary in his view to hold according to this opinion that the agent intelligence is nothing but a cause acting upon us only, and he said this clearly in his *Commentary on the Nicomachean Ethics*.[243] {486} This is contrary to his opinion in *The Letter on the Intellect*, for there he said that it is possible for the material intellect to understand separate things.[244] This is the opinion of Ibn Bâjjah. Those then are the questions for those who assert that the material intellect is generated and that the end is to be conjoined with separate things.

We also see that for those asserting it to be a separate power questions no less [challenging] than those follow. For if it is in the nature of that material intellect that it understands separate things, it is necessary that it be understanding them always, in the future and in the past. It is thought, therefore, that it follows upon this position that as soon as the material intellect is conjoined with us, the agent intellect too is conjoined with us, which is unthinkable and contrary to what people assert.

But that question can be resolved by what we said earlier, namely, that the material intellect is not united with us per se and initially but is united with us only in virtue of its uniting with the forms of the imagination. Since it is so, it is possible to say that the way in which the material intellect is united with us is different from the way in which it is united with the agent intellect. If it is different, then there is no conjoining at all.[245] If it is the same, but initially it is in some disposition and afterwards in another, what then is that disposition? If, however, we assert that the separate material intellect does not have the nature for understanding separate things, then the uncertainty will be greater. Those, therefore, are all questions which arise {487} for those asserting that human perfection is to understand separate things.

We must also recount the accounts on the basis of which it is thought to follow that we have a nature for understanding separate things ultimately. For these accounts are completely opposite to those and perhaps in virtue of this we will be able to see the truth. The reason for that uncertainty and labor, however, is that we find no account by Aristotle concerning this intention, although Aristotle did promise to explain this.[246]

Let us say, therefore, that Ibn Bâjjah investigated this question at length and worked to explain that this conjoining is possible in his treatise which he called, *On the Conjoining of the Intellect with Man*. In his *Book on the Soul* and in

243. Regarding this lost commentary, see n. 234.

244. Al-Fârâbî, *Letter on the Intellect* (1983), 17.9–22.8; (1973), 216–217; (1974), 98–101.

245. That is, if it is altogether different, then our conjoining is no literal and direct conjoining at all.

246. *De Anima* 3.7, 431b17–19.

many other books it will be seen that this question did not leave his mind nor over time did he take his eye off it. We already expounded that treatise to the extent that we could.[247] For this topic is extremely difficult, and since such was the case for Ibn Bâjjah in regard to this question, how much more [can be expected] of any one else?! The word of Ibn Bâjjah in regard to this is more firm than [that] of others, but nevertheless the questions which we recounted arise for him. We must recount here the methods of that man, but first what the commentators said in regard to this.

Let us say, therefore, that Themistius was supported in this by way of the major. For he says that since the material intellect has the power to separate forms from matters and to understand them, how much more [reasonable is it that] it has a natural disposition for understanding these which are from the outset free of matter.[248] That account will come about in such a way that the material intellect is either corruptible {488} or not corruptible, namely, separable or not separable.[249] But according to the opinion of those saying that the material intellect is a power in the body and generated, that account will be sufficient in a qualified respect [only], not probable [in its own right]. For it does not follow that what is visible in itself is more visible for us. For instance, considering color and the light of the sun, [we see that] color has less of the intention of visibility than does the sun, since color is visible only in virtue of the sun, but we cannot look upon the sun as [we do] color. This occurs for sight owing to the mixture of matter.

But if we assert that the intellect is not mixed with matter, then certainly that account will be true, namely, that what is more intelligible is apprehended more [perfectly]. For in the case of things capable of apprehending which are

247. "Ibn Bâjjah, however, expounded his own account and said that his opinion is the opinion of all the Peripatetics, namely that conjoining is possible and that it is the end [for human beings]" {433}. Averroes is likely referring to his summary of Ibn Bâjjah's *Treatise on the Conjoining of the Intellect with Man* in his *Short Commentary on the De Anima* (1950), 90–95; (1987), Spanish, 214–221. On the doctrine of Ibn Bâjjah, see the introduction, pp. xxv–xxvii and lxxxix–xciii. Also see Altmann (1965).

248. ὃς γὰρ καὶ τὰ ἔνυλα εἴδη χωρίζων τῆς ὕλης νοεῖ, δηλονότι πέφυκε μᾶλλον τὰ κεχωρισμένα νοεῖν (Themistius, *De Anima Paraphrase* [1899], 115.6–7; "For just as it also thinks the enmattered forms by separating them from matter, so is it clearly all the more naturally fitted for thinking the separate forms." (ibid. [1996], 141); فكما يعقل الصور المخالطة للهيولى بأن [يفرقها] من الهيولى فمن البين أنّه أحدى بأن يكون من شأنه أن يعقل الأشياء المفارقة (ibid. [1973], 210.6–8); "For as it thinks enmattered forms by separating them from matter, so it is clear all the more that it is of its nature to know separate things."

249. That is, that argument would hold regardless of whether the material intellect were corruptible or incorruptible, separate or not separate.

not mixed with matter, what apprehends the less perfect necessarily apprehends the more perfect and not the contrary. But if this is necessary from its nature and substance, then the aforementioned question arises, which is: how is [the agent intellect] not conjoined with us in the beginning, namely, immediately when the material intellect is conjoined with us? If, therefore, we assert that it is conjoined with us finally, not initially, we ought to give the reason.

On this topic, however, there is support for Alexander in what I say, and this is the fact that when every generated being reaches the end in generation and final actuality, then it will reach the completion and end of its activity, if it is among beings which act, or in its affection, if it is from among passible beings, or in both, if it is of both. For instance, one does not come to the end in the activity of walking except when he comes {489} to the end in generation.[250] And because the intellect which is in a positive disposition is one of the generable beings, it is necessary that when it will have come to the end in generation, it come to the end in its activity. Since its action is to create and to understand intelligibles, when it is in final actuality, it necessarily possesses these two activities actually. Actuality in creating intelligibles is to make all intelligibles in potency to be intelligibles in act. Perfection in understanding is to understand all things separate and not separate. It is necessary, therefore, that when the intellect which is in a positive disposition comes to perfection in its generation, it have these two activities.

In regard to this there are no few questions. For it is not self-evident that the perfection of the activity of understanding is to understand separate things, unless this term, *to imagine*,[251] were to be said of these things and material things in a univocal way, as this term, *to walk*, is said of the less actual and the more actual.

Also, how is the agent intellect's proper action, which is to make intelligibles, ascribed to a generable and corruptible intellect, namely, what is in a positive disposition? Unless [perhaps] one asserts that the intellect which is in a positive disposition is the agent intellect in composition with the material intellect, as Themistius says,[252] or asserts that the final form belonging to us by which we separate the intelligibles and understand is composed of the intellect which is in a positive disposition and the agent intellect, as Alexander and Ibn Bâjjah assert, and we also figured to be apparent from the account of Aristotle.

250. Walking is essentially a motion, and so it is an imperfect or incomplete activity. When its end is achieved, there is no motion.

251. *Ymaginari* here is surely تصور *taṣawwur*, which in the case of material entities is imagination but in the case of immaterial entities is conceptualization.

252. This is the point of an extended discussion by Themistius. See Themistius, *De Anima Paraphrase* (1899), 99.8ff; (1973), 179.6ff; (1996), 123ff.

Even if we had asserted this to be so, nothing would result from the perfection of this activity of creating intelligibles {490} except the perfection of the activity of understanding these things, not [perfection of the activity] of understanding separate things. For it is impossible that understanding these be ascribed to generation or to coming to be by some generated being (for instance, [to coming to be] by the intellect which is in a positive disposition), unless accidentally. If [it were] not [so], then the generable will be made eternal, as we said.

A question of great importance also arises in the case of the account saying that the form by which we extract intelligibles is the intellect which is in a positive disposition in composition with the agent intellect. For what is eternal does not need the generable and corruptible in its activity. How, then, is the eternal in composition with the corruptible in such a way that there comes to be from them one activity? But we will speak about this later.[253] For it seems that this position is, as it were, the starting point and foundation of what we want to say concerning the possibility of conjoining with separate things according to Aristotle, namely, the position that the final form belonging to us by means of which we extract and make intelligibles in virtue of our will is composed of the agent intellect and the intellect which is in a positive disposition. We see, therefore, from the account of the Peripatetic commentators directed toward this end that this is possible,[254] namely, to understand separate things ultimately.

Ibn Bâjjah, however, said a great deal on this matter, chiefly in the treatise which he called *On the Conjoining of the Intellect with Man*. What supported his position on this question is this: first he asserted that the theoretical intelligibles have come to be; then he asserted that everything which has come to be has a quiddity; then he asserted that for everything having a quiddity, the intellect is naturally constituted to extract that quiddity; and from these he concluded that the intellect is naturally constituted to extract the forms and quiddities of intelligibles.[255] Al-Fârâbî is in agreement with him on this in his book {491} *On Intellect and the Intelligible*[256] and it is from there that Ibn Bâjjah drew this. With this Ibn Bâjjah concluded that the intellect is naturally constituted to extract forms and quiddities of intelligibles.

He went about this in two ways, one in the *Treatise*[257] and a second in his

---

253. {497ff}.

254. I read *possibile* with manuscripts A, B, D, and G instead of *possibilem*.

255. This is the doctrine implicit in the account of the grasp of intelligibles given by Ibn Bâjjah in sections 9ff. of his *Treatise on Conjoining with the Intellect*. Ibn Bâjjah, *Treatise on the Conjoining of the Intellect with Man* (1942), 15ff.; Spanish, 33ff.; (1968), 163ff.; (1981), 188ff.

256. Al-Fârâbî, *Letter on the Intellect* (1983), 12.4–17.8; (1973), 215–216; (1974), 96–99.

257. That is, Ibn Bâjjah, *Treatise on the Conjoining of the Intellect with Man* (1942), (1968), (1981).

Book on the Soul,[258] and they are similar to one another. In the *Book on the Soul* he joined to this that multiplicity does not accrue for the intelligibles of things except in virtue of the multiplication of spiritual forms with which they will be sustained in each individual. According to this the intelligible of horse in me will be different from its intelligible in you. From this it follows by conversion of the opposite that for every intelligible not having a spiritual form by which it is sustained, that intelligible is one in me and in you.[259] Next he joined to this that the quiddity and form of the intelligible does not have an individual spiritual form by which it is sustained, since the quiddity of an intelligible is not the quiddity of a singular individual, be it spiritual or bodily, for it was explained that the intelligible is not an individual. From this it follows that the intellect is naturally constituted to understand the quiddity of the intelligible belonging to the intellect which is one for all human beings and what is such as this is a separate substance.[260]

In the *Book on the Soul* he first asserted in regard to the quiddity of an intelligible insofar as it is intelligible, [1] if it has not been conceded by us not to have a quiddity and [has not been conceded by us][261] to be simple but rather [is asserted to be] composed (as is the disposition in all quiddities which have come to be), and [2] [if] it has been said that the quiddity of that intelligible insofar as it is intelligible also has a quiddity, namely, the intelligible of that quiddity, {492} then that intellect [which considers these] will also be naturally constituted to revert and to extract that quiddity.[262]

If it has not been conceded by us that this quiddity is simple and that the being belonging to it is the same as the intelligible, then what occurs in the first case will occur in regard to this, namely, that it also has a quiddity which has come to be. It is then necessary either that this proceed into infinity, or that the intellect be stopped there [in its regress]. But because it is impossible for this to proceed into infinity (because it would make infinite quiddities and intellects infinitely diverse in species exist, namely, insofar as some of them

---

258. The incomplete extant text of this work ends abruptly in the course of a discussion of the rational faculty. See Book 3, n. 33, at {397}.

259. That is, the intelligible is one in itself, but it has distinct spiritual forms by which it is a particularized intention in each of us.

260. That is, the human intellect is naturally constituted to know the intelligible form in itself which exists in the separate agent intellect.

261. I follow de Libera in *Long Commentary, Book 3* (1998), 381, n. 820, in preferring manuscripts A, C, D, and G, which omit *non* here.

262. That is, if we say that each intelligible has a quiddity and is composed, not simple, then if the quiddity has a quiddity and it is the nature of the intellect to extract quiddities, then the intellect will aim to extract the ultimate quiddity. The unacceptable consequences of this position are immediately given by Averroes in what follows.

are more freed from matter than others), it is necessary that the intellect be stopped. It will come to a stop when it reaches either [1] a quiddity which does not have a quiddity, or [2] something having a quiddity but [one such that] the intellect does not have the natural ability to extract it, or [3] [when] it reaches something which neither has nor is a quiddity. But it is impossible to find a quiddity which the intellect is not naturally constituted to extract from a quiddity, for that intellect then would not be called intellect except equivocally, since it was asserted that the intellect is naturally constituted to separate the quiddity insofar as it is a quiddity. It is also impossible for the intellect to reach something which neither has a quiddity nor is a quiddity, for what is not a quiddity and does not have a quiddity is a privation without qualification. There remains, therefore, the third division, namely, that the intellect reaches a quiddity not having a quiddity,[263] and what is so is a separate form. He supported this by what Aristotle is accustomed to say in such demonstrations, namely, that when it is necessary to cut off an infinite regress, it is better to cut it off in the beginning.[264] {493}

The conclusion of that demonstration, therefore, will be the same as the conclusion of the aforementioned demonstration. For if he had not added this, someone would have been able to say that there are many intellects intermediate between the intellect which is in a positive disposition and the agent intellect, either one, as al-Fârâbî intends in his treatise *On Intellect and the Intelligible*, which he called there *acquired*,[265] or more than one. It is thought that al-Fârâbî concedes this in his *Commentary on [Aristotle's] On Generation and Corruption*, where he says, "How are those intermediate intellects exhausted?"[266] that is, those whose existence we asserted to be between the theoretical intellect and the agent intellect. Those, therefore, are the more firm ways by which that man [scil., Ibn Bâjjah] proceeded in regard to this intention.

Let us say, however: But if this name *quiddity* is said of the quiddities of material things and of the quiddities of separate intellects in a univocal way, then the proposition saying that the intellect is naturally constituted to separate quiddities insofar as they are quiddities will be true. Similarly, if saying that intelligibles are composite and individuals are composite were something univocally said, [the same would be the case]. If, however, [the predication] is equivocal, the demonstration will not be true. But how [this is so] is very difficult, for it is self-evident that this name *quiddity* is not said of these with pure

263. That is, it is the quiddity itself, not merely something having a quiddity.

264. *De Anima* 3.2, 425b17–18; *Metaphysics* 7.6, 1032a2ff.

265. Al-Fârâbî, *Letter on the Intellect* (1983), 21.8–22.6; (1973), 217; (1974), 100–101.

266. This work is not extant. What is at issue here is how the many intermediate stages of intellectual abstraction, the intermediate intellects, are traversed in order for the intellect to reach the complete grasp of the intelligible quiddity itself.

univocity nor with pure equivocation. But whether it is said in many ways because it is intermediate needs consideration.[267]

But if we concede this to be said in a univocal way, the aforementioned question will occur, [the question of] how what is corruptible understands what is not corruptible, according to the opinion of those saying that the material intellect is corruptible {494} (this is the opinion of Ibn Bâjjah); or how what is naturally constituted to understand these things in the future and in the past understands by virtue of a new intellection, according to the opinion of those saying that the material intellect is not generable or corruptible. Also, if we have asserted that to understand separate things is in the substance and nature of the material intellect, why, then, is that intellection not analogous to the material intellections belonging to us in such a way that this [sort of] understanding is one of the parts of the theoretical sciences and will be one of the things sought in theoretical science?

Ibn Bâjjah seems to be undecided in this passage. In the treatise which he called *Of Farewell* he said that possibility is of two sorts: natural and divine, that is, that the intellection of that intellect is of a divine possibility, not of a possibility of nature.[268] In the treatise *On Conjoining*, however, he said, "When the philosopher has ascended in another way to the contemplation of the intelligible insofar as it is intelligible, then he will understand separate substance." It is evident from this that [the activity of] understanding the intelligible according to him is part of the theoretical sciences, namely, natural science.[269] This also appeared in his investigation.

Since it is so, the ignorance of that science which occurs for all of us human beings either will be because still we do not know the propositions which lead us to this science, as it is said of many arts which seem to be possible but are of causes unknown, for instance, alchemy; or [it will be because] this understanding of this is acquired through exercise and use of natural things,

267. At issue here is whether intellectual understanding of composite material things of the sublunar world is the very same activity as intellectual understanding of immaterial incomposite substances, in particular the agent intellect.

268. Ibn Bâjjah, *Letter of Farewell* (1943), 38–39; Spanish, 84–85; (1968), 141.11–142.7. In this work Ibn Bâjjah holds that we are able to exercise a natural capacity for science but that the ability to know one's essence and to know separate intellect requires the help of God.

269. Ibn Bâjjah, *Treatise on the Conjoining of the Intellect with Man* (1942), 16ff.; Spanish, 35ff.; (1968), 164ff.; (1981), 189ff. There and in sections 12–15 of his *Letter of Farewell* ([1943], 24–30; Spanish, 59–69; [1968], 123–131), Ibn Bâjjah discusses the progression of abstraction through various levels, from that of the common folk to that of the natural philosopher concerned with material forms and finally to the highest level of abstraction which grasps the forms themselves.

but we have not yet had enough exercise and use to be able {495} to acquire this intellection; or this will be on account of a deficiency of our nature in a natural way.

If, then, this occurs on account of a deficiency in nature, then we and all who are naturally constituted to acquire this science are called human beings equivocally. If this occurs on account of ignorance of the propositions leading into this science, then theoretical science will not yet have been realized. Perhaps Ibn Bâjjah means this to be a view one cannot hold, but not [altogether] impossible. If this occurs on account of custom, then the account will be close to the account saying that the reason for this is ignorance of the propositions which lead to this science. All this is said while seen to be unlikely, although not impossible. How, therefore, can he evade those questions mentioned earlier?

Those, then, are all questions arising in this inquiry and they are as difficult as you see. We must say what has appeared to us to be the case regarding this. Let us say, therefore: the intellect existing in us has two activities insofar as it is ascribed to us, one of the genus of affection, namely, understanding, and the other of the genus of activity, namely, to extract forms and denude them of matters, which is nothing but making them intelligible in act after they were such in potency. [Hence] it is evident that after we have possessed the intellect which is in a positive disposition, it is in our will to understand any intelligible we wish and to extract any form we wish.

This activity, namely, to create and make intelligibles, is prior in us to the action which is understanding, as Alexander says.[270] For this reason he says that it is more appropriate to describe the intellect in virtue of this action, not in virtue of affection, since {496} in affection it shares in something else [also] belonging to the animal powers of the soul, but this is according to the opinion of those saying that affection in these is not said equivocally.

270. ἔτι καὶ πρότερον αὐτῷ τὸ ποιεῖν καὶ οὐσιῶδες. πρότερον γὰρ ποιεῖ τῇ ἀφαιρέσει νοητόν, εἶθ' οὕτως λαμβάνει τούτων τι ὃ νοεῖ τε καὶ ὁρίζεται, ὅτι τόδε τί ἐστι. καὶ γὰρ εἰ ἅμα χωρίζεται καὶ λαμβάνει, ἀλλὰ τὸ χωρίζειν προεπινοεῖται· τοῦτο γάρ ἐστιν αὐτῷ τὸ ληπτικῷ εἶναι τοῦ εἴδους (Alexander, *De Intellectu* [1887], 111.15–19). "Moreover, its producing is prior and [part of] its substance. First it produces by abstraction [something] intelligible, and then in this way it apprehends some one of these things which it thinks and defines as a this-something. Even if it separates and apprehends at the same time, nevertheless the separating is conceptually prior; for this is what it is for it to be able to apprehend the form." (ibid. [2004], 36; [1990], 54). وأيضاً. فإن الفعل فيه أقدم ، وهو ذاتي له ، لأنه أولاً [ولا] يوجد فاعلاً للمعقولات ثم حينئذ يأخذها إثر تعقلها ويحدها بأنها كذا ، فانه وإن كان أفراده الأشياء شيئاً شيئاً وأخذه إياها يكونان معاً ، فإن الأول ينفعل مقدماً للآخر ، فإن هذا هو أخذ الصورة (ibid. [1971], 38.15–18); cf. (1956), 193.1–4.

Owing to that activity, namely, extracting any intelligible we wish and making it in act after it was in potency, Themistius held that the intellect which is in a positive disposition is composed of the material intellect and the agent [intellect].[271] This is the same thing that made Alexander believe that the intellect which is in us is composed, or as it were composed, of the agent intellect and that which is in a positive disposition, since he holds that the substance of this [intellect] which is in a positive disposition ought to be different from the substance of the agent intellect.[272]

These two fundamental points have been asserted, namely, that the intellect which is in us has these two activities, namely, to apprehend intelligibles and to make them, while the intelligibles come to be in us in two ways: either naturally (they are the primary propositions with respect to which we do not know when, whence, and how they came forth) or voluntarily (they are intelligibles acquired on the basis of the primary propositions).[273] It was explained that it is necessary that the intelligibles possessed by us naturally be from something which is in itself an intellect freed from matter (this is the agent intellect). When this has been explained, it is necessary that the intelligibles possessed by us from the primary propositions be some product brought together from propositions known and the agent intellect. For we cannot say that the propositions do not enter into the being of acquired intelligibles; nor can we even say that they alone are agents of these (for it was already explained that the agent is one and eternal), as intended some of the Ancients who held that Aristotle meant these [primary propositions] by *agent intellect*.[274]

Since it is so, it is necessary that the theoretical intellect {497} be something

271. See Book 3, n. 233.

272. See Alexander, *De Anima* (1887), 89.11–91.6; (1979), 117–120, for his discussion of the separate productive intellect (agent intellect) in relation to our intellect and understanding. Cf. Alexander, *De Intellectu* (1887), 111.27–32; (1971), 39.6–10; (1956), 194.1–6. "The intellect that is by nature and from without will assist that in us, because other things too would not be intelligible, though being [so] potentially, if there did not exist something that was intelligible by its own peculiar nature. This, being intelligible by its own nature, by being thought comes to be the one who thinks it; it is intellect that has come to be in the one who thinks, and it is thought 'from without' and [is] immortal, and implants in the material [intellect] a disposition such that it thinks the things that are intelligible potentially." (ibid. [2004], 36–37; [1990], 54–55).

273. Cf. Book 3 {407} and {506}, as well as Book 3, n. 90.

274. The primary propositions gathered empirically are not themselves intelligibles, but they do contribute to the being of acquired intelligibles; nor are they the agents in the generation of acquired intelligibles since that agent is the separate agent intellect. Note that in the present context Averroes is using the same term, "primary propositions," sometimes to denote first principles of the understanding (cf. Book 3, n. 90) and

generated by the agent intellect and by primary propositions. That sort of intelligible happens to exist voluntarily, contrary to the way the first natural intelligibles exist. For with respect to every activity which has come to be from the
compound of two different things, it is necessarily the case that one of those two
be as it were matter and instrument and the other be as it were form or agent.
The intellect in us, therefore, is composed of the intellect which is in a positive
disposition and the agent intellect, either in such a way that the propositions are
as it were matter and the agent intellect is as it were form, or in such a way that
the propositions are as it were the instrument and the agent intellect is as it were
the efficient [cause]. For the disposition is similar in this case.

But if we have asserted that the propositions are as it were the instrument,
it will happen that an eternal activity arises from two things, one of which is
eternal and the other not eternal (or it may be asserted that the instrument is
eternal; and thus the theoretical intelligibles will be eternal). This will happen
all the more if we have asserted these propositions to be as it were matter. For
it is impossible for something generable and corruptible to be the matter of
something eternal. How, then, can we escape this question?

Let us say, therefore, that if what we said, that the propositions necessarily
are from the agent intellect either as matter or as instrument, if they enter into
the being of the theoretical intelligibles, then it was not the account of a necessary consequence insofar as matter is matter and instrument is instrument.
Rather, insofar as it is necessary here that there be proportion and disposition
between the agent intellect and the propositions {498} which are likened to
matter and an instrument in some way, not because it is true matter or a true
instrument, it then seems to us that we can know the way in which the intellect which is in a positive disposition is as it were matter and the subject of the
agent [intellect]. And when that way has been set forth by us, perhaps we will
be able to know easily the way in which [the intellect which is in a positive
disposition] is conjoined with separable intelligibles.

Let us say, therefore: the account, however, of one saying that if the conclusions are acquired by us from the agent intellect and the propositions, it is
necessary that the propositions be in relation to the agent intellect as it were
true matter and true instrument, that account, I say, is not necessary. But to an
extent it is necessary that there be [some] relation in which the intellect which
is in a positive disposition will be likened to matter and the agent intellect will
be likened to form. What, then, is that relation and from what does it arise for
the agent intellect that it has this relation to the intellect which is in a positive

---

sometimes to denote propositions known from experience which contribute to the
content of the theoretical intellect.

disposition, while one is eternal and the other generable and corruptible? For all of these [thinkers] concede this relation exists. That the theoretical intelligibles are existing in us from these two intellects, namely, from what is in a positive disposition and from the agent intellect, compels them [to accept this view], as it were.

But Alexander and all those holding that the material intellect is generable and corruptible are not able to provide the cause for this relation. For those, however, who assert that the operating intellect is the intellect which is in a positive disposition, it will happen that the theoretical intelligibles are eternal and many other impossible things following upon this position.[275] {499}

But for us who have asserted that the material intellect is eternal and the theoretical intelligibles are generable and corruptible in the way in which we mentioned, and that the material intellect understands both, namely, the material forms and the separate forms, it is evident that the subject of the theoretical intelligibles and of the agent intellect in this way is one and the same, namely, the material [intellect]. Similar to this is the transparent which receives color and light at one and the same time; and light is what brings color about.[276]

When this conjoining in us between the agent intellect and the material intellect has been established, we will be able to find out the way in which we say that the agent intellect is similar to form and that the intellect which is in a positive disposition is similar to matter. For in regard to any two things of which one is the subject and the second is more actual than the other, it is necessary that the relation of the more actual to the less actual be as the relation of form to matter.[277] With this intention we say that the proportion of the first actuality of the imaginative power to the first actuality of the common sense is as the proportion of form to matter.

We, therefore, have already found the way in which it is possible for that intellect to be conjoined with us in the end and the reason why it is not united with us in the beginning. For when this has been asserted, it will necessarily happen that the intellect which is in us in act be composed of theoretical intelligibles and the agent intellect in such a way that the agent intellect is as it were the form of the theoretical intelligibles and the theoretical intelli-

275. That is, given that eternal intelligibles are grasped in intellectual understanding, if the agent in the process is the intellect in a positive disposition (*intellectus in habitu*, العقل بالملكة) which resides in us, then the eternal intelligibles will reside in us.

276. The transparent receives actualization as transparent from light and at the same moment receives color thanks to the light which enables color in potency to become color in act. Likewise, the material intellect receives actualization as intellect from the agent intellect and at the same moment receives intelligibles thanks to the agent intellect, which enables what is intelligible in potency to become intelligible in act.

277. Cf. *De Anima* 3.5, 430a10–11, and above {436–437}.

gibles are as it were matter. In this way we will be able to generate intelligibles when we wish. For because that in virtue of which something carries out its proper activity is the form, while we carry out {500} our proper activity in virtue of the agent intellect, it is necessary that the agent intellect be form in us.

There is no way in which the form is generated in us except that. For when the theoretical intelligibles are united with us through forms of the imagination and the agent intellect is united with the theoretical intelligibles (for that which apprehends [theoretical intelligibles] is the same, namely, the material intellect), it is necessary that the agent intellect be united with us through the conjoining of the theoretical intelligibles. It is evident [then] that when all the theoretical intelligibles exist in us in potency, it will be united with us in potency. When all the theoretical intelligibles exist in us in act, it will then be united with us in act. And when certain [theoretical intelligibles] exist in potency and certain in act, then it will be united in one part and not in another. Then we are said to be moved to conjoining.

It is evident that when that motion is complete, immediately that intellect will be conjoined with us in all ways. Then it is evident that its relation to us in that disposition is as the relation of the intellect which is in a positive disposition in relation to us. Since it is so, it is necessary that a human being understand all the intelligibles through the intellect proper to him and that he carry out the activity proper to him in regard to all beings, just as he understands by his proper intellection all the beings through the intellect which is in a positive disposition when it has been conjoined with forms of the imagination. {501}

In this way, therefore, human beings, as Themistius says, are made like unto God in that he is all beings in a way and one who knows these in a way, for beings are nothing but his knowledge and the cause of beings is nothing but his knowledge.[278] How marvelous is that order and how mysterious is that mode of being!

---

278. διὸ καὶ θεῷ μάλιστα ἔοικε· καὶ γὰρ ὁ θεὸς πὼς μὲν αὐτὰ τὰ ὄντα ἐστί, πὼς δὲ ὁ τούτων χορηγός. τιμιώτερος δὲ ὁ νοῦς καθὸ δημιουργεῖ μᾶλλον ἢ καθὸ πάσχει· πανταχοῦ γὰρ ἡ ποιητικὴ ἀρχὴ τῆς ὕλης τιμιωτέρα, καὶ γίνεται μέν, ὥσπερ ἔφην πολλάκις, ὁ αὐτὸς νοῦς καὶ νοητός, ὥσπερ ἡ ἐπιστήμη ἡ κατ᾽ ἐνέργειαν αὐτό ἐστι τὸ ἐπιστητόν. (Themistius, De Anima Paraphrase [1899], 99.23–28); "That is why it also most resembles a god; for god is indeed in one respect [identical with] the actual things that exist, but in another their supplier (khorêgos). The intellect is far more valuable insofar as it creates than insofar as it is acted on; that is because the productive first principle is always more valuable than the matter [on which it acts]. Also, as I have often said, the intellect and the object of thought are identical (just as are actual knowledge and the very object of knowledge)" (ibid. [1996], 124–125). ولذلك قد يشبه خاصّه

In this way will be established the opinion of Alexander, according to which he says that to understand separate things comes about through conjoining of that intellect with us. This is not because understanding is found to exist in us after previously it did not, which is the cause in the conjoining of the agent intellect with us, as Ibn Bâjjah intended, but rather [it is because] the cause of intellection is conjoining, not the contrary.[279]

In virtue of this the question of how it understands what has long existed with a new intellection is solved. It is also evident from this why we are not conjoined with this intellect in the beginning but rather in the end. For so long as the form is in us in potency, it will be conjoined with us in potency and for so long as it is conjoined with us in potency, it is impossible for us to understand something in virtue of that. But when the form is made to exist in act in us (this will be in its conjoining in act), then we will understand all the things which we understand in virtue of [this intellect] and we will bring about the activity proper to ourselves in virtue of it.

From this it appears that its intellection is not something which belongs to the theoretical sciences but rather is something analogous with a thing {502} generated naturally by the learning of the theoretical sciences. For this reason it is not far-fetched that human beings help themselves in regard to this intention, just as they help themselves in the theoretical sciences. But it is necessary for there to be found what arises from the theoretical sciences, not from others. For it is impossible for false intelligibles to have conjoining, since they are not something occurring naturally, but are things unintended, such as a sixth finger and a monster in creation.[280]

إلها فإنّ الله هو بجهة ما الموجودات أنفسها وبجهة ما المنعم بها. والعقل من طريق ما هو يصوغ
أحرى بأن يكون أشرف منه من طريق ما ينفعل فإنّ في كلّ شيء المبدأ الفاعل أشرف من الهيولى
ويصير كما قلت مرارا كثيرة هو بعينه عقلا ومعقولا كما أنّ العلم بالفعل هو المعلوم نفسه .ibid)
[1973], 180.6–10). In his *Long Commentary on the Metaphysics*, Averroes also speaks of God's knowledge as the cause of being: "The truth is that because it knows only itself, it knows the existents through the existence which is the cause of their existences. . . . For His knowledge is the cause of being and being is the cause of our knowledge." *Long Commentary on the Metaphysics* (1952), 1707–1708; (1962), 337 A–B. (1984), 197. Also see Druart (1995b).

279. Conjoining is a necessary condition for knowing. We do not have understanding so that we may conjoin with the separate agent intellect, as Ibn Bâjjah has it, but rather we conjoin with the separate agent intellect so that we may have understanding. The end, then, is intellectual understanding, which fulfills our natures as rational beings, and this is not a means to a greater end beyond our intellectual fulfillment.

280. The agent intellect brings to actuality as intelligibles only those which truly are naturally occurring intelligibles in potency, the images of which are formed thanks to the individual internal powers of imagination, cogitation, and memory and presented to the agent intellect. On the issue of "fictional forms" in Avicenna, see Black (1997).

It is also evident that when we assert that the material intellect is generable and corruptible, we will then find no way in which the agent intellect will be united with the intellect which is in a positive disposition by a uniting proper to it, namely, with a uniting similar to the conjoining of forms with matters.

When that conjoining has not been asserted, there will be no difference between relating it to a human being and relating it to all beings except in virtue of the diversity of its activity in them.[281] In this way its relation to a human being will be only the relation of the agent to the human being, not a relation of form, and the question of al-Fârâbî which he voiced in his *Commentary on the Nicomachean Ethics* arises. For assurance of the possibility of the conjoining of the intellect with us lies in explaining that its relation to a human being is a relation of form and agent, not a relation of agent alone. This, therefore, appeared to us in regard to the way sought after. If more appears to us later on, we will write [it].[282] {503}

37. Let us, therefore, gather by way of summary the things which have been said in regard to the soul. Let us, therefore, say that the soul is in some way all beings. For beings are either intelligible or sensible. But knowing intelligible things is after the manner of sensing a sensible thing. (3.8, 431b20–23)

Since it has been explained what are the kinds of apprehensive powers of the soul and that they are of two sorts, namely, of sense and of intellect, it is necessary for us now to make a summary [account] concerning the soul and to say descriptively that it is in a way all beings. For all beings are either sen-

281. Cf. {454}.

282. On this account, the agent intellect is our "form" in its actualization of the theoretical intelligibles in the individual human being's theoretical intellect. Because of the nature of this relationship of what is analogous to form (agent intellect) and what is analogous to matter (the individual's theoretical intellect), there are no grounds here for the assertion of personal immortality for individuals. While the agent intellect is the form and actuality of our intellects and understanding—that is, of our individual perishable theoretical intellects and of our imperishable shared material intellect—there is no substantial change transforming our individual generable and corruptible intellects into eternal substances, as al-Fârâbî had it. Nor is there here the denial of conjoining with the agent intellect and pessimism about the attainment of knowledge as a consequence of a denial of substantial conjoining, as al-Fârâbî is reported to have held in his late lost *Commentary on the Nicomachean Ethics*. See n. 243.

In *Epistle 1 On Conjunction*, Averroes writes, "It is clear . . . that the agent intellect is not cause of the material intellect in as much as it is agent cause alone but in a way such that it is also its final perfection according to the mode of formal and final [cause], as is the case for sense in relation to what is sensed. This is one of the things which deceived al-Fârâbî, when he thought that [the agent intellect] was only the agent cause, as are material movers." Geoffroy and Steel (2001), 216. My translation of the French.

sible or intelligible. The disposition of sensibles to sense, however, is just as the disposition of intelligibles to intellect and + sense to the sensible +.[283] It happens, therefore, necessarily that the soul is all beings in one of the ways in which it is possible to say that the soul is all beings.

38. **And it should be known how. Let us say, therefore, that knowing and sensing are divided according to the division of beings. If, therefore, [knowing and sensing] are in potency, the intelligible and the sensible will be in potency, if in act, in act.[284] For it is necessary that they be either those beings or [their] forms. They are not those beings, for the stone does not exist in the soul but rather the form. For this reason the soul is like the hand, for the hand is an instrument for instruments and intellect is a form for forms and sense a form for sensibles.** (431b23–432a3)

After he had explained that the soul is in a way all beings, he began to explain that way. He said: **Let us say, therefore, that knowing,** etc. That is, the differences belonging to the beings in virtue of which they are divided are {504} the same as the differences belonging to the soul. These are potency and act. For just as sense and intellect are either in potency or in act, so too every sensible and intelligible is either in potency or in act. Since it is so, if that which senses is in potency, the sensible will be in potency, and if it is in act, the sensible will be in act. It is similarly so for the intellect with respect

283. *Sensus ad sensatum.* Crawford marks this text as corrupt.

284. The Text here omits the following Greek at 431b26–28: τῆς δὲ ψυχῆς τὸ αἰσθητικὸν καὶ τὸ ἐπιστημονικὸν δυνάμει ταῦτά ἐστι, τὸ μὲν <τὸ> ἐπιστητὸν τὸ δὲ <τὸ> αἰσθητόν. "Within the soul the faculties of knowledge and sensation are *potentially* these objects, the one what is knowable, the other what is sensible." Aristotle, *De Anima* (1984). The alternate translation retains this text to some extent: وقوة النفس الحاسة والعلامة هما شيء واحد إذا حُملا على المعلوم والمحسوس (ibid. [1954]; "With respect to the soul's power for sensing and cognizing, these two are one when they are related to what is known and what is sensed." In his *Middle Commentary* Averroes seems to give evidence of knowing the correct text: و ذلك أنه إن كانت الموجودات المعقولات موجودة بالقوة فالمعقولات هى معقولة بالقوة وإن كانت المعقولات بالفعل فالموجودات بالفعل ، وكذلك الأمر فى المحسوسات مع الحواس; "For, if the intelligible existents are in potentiality, the intelligibles are, too; while, if the intelligibles are in actuality, so are the existents; and likewise for sensible objects with the senses" (*Middle Commentary* [2002], 122.11–14). The corruption could have been in the Arabic manuscript of the Latin translator, or early in the transmission of the Latin text. Another possible alternative is that when composing the *Long Commentary*, Averroes may have known this text by way of Themistius. Cf. Themistius, *De Anima Paraphrase* (1899), 115.12–13; (1973), 210.13–15. "That is because existing objects are either objects of perception or objects of thought, and actual knowledge is [identical with] the objects of knowledge, while actual perception is [identical with] the objects of perception." (ibid. [1996], 141).

to the intelligible. [Hence,] it must be truly said that this part belonging to the soul is that part belonging to the beings.[285] For things which have differences which are the same are themselves the same in that way in which they have the same differences. Intellect, therefore, is the intelligible and sense is the sensible. Next he said: **For it is necessary**, etc. That is, there are only the two modes, so that the intellect is the intelligible existing outside the soul or its form, and likewise sense with the sensible. It is impossible for the being itself to be intelligible or sensible,[286] namely, through its form and its matter, as the ancients held, for then, when it would understand a stone, the soul would be a stone, and if wood, it would be wood. It remains, therefore, that what exists in the soul with reference to beings is the form alone, not matter. He meant this when he said: **for the stone**, etc. That is, for the stone does not exist in the soul but rather only its form. Next he reported that this is the reason why the soul takes on many different forms, like the hand which is an instrument which takes on all instruments. He said: **For this reason the soul is like the hand,** etc.

39. **And because, as is thought, magnitude is + to exist as sensibles of sensible things + and it is the species of sensible things {505} individually,[287] while intelligibles are those things which are said by way of what is fleeting, while things existing in sensibles are according to the mode of positive disposition and affection. For this reason he who senses nothing, learns nothing and understands nothing. If, therefore, one sees, one will necessarily see[288] some images, for images are similar to sensibles but without matter.[289] For imagination is different from affirmation and negation. For assent**

285. The use of *pars*, "part," here is awkward since what is at issue is the *mode* of existence (potential or actual) of the object and its respective apprehending faculty, as Averroes makes clear in the lines which follow. The term denotes the intention. The problem is with the Latin translation, rather than the Arabic, in all likelihood.

286. That is, it is impossible for it to be per se intelligible in act or per se sensible in act since that would mean that it is per se apprehensive. Rather, it is something intelligible or sensible in potency only by reference to a distinct apprehending power, that of the soul or that of the intellect.

287. *Singulariter*: κεχωρισμένον, "separate in existence." Aristotle, *De Anima* (1984).

288. *Viderit . . . videt* corresponds to the Greek θεωρῇ . . .θεωρεῖν, but Averroes' Comment makes it clear that he understands it to refer to intellectual understanding. See below {506}.

289. Crawford marks part of this problematic passage as corrupt: *Et quia, secundum quod existimatur, magnitudo est + esse sensibilia sensibilium +, et est species sensibilium singulariter, intelligibilia autem sunt que dicuntur modo velocis, res autem existentes in sensibilibus sunt secundum modum habitus et passionis.* The Greek here at 432a2–10 is rendered, "Since it seems that there is nothing outside and separate

and non-assent are found in virtue of the composition of certain beliefs with certain others. In virtue of what, however, are primary beliefs discerned in such a way that they are not images? For if they are not images, they nevertheless do not come to be without images. (432a3–14)

Because, as is thought, body, which is the more universal genus of sensible things, exists in sensible things, it is also a universal form for sensible things insofar as the intellect discerns and separates it from sensibles. Next he said: **and intelligibles are**, etc. That is, and since body, which is the more universal of intelligibles, is separated by intellect but is existing in sensible things, it is necessary that the forms existent in the intellect be in accord with fleeting movement and the nature of fleeting change,[290] not stable, and that those same forms be existent outside the soul in sensible things in accord with the fact that the positive disposition exists in what has the positive disposition and the thing which is stable [exists] in the thing affected.[291] {506} Next he said: **For this reason he**

---

in existence from sensible spatial magnitudes, the objects of thought (τὰ νοητά) are in the sensible forms, viz. both the abstract objects and all the states and affections of sensible things. Hence no one can learn or understand anything in the absence of sense, and when the mind is actively aware of anything it is necessarily aware of it along with an image; for images are like sensuous contents except in that they contain no matter." Aristotle, *De Anima* (1984); Greek added. The alternate translation is also problematic: وجب أن يكون المعقول : إما واحداً من الأشياء المقولة بالتعرى من الهيولى، أو ما كان من غير أمر المحسوسة والآفات المعترية لها (ibid. [1954]); "It is necessary that the intelligible be either one of the things said by abstraction from matter or what is without the character of the sensible and the abstracted affections belonging to it." Note that *modo velocis* fails to render correctly the corresponding Greek ἐν ἀφαιρέσει, "in abstraction." The precise nature of the error here is not completely clear, but perhaps it is one of scribal errors in the Arabic transmission of the text with مسيل (which is found in Themistius; see the following note) or a form from the root سرع (which is found in the corresponding passage of the *Middle Commentary*, in the phrase وجود الأشياء السريعة الزوال, "the existence of fleeting things" [*Middle Commentary* (2002), 122.24], which Ivry renders as "the kind of transitory existence") substituted for what may have been an original translation using a form of سلب.

290. Averroes, challenged by his corrupt Text, appears to have drawn on the work of Themistius for assistance where mention is made of ἡ μὲν γὰρ ἄπαυστος ῥοὴ τῶν σωμάτων (Themistius, *De Anima Paraphrase* [1899], 115.21); مسيل الأجسام الذى لا فتور له (ibid. [1973], 211.3–4); "the incessant flux of bodies." (ibid. [1996], 142).

291. "The difference between the two types of existence is that the existence of forms in the intellect and sense is of the kind of transitory existence which is called 'disposition (الاحوال),' while the forms' existence outside the soul is of the kind of stable existence which is called 'habit (ملكة).'" *Middle Commentary* (2002), 122.23–123.1; Arabic added. The existence of forms in the soul or in the senses is not one of fixity or stability, but

who senses nothing, learns nothing. That is, because the intelligible intention is the same as the thing which sense apprehends in the sensible, what senses nothing necessarily learns nothing by way of knowledge and discernment by intellect. Next he said: **If, therefore, one sees**, etc. That is, that same thing is the reason why, when the intellect which is in us has seen and understood something, it will not understand it unless it is joined with its image. For images are certain sensibles for the intellect and exist for it in place of sensibles during the absence of sensibles, but they are immaterial sensibles. Next he said: **For** the image **is different**, etc. That is, we said that the images are of the genus of sensible things and are not of intellect because intellect has its own affirmation and negation, but affirmation and negation are different from imagination. But assertion and non-belief,[292] existing in the intellect not from sense but from reason, come to be in the composition of beliefs which are had in turn from sense. He said this because there is uncertainty concerning natural propositions (which are such that we do not know whence they come or when) as to whether or not they arise from sense.[293] It is said: perhaps they do not arise from sense as [so] many conclusions. Next he said: **In virtue of what, however, are primary beliefs discerned?** That is, as it seems to me, in virtue of what, therefore, can someone say that the first propositions are discerned from sensibles and do not need them at all, and for this reason are different from imagination? For if we concede that the first propositions are not imagination, nevertheless, they seem {507} to exist with the imagination, and this shows that they need sense. This completes the account of the rational [part of the soul].

40. **Because the souls of animals are defined in virtue of these two powers, of which one is a discerning [power], because it is for the activity of sense and intellect, and the other [a power] for local motion, and we already settled the account of sense and intellect, now it is necessary to say in regard to the mover what [part] of the soul it is and whether it is a part distinct in magnitude or in definition, or whether it is the whole soul. And if it is a part of it, [we must say] whether it is something in its own right different from those customarily mentioned, or those things mentioned are not one of those.**[294] (3.9, 432a15–22)

---

rather one of transitory internal intellectual or sensory "dispositions" or "states." In contrast, the existence of forms in things external to the soul and its powers is one of independent fixity and stability called ملكة, which in the present context might be better rendered "[external] disposition."

292. *Incredulitas*. That is, assertation of negation.

293. Cf. Book 3 {407} and {496}.

294. The Text is slightly corrupt in the version Averroes used here. The Greek has κἂν εἰ μόριόν τι, πότερον ἴδιόν τι παρὰ τὰ εἰωθότα λέγεσθαι καὶ τὰ εἰρημένα, ἢ

After he had completed the account of the discerning powers, he returned to the account of the power for motion in place and he began to give the reason why he began to speak about this power. He said: **Because the souls of animals**, etc. That is, because the ancients were accustomed to define the souls of animals by two powers, one of which is an apprehensive and discerning power, while the other is for motion in place (we already completed the account of the discerning power with what we said about the power of sense and intellect), it is necessary for us to say now about the mover in place just what [part] of the soul it is. Next he said: **whether it is one part**, etc. That is, it should also be sought out with respect to this power whether it is a part of the soul or the whole soul and, if it is a part of the soul, whether it is separate from the others in quiddity and place, as many ancients held, or it differs only in quiddity and definition. Next he said: **And if it is a part of it**, etc. That is, and if that power is {508} part of the soul, whether it is one of these parts mentioned by the ancients or [whether] it is not one of those but rather a different one.

41. **With this account there also arises a question and it is how there are parts of the soul and how many they are. For they seem in a way to be infinite and [it seems] that they are not those parts which people count in the definition, namely, the rational, the emotional, and the desiderative. Some divide it into rational and irrational. For it seems to be divided according to differences dividing it also into different parts among which there exists greater diversity than among those of which even we speak, namely, the nutritive power existing in plants[295] and the sensitive power which no one wishes to count, for it is neither non-rational nor rational. Also the power in virtue of which imagination comes about differs per se from the others.** (432a22–b1)

τούτων ἕν τι. "If it is a part, is that part different from those usually distinguished or already mentioned by us, or is it one of them?" Aristotle, *De Anima* (1984). In composing his *Middle Commentary*, Averroes may have had a different version of the same translation of the *De Anima*, one in accord with the Greek: وإن كان جزءا منها أهو شيء غير الأجزاء; التى جرت العادة بذكرها للنفس أو جزء واحد منها, "Moreover, if it is part of the soul, is it something other than the parts which are customarily mentioned, or one of them?" *Middle Commentary* (2002), 123.17–18. Although it is far from certain, he may have been working with the alternate translation, which has some similarities: وإن كان المحرك جزءا (Aristotle, *De Anima* [1954]); من أجزاء التى من مرادنا أن نقول بها ، وهى غير التى ذكرنا؟ "And if the mover is one of [the soul's] parts, is it distinctly other than the parts we sought to mention and [parts] other than those we mentioned?"

295. The Text here omits the Greek καὶ πᾶσι τοῖς ζῴοις, "the nutritive, which belongs both to plants *and to all animals*." Aristotle, *De Anima* (1984); my emphasis. As Badawi notes (ibid. [1954], 80, n. 3), the alternate translation is corrupt with الزمان, "time," in place of the expected الحيوان, "animals" النامية فى جميع الزمان وفى جميع النامية; "in regard to all time and in regard to all growth."

There arises in this investigation a question common to all the powers of the soul, namely, how the parts of the soul are many and one and how many they are. Next he gave the reason why it is difficult to know how many its parts are. He said: **For they seem**, etc. That is, for when someone wishes to count them, they seem to be infinite rather than finite, for its parts are not those parts which human beings have been accustomed to count {509} when they define the soul. He said **in a way** because if someone wished to count the concupiscible soul by the number of things which it desires, then it seems that it is infinite. He cites Plato for saying that the parts of the soul are three: rational, emotional, and desiderative. He asserted that the emotional and desiderative are two and [yet] they belong to one power, namely, to the concupiscible soul. Next he said: **Some divide**, etc. That is, in this they make an error and mistake. For it seems that according to the differences it should have, the soul is divided into parts which are more diverse than those parts into which they divide the soul. Next he enumerated those parts. He said: **namely, the nutritive power,** etc. That is, for instance, the soul is divided into the nutritive power and the sensitive [power]. For no one can put the sensitive soul into the rational power nor into the irrational power. It is not among those things which lack reason because it is something which has apprehension, nor is it among things having reason, for reason does not exist in all animals. He meant by this to make known the error of the two [sorts of] division, namely, of one division of it into rational, emotional, and desiderative, and of the other division of it into rational and non-rational. For one who divides it into these two finds it difficult to be able to put many powers into both of those, for instance, sense and imagination. But one who divides it into those three has erred in two ways. He sets aside many differences, for instance, to take nourishment and to imagine, {510} and he even has divided the same power, the concupiscible, into more than one. When the soul is divided in such a way, then the parts of the soul will be infinite, as he indicates at the beginning.

42. **An important question arises regarding in which of those [parts imagination] is taken to be and whether it is the same or different, and chiefly if someone has asserted that the parts of the soul are different.[296] It is unthinkable also, in light of what we said, to distinguish this which is**

296. The Text here omits πρὸς δὲ τούτοις τὸ ὀρεκτικόν, ὃ καὶ λόγῳ καὶ δυνάμει ἕτερον ἂν δόξειεν εἶναι πάντων; "and lastly the appetitive, which would seem to be distinct both in definition and in power from all hitherto enumerated." Aristotle, *De Anima* (1984). Averroes' alternate translation, while obviously corrupt, does contain some remnants of this passage: ومع هذا فانا نجد الشوق وهو الأرب غير هذه الأجزاء جميعاً بالمعنى وبالقوة (ibid. [1954]); "Then we find desire, which is the end wholly other than these parts in intention and power."

thought to be different from all things in definition and activity. For what
governs exists in the cogitative part,²⁹⁷ while desire and anger are found in
the non-rational. If, therefore, the soul has three parts, then desire is found
in each of those.²⁹⁸ (432b1–7)

There arises for us a question in regard to which of those three or two
powers we have counted as having the power of imagination, namely, whether
this power is one of those powers into which we divided the parts of the soul
or [whether] it is different from them, chiefly if someone asserts that the parts
of the soul are different in definition and place. Next he said: **It is unthinkable**, etc. That is, it is unthinkable to divide this power which is thought to
be different from all in definition and activity (he means the desiderative
power) and to put it both in what has reason and in what lacks reason and
not to assert it as something proper to one of the two modes, as is the case
with other powers of the soul, but [to put it] in both. For the governing power
exists only in the rational soul (he meant this when he said **in the cogitative
part**) {511} and a non-governing [power], such as desire and anger, exists in
the non-rational. But we see that power to be enumerated according to the
number of powers in such a way that if the parts of the soul are three, then
desire will be found in all of them. He meant this when he said: **If, therefore,
the soul**, etc.

43. **What, however, we have reached in the account is [the issue of] what
it is which moves animals from place to place. It is thought that motion,
which involves growth and deterioration, exists in all animals and what
exists in all animals is what the generative and nutritive are thought to move.
Later on we will consider breathing,²⁹⁹ sleep, and wakefulness, for in regard
to those there are many questions.** (432b7–13)

297. ἔν τε τῷ λογιστικῷ γὰρ ἡ βούλησις γίνεται; "for wish is found in the calculative
part" (Aristotle, *De Anima* [1984]); الروية في الفكر (ibid. [1954]); "wish is in cogitation." In
the *Middle Commentary* (2002), 124.12–13, we find, "The principal expression of this
part, which is called choice (اختيارا), occurs in the cogitative faculty (في الفكر)"; Arabic
added.

298. The Greek has: "It is absurd to break up the last-mentioned faculty: for wish is
found in the calculative part and desire and passion in the irrational; and if the soul is
tripartite appetite will be found in all three parts." Aristotle, *De Anima* (1984). Corresponding to the Latin's *inopinabile*, "unthinkable," the *Middle Commentary* (2002), 124.10,
has ومن العسير, "difficult," while the alternate translation has ومن القبيح, "repugnant"
(ibid. [1954]).

299. The Text drops καὶ ἐκπνοῆς, "and [breathing] out." Aristotle, *De Anima* (1984);
my addition. This is not dropped from Averroes' alternate translation (ibid. [1954]):
إخراج, nor from the *Middle Commentary* (2002), 124.19: وإخراجه.

But we did not intend [to take up] those questions in this place. For our intention is to investigate the nature of what it is which moves the animal in place. Next he said: **It is thought that the motion,** etc. That is, it is thought that motion of an animal in growth and deterioration exists in all animals and what is such is ascribed to the power which moves [the animal] to generating and to taking nutrition. He intended with this to make it known that this motion is different from local motion existing in what is moved in a local way, although each is in place, and that the mover in these is different. Next he said: **Later on we will consider,** etc. That is, after we have spoken concerning this power, we will consider breathing, sleep, and wakefulness, since each is a motion by the soul and involves many questions.

44. **Let us, therefore, consider local motion and what it is which moves animals by local motion.** {512} **It is evident that this [motion] is not by the nutritive power, for [the nutritive] power is always ascribed to those, while [local motion] is either with imagination or with desire.**[300] **For nothing is moved except either by desire for something or by flight from something, unless its motion is violent. If that were also a disposition of plants, they would be moved and they would have an organic part assisting this motion.** (432b13–19)

The activity of the nutritive power is always [present] and is ascribed to plants, while the activity of that [other] power is not always [present] nor is it in plants. And that motion which is in place always involves imagination and desire for something, for nothing is voluntarily moved except either out of desiring or out of fleeing something. Consequently, if that motion were from the nutritive soul, it would occur that this soul would be desiring and imagining. If the nutritive power were something which moves in place, it would happen that plants would be moved in place. And if plants were moved in place, then they would have this disposition, namely, imagination and desire, and they would also have an organic member in virtue of which motion comes to be.

45. **It is different from sense in this way too. For many animals have sense and are motionless in the same place and completely unmoving. If, then, nature does nothing in vain and works in a complete way in the cases of necessary things, unless it is in reference to things that are monstrosities which are not complete (for such animals are complete, not monstrosities, and the indication of it is that they generate and have {513} maturation and**

300. The Text here carries a sense different from the Greek: "for this kind of movement is always for an end and is accompanied either by imagination or by appetite." Aristotle, *De Anima* (1984). The alternate translation is awkward but closer to the Greek: من أجل شيء واحد (ibid. [1954]); "for the sake of one thing."

decline), then for this reason they do not have organic members through which there comes to be local motion. (432b19–26)

It is also necessary in this way for that power moving in place to be different from sense. For many animals have sensation but are completely unmoving. It is necessary that those animals not move at all. For since nature does nothing in vain, that is, it makes no member without benefit nor does it lack necessary things, that is, nor does it abstain from providing an animal with a member in which there is a necessary benefit (unless this is due to occurrences happening infrequently, as a sixth finger). Those unmoved animals do not have an instrument for walking and they are still complete, not monstrous. The indication of it is that they generate [animals] like themselves and also have maturation and decline in their lives as do other natural beings whose being is natural. Hence it is necessary that those animals be unmoved and for this reason they do not have members for motion. You ought to know that he employs the argument from concomitance to refute [the position] that these powers are causes of motion only in this way because what is at issue is the proximate cause of motion. If not, then sense is one of the causes of that motion, but a remote cause.[301]

46. **But what causes motion is neither the cogitative part nor that which is called intellect. For the cogitative part[302] does not see what it does nor does it say anything in regard to what is fled or in regard to what is pursued.**

301. The argument from concomitance is that of the second figure of the syllogism in the affirmative, which does not yield a necessary conclusion. Cf. {416}, Book 3, n. 128. Here the argument would be that because one kind of animal has sensation and another kind has sensation, then whatever other characteristics the first has (here, local motion), the second must have. The argument would then be that the cause of local motion is the possession of sensation. But this conclusion is not necessary. If it were, one would conclude that everything having sensation has local motion, which is not the case. Consequently, the proximate cause of local motion is not sensation and so must be attributed to another power of the soul. Nevertheless, the remote cause of local motion for those things which have local motion is indeed sensation since appetite and desire, which arise because of sensation, move what has local motion.

302. This is a significant corruption of the text of Aristotle, for which the corresponding Greek here is ὁ θεωρητικὸς <νοῦς>, "mind as speculative." Aristotle, *De Anima* (1984). The alternate translation has النظر فى العقل (ibid. [1954]); "theoretical contemplation in the intellect," and it was consulted by Averroes, as is evident in his Comment. Without mentioning his source, Averroes seems to correct this text in his Comment at Book 3 {46.12}ff., using Themistius, *De Anima Paraphrase* (1899), 118.8–9. There Themistius writes of the first theoretical intellect: ἐπεὶ γὰρ διττὸς ὁ νοῦς, ὁ μὲν θεωρητικὸς οὐδὲν θεωρεῖ τῶν πρακτῶν οὐδὲ περὶ φευκτοῦ καὶ ὀρεκτοῦ διανοεῖται. "For there are two kinds of intellect: the contemplative <and the practical>. <The contemplative

Motion, however, is always found either in what flees or in what pursues. It is also not among the things which, when they have seen {514} such a thing, they set forth in pursuit or flight, as frequently we hold something to be desirable or fearful and are not sent into fear. The heart, however, is moved when a different member is enticed.[303] (432b26–433a1)

By **the cogitative part** one can understand the theoretical intellect and by the part **which is called intellect** the practical intellect. For this reason he said: **For the cogitative part does not see**, etc. That is, for the theoretical [intellect] does not consider practical things nor anything useful and pursued nor anything harmful and fled. Motion in place, however, is found only either in what pursues or in what flees. Next he said: **It is also not among the things**, etc. That is, neither is it also a part of the intellect which is naturally constituted to consider what is pursued and what is fled and which excites a movable member to motion toward the desirable thing or [which excites] a movable member in fear to motion [away from a fearful thing]. [This is what] happens for us when we imagine something desirable or fearful because the member proper in reference to that desirable thing is moved in us and the heart is constrained then by that fearful object. The intellect sees nothing of this, but we see it to be unmoved from that fearful object or to that which is desirable. He meant this when he said: **The heart, however,** etc. It is this way in the manuscript. [But] perhaps there is missing from this only that the intention was this, namely: the heart, however, is moved out of fear or out of desire when another member is moved from desire. What we find in the other translation shows

[intellect]> does not contemplate about what has to be done, nor think discursively about what is to be avoided and desired" (ibid. [1996], 144);وليس أيضاً النطقيّ الذى يقال له العقل هو المحرّك فإن العقل ضربان أحدهما نظريّ والآخر عمليّ فأمّا النظريّ فليس ينظر فى المعمولات و لا يميّز شيئًا من أمر المهروب منه والمطلوب (ibid. [1973], 217.9–12); "Moreover, it is not the case that the rational part which is called the intellect is the mover, for intellect is of two sorts, one theoretical and the other practical. The theoretical does not contemplate *intelligibles* (!) and does not discern anything to be fled or pursued." Cf. Book 2, Text 32 {177}, at 415a11–12, where τοῦ θεωρητικοῦ νοῦ is rendered *Intellectus . . . speculativus et cogitativus*.

303. "Further, neither can the calculative faculty or what is called thought be the cause of such movement; for mind as speculative (ὁ . . . θεωρητικὸς) never thinks what is practicable, it never says anything about an object to be avoided or pursued, while this movement is always in something which is avoiding or pursuing an object. No, not even when it is aware of such an object does it thereby enjoin pursuit or avoidance of it; e.g. the mind often thinks of something terrifying or pleasant without enjoining the emotion of fear. It is the heart that is moved (or in the case of a pleasant object some other part)." Aristotle, *De Anima* (1984); Greek added.

this, namely: "Frequently the intellect cogitates regarding something fearful or something desirable, but there will not be fear or desire on account of this. The heart, however, is moved with the motion of fear {515} but not from the intellect. When it cogitates regarding something desirable, then a member different from the heart is moved with the motion of desire."[304]

47. **When the intellect has commanded and cogitation has affirmed to flee something or to pursue it, [the heart] will not be moved, but it does what is in concert with desire, just as one who cannot restrain himself. Generally we see he who has the art of medicine does not [always] cure because there is something else which governs activities which come about through knowledge.** (433a1–5)

We see also that the intellect frequently commands that something be pursued or fled, but nevertheless people are not moved by the fact that the intellect gives its assent but from the fact that it is in concert with desire, as happens for a human being seeking pleasure who does not restrain himself. Next he said: **Generally,** etc. That is, generally we see frequently that many people who know some art do not act in virtue of that art, as we see many physicians not cure themselves when they are ill. This is only because there is another mover governing the activity of those activities which are carried out through knowledge and art. If it were not so, it would happen that everyone having knowledge of some operation would do that thing which he knows.

48. **Governance in regard to this motion does not belong to knowledge. Nor does it even belong to desire. For hermits**[305] **have desire and longing, but they do not do these things toward which they are moved by desire, because they follow intellect.** (3.10, 433a10) **It appears, therefore, that** {516}

---

304. The corresponding Arabic in Badawi's edition is: وكثيراً ما يتفكر العقل في شيء مخيف أو في شيء مُلِذّ فلا يكون الخوف عن أمر ولا للذة حركة ؛ فإن القلب يتحرك حركة الخوف ـ وليَس ذلكَ عن العقل ؛ وإذا تفكر في شيء ملذ كان عضواً غير القلب المتحرك حركة اللذة. (Aristotle, *De Anima* [1954]); "Oftentimes the intellect cogitates about something dreadful or something desirable, though there is no dread involved and no movement of desire. The heart is moved by the motion of fear—and this is not from the intellect. When it cogitates about something desirable, what is moved by the notion of desire is a part other than the heart." The final part of this citation of the alternate translation corresponds to the beginning of Book 3, 47.1–4 {515}: *Et cum intellectus miserit et cogitatio affirmaverit fugere aliquid aut querere aliquid, non movebitur, sed facit illud quod convenit delectationi, sicut qui non potest se retinere.* There is no mention of heart in the corresponding section of the *Middle Commentary* (2002), 125.14–17.

305. *Heremite*: The corresponding Greek, οἱ . . . ἐγκρατεῖς, is rendered "those who successfully resist temptation." Aristotle, *De Anima* (1984).

the causes of the motion are these two, namely, desire and intellect, even if someone asserts that imagination is similar to intellect. For in most things we follow imagination without knowledge, for other animals do not have opinion or cogitation,[306] but only imagination. These two, therefore, namely, desire and intellect, are what cause motion from place to place. (433a5–13)

What, therefore, predominates in regard to that motion and is proper to this is not knowledge, since we are frequently moved by desire, although the intellect sees that we ought not to be moved. Nor is what predominates in that motion even desire, because many human beings have desires but do not follow desire, but rather [follow] intellect. When he had explained that it is impossible for local motion to be ascribed to one of those powers individually, and it also appears that each of those takes part in causing the motion (for motion does not come about without desire nor without intellect or imagination), he said: **It, therefore, appears**, etc. That is, it therefore appears from what we said that what causes the motion is two, namely, intellect and desire, or imagination, which is similar to intellect. For in most matters we are moved by imagination without knowledge, as animals are moved. For other animals do not have knowledge, but in place of it they have imagination. Those two powers, therefore, are what cause motion from place to place, namely, desire and intellect or imagination.

49. **And the practical intellect (this is what cogitates concretely) differs from the theoretical [intellect] in actuality.[307] For every {517} desire is a desire for something. For desire is not the principle of the practical intellect, but that particular thing is a principle of the intellect.[308] For this reason it neces-**

---

306. *Sine cognitione . . . non habent estimationem neque cogitationem*: παρὰ τὴν ἐπιστήμην . . . οὐ νόησις οὐδὲ λογισμὸς ἔστιν; 433a10–12; "(for many men follow their imaginations *contrary to knowledge*, and in all animals other than man *there is no thinking or calculation*)." Aristotle, *De Anima* (1984); emphasis added. While *cogitatio* is reasonable as ultimately derived from λογισμός, *estimatio* is far from νόησις. The alternate translation is also problematic here: (فى سائر الحيوان ليس الادراك إلا بالتوهم و بالفكر) (ibid. [1954]); "in the other animals there is no apprehension except by imagination and cogitation."

307. "It differs from speculative thought in the character of its end (τῷ τέλει)" Aristotle, *De Anima* (1984); Greek added.

308. It appears that the Greek οὐ γὰρ ἡ ὄρεξις at 433a15–16 was read as οὐ γὰρ ἡ ὄρεξις, "For desire is not . . . " for the original Arabic translation from Greek. The Greek is rendered: "for that which is the object of appetite is the stimulant of practical thought; and that which is last in the process of thinking is the beginning of the action." Aristotle, *De Anima* (1984). ἀρχὴ τῆς πράξεως , here rendered "the beginning of the action," is not soundly reflected in *principium intellectus*. The alternate translation suffers from

sarily appears that these two are what cause motion, namely, desire and cogitation in reference to action. For the object of desire causes motion and for this reason cogitation causes movement, because it is a desiderative [power].[309] (433a14–19)

The intellect in virtue of which there is activity (this is the cogitative practical [intellect]) differs from the theoretical [intellect] in actuality and end. For the end of the theoretical [intellect] is just to know, while that of the practical [intellect] is to act. Next he said: **every desire**, etc. That is, because every desire is desire for something, for this reason desire is not the principle moving the practical intellect, but that desired object moves the intellect. Then the intellect will desire and when it has desired, then the human being will be moved, namely, by the desiderative power, which is the intellect or imagination.[310] Next he said: **For this reason it necessarily**, etc. That is, because the principle of motion is from the desired object, it appears that these two move the human being, namely, desire and belief which exist in reference to operation, in this way, namely, that what causes desire and what causes movement (which is intellect) are the same, but it is the cause of movement because it causes desire

---

textual difficulties here also, reading οὗ as οὐ and rendering the last part of the sentence less that soundly: وليس هذه الشهوة بدء العقل الفعال ، بل أجزاء العقل الفعال بدء العقل (ibid. [1954]); "and this desire is not the starting point of the active understanding but rather parts of active understanding are the starting point of the intellect." Some of the Greek manuscripts, however, do have οὐ. See ibid. (1956). Note that العقل الفعال, "active understanding," is here a term carrying the sense of "the intellect which is active in practical action."

309. The Greek text has: τὸ ὀρεκτὸν γὰρ κινεῖ, καὶ διὰ τοῦτο ἡ διάνοια κινεῖ, ὅτι ἀρχὴ αὐτῆς ἐστι τὸ ὀρεκτόν. καὶ ἡ φαντασία δὲ ὅταν κινῇ, οὐ κινεῖ ἄνευ ὀρέξεως; "for the object of appetite starts a movement and as a result of that thought gives rise to movement, the object of appetite being to it a source of stimulation. So too when imagination originates movement, it necessarily involves appetite." Aristotle, *De Anima* (1984). ἀρχὴ seems perhaps to have been moved toward the end of the sentence so as somehow to be read with the sentence which follows. See Text 50 below. The alternate translation is sound: المشتهىَ بَدْءُ حركة الفكر. – والتوهم إذا حرك لا يحرك بغير شهوة (ibid. [1954]); "That which is desired is the beginning of the motion of cogitation. And when imagination causes motion, it does not cause motion in the absence of desire."

310. Ivry (*Middle Commentary* [2002], 208, n. 7) notes that this sentence appears in the *Middle Commentary*, which has فإذا حركه اشتهى العقل أو التخيل وإذا اشتهى تحرك الإنسان به ، أعنى عن القُوة المشتهية التى هى العقل والتخيل; "When it elicits motion, the intellect or imagination desires [the object]; and when desiring, the person moves due to it—that is, due to the appetitive faculty which is the intellect and imagination." Ibid., 126.6–8.

for the thing.[311] He meant this when he said: **For the object of desire**, etc. That is, for because the object of desire is itself what moves that which apprehends (this is the practical intellect or imagination) and when the intellect apprehends something, it will desire in virtue of knowledge and will move in virtue of desire, it is necessary that the intellect itself be a cause of motion insofar as it is what desires, not insofar as it is what apprehends, and not insofar {518} as desire is a power different from the intellect which is also a cause of motion, as he himself will explain later. What he said concerning the practical intellect should be understood concerning the imagination, for animals universally are moved by imagination. If, therefore, form is imagined on the basis of cogitation, then motion will be ascribed to the practical intellect. If it is not on the basis of cogitation, then it will be ascribed to the imaginative power itself.

50. **The beginning of this will be at the time at which imagination is moved. There is, therefore, no motion in the absence of desire. There is therefore one mover, namely, what desires. For if the mover were two, namely, intellect and desire, then it would move in a common way. But the intellect does not seem to cause motion at all in the absence of desire. For when will and desire are moved in cogitation, then will causes motion.[312] Desire moves with motion which does not involve cogitation. Desire is a certain kind of appetite.** (433a19–26)

The beginning of this motion which is from the thing desired will be at the time at which the imagination is moved by the thing desired without appetite. For imagination first apprehends the object of desire, namely, it is affected by it by way of apprehension; when it apprehends it, it will perhaps desire [it]; and when it has desire and there is there no different contrary desire nor a different contrary power {519} of soul, then the animal will move in place toward that object of desire. Next he said: **There is therefore one mover**. That is, for because the mover, therefore, which is the object of desire, is one, it will

---

311. The corresponding sentence in the *Middle Commentary* helps elucidate what we have in the Latin of the *Long Commentary*. ومن قبل أن مبدأ الحرك يظهر أنها من المشتهية "As it يظهر أيضا أن هذين هما الذان يحركان الإنسان ، أعني الشهوة والاعتقاد أو التخيل is evident that the principal factor of motion derives from the desired object, it is also evident that both these—namely, desire and belief or imagination—are the factors which move a person." *Middle Commentary* (2002), 126.9–11.

312. (ἡ γὰρ βούλησις ὄρεξις, ὅταν δὲ κατὰ τὸν λογισμὸν κινῆται, καὶ κατὰ βούλησιν κινεῖται); "(for wish is a form of appetite; and when movement is produced according to calculation it is also according to wish)." Aristotle, *De Anima* (1984). The alternate translation also varies from the Greek: وذلك أن الروية أرب وشهوة ، وتحرك العقل بالفكر فإنما يتحرك بالروية (ibid. [1954]); "For will is wish and desire and moves the intellect by cogitation. So, then, it is moved only by will."

happen that what is moved by it, which is what moves the animal, namely, the
power of desire, is one also. This is either intellect or imagination insofar as
each is what has desire. If what moves the animal were two, namely, intellect
per se and the desiring power per se insofar as they are different, then the
motion of the animal would not proceed from them except incidentally,[313]
namely, in virtue of a nature common to those two powers which would be
different from each of those. Next he said: **But the intellect**, etc. That is, if it
were so, then it would happen that the intellect per se and also desire per se
would move the animal, and it is not so. For intellect does not seem to cause
motion except voluntarily, just as imagination does not seem to cause motion
without desire. The difference between will and desire is that when will and
desire cause motion, then will moves in virtue of cogitation, while desire moves
[but] not in virtue of cogitation.[314] Next he said: **Desire is a certain kind of
appetite.** This is how it stood in the manuscript and it is wrong and should be
read: **Appetite is a certain kind of desire.**[315] That is, that the part of the soul
which desires is what causes motion universally. If, therefore, it desires in
virtue of cogitation, it will be called will and if it is without cogitation, it will
be called appetite. This error is shown in the other translation, in which it is
said: "Appetite, however, causes motion without cogitation, because appetite
is a kind of desire."[316]

51. **All intellectual understanding, therefore, is correct, while appetite
and imagination are sometimes correct and sometimes not. For this reason
the appetitive part always causes motion, but this[317] either {520} will be good
or will be thought to be good. But [this does] not [occur] in regard to all**

313. ولو كان المحرك للحيوان اثنان أعني العقل على حدة والشهوة على حدة، لكان تحرك
الحيوان عن كل واحد منهما عارضا; "Were an animal to have two [independent] sources
of motion—the intellect by itself and desire by itself—then the motion induced by each
one would be an incidental sort." *Middle Commentary* (2002), 126.20–21.

314. With the exception of the lemmata and this last sentence, the content of what
Averroes says here is virtually identical with what he says in the *Middle Commentary*
(2002), at 126.11–127.5. What is different is the explanation of the role of cogitation as a
power involved with the will. There is no mention of cogitation in this context in the
Middle Commentary.

315. Averroes here suggests rightly that an error has occurred in the transmission
of Aristotle's text. The Greek has ἡ γὰρ ἐπιθυμία ὄρεξίς τίς ἐστιν; "for wish is a form
of appetite." Aristotle, *De Anima* (1984). His view, like that of the English translators, is
based on the understanding that ἐπιθυμία is a species of the genus ὄρεξις. The same
view is found in the alternate translation. See the following note for that text.

316. وأما الشهوة فإنما تحرك بغير فكر – لأن الشهوة إنما هى ضرب من الشوق (Aristotle, *De
Anima* [1954]).

317. *Hoc*: a particular object of appetite.

[goods], for that [good] as actual is praiseworthy,[318] **and the actual**[319] **[good] is that for which it is possible that it can be otherwise.** (433a26–30)

Every activity of intellectual understanding is correct, while activities which come about from appetite and imagination are sometimes correct and sometimes not. For this reason the appetitive part always causes motion, because it causes motion toward what is correct and toward what is not correct. Intellectual understanding, however, causes motion only toward what is correct alone, and for this reason it does not always cause motion. Next he said: **but this either is good**, etc. That is, but this toward which the appetitive power causes motion either is good or is thought to be good but is not. This good toward which that power is moved is not the good common to all, for that good which is always in act is praiseworthy without qualification. He meant this when he said: **But [this does] not [occur] in regard to all [goods], for that [good] as actual is praiseworthy**, that is, that good existing in all things, for that good which is always actual is praiseworthy.[320] Next he said: **and the actual is that which [. . .] is otherwise**. That is, and the good which is pure activity is the good which moves in a way different from the way in which those goods which sometimes are in potency and sometimes in act move. This

318. The sense requires that we understand that what is praiseworthy is something which is attractive for us. That is, it is deemed praiseworthy because we find some good in it to be desirable.

319. The Latin *actuale* here may reflect a corruption of عملي, "practical," into فعلي, "actual," with the loss of the notion of practical doing contained in the Greek πρακτόν. Or it may reflect difficulty in understanding المعمول, which in fact appears in the corresponding passage of the alternate translation. Aristotle, *De Anima* (1954). The latter is likely the case since, as indicated in the next note, Averroes gives two interpretations of this text corresponding to two senses of المعمول, "active" or "actual" and "practiced" or "practical." The Greek here is rendered: "Now thought is always right, but appetite and imagination may be either right or wrong. That is why, though in any case it is the object of appetite which originates movement, this object may be either the real or the apparent good. To produce movement the object must be more than this: it must be good that can be brought into being by action; and only what can be otherwise than as it is can thus be brought into being." Ibid. (1984). In the *Middle Commentary* Averroes writes only of الخير العملي, "the practical good," and says nothing of the "actual good." *Middle Commentary* (2002), 127.14.

320. In what follows Averroes gives two interpretations of this Text and finds more suitable the second, which is in fact more in accord with the original text of Aristotle. Here in the first interpretation Averroes is uncertain about المعمول as used in the Arabic Text. That is, he understands it here as concerning the value of what is in actuality over what is in potentiality rather than concerning what is actual as practical. See the previous note. This also affects the comments of Averroes in the lines which follow here.

can be understood in light of his having said **But not in regard to all [goods]**, that is, but not universally. That is, the good toward which that power is moved is not wholly good, that is, always and without qualification, for that good which is in act is asserted to be praiseworthy. Or another way: **But not in regard to all [goods]**, that is, but a good which that power apprehends is not the good existing as praiseworthy by all, but rather it is a good for the practical intellect as something praiseworthy for that power and [also] a good which {521} can be found in a way different from the one in which it is a good. The common good for all, however, is the pure good. The intention in those is fairly similar and the latter [intention] seems, as it were, more fitting.

52. **It already appeared, therefore, that such a power of the soul causes motion and it is what is called the appetitive [power]. If those who divide the soul [into parts], divide it according to powers, then they will find a great many parts, namely, the nutritive, the sensitive, the understanding, the cogitative,**[321] **and the desiderative. For those are distinct from one another and more so than are the desiderative and likewise the irascible.**[322] (433a31–b4)

It already appeared from this account that such a power from among the powers of the soul, which apprehends and desires a thing, is a power moving the animal and that it is what is called the appetitive [power]. For those who are accustomed to dividing the soul into three parts or into two parts, it was necessary for them, if they intended to divide that according to the powers it should have, that they divide it into more parts, since it has more parts than those three, for instance, the nutritive, the sensitive, the understanding, and the cogitative.

53. **Owing to diversity, appetites are contrary to one another. This happens when the sorts of appetite are opposed,**[323] **and this will be only for what has sense through time. Intellect compels us to resist for the sake of a future thing and appetite [compels us to motion] for the sake of the reality of a present pleasure. It is thought, therefore, that the thing providing present**

---

321. Here *cogitantem* corresponds to the Greek βουλευτικόν. However, the *Middle Commentary* (2002), 128.20, has المروية, "deliberative."

322. ταῦτα γὰρ πλέον διαφέρει ἀλλήλων ἢ ἐπιθυμητικὸν, καὶ θυμικόν; "for these are more different from one another than the faculties of desire and passion." Aristotle, *De Anima* (1984).

323. τοῦτο δὲ συμβαίνει ὅταν ὁ λόγος καὶ αἱ ἐπιθυμίαι ἐναντίαι ὦσι; "which happens when a principle of reason and a desire are contrary." Aristotle, *De Anima* (1984). Note that the plural αἱ ἐπιθυμίαι is rendered singular by Smith and Barnes in this edition. The alternate translation also has the singular: ويعرض ذلك إذا اختلف الفكر والشهوة (ibid. [1954]).

pleasure {522} is pleasure without qualification, because it does not refer to a future thing. (433b5–10)

It can be understood: on account of the diversity of the appetites which are in the concupiscible soul, they contradict one another in regard to motion. Or [it can be understood] in another way: that is, on account of the diversity of the appetite of the concupiscible soul from the intellect, they contradict one another. This latter is the more evident. Next he said: **This happens**, etc. That is, this happens in one and the same thing[324] when the sorts of the appetites in it are opposed. That sort of contrariety is found only in an animal which apprehends time, because in the present it apprehends with respect to the thing something different from that which [it apprehends with respect to the thing] in the future, for instance, to judge that now it is something pleasurable and in the future painful.[325] Next he said: **Intellect compels [us] to resist**. He meant to show the diversity of the two sorts in reference to appetite, namely, the appetite of intellect and the appetite of the concupiscible soul. For the concupiscible soul causes movement toward a thing which is pleasurable in act. The rational soul, however, frequently resists this on account of future harm, for instance, [regarding] intercourse and intoxication.[326] Next he said: **It is thought, therefore**, etc. That is, many therefore think that the thing presently pleasurable is pleasurable without qualification and never painful, because the concupiscible power does not see the pain occurring in the future.[327]

324. That is, in one and the same soul.

325. This sentence is found in the *Middle Commentary* (2002), 127.23–128.2: وهذا النحو من التضاد إنما يوجد من الحيوان فى الحيوان الذى يدرك الزمان وهو الناطق ، لأنه يدرك من الشئ فى الزمان الحاضر غير ما يدرك منه فى الزمان المستقبل ، مثل أن يدرك أنه لذيذ فى الحاضر مؤذ فى المستقبل "This sort of contrariety occurs to an animal who apprehends time—namely, a rational animal—for he apprehends in the present something in the object other than that which he apprehends in it in the future. For example, he apprehends that the object is pleasant now, but injurious in the future."

326. This sentence is also found in the *Middle Commentary*: والنفس النزوعية هى التى تحرك إلى اللذيذ الحاضر والعقل هو الذى يحكم بمضرة ذلك فى المستقبل، مثل الحال فى الجماع والتفنق فى المطاعم; "It is the appetitive faculty which moves toward present pleasure and the intellect which judges its future harm, as occurs with copulation and gourmandizing." *Middle Commentary* (2002), 128.2–4.

327. This sentence too is found in the *Middle Commentary*, although the difference should be noted. The *Middle Commentary* has mention of the intellect failing to consider future harm, while the *Long Commentary* has "the concupiscible power." وقد يظن كثير من الناس أن اللذيذ الحاضر لذيذ بإطلاق من قبل أنه لا يلحظ العقل فيهم ما يعرض من ذلك فى المستقبل من الأذى; "Many people think that the currently pleasant is absolutely pleasant, because their intellect does not consider the injury which will be incurred by it in the future." *Middle Commentary* (2002), 128.4–6.

54. **The cause of motion is the object of appetite inasmuch as it is an object of appetite. For the object of appetite precedes the others, for this causes motion and is [itself] unmoved, because it moves imagination and intellect.**[328] **Things causing motion, however, are many in number because the things in virtue of which motion comes about** {523} **are three, one is the mover, another is the thing in virtue of which it causes motion, and the third is what is moved. The mover exists in two ways: one is as immovable, while the other is as movable.**[329] **What is unmoved is that which is understood to be good.**[330] **But the appetitive part is mover and moved. (For it moves what is moved insofar as it is an object of appetite, because appetite is a kind of motion, namely, [appetite] which is in act.) What is moved is the animal. The instrument causing motion is appetite. Those are bodily things, and for this reason they should be investigated in the context of actions common to the soul and to the body.** (433b10–21)

The first mover in this motion is the thing which is the object of appetite insofar as it is an object of appetite. For the thing which is the object of appetite precedes the other things which move the animal in this motion because it moves and is not moved, and that is the disposition of a first mover.[331] Next he said: **because it moves imagination and intellect.** That is, it is a

328. The beginning of this Text fails to reflect εἴδει μὲν ἓν ἂν εἴη, with the result that the sentence is construed differently. "*It follows that while that which originates movement must be specifically one, viz.* the faculty of appetite as such (or rather farthest back of all the object of that faculty; for it is it that itself remaining unmoved originates the movement by being apprehended in thought or imagination), the things that originate movement are numerically many." Aristotle, *De Anima* (1984); emphasis added to indicate omitted text. The alternate translation differs from the Greek: فيرى الشوق محركاً بالصورة أولى هذه (ibid. [1954]); "So desire accounts for motion by form المحركات ، وهو الشيءوالمشتهى المطلوب as prior to these movers. This [mover] is the thing desired and sought after."

329. The Text here may be faulty. The Latin's *mobilis* corresponds to τὸ δὲ κινοῦν καὶ κινούμενον, "or that which at once moves and is moved." Aristotle, *De Anima* (1984); emphasis added. The alternate reflects the Greek well with أحدهما لا يتحرك فى نفسه والآخر متحرك منتقل ، (ibid. [1954]); "One of the two is unmoved in itself and the other causes motion and is moved."

330. *Bonum intellectum* corresponds to the Greek τὸ πρακτὸν ἀγαθόν, "the realizable good." Aristotle, *De Anima* (1984).

331. These initial sentences of this Comment are virtually identical to what Averroes writes in the *Middle Commentary*: والمحرك الأول فى هذه الحركة هو الشيء المشتهى بما هو مشتهى، وذلك أن الشيء المشتهى يتقدم سائر الأشياء المحركة للحيوان فى هذه الحركة ، لأن هذا هو الذى يحرك فى هذه الحركة ولا يتحرك وهذه هى صفة المحرك الأول؛ "The prime mover in this motion is the object of desire qua desideratum. It is prior to other things which move an animal in this [sort of] motion, for it causes motion of this sort and is not

mover because it moves imagination when appetite belongs to the imaginative part or intellect if appetite belongs to that part of the soul.[332] Next he
said: **The things causing motion, however, are many in number.** That is,
the things causing motion, however, by which that motion comes to be are
more than one.[333] Next he said: **because the things in virtue of which motion comes about,** etc. That is, it happens that the mover is more than one on
account of what was explained in the general accounts,[334] namely, that every
motion comes about through three things, of which one is the mover which
is unmoved, another that in virtue of which it moves (this is the mover and
moved), and the third is what is moved and not a mover.[335] Next he said: **The
mover** {524} **exists in two ways,** etc. That is, it was explained there that the
mover exists in two ways, namely, as unmoved mover (this is the first) and
as mover which is moved (it is this in virtue of which the first mover causes
motion). Next he showed what each of those three is in regard to this motion.
He said: **What is unmoved is that which is understood to be good** , etc. That
is, what is mover and unmoved in this motion is what is thought good and
what the appetitive soul apprehends. The mover and the moved is the thing

---

moved, which is the attribute of a prime mover." *Middle Commentary* (2002), 128.6–9. In
the *Middle Commentary* this text is continuous with the texts cited in the following notes
for much of the rest of this Comment. Averroes has broken that continuity here in the
Long Commentary with citations of the relevant Text of Aristotle.

332. Again, this sentence is virtually identical to what Averroes writes in the *Middle
Commentary:* وإنما صار محركا أولا من قبل أنه يحرك المتخيل إذا كانت الشهوة للجزء المتخيل
أو يحرك العقل إذا كان الشهوة لهذا الجزء من النفس أيضا; "It is indeed a prime mover,
since it moves the imagination when desire occurs to the imaginative part of the soul,
or it moves the intellect when desire occurs to it also." *Middle Commentary* (2002),
128.9–11.

333. Again, this sentence is virtually identical to what Averroes writes in the *Middle
Commentary:* فإن المحركون الذين يلتئم بهم هذه الحركة فهم أكثر من واحد; "The moving
agents in which this motion is coordinated are more than one." *Middle Commentary*
(2002), 128.12–13.

334. *Physics* 8.5, 256b14ff.

335. Again, this sentence is virtually identical to what Averroes writes in the *Middle
Commentary:* وذلك أنه قد تبين فى الأقاويل الكلية أن كل حركة فهى تلتئم من ثلاثة أشياء
أقل ذلك أحدها المحرك الذى لا يتحرك، والآخر الشيء الذى به يحرك وهذا هو متحرك محرك
ومجموعهما هو الذى يسمى المتحرك من تلقائه والثالث الممتحرك الغير محرك; "this, in
that it has been explained in general terms that every motion is coordinated by three
things, at least: one is the mover which is not moved; another, that with which it moves,
which is moved, moving, and a combination of both and is called self-moved; and the
third is the moved object which does not cause motion." *Middle Commentary* (2002),
128.13–16.

which has appetite,[336] that is, the member of the body in which that part of the soul exists, while appetite is the motion which arises from the thing which is the object of appetite in virtue of what is understood in act.[337] Perhaps he meant this when he said: **because appetite is a motion, namely, [motion] which is in act**, that is, appetite which arises from the thing which is the object of appetite in act. Or alternatively: that is, the appetite which is appetite in act. What is moved and not a mover, which is a third thing in regard to this motion, is the animal.[338] Next he said: **The instrument . . . is appetite**, etc. That is, because that in virtue of which the first mover moves is necessarily a body, since it is moved, as was explained in the general accounts,[339] and appetite here is that in virtue of which the first mover causes motion, therefore the thing which has appetite in virtue of which the animal is moved is the body and appetite is its form. For this reason it is necessary to seek out these things in virtue of which that motion comes about where he speaks about actions common to soul and body, that is, in the part of natural science in which he speaks about those common actions, such as sleep and wakefulness. He had spoken about this in the treatise which he wrote *On the Motion of Animals*,[340] but that treatise has

336. Again, this part of this sentence is virtually identical to what Averroes writes in the *Middle Commentary*: فأما الشيء الذى هو فى هذه الحركة محرك غير متحرك فهو الخير; المعقول، وأما المحرك المتحرك فهو الجزء الشهوانى من البدن "That which moves and is not moved in the motion under discussion is the intelligible good; the moving and moved thing is the desiderative part of the body." *Middle Commentary* (2002), 128.16–18.

337. That is, appetite as mover results from actual thought of the desired object.

338. Again, this sentence is virtually identical to what Averroes writes in the *Middle Commentary*: وأما المتحرك الغير محرك فهو الحيوان; "and that which is moved and does not cause motion is the animal." *Middle Commentary* (2002), 128.18–19.

339. *Physics* 8.5, 256b15–19.

340. Again, these sentences are virtually identical to what Averroes writes in the *Middle Commentary*: ولما كان الشيء الذى به يحرك المحرك الأول واجبا أن يكون جسما إذ كان متحركا حسيما تبين فى الأقاويل الكلية، وكانت الشهوة هاهنا هى الذى به يحرك المحرك الأول فى هذه الحركة، فالشيء الشهوانى الذى به يتحرك الحيوان هو جسم و الشهوة هى صورته. ولهذه العلة ينبغى أن نلتمس معرفة الأجسام التى بها تلتئم هذه الحركة حيث نتكلم فى تلخيص الأشياء التى تلتئم بها الأفعال الموجودة للنفس والبدن. وذلك فى الجزء من العلم الطبيعى الذى نتكلم فيه فى الأفعال المشتركة للنفس والبدن وهو الكتاب المعروف بحركة الحيوان المكانية; "As the object in which the first mover acts has to be a body, since it is moved (as has been explained in the [preceding] general remarks), and as it is actual desire with which the first mover performs this motion, the desiderative faculty whereby the animal moves is corporeal, and desire is its form. It is appropriate, for this reason, to seek knowledge of the bodies with which this motion is coordinated when we engage in explaining the factors whereby the activities common to soul and body are coordinated. This is that part of natural science in which we speak [of such activities], which is the book known as *De motu animalium*." *Middle Commentary* (2002), 128.19–129.5.

not come down to us, but what was transmitted to us was a part of the summary of Nicolaus.[341] {525}

55. I say now generally that the body is moved by motion of a very similar sort. For where the starting point is, there also is the end, as circular motion.[342] For in this convexity and concavity are found one as end and the other as starting point. For this reason one is at rest while the other is moved, although in definition they are different; in spatial magnitude, however, they are not distinct. For everything which is moved is moved by pushing and pulling. Hence it is necessary that the thing be at rest, as what happens in the case of a wheel, and that the starting point of motion be from this. (433b21–27)

After he had made it known that the inquiry concerning things in virtue of which that motion comes about is more fitting elsewhere, he began here to recount something general. He said: **I say now generally,** etc. That is, I say now that the body is moved by the first instrument in such a way that the first instrument which moves it, which is the subject of the desiderative soul, is in the body of the animal in one place from which the parts of the moved part of the animal are pushed and toward which the parts of that part are pulled by that instrument.[343] For in the case of every motion composed of pulling and push-

---

341. Drossaart Lulofs speculates that this may be a reference to a section of the zoological part of the compendium *On the Philosophy of Aristotle* by Nicolaus. See (in the primary sources) Nicolaus of Damascus (1965), 39 and 11. Also see Peters (1968), 48. Cf. Aristotle, *Movement of Animals*, ch. 10, 703a4ff., as Ivry suggests at *Middle Commentary* (2002), 209, n. 16, and ch. 6, 700b4ff.

342. This Text significantly fails to reflect the corresponding Greek: "To state the matter summarily at present, that which is the instrument in the production of movement is to be found where a beginning and an end coincide as e.g. in a ball and socket joint." Aristotle, *De Anima* (1984). The corresponding text in the alternate translation is cited by Averroes in his Comment. For that Arabic text, see below.

343. This sentence is found in the *Middle Commentary* with only slight variations. إن البدن يتحرك عن الآلة الأولى المحركة له التي هي موضوع النفس المتشوقة ، و هي من بدن الإنسان في موضع واحد منه تندفع عنها جميع أجزاء الجهة المنبسطة من الحيوان واليه تنجذب جميع أجزاء الجهة المنقبضة منه؛ "the body is moved by the first organ which moves it, which is the substrate of the desiderative soul. It is a place in the human body from which all parts of its constricting aspect are pulled." *Middle Commentary* (2002), 129.6–9. Differences in the Arabic are indicated by the overbar. Comparison of this with the extant Arabic fragment in the next note indicates support for the reading على in ان الآلة الأولى in the *Middle Commentary*'s Modena manuscript. See *Middle Commentary* (2002), 129, n. 2. The first half of the sentence following immediately here is also identical with ibid., 129.12–13: وذلك أن كل حركة مؤلفة من جذب ودفع لا بد, which is exactly what is found in the extant fragment. See the following note.

ing, it is necessary that the starting point from which the pushing exists be the end toward which there is pulling. For this reason he said: **as circular motion.**[344] For circular motion is composed of pulling and pushing. However, that the motion of an animal is composed of pulling and pushing is evident. For when the right part is moved by us and we are held stable on the left, then certain parts of that part will be {526} pushed toward the front and certain parts pulled, and they are the parts which are farther back. The pulling and pushing of these is not in a straight line but in lines not straight, more curved than straight, and for this reason it is likened to the circle. The instrument in virtue of which the body desires first and generally is not known by us. In place of this account we find a clearer account in the other translation as follows: "Let us, therefore, say briefly that the mover is, as it were, something possessing this disposition in its starting point and in its end, just as what is called in Greek *gigglimus*.[345] For there is convexity and concavity in it, and one of these is the end and the other the starting point."[346] Next he said: **For in this convexity and concavity are found.** That is, for in everything which is moved by pushing and pulling, not in a straight way, there happens to exist concavity and convexity in such a way that what is convex is unmoving from what will be the starting point of the pushing and to what is the end of pulling, and what is concave is moved, as is the case for a body moved in a circular way. For the motion of every body which is moved in a circular way is composed of pulling and pushing, as was said in the Seventh Book of the *Physics*.[347] Next he said:

---

344. Arabic fragments correspond to Book 3, 55.16–24: ان البدن يتحرك عن الآلة الأولى، على ان الآلة الأولى المحركة له والتي هي موضوع النفس المتشوقة هي في بدن ⟨الحيوان⟩ في موضع واحد ، منه تندفع عنها جميع أجزاء الجهة المنبسطة من الحيوان واليه تنجذب ⟨الأجزاء⟩ الأخرى ⟨. .⟩. وذلك أن كل حركة مؤلفة من جذب ودفع لا بد ⟨أن يكون⟩ لها مبدأ منه تندفع ونهاية اليها تنجذب ويعني بقوله : بمنزلة الحركة اللولبية (*Long Commentary* Fragments [1985], 45). Perhaps due to the omission of و, the Latin translator understood the last portion of this text differently from what we have in the fragments. The Arabic has "<it is necessary that> it have a starting point from which it is pushed and an end toward which it is pulled." Cf. the previous note regarding this text in the *Middle Commentary*. Ben Chehida's conjecture of <الحيوان> may be corrected with the *Middle Commentary*'s الإنسان. *Middle Commentary* (2002), 129.8.

345. ὁ γιγγλυμός: a ball-and-socket joint.

346. فأما الآن فإنا نختصر بايجاز فنقول إن المحرك كآلة هو الذي بحال واحدة من بدئه ونهايته ، مثل الذى يسمى باليونانية جنجلموس فان فيه أحد وثنية : فأحد هذين نهايته والآخر بدؤه (Aristotle, *De Anima* [1954]). This text is apparently quoted in the Arabic fragments at *Long Commentary* Fragments (1985), 45. Note that أحد is missing in the fragments. In its place Ben Chehida suggests <تحدب>.

347. Averroes seems to have in mind *Physics* 8.10, 267b9–17 and perhaps also *Physics* 7.2, 243a15ff.

one is **as end and the other as starting point**, etc. That is, one part is unmoving in virtue of the motion of the pulling of the end and [the other] in virtue of the motion of the pushing [is] the starting point. For this reason it is necessary that what is convex, or what is in place of the convex, be unmoving and that what is concave, or what is in place of the concave, be moved. Still, the starting point and the end in this motion are different in definition, while they are the same in spatial magnitude, as the center of a circle. And this is the contrary of straight motion, namely, that the starting point and the end are in it as different in definition and in magnitude. The member [of the body] which is such as this in the animal is the heart, according to him.[348]
Next he said: **For everything {527} which is moved is moved according to a certain convexity**. That is, it was necessary that in the animal there be such a member at rest because it is the starting point of the motion of pushing and the end of pulling because everything which is moved by pulling and pushing is necessarily by way of some unmoving convexity toward which the pulling motion reaches and from which the pushing motion begins. For this reason it is necessary that in every such case there be something stable which is the starting point and the end, as the center in a wheel. That account is founded on two propositions, one that the motion of an animal in place is composed of pushing and pulling and the other that every motion composed of pulling and pushing has an unmoving thing from which there is a starting point of pushing motion and toward which there is an end of attractive [motion]. For it appears that it is necessary in regard to every motion that this from which there is motion and toward which there is motion is at rest. Since, therefore, motion is composed of pushing and pulling, it will happen that what is at rest is the same. When, therefore, these two propositions have been conceded, it will follow from these that in the animal there is a member at rest from which the motion of pushing begins and toward which it reaches. Because we see that the final member which is at rest in local motion is the

348. Arabic fragments correspond to Book 3, 55.42–59: ‹يعني ان كانت كل حركة مؤلفة من الجذب والدفع على غير استقامة لزم ان توجد في شيء فيه تحديب وتقعير حتى يكون المحدب الذي فيه ساكن ومنه مبدأ حركة الدفع واليه نهاية حركة الجذب ، والمقعر متحرك كالحال في الجسم المتحرك ‹حركة› دورة. فان كل جسم متحرك دورة فحركته مؤلفة من جذب ودفع كما قيل ‹في السابعة من السماع ثم قال : كما كان ذلك نهاية فهذا أيضا له مبدأ› فيلزم ان يكون هذا الجزء الساكن أما بحركة الجذب فنهاية وأما بحركة الدفع فمبدأ ولذلك يجب ان يكون المحدب أو الشيء الذي يتنزل منزلة المحدب فساكن ، فأما المقعر او الذي ينزل منزلة المقعر فمتحرك ، على انّ المبدأ والنهاية في هذه الحركة هما مختلفين في الحدّ وإما في العظم فواحد بمنزلة المركز وهذا بخلاف ما عليه الأمر في الحركة المستقيمة – أعني ان المبدأ فيها والنهاية مختلفين بالحد والعظم ، والعضو الذي بهذه الصفة في الحيوان هو القلب عنده (*Long Commentary* Fragments [1985], 45). Note that Ben Chehida fails to provide the location of the closing brackets <following يعني›.

heart,[349] it is necessary that its starting point be from this. That passage, therefore, should be understood in this way. And those propositions are evident and apparent but to verify them through induction and to give the causes of appearances in this matter is proper to an account concerning the local motion of animals.

56. Generally, as we said, because the thing, insofar as it is an animal, has appetite, so in virtue of that intention it moves itself. There is no desire {528} in the absence of imagination, for everything imagined is either sensible or an object of cogitation (for this is found in other animals). (3.11, 423b31) Let us, therefore, consider in regard to imperfect animals what moves those in which sensation is only through touch alone.[350] Let us say, therefore: is it possible for them to have pain and pleasure? If they have these two, they necessarily have appetite. How, then, will there be imagination? Or perhaps, as they are moved by indeterminate motion, does it also exist in this way in them? For it is in them, as we said, with imagination of the indeterminate sensible. (433b27–434a6)

Because the thing, insofar as it is an animal, has appetite, it is necessary that it move itself in virtue of that intention. No appetite exists without imagination, for every thing which imagines either has that imagined form by which it is moved from sense, or it has it from cogitation. In human beings, however, it is had from cogitation, while in other animals from sense. Since we assert that every appetite comes about from imagination, while imagination comes about from the five senses in perfect animals, it is necessary to consider how imperfect animals, which have only touch alone, are moved. It is evident that if those have pleasure and pain, it is necessary that they have appetite. But if we assert that these have appetite, it will be necessary that they have imagination.[351] But those are thought not to have imagination since they

349. Arabic fragments correspond to Book 3, 55.80–81: وذلك أننا نرى ان آخر كل عضو سكن في الحركة في المكان هو القلب (*Long Commentary* Fragments [1985], 45).

350. The Text here fails to render the Greek πότερον ἐνδέχεται φαντασίαν ὑπάρχειν τούτοις, ἢ οὔ, καὶ ἐπιθυμίαν. "Can they have imagination or not? or desire?" Aristotle, *De Anima* (1984). The Greek is reflected in the alternate translation: وهل يمكن أن يكون لمثله توهم وشهوة أم لا يمكن؟ (ibid. [1954]); "Can its like have imagination and desire or not?"

351. With only minor variations, the entire Comment up to this point is also found in the *Middle Commentary*: ولما كان الحيوان بما هو حيوان له شهوة فواجب أن يكون بذلك المعنى يحرك ذاته. وكل شهوة فهى غير عرية من التخيل، وذلك أن كل متخيل فإما أن تكون الصورة الخيالية المحركة له حاصلة عن الحس ،إما أن تكون حاصلة عن الفكر. فأما الحاصلة عن الفكر فهى للإنسان ، وأما الحاصلة عن الحس فهى للحيوانات الآخر.(!) (327) وإذا فرضنا أن كل شهوة إنما توجد عن تخيل والتخيل يكون عن الحواس الخمس فى الحيوانات الكاملة، فقد يجب أن

are moved toward sensibles only in the presence of those [sensibles] or are moved with indeterminate motion. But whatever way it may be, let us say that just as they are moved with indeterminate motion, {529} that is, toward an indeterminate intention, so too it seems that they imagine with an indeterminate imagination, since they sense with indeterminate sensation.[352]

57. This is also found in other animals. The cogitative power, however, is in rational [animals] alone. To choose to do this or that belongs to cogitative activity.[353] **It figures itself one of necessity,**[354] **for it is moved toward the**

ننظر كيف الأمر في حركة الحيوانات الغير كاملة وهي التي ليس يوجد لها إلا حس اللمس. والأمر في هذه بين أنّه إن كان توجد لها اللذة والأذى فقد يجب أن توجد لها الشهوة. قإن كان ذلك كذلك فواجب أن يكون لها تخيل; "As, moreover, the animal qua animal has desire, there must be something here which moves itself. Every desire, furthermore, is not free of imagination, since the imaginative form which moves everything imagined occurs because of either perception or cogitation. That which occurs due to cogitation belongs to man, while that which occurs due to perception belongs to the other animals [also]. (327) Having posited that imagination is the source for the occurrence of every desire and that imagination derives from the five senses in perfect animals, we ought to see what the situation is in the motion of imperfect animals, those which have only the sense of touch. In this case, it is clear that, if pleasure and harm occur to them, then such animals must have desire and, hence, imagination. It might seem that those animals do not have imagination, since they are moved only in a vague and indeterminate way." *Middle Commentary* (2002), 129.18–130.8.

352. Part of this sentence is quite similar but not identical to what is found in the *Middle Commentary:* ولكن نقول إنه كما قد تتحرك حركة غير محدودة ولا محصلة كذلك يوجد لها تخيل غير محصل ولا محدود; "We say, however, that, just as an animal may be moved in an indeterminate and vague way, so can a vague and indeterminate imagination be found in it." *Middle Commentary* (2002), 130.9–10.

353. *Virtus autem cogitativa est in rationabilibus . . . de actione cogitativa.* ἡ δὲ βουλευτικὴ ἐν τοῖς λογιστικοῖς . . . λογισμοῦ ἤδη ἐστὶν ἔργον; "Sensitive imagination, as we have said, is found in all animals, deliberative imagination only in those that are calculative: for whether this or that shall be enacted is already a task requiring calculation" (Aristotle, *De Anima* [1984]); فالتوهم الحواسي ، كالذي قيل ، موجودٌ في سائر الحيوان وأما التوهم الذي يكون على الروية فإنما هو لذي النطق ، فإن الاختيار من فعل الفكر (ibid. [1954]); "For sensitive imagination, as was said, exists in the rest of the animals. The imagination which is deliberative belongs only to what has reason, for choice is from an activity of cogitation." Comparison of this Text of the *Long Commentary* with what we find in the *Middle Commentary* (2002), at 130.11–12 (where الرأى, "deliberation," not الفكر, "cogitation," corresponds to ἡ βουλευτικὴ) supports the view that Averroes was using different versions of the same translation of the *De Anima* when he composed these two works. See the introduction pp. lxxvii–lxxix.

354. This fails to render clearly the Greek καὶ ἀνάγκη ἑνὶ μετρεῖν, "and there must be a single standard to measure by." Aristotle, *De Anima* (1984). The alternate translation

greater in such a way that it is able to act from many imaginings. This is the cause of opinion.[355] **For it does not have cogitation because it does not involve something which comes about from reason.**[356] **This is something which is so on account of pleasure, because it does not have the cogitative power.**[357] **It, therefore, commands and moves sometimes this and sometimes that. For the appetite moves the appetite, just as a sphere, when it has the intention of containment.**[358] **For according to nature it is prior and a mover, in such a way that they are moved to motion.** (434a6–15)

Imagination exists in other animals, while cogitation exists in rational animals. For choosing to do this imagined thing and not another belongs to the activity of cogitation, not to the activity of imagination. For what judges that this imagined thing is more pleasant than another ought to be of necessity the same power which reviews imaginings in which it judges what is more pleasurable. He meant this when he said: **It figures itself one of necessity.** {530} That is, as I figure, it is necessary that one power review those imaginings until it apprehends what is more pleasant among them, as one thing reviews unequal numbers until it apprehends which is comparatively greater. Likewise, cogitation reviews imaginings and compares them until it is able to be affected by the imagination of some one of these. This is the reason why a rational animal has opinion, for opinion is belief which arises from cogitation. Next he said: **For it does not have cogitation**, etc. That is, aside from the rational animal, none has cogitation because none has reason. The motion of animals is due to pleasure and it is simple motion, not complex [motion]. This is because it does not have the cogitative power together with appetite in such a way that these two powers command one another to the extent that the animal is moved sometimes on account of will as [is the case] in regard to the rational animal.

---

has أحد الأمرين إلى المثل فى مضطر وهو (ibid. [1954]); "It is compelled toward one of two in the case of what is similar."

355. The Text fails to render the Greek μὴ δοκεῖν ἔχειν, "is held not to involve." Aristotle, *De Anima* (1984). The alternate translation omits this sentence.

356. The Text fails to render the Greek <αὕτη δὲ ἐκείνην>, which Ross brackets in Aristotle, *De Anima* (1956). This is rendered "though opinion involves imagination" in ibid. (1984). The alternate translation has القياس عن الكائن العزم له ليس أنه ذلك وعلة (ibid. [1954]); "The reason for this is that it does not have decision existing on the basis of reasoning."

357. This is an interpretive translation which adds to the Greek a reference to pleasure. The Greek is rendered, "Hence appetite contains no deliberative element." Aristotle, *De Anima* (1984). The alternate translation reflects the Greek.

358. *Continentie*: ἀκρασία, "moral weakness" (Aristotle, *De Anima* [1984]); تهتك (ibid. [1954]); "degradation." Crawford notes that manuscript D adds *non*.

Next he said: **For the appetite moves the appetite**, etc. That is, for it happens in what has more than one appetite that the animal may be moved in certain situations by two appetites at the same time, when it happens that one appetite is predominant and contains the second. For then it will lead it toward its motion, when the commanded appetite remains moved in its proper motion, as happens in the case of celestial bodies. For any given one of the orbs of the wandering stars seems to be moved with diurnal motion in virtue of an appetite of the orb of the fixed stars, although with its appetite it is moved by its proper motion. Next he said: **For according to nature it is**, etc. That is, this happens to this sphere which contains others, namely, to be in command over these {531} on account of this because it is prior by nature to the others and is what moves them, in such a way that in virtue of this it happens that the others are moved by it.

58. **The cognitive power, however, is not moved, but is at rest, because in one case [the premise] involves at once opinion and judgment of the universal,**[359] **while in the other it is of particulars. For this makes it such that such a thing must do such an action, while that is such that because that thing is so, I also am so. For this latter also causes motion, but the universal does not. Or [it is] both, but one is at rest, while the other is not.** (434a16–21)

The power, however, which apprehends the universal is not moved to the object apprehended, because it is a power which is only of opinion and of apprehension of a universal thing. The universal thing, however, does not cause motion at all, since it is not some singular thing. The power, however, which apprehends the particular is among particulars and is moved when [a particular] causes motion. He meant here, therefore, by **cognitive power** the power apprehending the universal thing. Next he said: **For that makes**, etc. That is, for the power which apprehends the universal affirms that every such thing must carry out such an activity, while the particular power is what apprehends an instance for itself according to the disposition which it affirmed, if it were to be knowing, so that it carries out that activity. The composition in virtue of which the activity comes about will, therefore, arise from apprehension on the part of those two powers. Next he said: **For this latter causes motion**, etc. That is, for the intention of the particular causes motion, while motion in reference to the universal either is not due to this or we should say that {532} motion is due to both, but is due to the universal because it is at rest and due to

---

359. *Quia illa est existimationis et iudicii universalis insimul*: ἐπεὶ δ' ἡ μὲν καθόλου ὑπόληψις καὶ λόγος; "Since the one premiss or judgement is universal. . . ." Aristotle, *De Anima* (1984). The *Middle Commentary* (2002), 131.5–6, has لأن هذه القوة إنما ;هى للعلم وإدراك الأمر الكلى فقط "since that faculty belongs solely to cognition and the apprehension of universals."

the particular because it is what is moved.[360] He meant this when he said: **but one is at rest, while** the other **is not.** That is, but if the universal is the mover, it will be so insofar as it is at rest, while the other particular will be so insofar as it is moved.

59. **It is necessary, therefore, that the nutritive soul be in every one and that the soul exist in these from generation until corruption. For it is necessary that everything generated have a beginning**[361] **and an end and decline, which cannot exist without food. Therefore the nutritive power necessarily exists in all things capable of growth and decline.** (3.12, 434a22–26)

Since he completed the account of all the universal powers of the soul, he wants to show what exists of necessity among these in animals and what exists for betterment. He said: **It is necessary, therefore, that the nutritive soul be in every** living thing . . . **from** first **generation until corruption.** For it is necessary that everything having soul have growth and decline, since it is impossible for it to come immediately to its final actuality, but [it does so] by gradually declining and entering into old age. Since the cause of growth is nothing but nutrition and the cause of decline is nothing but lack and scarcity of food,[362] it is necessary that the nutritive soul be in everything which is such that it grows and ages. Since every living thing is such as this, it is necessary that every living thing be capable of nutrition.

60. **It is not necessary that the power of sensation exist without qualification. It is not possible for an animal to live without that, nor also in the case of things which do not receive {533} form without matter.**[363] **It is necessary,**

---

360. This sentence is nearly the same as that in the text of the *Middle Commentary*:
وإذا كان هذا هكذا فبين أن الأمر الجزئي يحرك، وأما الكلى فإما أن نقول إنه ليس له تحريك على حدته أو نقول إن التحريك لهما جميعا لكن الكلى من قبل أنه ساكن والجزئي من قبل أنه يتحرك; "This being the case, it is clear that the particular causes motion, whereas we can say either that the universal has no motion of its own or that motion belongs to both: the universal in that it is stationary, the particular in that it is moved." *Middle Commentary* (2002), 131.12–15.

361. *Principium* does not render the Greek αὔξησιν, "For what has been born must grow." Aristotle, *De Anima* (1984). The alternate translation is in accord with the Greek.

362. This is certainly an odd statement, perhaps a result of a problem in the Latin translator's Arabic manuscript. In the *Middle Commentary* (2002), 131.18–132.1, he writes, "It certainly must be the case that every mortal being has a beginning, acme, and decline; the acme is due to growth, the decline to decay, and none of this is possible without nutrition."

363. The Text fails to render the Greek οὔτε γὰρ ὅσων τὸ σῶμα ἁπλοῦν ἐνδέχεται ἁφὴν ἔχειν "But sensation need not be found in all things that live. *For it is impossible for touch*

therefore, that sense be in animals, if nature does nothing in vain. For all things existing by nature either are for the sake of something or are accidents consequent upon things which are for the sake of something. For every body which moves about without sense suffers corruption and does not come to [its natural] end, although it was of the activity of nature. It is known, therefore, that the power of sensation will necessarily be found in animals, since in this way there is motion without sense. But that also is the case in the things which have been naturally constituted to be at rest.[364] (434a27–b2)

It is not necessary that the power of sensation exist without qualification, that is, in all things which grow and suffer corruption; but in animals alone is it necessary that there be power of sensation. For it is impossible for something to be an animal without this power. This is [in fact] the case in regard to things which receive [life] immaterially, for the term life is said of these and those equivocally. He is making reference to celestial bodies. Next he said: **It is necessary, therefore, that sense be in animals**, etc. That is, it is apparent that it is necessary that sense be in every animal; and this is because nature does noth-

---

to belong either to those whose body is uncompounded or to those which are incapable of taking in forms without their matter." Aristotle, De Anima (1984); emphasis added. The alternate translation reflects the Greek poorly: لأنه لا يمكن لما كان جسمه مبسوطاً أن يصير ذا حس ؛ ولا يمكن أيضاً الحيوان أن يكون بغير هذا الحس ولا ما كان قابلا للصور يمكنه أن يكون بغير هيولى (ibid. [1954]); "Because it is not possible for what has a simple body to come to possess sense. And it is not possible as well for the animal to be without this sense nor can what is receptive of forms be without matter."

364. Averroes' Text of Aristotle suffers from several corruptions and difficulties. Among those is the omission of Text corresponding to the Greek πῶς γὰρ θρέψεται; τοῖς μὲν γὰρ μονίμοις ὑπάρχει τοῦτο ὅθεν πεφύκασιν. Starting at the text corresponding to "although . . ." above, the Greek has: "which is the aim of Nature; for how could it obtain nutriment? Stationary living things, it is true, have as their nutriment that from which they have arisen." Aristotle, De Anima (1984); emphasis added. As is evident in the Comment, Averroes understood Aristotle's intention here to be a discussion of celestial bodies. The same is the case for the corresponding passage in the Middle Commentary (2002), at 132.11–13. The alternate translation has ما يفسد قد وتنقل سير ذى جسم فكل لم يكن له حس ؛ ثم لا ينتهى إلى الغاية التى يقصد إليها الطباع. وإلا فكيف يجوز أن يكون مغتذياً؟ فأما راسية الأجسام والنامية منها فجائز أن لا يكون لها حس وأن تكون ثابتة عنها منتقلة غير أماكنها فى (Aristotle, De Anima [1954]); "For every body possessing movement and motion which may suffer corruption is something which does not have a sense. Then it does not reach the end which nature has intended. But how is it possible for it to be nourished? As for the stationary character of bodies and plants among them, it is conceivable that it does not have a sense and that there be a stabilization in their places without local movement on their parts."

ing in vain. For all natural things either are for the sake of something or are accidents which must be consequent upon the nature and not intended, for instance, hairs which spring up indiscriminately on the body. Since it is so, if the animal were not to have sense and yet it were to move about, immediately it would suffer corruption before reaching completeness. Then nature would act in vain, since it began to generate beings which cannot reach the end for the most part or at all. It is known, {534} therefore, that it is necessary for the power of sensation to exist of necessity in animals which move about, namely, in those which search for food. Next he said: for **in this way there is motion without sense**. That is, since if something were found to be moved in place without [possessing] the power of sensation, then its being is of a different kind from the being of generable and corruptible things. He is making reference to the celestial bodies, for those, because they are neither generable nor corruptible, if they were to have sense, then nature would act in vain, just as, if those movable generable and corruptible things were not to have sense, then nature would act in vain. Next he said: **But** this **is also the case for things which have been naturally constituted to be at rest**. That is, but the privation of sense ought to exist with respect to generable and corruptible things in those which are naturally constituted to be at rest and not to be moved toward food, namely, in plants.

61. **It is impossible for a body having soul, intellect, and judgment**[365] **to be without sense since it is not stationary, whether it is generated or not generated. For the reason why [what does not move about] does not have this is that neither its body nor its soul derives benefit from it. Now, however, neither of those is the case: the first because for the most part it does not have understanding, the second because for the most part it is not.**[366] (434b3–7)

365. ἔχειν μὲν ψυχὴν καὶ νοῦν κριτικόν, "have a soul and a discerning mind." Aristotle, *De Anima* (1984). The alternate translation is in accord with the Greek: ذا نفس وعقل مميز (ibid. [1954]).

366. Apparently the corresponding Greek was not soundly rendered into Arabic. (διὰ τί γὰρ οὐχ ἕξει) ἢ γὰρ τῇ ψυχῇ βέλτιον ἢ τῷ σώματι, νῦν δ᾽ οὐδέτερον· ἡ μὲν γὰρ οὐ μᾶλλον νοήσει, τὸ δ᾽ οὐθὲν ἔσται μᾶλλον δι᾽ ἐκεῖνο)—οὐθὲν ἄρα ἔχει ψυχὴν σῶμα μὴ μόνιμον ἄνευ αἰσθήσεως. The sense of the Greek is different: "Why should it not have sensation? It would have to be better either for the soul or for the body; but in fact it is neither—for the absence of sensation will not enable the one to think better or the other to exist better. Therefore no body which is not stationary has soul without sensation." (Aristotle, *De Anima* [1984]). The alternate translation is problematic: (فلم يكون له حس فيكون أكرم إما بالنفس وإما بالجسم؟ فانه متى لم يكن له حس ، لم يكن باحدى هاتين الحالتين ، وذلك أن النفس لا تدرك شيئاً بفعلها ، والجسم من أجل هذه العلة التى هى عدم والحس لا يساوى شيئاً) (ibid. [1954]); "(For why does it have sense? Is it

It is impossible for the body to have soul and intellect without sense when that body is not stationary but generable and corruptible, whether it be simple {535} or composite. He meant this when he said, as I figure, **generated or not generated.** For the reason why there ought to be an animated intelligent body without sense, if there can be, is because that animated body does not derive benefit from sense, neither in soul nor in body. But if we assert there is an animated intelligent body which is neither generable nor corruptible, it is evident that it does not need sense, since sense would not provide any benefit for it. For it does not have any benefit which is through the soul because the sensitive soul impedes the intellect for the most part. He meant this when he said: the first **because for the most part it does not have understanding,** that is, the power of sensation, however, for the most part is not involved in understanding in an intelligent animal.[367] But it also does not provide the benefit attributed to the power of sensation which exists through the body, because sense for the most part is not a cause of length and duration of life. He meant this when he said: the second **because for the most part it is not.** That is, sense for the most part is the reason why the thing is not, that is, that it is corrupted, and for this reason things having sensation are of shorter life than many plants.[368]

62. **In light of this, is there no moved body having soul without sense? But if it has sense, then necessarily either it will be simple or composite. It is impossible for it to be simple because [the simple] does not have touch, and it is necessary for it to have this.** (434b7–11)

In light of what was explained, if there is some moved body having soul and neither generable nor {536} corruptible, then that body will not need sense. Then it should now be asked whether there is a moved body having soul without sense or whether there is no such body. He indicates that one should inquire elsewhere concerning this.[369] Next he said: **But if it has sense,** etc. That is, but it is evident that if the power of sense is in some body, it is necessary that this body be either simple, that is, one of the four simple [elements], or a composite

---

then better either in soul or in body? When it does not have a sense, it is not in one of these two dispositions. For [then] the soul does not apprehend anything by its activity, and the body is for the sake of this cause which is a privation and the sense is not equal to a thing.). . . ."

367. That is, animals having the power of sensation for the most part do not also have the power of understanding found in intelligent animals.

368. Averroes also expresses this view of sensation as requisite for animal existence but potentially detrimental to well-being and long life in the *Middle Commentary*. See *Middle Commentary* (2002), 132.20–21.

369. For the view of Averroes, see his *De Substantia Orbis* (1986) and Endress (1995).

of them because it is generable and corruptible. It is impossible for the body to be simple, for it is impossible for a simple body to have the sense of touch and it is necessary for touch to be in everything having sense.

63. **This is known concerning those things: that an animal is an animated body and every body is tangible, and everything tangible is perceptible by touch; therefore, the body of an animal is necessarily capable of touch, if animals are naturally constituted to avoid [certain things]. The other remaining senses sense through other mediating things, for instance, smell, sight, and hearing. If, therefore, what is capable of touch is not found with sense, it is impossible for it to take in certain things and to flee from others, and so it is impossible for the animal to survive. For this reason, taste is as touch, for it concerns food and food concerns tangible body.** (434b11–19)

This is known from these propositions: since every animal is an animated body, and every body is tangible, and everything tangible is perceptible through touch, therefore, if the body of an animal ought to be preserved and ought to avoid accidents, {537} it is necessary that it have touch.[370] The other remaining senses which it has apprehend the other sensibles through mediating bodies different from their proper sensibles,[371] for instance, the senses of hearing, smell, and sight. If, therefore, the animal does not sense tangible bodies, then it is impossible for it to come to certain bodies and use them to some benefit or to flee from certain harmful things. Since it is so, it is impossible for the animal to survive.[372] Next he said: **For this reason**, etc. That is, on account of this necessity the sense of taste is more necessary in animals just as is touch.

---

370. Cf. *Middle Commentary* (2002), 133.5–8: وقد يوقف على ضرورة وجود الحس للحيوان من هذا الذى أقوله. وذلك أنه لما كان كل حيوان كائن فاسد جسما ملموسا وكل ملموس محسوس بحاسة اللمس، فبدن الحيوان من الاضطرار بأن يكون ملموسا; "That the existence of this sense is necessary for an animal can be shown by the following remarks: As every mortal animal is a tangible body, and everything tangible is perceptible by the sense of touch, then, necessarily, the body of an animal is tactile."

371. Cf. *Middle Commentary* (2002), 133.11–12: ويكون باقى الحواس الموجودة له يدرك بها سائر المحسوسات بتوسط أجسام أخر (!) هى غير المحسوسات التى يدركها; "The rest of the senses found [in an animal] apprehend the remaining objects of sensation by means of other bodies different from the sensible objects being apprehended."

372. Cf. *Middle Commentary* (2002), 133.12–15: فإن كان الحيوان ليس يوجد له الحس بالأجسام الملموسة فليس يمكن أن يقبل على بعض الأجسام التى ينتفع بها ولا يهرب من التى تضره وتفسده، ولو كان ذلك كذلك لم يمكن أن يسلم الحيوان; "Were an animal not to have the sense [of touch] for tangible bodies, it would not be able to accept those bodies from which it benefits nor flee from those which damage and corrupt it; and, were this the case, the animal would not be able to be safe."

For taste is for the sake of food, namely, for knowing the fit from the unfit, and food is in a tangible body. For this reason it is necessary that what has the sense of taste have the sense of touch, as we explained earlier.[373]

64. **However, sound, color, and odor do not nourish, nor does any growth or decline come from these. For this reason taste was necessarily a kind of touch, because it senses only what is tangible and nutritious. Those, however, also necessarily belong to animals and it is evident that it is impossible for an animal to exist without sense. Those other [senses], however, exist for betterment and this does not happen for every genus of animals, but [only] for certain genera. Just as that [animal] must be something which moves about if it is naturally constituted to survive, [it must] not [be the case] that it senses only when it touches, but [that it does so] also from a distance.** (434b19–27)

However, sound, color, and odor do not nourish the body when they come to it, nor do they cause in the body {538} gain or loss as food does. For this reason which I mention, taste is necessarily a kind of touch, that is, because the sense of taste is of some tangible nutrient.[374] He meant this when he said: **because there is sensation only of what is tangible.** Next he said: **Those, however, belong to animals . . . necessarily.** He meant the sense of touch and the sense of taste. Next he said: **Those others, however,** that is, the three other senses. Next he said: **and this does not happen,** etc. That is, and those three senses are not found in every genus of animals but in certain genera. Next he said: **Just as that [animal] must be something which moves about,** etc. That is, thus, when it is necessary for an animal to move about if it is naturally constituted to survive, it is more perfect for it not just to apprehend harmful and useful sensibles nearby only and through touch, but also from a distance, since by those two ways of sensing it will be more perfectly and better preserved.

---

373. {171}.

374. Cf. *Middle Commentary* (2002), 133.19–134.2: قال : وأما القرع واللون والرائحة فليست واحدة منها تغذوا جسم الحيوان إذا وردت عليه، أعنى أنه ليس الجسم بغاذ ما هو ذو لون ولا قرع إلا بالعرض، ولذلك لا يحدث عنها فى الجسم زيادة ولا نقصان كما يحدث عن الغذاء. ولهذه العلة كان الذوق من الاضطرار لمسا ما، أى من قبل أن حس الذوق إنما يكون لشيء ملموس غاذ (334) "He said: *Neither sound, color, nor smell nourish the body of an animal when they reach it*—that is, the body is not nourished other than incidentally insofar as it is capable of [receiving] color and sound. Therefore, *neither increase nor diminution will occur to the body from them, as will happen because of food. Accordingly, taste is necessarily a kind of touch—that is, because the sensation of taste occurs only in relation to a tangible, nourishing object.*" Emphasis added to indicate portions of the *Middle Commentary* text related to the *Long Commentary* text.

65. This will be so only when the sensible is through a medium, because [the medium] is affected and moved by the sensible, while [the animal is affected and moved] by [the medium]. Just as what causes motion in place does so up to the point that there is change, likewise what impels something else does so until [that] is impelled. The motion will be through a medium. (The first causes motion or impels without being impelled and the other is impelled only and does not impel, while the medium has both [properties] and the intermediates[375] are many.) This is similarly the case too for alteration, but [this involves] what is resting in the same place.[376] [This is] just as one who presses [something] in wax, presses as long as he moves [the thing] and so far as {539} the impression reaches. In the case of stone, however, there is no impression at all, while water is affected by impression to a great distance. Air, too, is moved a great deal and acts and is affected, if it remains and is the same. For this reason it is better [to hold] that air is affected in virtue of reflection by body and color, than that it may be possible that sight [itself be affected directly] through change and reflection [by body and color].[377] It is the same in the case of smooth things. For this reason this [medium] moves sight also, just as the impression in the wax is brought through to its end points. (434b27–435a10)

Sensing what is at a distance comes about when the sensible moves what senses through a medium, since when what acts as a medium is affected and moved by the sensible, also this which belongs to the sense[378] is affected by the medium. Next he said: Just as **what causes motion in place**, etc. That is, just as a body moving in place, insofar as it moves, needs to do so up to the point that it is moved and is changed, similarly what impels another thing

375. The Latin *meaia* here is a typographical error in the Crawford edition for *media*.

376. This Text is less clear than the Greek. "Just as that which produces local movement causes a change extending to a certain point, and that which gave an impulse causes another to produce a new impulse so that the movement traverses a medium—the first mover impelling without being impelled, the last moved being impelled without impelling, while the medium (or media, for there are many) is both—so it is also in the case of alteration, except that the agent produces it without the patient's changing its place." Aristotle, *De Anima* (1984).

377. The Greek is clearer. "That is why in the case of reflection it is better, instead of saying that the sight issues from the eye and is reflected, to say that the air, so long as it remains one, is affected by the shape and colour." Aristotle, *De Anima* (1984). Aristotle here is referring to Empedocles' theory of effluences and vision, which Plato espouses at *Timaeus* 45b2–46c6. On this account, vision is the result of an internal fire proceeding from the eyes to the seen object.

378. That is, the physical organ is moved or affected.

needs to be impelled, and then it impels. Thus, motion in such things has at least three components, namely, the first mover, the intermediate, and the final moved thing. The first mover impels and causes motion and is not moved, the final moved thing is impelled and moved and does not cause motion, while the intermediate does both, namely, it causes motion and is moved. The intermediate, however, can be one and can be more than one. Next he said: **This is similarly the case too for alteration**, etc. That is, according to the disposition which we recounted concerning motion in place, namely, that it is composed of three things in such a way that it relates to this change which comes about from sensibles grasped by the senses through intermediaries. For sensibles cause motion and are not moved and intermediates between these move the senses and are moved by the sensibles, {540} while the senses are moved and do not cause motion. But there is a difference between these because that change which is in those things is through a medium and a medium remaining in the same place is also not [in itself] altered by this. But in the case of motion in place the medium is altered, and similarly for the final moved thing. When he had explained these things which that change has in common with change in place and in virtue of what things it is distinguished from it, he gave an example of this. He said: **[This is] just as one who presses** wax, etc. That is, that motion belonging to the medium in its parts from the sensible is exactly like the impression of a seal in wax. Just as the wax is moved with its parts by the seal and that motion reaches into the wax so far as the power of the one impressing is able to reach, and the wax remains [a unitary whole] in all its parts, so is this the disposition in the motion of the medium with the sensibles, namely, that [the medium] is pressed by these and impelled toward everything toward which the power of the pressing reaches and [the medium as a whole] remains in its place unmoved.[379] Next he said: **In the case of a stone**, etc. That is, that motion is not accommodated in every body, for a stone and its like cannot at all be pressed but rather what can be pressed is akin to water. For water

---

379. Cf. *Middle Commentary* (2002), 134.21–135.2: قال : وهذه الحركة التى تكون للمتوسط فى أجزائه عن المحسوسات هى أشبه شىء بمن يغمز على الشمع بطابع. وذلك أنه كما أن الشمع يتحرك فى أجزائه عن شكل الطابع وتنتهى تلك الحركة إلى حيث انتهت قوة الغامز والشمع ثابت بجملة أجزائه، كذلك الحال فى حركة المتوسط مع المحسوسات. أعنى أنه يتغمز عنها ويندفع إلى حيث انتهت قوة تحريك المحسوسات وهو ثابت بعينه; "He said: This motion which is induced in the parts of the medium by the objects of sensation most resembles the situation which obtains when one impresses a seal upon wax. Just as the parts of the wax are moved by the shape of the seal—the motion extending to the part where the impressing force terminates, while the wax remains stationary in its parts— such is the situation in the motion of the medium with objects of sensation: the medium, while remaining stationary in itself, is impressed and driven by them to the point where their motive force terminates."

seems to be pressed over a distant space. Likewise for air, for it frequently seems to act and be affected by pressing, when it is stable as a whole, unmoved and undivided.[380] Next he said: **For this reason it is better [to hold] that air is affected**, etc. That is, because in the case of a medium this impression is possible, for this reason it is better to say, in the case of the reflection which comes about in things which can be heard and in things which can be seen, that it is nothing other than that the air is reflected by that motion which is in it and by that affection which comes about from sensibles, when {541} it has encountered something which that motion cannot pass through soundly in reference to the senses.[381] This is better than to say that there is a reflection of bodies outside sight, as certain of the ancients say, and the empiricists[382] concede, when there may be no external bodies there. Next he said: **It is . . . in the case of smooth things**, etc. That is, that motion is in wet things. He meant this by **same** for **smooth things**. For this reason air also will move sight, just as a seal existing in wax is pushed to the extreme end to the extent that it moves air in a second part, so too in this way the sensible will move air in such a way that it is carried through it to the surface touching the sense, and in this way it moves the sense.[383]

---

380. Cf. *Middle Commentary* (2002), 135.2–6: وهذا النحو من الحركة ليس يتأتى في كل جسم وذلك أن الحجر وما أشبهه لا ينغمز البتة وإنما ينغمز مثل الماء والهواء، فإنا نجدهما كثيرا ما ينفعلان عن التحريك مسافة بعيدة إذا كان كل واحد منهما ثابتا بجملته غير متحرك ولا متشذب; "This kind of motion does not come about in every body, for the stone and its like are not impressionable at all, while things like water and air are. We often find them affected by motion over an extensive distance, each one being stationary in its entirety, unmoved [as such], and undispersed."

381. That is, the medium bearing sound or light can affect the quality of sound or sight. For example, an intervening wall affects the medium between persons and thereby affects their ability to hear one another, or fog can affect the medium such that sight is affected.

Cf. *Middle Commentary* (2002), 135.7–11: (733) ولكون المتوسط يمكن فيه هذا الانغماز والتحريك والتحرك كان الأفضل أن نقول في الانعكاس الذي يكون في المسموعات وفي المرئيات أنه ليس هو شيئا إلا أن الهواء ينعكس بتلك الحركة التي فيه عن المحسومات إذا صادفت تلك الحركة شيئا لا يمكن أن تنفذ فيه على استقامة إلى الحواس أنفسها; "As it is possible of the medium to experience impression and motion [in an active and passive way], it is better to say that the reflection which occurs with audible and visible objects is nothing other than the air reflecting the objects of sense by its motion, when that motion meets something which it cannot traverse directly en route to the senses themselves."

382. *Perspectivi*.

383. Cf. *Middle Commentary* (2002), 135.16–17: المحسوس يحرك الهواء حتى ينفذ فيه إلى السطح الخاص بجسم الحاسة فيحرك الحاسة; "the sensible object moves the air until it penetrates through it to the particular surface of the corporeal sense organ and moves it."

66. **It is, therefore, evident that it is impossible for the body of an animal to be simple as fire or air [are]. For it is impossible to have one of the other senses without touch, for every animated body is capable of touch, as we said. Those other [elements] are instruments of sense, except earth. For all cause sensations because they sense through another and through a medium.**[384] **Touch, however, comes about in touching and for this reason is called by this name. This is because other instruments of sense do not sense except through the mediation of touch (but this is with other things mediating), while that [sense of touch] is thought to be sufficient per se. For this reason the body of an animal is not one of those elements. Nor is it earth. For touch is, as it were, intermediate in relation to the other sensibles and an instrument {542} of sense. And the recipient thing does not include only changes which involve earth but also those which involve hot and cold and other tangibles. For this reason we do not sense through bones, hairs, and other such parts.**[385] **For this reason plants do not have any of these senses, because they are [composed] of earth. For it is impossible for there to be another sense without touch, and this instrument which belongs to sense is not composed of fire**[386] **or any of those other elements.** (3.13 435a11–b4)

It is impossible, therefore, for the body of an animal to be simple. For it is impossible for the animal to have any of these three senses without touch, for every animated thing must be something which has the sense of touch. Next he said: **Those other [elements]**, etc. That is, the simple bodies are instruments of these three senses, except for earth, which is not an instrument of any sense. This was because all those senses, namely, the three, cause sensation because they need simple instruments and an extrinsic medium, that is, things devoid of sensibles, namely, so that the instrument and medium in sight do not have color nor [is there] odor in the olfactory sense nor [is there] sound in

384. The Text has lost the sense of the Greek, which has τὰ δὲ ἄλλα ἔξω γῆς αἰσθητήρια μὲν ἂν γένοιτο, πάντα δὲ τῷ δι᾽ ἑτέρου αἰσθάνεσθαι ποιεῖ τὴν αἴσθησιν, καὶ διὰ τῶν μεταξύ. "All the other elements with the exception of earth can constitute organs of sense, but all of them bring about perception only through something else, viz. through the media." Aristotle, *De Anima* (1984). The alternate translation, though imperfect, is somewhat closer to the Greek: تكون ، ما خلا الأرض ، والجميع (ibid. [1954]); حاسة . إلا أن تكون كلها تفعل حساً وتدرك ما كان الهواء لها بالمتوسط بينهما "All, with the exception of earth, may be involved in sensing but they all bring about sensation and perceive what is air for them through what is intermediate between them."

385. The Text here fails to reflect ὅτι γῆς ἐστίν, 435a25, "because they consist of earth." Aristotle, *De Anima* (1984). The alternate translation is in accord with the Greek: لأنها من الأرض وحدها.

386. The Greek has γῆς, "earth," instead of "fire." The alternate translation is in accord with the Greek.

hearing. What are devoid of those either are the simple bodies or that in which the simple bodies predominate. But touch differs from those senses because it apprehends its sensible without a medium and for this reason it uses no intermediate element in regard to what is extrinsic. When this has been explained concerning the sense of touch, it is necessary that its instrument not be simple. Generally he wants to explain here that touch differs from the other senses in this regard. For if the other senses can be devoid of touch, then it would be possible for the body of an animal having those senses to be {543} simple, while for touch it is the contrary, namely, that it is impossible for its instrument to be simple. For every instrument ought to be devoid of sensible. Because it is impossible that any body be devoid of the four qualities, it is necessary that the instrument of that sense be intermediate, that is, a mixture of the elements. Since it is so, it happens that this power is the essential reason why the body of an animal is composite. Next he said: since it is the case that **other instruments of sense**, etc. That is, since the other senses use the three elements for instruments and media, it is necessary that touch not use any of them and that its instrument be composite, not simple. Still, the instruments which those use cannot be devoid of touch and on this basis they are composite. If this were not [the case], it would be necessary that they be simple things. Next he said: **but this is** through other mediating things. That is, but their lack of touch is not a lack belonging to what apprehends its sensible directly without a medium, but [something which characterizes what apprehends] through other media and through other instruments. Next he said: **For this reason the body of an animal is not one of those elements**, etc. That is, on account of what we said, none of those elements is the body of an animal. Not even earth, insofar as it is simple or nearly simple, since the other senses use the elements as instrument and medium, and [touch] is a power other than those. Hence, it does not use the elements as instrument, since its instrument ought to be the medium between tangible things, since it cannot be made devoid of tangible qualities nor can it apprehend tangible things if it were a simple tangible, that is, some perfect tangible quality. Next he said: **And the recipient . . . does not include**, etc. That is, what is receptive of touch does not necessarily {544} have qualities which involve earth alone, but hot and cold and other tangible qualities. For this reason it was necessary that what receives a tangible be a mean, since it cannot be devoid of all things nor even can it sense if any of the tangible qualities predominates in it. For this reason we do not sense through bones or through hairs, on account of the predominance in these bodies of the qualities which involve earth. For this reason plants do not have the sense of touch. Hence, neither do they have other senses, because it is impossible for the other senses to be found without touch. And the instrument of touch is neither fire nor some other body which is among the elements, nor is it a body ascribed to these predominantly.

67. It was explained, therefore, that animals necessarily die when they cease to have this sense alone and also that it is impossible for it not to be in animals. For animals do not necessarily have any other sense but this. For this reason other sensibles do not corrupt animals by predominating excess, for instance, color, sound, and smell, but rather they only corrupt the instruments of sense, except accidentally. (For instance, when there is a great blow together with sound, for all those cause corruption in animals, but accidentally.)[387] **For this reason flavors also harm animals through the mediation of taste, for taste is a kind of touch.**[388] **Predominating excess, however, of what is tangible, for instance, of hot and cold and hard, corrupts animals.** (435b4–14) {545}

It was already explained from this account that animals die when they have lost touch and that it is impossible for that sense not to exist in an animal while the animal is an animal, which is not the case for the other senses. For it is not necessary for an animal to have any sense except touch. On account of this, predominating excess and strength of the other sensibles do not corrupt an animal, for instance, strong color, strong sound, and strong odor, but they only corrupt their proper instruments, except accidentally (for instance, when with sound there has been a great blow, and likewise for color and odor). Flavors, however, do harm animals in an essential way, through the mediation of taste, for taste is a kind of touch. But the qualities corrupting animals are tangible, for instance, hot, cold, and hard.

68. The predominant excess of any sensible expels the instrument of sense, and for this reason what is tangible expels touch. Life is defined in virtue of touch, for it is impossible for an animal to exist without touch. For this reason the predominant excess of what is tangible not only corrupts the instrument of sense but also even the animal, because it is necessary for the

387. Averroes' Text of Aristotle omits part of the Greek: οἷον ἂν ἅμα τῷ ψόφῳ ὦσις γένηται καὶ πληγή· καὶ ὑπὸ ὁραμάτων καὶ ὀσμῆς ἕτερα κινεῖται, ἃ τῇ ἁφῇ φθείρει; "as when the sound is accompanied by an impact or shock, *or where through the objects of sight or of smell certain other things are set in motion,* which destroy by contact." Aristotle, *De Anima* (1984); my emphasis. The alternate translation reflects the Greek: فتتحرك أشياء أُخَر مع الرائحة واللون (ibid. [1954]); "for other things are set in motion by odor and color."

388. "Flavour also destroys only in so far as it is at the same time capable of contact." Aristotle, *De Anima* (1984).

animal that it be a being, not that it be in a better disposition. Those other senses, however, are in the animal for the better, sight so that it may see in air and water; taste so that it may sense the pleasant and unpleasant and that it may have appetite and be moved; and likewise for smell; hearing that it may hear a thing; and tongue that it may signify something in another way.[389] (435b15–25) {546}

The predominant excess of every sensible, when it is intense, corrupts its proper instrument, whether it is touch or something else. Next he said: **In virtue of that it was defined**, etc. That is, through that power, namely, touch, animal is defined. The reason for this is that it is impossible for the animal to exist without touch. For this reason it happens that an intense tangible corrupts not only the instrument of sense but also the animal in an essential way, because the sense of touch is among things necessary for the animal, namely, for it to be a being, not insofar as it is better for it, as it is in the case of the other remaining senses. Next he said: **sight so that it may see in air and water**. Likewise concerning smell, namely, that primarily it is for the sake of appetite for food. Hearing, however, so that it may hear a thing, that is, sounds, and understand in virtue of those, in rational animals and in brute animals. In rational animals [this is] so that they may understand the intentions which the words signify. Tongue, however, so that it may signify the thing in another way. He is indicating, as I believe, the help which it affords in regard to words, not taste. For this help appears to be more for betterment than taste, since taste is thought to be more necessary on account of its nearness to touch. The other senses, however, are for the sake of betterment, chiefly sight and hearing. This is evident.

389. The Greek has <γλῶτταν δὲ ὅπως σημαίνῃ τι ἑτέρῳ>, "and a tongue that it may communicate with its fellows." Aristotle *De Anima* (1984). The alternate translation has وكذلك صار اللسان فيه ليجيب به غيره بالكلام والحديث (ibid. [1954]); "And likewise there comes to be a tongue in it so that by it it may communicate with another by speech and talk."

Bibliography

Primary Sources, including translations

Averroes

Against the Avicennians on the First Cause (1997). "An Unknown Treatise of Averroes Against the Avicennians on the First Cause. Edition and Translation," Carlos Steel and Guy Guldentops (eds. and trans.). *Recherches de théologie et philosophie médiévales* (formerly *Recherches de théologie ancienne et médiévale*) 64 (1997): 86–135.

Commentaria Averrois in Galenum (1984) (1998). *Commentaria Averrois in Galenum*, Maria Concepción Vázquez de Benito (ed.). Madrid: Consejo Superior de Investigaciones Científicas, Instituto "Miguel Asín," Instituto Hispano-Árabe de Cultura, 1984. *Averroes, Obra Médica*, María Concepción Vázquez de Benito (trans.). Seville: Universidad de Córdoba, 1998.

Commentary on the De Intellectu of Alexander (2001). "La Tradizione Guideo-Araba ed Ebraica del *De Intellectu* di Alessandro di Afrodisia e il Testo Originale del *Commento di Averroè*," Mauro Zonta (ed.), *Annali di Ca' Foscari. Rivista della Facoltà di Lingue e Letterature Straniere dell' Università di Venezia* 40.3 (2001) (Serie orientale 32): 17–35; Arabic text of Averroes' *Commentary on the De Intellectu of Alexander*, 27–34. A Hebrew translation of this work was edited by Herbert Davidson in "Averroes' Commentary on the *De Intellectu* Attributed to Alexander" (in Hebrew), *Shlomo Pines Jubilee Volume*, M. Idel et al. (eds.), v. 1, 205–217. Jerusalem: Jerusalem Studies in Jewish Thought, 1988.

Decisive Treatise (1959) (1961) (2001). Averroes, *Kitâb faṣl al-maqâl with Its Appendix (Ḍamîma) and an Extract from Kitâb al-kashf ʿan al-manâhij al-adilla*, George F. Hourani (ed.). Leiden: Brill, 1959. *Averroes. On the Harmony of Religion and Philosophy. A Translation, with Introduction and Notes, of Ibn Rushd's Kitâb faṣl al-maqâl with Its Appendix (Ḍamîma) and an Extract from Kitâb al-kashf ʿan manâhij al-adilla*, George F. Hourani (trans.). London: Luzac, 1961. *Averroes. The Book of the Decisive Treatise Determining the Connection between the Law and Wisdom and Epistle Dedicatory*, Charles E. Butterworth (trans.). Provo, Utah: Brigham Young University Press, 2001.

De Substantia Orbis (1986). *Averroes' De Substantia Orbis. Critical Edition of the Hebrew Text with English Translation and Commentary*, Arthur Hyman (ed. and trans.). Cambridge, MA, and Jerusalem: Medieval Academy of America and Israel Academy of Sciences and Humanities, 1986.

Epistle 1 On Conjunction. See Geoffroy and Steel (2001).

Epistle 2 On Conjunction. See Geoffroy and Steel (2001).

Epistle on the Possibility of Conjunction (1982). *The Epistle on the Possibility of Conjunction with the Active Intellect by Ibn Rushd with the Commentary of Moses Narboni. A Critical Edition and Annotated Translation*, Kalman P. Bland (ed. and trans.). New York: Jewish Theological Seminary of America, 1982.

Explanation of the Sorts of Proofs in the Doctrines of Religion (1998) (1947) (2001). Ibn Rushd, *al-Kashf 'an al-manâhij al-adillah fî 'aqâ'id al-millah*, Muḥammad 'Âbid al-Jâbrî (ed.). Beirut: Markaz Dirâsât al-Wahdah al-'Arabîyah, 1998. A complete Spanish translation of this is found in Alonso (1947). An English translation is now available: *Faith and Reason in Islam. Averroes' Exposition of Religious Arguments*, Ibrahim Najjar (trans.). Oxford: One World, 2001. The discovery of a new manuscript version of this work has been announced by Marc Geoffroy. See Geoffroy (2001).

Incoherence of the Incoherence (1930) (1969). *Averroès. Tahafot at-Tahafot*, Maurice Bouyges, S.J. (ed.). Beirut: Imprimerie Catholique, 1930. *Averroes' Tahafut al-Tahafut (The Incoherence of the Incoherence)*, Simon Van Den Bergh (trans.). 2 vols. London: Luzac, 1969.

Kitâb al-Kullîyât (2000). *Kitâb al-Kullîyât: Les Généralités d'Ibn Rochd.*, M. Belkeziz Ben Abdeljalil (ed.). Casablanca: Imprimerie Najah al-Jadida, 2000.

Long Commentary (1953). *Averrois Cordubensis Commentarium Magnum in Aristotelis De Anima Libros*, F. Stuart Crawford (ed.). Cambridge, MA: Mediaeval Academy of America, 1953. Pagination for this work is given in curly brackets { } throughout. Selections of this work are translated into Spanish in Martínez Lorca (2004) and Puig (2005). Substantial portions of Book 3 are translated in the next two items in this bibliography. For a modern translation from Latin into Arabic, see *Long Commentary Modern Arabic Trans.* (1997).

Long Commentary. Book 3 (1980–1981, 1982–1983). "Livre III du *Grand Commentaire* d'Averroès sur le *Traité de l'âme d'Aristote*," Alain Griffaton (trans.), *Majallat Kullîyat al-'Adab wa-l-'Ulûm al-Insânîyah* (Fez) 4–5 (1980–1981): 741–721; 6 (1982–1983): 63–88. This is a partial translation of *Long Commentary* (1953) Book 3, corresponding to {379–454}.

Long Commentary. Book 3 (1998). *Averroès. L'intelligence et la pensée. Grand commentaire du De anima, Livre III (429a10–435b25)*, Alain de Libera (trans.). Paris: Flammarion, 1998. This is a translation of Book 3 Texts and Comments for 3.1 429a10–3.8 432a15, omitting Texts and Comments 40–67, *Long Commentary* (1953) {507–546}.

Long Commentary Fragments (1985) (2005). Fragments of the *Long Commentary on the De Anima* in Arabic, edited by Abdelkader Ben Chehida in "Iktishâf al-naṣṣ al-'arabî li-ahamm ajzâ' al-shar al-kabîr li-*kitâb al-nafs* ta'lîf Abî al-Walîd ibn Rushd," *Al-Ḥayât al-Thaqâfiyya* 35 (1985): 14–48. These fragments, in Hebrew script now published by Ben Chehida in Arabic script, are found among marginal notes to the Modena manuscript of the *Middle Commentary on the De Anima*. This manuscript, Modena, a.j.6.23, is one of the two primary manuscripts used by Alfred L. Ivry in his critical edition in *Middle Commentary* (2002). In addition to *Long Commentary* Fragments (1985), see *Middle Commentary* (2002), xxviii–xxix, and *L'original arabe du Grand commentaire d'Averroès au De anima d'Aristote. Prémices d'édition*, C. Sirat and M. Geoffroy. Paris: J. Vrin, 2005. Only when it seems necessary have I included in my citations Ben Chehida's reconstructions from the Latin of portions of the context of the fragments. Those reconstructions are enclosed in angle brackets < >. The admittedly preliminary study of Sirat and Geoffroy appeared only after the completion of my translation. Still, in the notes I have cited their work on nine fragments from the end of Book 2 and from Book 3. In citations of texts from *Long Commentary* Fragments (2005), Sirat and Geoffroy use curly brackets { } to indicate conjectured text where margins have been cut off.

Long Commentary Modern Arabic Trans. (1997). *Averroes. Grand commentaire sur le Traité de l'âme d'Aristote.* Translated from Latin into Arabic by B. Gharbi. Tunis: Académie Tunisienne des Sciences, des Lettres et des Arts "Beit Al-Hikma," 1997. [Ibn Rushd, *al-Sharḥ al-kabîr li-Kitâb al-nafs li-Aristû*, Ibrâhîm al-Gharbî (trans.). Tunis: al-Majmaʿ al-Tûnisî li-l-ʿulûm wa-l-âdâb wa-l-funûn, 1997]. The second volume of this work is a reprint of *Long Commentary* (1953).

Long Commentary on the De Caelo (2003) (1994). *Averrois Cordubensis commentum magnum super libro De celo et mundo Aristotelis*, Francis James Carmody and Rüdger Arnzen (eds.). 2 vols. Louvain: Peeters, 2003. One-third of the Arabic text is extant. See *Commentary on Aristotle's Book on the Heaven and the Universe, by Ibn Rushd. Sharḥ Kitâb al-Samâʾ, wa-l-ʿâlam*, facsimile of the unique Tunis manuscript, prepared by Gerhard Endress. Frankfurt am Main: Institute for the History of Arabic-Islamic Science at Johann Wolfgang Goethe University, 1994.

Long Commentary on the Metaphysics (1952) (1962) (1984). *Averroès Tafsîr mâ baʿd aṭ-Ṭabîʿat*, Maurice Bouyges (ed.). 4 vols. Beirut: Imprimerie Catholique, 1938–1952. Volumes 2 and 3 of this work were reprinted by Dâr al-Machreq in Beirut in 1967. *Aristotelis Metaphysicorum Libri XIIII cum Averrois Cordubensis in eosdem commentariis et epitome*, in *Aristotelis Opera Cum Averrois Commentariis*. Venice: Apud Iunctas, 1574, v. 8. These Latin texts are cited here according to the 1962 Minerva (Frankfurt am Main) reprint. *Ibn Rushd's Metaphysics. A Translation with Introduction of Ibn Rushd's Commentary on Aristotle's Metaphysics, Book Lâm* by Charles Genequand. Leiden: E. J. Brill, 1984.

Long Commentary on the Physics (1962). The *Long Commentary on the Physics* in the translation attributed to Michael Scot is found in the 1962 Minerva (Frankfurt am Main) reprint of *Aristotelis Opera Cum Averrois Commentariis*. Venice: Apud Iunctas, 1562–1574, v. 4. On this and the possibility of another translation by Herman the German, see Schmieja (1999).

Long Commentary on the Posterior Analytics (1962) (1984). The *Long Commentary on the Posterior Analytics*, partially extant in Arabic, was translated during the Renaissance from Hebrew into Latin in two complete versions by Abram de Balmes and Jo. Francisco Burana and one incomplete version by Jacob Mantino. These Latin texts are cited here according to the 1962 Minerva (Frankfurt am Main) reprint of *Aristotelis Opera Cum Averrois Commentariis*. Venice: Apud Iunctas, 1562–1574, v. 1, pt. 2a. The extant Arabic is published in *Ibn Rushd. Sharḥ al-Burhân li-Aristû wa talkîṣ al-Burhân (Ibn Rushd. Grand commentaire et paraphrase des Seconds analytiques d'Aristote)*, ʿAbdurraḥmân Badawi (ed). Kuwait: al-Majlis al-Waṭanî lil-Thaqâfah wa-al-Funûn wa-al-Âdâb, Qism al-Turâth al-ʿArabî, 1984.

Medical Manuscripts of Averroes (1986). *Medical Manuscripts of Averroes at El-Escorial*, G. C. Anawati and P. Ghalioungui (trans. and eds.). Cairo: al-Ahram Center for Scientific Translations, 1986. This work contains translations of nine commentaries by Averroes on medical treatises by Galen.

Middle Commentary (2002). *Averroës. Middle Commentary on Aristotle's De Anima. A Critical Edition of the Arabic Text with English Translation, Notes and Introduction,* Alfred
   L. Ivry (ed. and trans.). Provo, Utah: Brigham Young University Press, 2002. References to the Text are to the page and line of the Arabic even when the facing page
   English is cited. The Arabic text was first published as *Averroes. Middle Commentary
   on Aristotle's De Anima,* Alfred L. Ivry (ed.). Cairo: Dâr al-Kutub, 1994. The section on
   the rational faculty is translated into French in Elamrani-Jamal (1997). A Spanish
   translation of the French is found in Martínez Lorca (2004).

Middle Commentary on the Prior Analytics (1982). *Talkhîs kitâb al-qiyâs,* in *Talkhîs mantiq
   Aristû,* vol. 1 of 3, Jîrâr Jihâmî (ed.). Beirut: al-Jâmi'ah al-Lubnânîyah, 1982.

On Plato's Republic (1974). *Averroes on Plato's "Republic,"* Ralph Lerner (trans.). Ithaca and
   London: Cornell University Press, 1974. This translation is based on the Hebrew text
   edited in *Averroes' Commentary on Plato's "Republic,"* E. I. J. Rosenthal (ed. and trans.).
   Cambridge: Cambridge University Press, 1956; reprint with corrections, 1966 and
   1969. While Rosenthal uses manuscript B as the base for his text, Lerner relies on
   manuscript A and other sources for his translation. See *On Plato's Republic* (1974),
   preface, vii–ix. A German translation is also available: *Kommentar des Averroes zu
   Platons Politeia,* Simon Lauer (trans.), with introduction by Friedrich Niewöhner.
   Zurich: Spur Verlag, 1996. (Translated from the Hebrew edition of E. I. J. Rosenthal
   utilizing Rosenthal's English translation and Lerner's English translation.) The Latin
   translation of Elia Delmedigo is in *Averroè. Parafrasi della "Republica" nella traduzione
   latina di Elia del Medigo,* Annalisa Coviello and Paulo Edoardo Fornaciari (eds.). Florence: L. S. Olschki, 1992.

Short Commentary on the De Anima (1950) (1985) (1987). تلخيص كتاب النفس, *Talkhîs Kitâb
   al-Nafs,* Ahmed Fouad El-Ahwani (ed.). Cairo: Imprimerie Misr, 1950. This edition
   contains the original version with Averroes' summary of Ibn Bâjjah's اتصال العقل
   بالإنسان *Risâlat Ittisâl al-'Aql bi-l-Insân (Treatise on the Conjoining of the Intellect with Man),*
   omitted in the edition of Gómez Nogales. *Epitome de Anima* تلخيص كتاب النفس,
   Salvador Gómez Nogales (ed.). Madrid: Consejo Superior de Investigaciones Científicas, Instituto "Miguel Asín," Instituto Hispano-Arabe de Cultura, 1985. This latter
   edition contains the later version of the *Short Commentary* with Averroes' revisions
   and reference to his *Long Commentary on the De Anima* and is translated in *La Psicología
   de Averroes. Comentario al Libro sobre el alma de Aristóteles,* Salvador Gómez Nogales
   (trans.). Madrid: Universidad Nacional de Educación a Distancia, 1987. This translation renders texts excised by Averroes found in the (1950) edition but not printed in
   the (1985) edition. Note that both of those Arabic editions incorrectly title the text as
   a تلخيص *talkhîs,* the term used for a middle commentary. The *Short Commentary on
   the De Anima* is also published in *Rasâ'il Ibn Rushd* (Hyderabad, 1947), which I do not
   cite here. Regarding the problems of the editions of the *Short Commentary,* see al-
   'Alawî (1986), 53, n. 8, and (1992), 807–811. Selections from Gómez Nogales' translation
   of the *Short Commentary* are also published in Martínez Lorca (2004).

Short Commentary on the Parva Naturalia (1949) (1961) (1972). *Averrois Cordubensis compen-
   dia librorum Aristotelis qui Parva Naturalia vocantur,* A. L. Shields and H. Blumberg
   (eds.). Cambridge, MA: Mediaeval Academy of America,1949. *Averroes. Epitome of*

Parva Naturalia. Translated from the Original Arabic and the Hebrew and Latin Versions, Harry Blumberg (trans.). Cambridge, MA: Mediaeval Academy of America, 1961. *Abû al-Walîd Ibn Rushd. Talkhîs Kitâb al-Hiss wa-l-Mahsûs*, Harry Blumberg (ed.). Cambridge, MA: Mediaeval Academy of America, 1972.

Other Primary Sources

Abû Muhammad 'Abdallâh Ibn Rushd (Averroes' son)

Burnett and Zonta (2000). Charles Burnett and Mauro Zonta (eds. and trans.), "Abû Muhammad 'Abdallâh Ibn Rushd (Averroes junior), *On Whether the Active Intellect Unites with the Material Intellect Whilst It Is Clothed with the Body*: A Critical Edition of the Three Extant Medieval Versions, together with an English Translation," *Archives d'histoire doctrinale et littéraire du Moyen Âge* 67 (2000): 295–335.

Albertus Magnus

Albertus Magnus, *De Anima* (1968). Albertus Magnus, *De Anima*, Clemens Stroick, O.M.I. (ed.). [Alberti Magni Opera Omnia VII, pars I]. Aschendorff: Monasterii Westfalorum, 1968.
Albertus Magnus, *De unitate* (1975). Albertus Magnus, *Libellus de unitate intellectus contra Averroistas*, Alfonsus Hufnagel (ed.) [Alberti Magni Opera Omnia XVII, pars I]. Aschendorff: Monasterii Westfalorum, 1975.

Alexander

Alexander, *De Anima* (1887) (1979). Alexander, *De Anima*: Alexander of Aphrodisias, *De Anima Liber Cum Mantissa*, Ivo Bruns (ed.). Berlin: Typis et Impensis Georgii Reimer, 1887. [Commentaria in Aristotelem Graeca, Suppl. II, pt. 1]. *The De Anima of Alexander of Aphrodisias: A Translation and Commentary*, Athanasios P. Fotinis (Washington, D.C.: University Press of America, 1979). The Arabic text is not extant. A new English translation is in preparation by Victor Caston.
Alexander, *De Intellectu* (1887) (2004) (1990) (1971) (1956). Alexander of Aphrodisias, *De Anima Liber Cum Mantissa*, ed. Ivo Bruns. Berlin, 1887. [Commentaria in Aristotelem Graeca, Suppl. II, pt. 1], 106–113. *Two Greek Aristotelian Commentators on the Intellect*, Frederic M. Schroeder (trans.), in Frederic M. Schroeder and Robert B. Todd (trans.). Toronto: Pontifical Institute of Mediaeval Studies, 1990. *Alexander of Aphrodisias. Supplement to On the Soul*, R. W. Sharples (trans.). London: Duckworth, 2004. Arabic text edited by J. Finnegan, S.J., in "Texte arabe du ΠΕΡΙ ΝΟΥ d'Alexandre d'Aphrodise," *Mélanges de l'Université Saint Joseph* (Beirut) 33 (1956): 159–202, and by Badawi,

pp. 31–42, in *Commentaires sur Aristote perdus en grec et autres épîtres*, ʿAbdurrahman
Badawi (ed.). Beirut: Dâr el-Mashriq, 1971.

Aristotle

Note: Unless otherwise noted, all English translations of Aristotle are taken from *The
Complete Works of Aristotle. The Revised Oxford Translation*, Jonathan Barnes (ed.), 2 vols.
Princeton: Princeton University Press, 1984.

Aristotelis Opera Cum Averrois Commentariis (1562). *Aristotelis Opera Cum Averrois Commentariis.* Venice: Iunctas, 1562 reprint Frankfurt am Main: Minerva, 1962.

De Anima (1862). *Aristotle, De anima libri III*, Adolphus Torstrik (ed.). Berolini: Apud
Weidmannos, 1862; reprint Hildesheim and New York: G. Olms, 1970.

De Anima (1900). Aristote, *Traité de l'âme*, G. Rodier (trans. with notes), 2 vols. Paris: E.
Leroux, 1900; reprint of the original French, Dubuque, Iowa: W. C. Brown, 1964.

De Anima (1954). *Aristotelis De Anima (Arisṭûṭâlîs fî an-Nafs)*, Abdurrahman Badawi (ed.).
Cairo: Imprimerie Misr S.A.E., 1954; reprint Beirut and Kuwait, 1980). All citations
of the *De Anima* in Arabic are from this work.

De Anima (1956). All citations of the Greek Text of the *De Anima* of Aristotle are taken
from *Aristotelis De Anima*, W. D. Ross (ed.). Oxford: Clarendon, 1956. Scriptorum
Classicorum Bibliotheca Oxoniensis/Oxford Classical Texts Series.

De Anima (1961). *Aristotle. De Anima*, edited with introduction and commentary by
David Ross. Oxford: Clarendon Press, 1961; reprint 1967.

De Anima (1965). *De Anima* with translation, introduction, and notes by R. D. Hicks.
Amsterdam: A. M. Hakkert, 1965. This is a reprint of the original published at Cam-
bridge: Cambridge University Press, 1907. There is also a more recent reprint: New
York: Arno Press, 1976.

De Anima (1984). The translation of the *De Anima*, J. A. Smith (trans.), revised by J. Barnes
in *The Complete Works of Aristotle. The Revised Oxford Translation.*

De Anima (1994). *Aristotle's "De Anima." Translated into Hebrew by Zerahyah Ben Isaac Ben
Shealtiel Hen. A Critical Edition with an Introduction and Index*, Gerrit Bos (ed.). Leiden,
New York, and Cologne: E. J. Brill, 1994.

Generation of Animals (1984) (1965). *Generation of Animals*, A. Platt (trans.), in *The Complete
Works of Aristotle. The Revised Oxford Translation*, Jonathan Barnes (ed.). *Aristotelis De
generatione animalium*, H. J. Drossaart Lulofs (ed.). Oxford: Oxford University Press,
1965.

Metaphysics (1984). "Aristotle's *Metaphysics*," W. D. Ross (trans.), in *The Complete Works
of Aristotle. The Revised Oxford Translation*, Jonathan Barnes (ed.).

Physics (1984). "Aristotle's *Physics*," R. P. Hardie and R. K. Gaye (trans.), in *The Complete
Works of Aristotle. The Revised Oxford Translation*, Jonathan Barnes (ed.).

Posterior Analytics (1941). "*Posterior Analytics*," G. R. G. Mure (trans.), in *The Basic Works
of Aristotle*, Richard McKeon (ed.). New York: Random House, 1941.

Prior Analytics (1948). "Aristotle's *Prior Analytics*," in *Mantiq Aristu*, A. Badawi (ed.), vol. 1.
Cairo: Maṭbaʿah Dâr al-Kutub al-Misrîyah.

Prior Analytics (1984). "Aristotle's *Prior Analytics*," A. J. Jenkinson (trans.), in *The Complete Works of Aristotle. The Revised Oxford Translation*, Jonathan Barnes (ed.).

al-Fârâbî

al-Fârâbî, *Book of Sophistic Refutations* (1986). al-Fârâbî, *Kitâb al-Amkinah al-Maghlaṭah*, Rafîq al-ʿAjam (ed.), in *al-Manṭîq ʿinda al-Fârâbî*, vol. 2. Beirut: Dâr al-Mashriq, 1986.

al-Fârâbî, *Letter on the Intellect* (1983) (1973) (1974). al-Fârâbî, *Alfarabi. Risâlah fî al-ʿaql*, ed. Maurice Bouyges, S.J. Beirut: Dâr el-Mashriq Sarl, 1983, 2nd ed. Partial English translation by Arthur Hyman in *Philosophy in the Middle Ages*, Arthur Hyman and James J. Walsh (eds.). Indianapolis: Hackett Publishing, 1973, 2d ed., 215–221. Italian translation by Francesca Lucchetta in *Farabi. Epistola sull'intelletto*. Padua: Antenore, 1974.

al-Fârâbî, *The Political Regime* (1964). *Al-Fârâbî's The Political Regime (al-Siyâsa al-Madaniyya, also known as the Treatise on the Principles of Beings)*, Fauzi M. Najjar (ed.). Beirut: Imprimerie Catholique, 1964.

al-Fârâbî, *Principles of the Opinions of the People of the Virtuous City* (1985). *Al-Farabi on the Perfect State. Abû Naṣr al-Fârâbî's Mabâdi' ârâ' ahl al-madîna al-fâḍila*, Richard Walzer (ed. and trans.). Oxford: Clarendon Press, 1985.

Galen

Galen's Compendium of Plato's Timaeus (1951). *Galeni Compendium Timaei Platonis*, Richard Walzer and Paul Kraus (eds. and trans.). London: Warburg Institute, 1951.

Galen on Respiration and the Arteries (1984). *Galen on Respiration and the Arteries. An Edition with English Translation and Commentary of De usu respirationis, An in arteriis natura sanguis contineatur, De usu pulsuum, and De causis respirationis*, David J. Furley and J. S. Wilkie (eds. and trans.). Princeton: Princeton University Press, 1984.

Ibn Bâjjah

Ibn Bâjjah, *Book on the Soul* (1960) (1961). Ibn Bâjjah, *Kitâb al-nafs*, M. S. Hasan al-Maʿsumi (ed.). Damascus, 1960. English translation: *Ibn Bajjah's ʿIlm al-Nafs*, M. S. Hasan al-Maʿsûmî (trans.). Karachi: Pakistan Historical Society, 1961. The Arabic text and translation are incomplete in these. Professor Gerhard Endress of Bochum discovered the lost Berlin manuscript of this work at the Jagellonian Library of Krakow in Poland. A Spanish translation of the complete book using this manuscript and the Oxford manuscript is being made by Joaquín Lomba.

Ibn Bâjjah, *The Governance of the Solitary* (1968, 1991) (1983) (1997). Ibn Bâjjah, *Tadbîr al-Mutawaḥḥid*, in *Risâ'il Ibn Bâjjah al-Ilâhîyah (Ibn Bâjjah [Avempace]. Opera Metaphysica*),

Majid Fakhry (ed.), 37–96. Beirut: Dâr an-Nahâr, 1968; 2nd ed. 1991. *The Governance of the Solitary*, partial translation by Lawrence Berman, in *Medieval Political Philosophy*, Ralph Lerner and Muhsin Mahdi (eds.). Ithaca, NY: Cornell University Press, 3rd ed., 1983. For a full Spanish translation, see *El Régimen del solitario, Ibn Bâyya (Avempace)*, Joaquín Lomba (trans.). Madrid: Editorial Trotta, 1997.

Ibn Bâjjah, *Letter of Farewell* (1943) (1968). Ibn Bâjjah, *Risâlat al-Wadâ'*, Miguel Asín Palacios (ed. with Spanish trans.), in "La 'Carta de Adiós' de Avempace," *al-Andalus* 8 (1943): 1–87. The Arabic text is also available in *Risâ'il Ibn Bâjjah al-Ilâhîyah* (*Ibn Bâjjah [Avempace]. Opera Metaphysica*), Majid Fakhry (ed.), 113–143. Beirut: Dâr an-Nahâr, 1968; 2nd ed. 1991.

Ibn Bâjjah, *Treatise on the Conjoining of the Intellect with Man* (1942) (1968) (1981). Ibn Bâjjah, *Risâlat Ittisâl al-'Aql bi-l-Insân*, Miguel Asín Palacios (ed. and trans.), in "Tratado de Avempace sobre la unión del intelecto con el hombre," *al-Andalus* 7 (1942): 1–47. The Arabic text is also available in *Risâ'il Ibn Bâjjah al-Ilâhîyah* (*Ibn Bâjjah [Avempace]. Opera Metaphysica*), Majid Fakhry (ed.), 153–173. Beirut: Dâr an-Nahâr, 1968; 2nd ed. 1991. French translation by Vincent Lagardère in "L'Epître d'Ibn Bâjja sur la conjonction de l'intellect avec l'esprit humain," *Revue des études islamiques* 49 (1981): 175–196.

Ibn al-Haytham

Ibn al-Haytham, *Optics* (1983) (1989). al-Hasan Ibn al-Haytham, *Kitâb al-Manâzir*, Abdelhamid I. Sabra (ed.). Kuwait: National Council for Culture, Arts, and Letters, 1983. *The Optics of Ibn al-Haytham*, A. I. Sabra (trans.). 2 vols. London: Warburg Institute, University of London, 1989. The Latin version of this work has been published with English translation in two volumes. See *Alhacen's Theory of Visual Perception. A Critical Edition, with English Translation and Commentary, of the First Three Books of Alhacen's* De Aspectibus, *the Medieval Latin Version of Ibn al-Haytham's* Kitâb al-Manâzir, A. Mark Smith. 2 vols. [Transactions of the American Philosophical Society Held at Philadelphia for Promoting Useful Knowledge, vol. 91, pts. 4 and 5.] Philadelphia: American Philosophical Association, 2001.

Ibn Sînâ / Avicenna

Ibn Sînâ, *Kitâb al-Nafs* (1959) (1968) (1972). *Avicenna's De Anima (Arabic Text) Being the Psychological Part of the Kitâb al-Shifâ'*, F. Rahman (ed.). London: Oxford University Press, 1959. *Avicenna Latinus. Liber De Anima seu Sextus de Naturalibus I-II-III*, S. Van Riet (ed.). Louvain: E. Peeters, and Leiden: E. J. Brill, 1972; *Avicenna Latinus. Liber De Anima seu Sextus de Naturalibus IV-V*, S. Van Riet (ed.). Louvain: Editions Orientalistes, and Leiden: E. J. Brill, 1968.

Ibn Sînâ, *Interpretation* (1970). Ibn Sînâ, *Al-Shifâ': al-Mantiq* 3 - *al-'Ibârah*, M. El-Khodeiri and I. Madkour (eds.). Cairo: Dar el-Katib al-'Arabî, 1970.

Ibn Sînâ, *Notes on the De Anima* (1947). *Aristû 'inda al-'Arab*, A. Badawi (ed.), 75–116. Cairo: Maktabat al-Nahḍah al-Miṣrîyah, 1947.

al-Kindî

al-Kindî, *On the Causes of Differences of Perspective* (1997). al-Kindî, *Liber Jacob al-Kindi de causis diuersitatum aspectus et dandis demonstrationibus geometricis super eas*, H. Hugonnard-Roche (ed.), J. Jolivet, H. Sinaceur, and H. Hugonnard-Roche (trans.), R. Rashed (rev.), 437–534, in *Oeuvres philosophiques et scientifiques d'al-Kindi*, vol. 1: *L'Optique et la catoptrique*, Roshdi Rashed et al. (eds.). Leiden: E. J. Brill, 1997.

Liber de causis (1882). *Die pseudo-aristotelische Schrift ueber das reine Gute bekannt unter dem Namen Liber de causis*, Otto Bardenhewer (ed.). Freiburg im Breisgau: Herdersche Verlagschandlung, 1882. An Arabic text of this work from the same manuscripts was published by Badawi in *Al-Aflâṭûnîyah al-muḥdathah 'inda al-'arab (Neoplatonici apud Arabes)*, 'Abdurrahman Badawi (ed.). Cairo, 1955; reprint Kuwait, 1977. The *Liber de causis (Kalâm fî maḥḍ al-khair):* A Study of Medieval Neoplatonism," Richard C. Taylor, doctoral dissertation, University of Toronto, 1981, contains a critical edition of the Arabic text of this work from additional manuscript materials with notes, English translation, and appendices.

Nicolaus of Damascus

Nicolaus of Damascus (1965). *Nicolaus Damascenus on the Philosophy of Aristotle. Fragments of the First Five Books Translated from the Syriac with an Introduction and Commentary*, H. J. Drossaart Lulofs (ed.). Leiden: E. J. Brill, 1965.

Proclus

Proclus (1963, 2nd ed.). *Proclus. The Elements of Theology*, E. R. Dodds (ed. and trans.). Oxford: Clarendon Press, 1963, 2nd ed. Originally published in 1933.

Themistius

Themistius, *De Anima Paraphrase* (1899) (1973) (1996) (1990) (1957). Themistius, *In Libros Aristotelis De Anima Paraphrasis*, R. Heinze (ed.). Berlin: G. Reimeri, 1899) [Commentaria in Aristotelem Graeca, 5.3]. *An Arabic Translation of Themistius' Commentary on Aristotle's De Anima*, M. C. Lyons (ed.). Columbia, SC, and Oxford, England: Bruno Cassirer, 1973. This text, based on an incomplete manuscript, is missing Berlin 1899 pp. 2–22 and some other passages. *Themistius, On Aristotle's On the Soul*, Robert B. Todd (trans.). Ithaca, NY: Cornell University Press, 1996. Todd also translated this text in *Two Greek Aristotelian Commentators on the Intellect*, Frederic M. Schroeder and Robert B. Todd (trans.). Toronto: Pontifical Institute of Mediaeval Studies, 1990. I reference the 1990 translation by Todd only when there is a significant variation from his 1996 translation. *Themistius. Commentaire sur le Traité de l'âme d'Aristote. Traduction de Guillaume de Moerbeke. Edition critique et étude sur l'utilisation du commentaire dans l'oeuvre de saint Thomas*, G. Verbeke (ed.). Louvain: Publications Universitaires de Louvain, 1957.

Thomas Aquinas

Thomas Aquinas, *De unitate* (1976). Thomas Aquinas, *De unitate intellectus contra Averroistas*, in *Opera omnia*, v. 43, 243–314. Rome: Editori di San Tommaso, 1976.

Thomas Aquinas, *Sententia libri De anima* (1984). Thomas Aquinas, *Sententia libri De anima*, in *Opera Omnia*, v. 45, 1. R.-A. Gauthier (ed.). Rome: Commissio Leonina; Paris: Librairie Philosophique J. Vrin, 1984.

Thomas Aquinas, *Quaestiones disputatae de anima* (1996). Thomas Aquinas, *Quaestiones de anima*, in *Opera Omnia*, v. 24.1, B.-C. Bazán (ed.). Rome: Commissio Leonina; Paris: Les Editions du Cerf, 1996.

Secondary Sources

al-ʿAlawî (1986). Jamâl al-Dîn al-ʿAlawî, *al-Matn al-Rushdî*. Casablanca: Dâr Touqbal li-n-nashr, 1986.

al-ʿAlawî (1992). Jamâl al-Dîn al-ʿAlawî, "The Philosophy of Ibn Rushd. The Evolution of the Problem of the Intellect in the Works of Ibn Rushd: From Philological Examination to Philosophical Analysis." In *The Legacy of Muslim Spain*, Salma Khadra Jayyusi (ed.), 804–829. Leiden, New York, and Cologne: E. J. Brill, 1992.

Alonso (1947). Manuel Alonso, S.I., *Teología de Averroes*. Madrid and Granada: Imprenta y Editorial Maestre, 1947. Reprinted with an introduction and summary bibliography, Rafael Ramón Guerrero, ed. Sevilla: 1998.

Altmann (1965). Alexander Altmann, "Ibn Bajja on Man's Ultimate Felicity," in *Harry Austryn Wolfson Jubilee Volume*, vol. 1, 47–87. Jerusalem: American Academy for Jewish Research, 1965.

Anawati (1978). G. C. Anawati, *Bibliographie d'Averroès (Ibn Rushd)*. Algiers: Organisation Arabe pour l'Education, la Culture et les Sciences, 1978.

Arnaldez (1998) (2000). Roger Arnaldez, *Averroès. Un rationaliste en Islam*. 2nd ed. Paris: Editions Balland, 1998; *Averroes. A Rationalist in Islam*, David Streight (trans.). Notre Dame, IN: University of Notre Dame Press, 2000.

Arnzen (1998). Rüdiger Arnzen (ed.), *Aristoteles' De anima: Eine verlorene spätantike Para-*

phrase in arabischer und persischer Überlieferung: Arabischer Text nebst Kommentar, quel-lengeschichtlichen Studien und Glossaren. Leiden and New York: E. J. Brill, 1998.

Bach (1881). Josef Bach, *Des Albertus Magnus Verhältniss zu der Erkenntnisslehre der Griechen, Lateiner, Araber und Juden. Ein Beitrag zur Geschichte der Noetik.* Vienna, 1881; reprint. Frankfurt am Main: Minerva, 1966.

Badawi (1972). Abdurrahman Badawi, *Histoire de la philosophie en Islam.* 2 vols. Paris: J. Vrin, 1972.

Ballériaux (1989). Omer Ballériaux, "Themistius et l'exégèse de la noétique aristotélici-enne," *Revue de philosophie ancienne* 7 (1989): 199–233.

Bauloye (1997). Laurence Bauloye, *La question de l'essence. Averroès et Thomas d'Aquin, com-mentateurs d'Aristote,* Métaphysique *Z1.* Louvain-la-Neuve: Editions Peeters, 1997.

Bazán (1972). Bernardo Carlos Bazán, "La noetica de Averroes (1126–1198)," *Philosophia* 38 (1972): 19–49.

Bazán (1985). Bernardo Carlos Bazán, "Le commentaire de S. Thomas d'Aquin sur le *Traité de l'âme.* Un événement: l'édition critique de la Commission Léonine." *Revue des sciences philosophiques et théologiques* 69 (1985): 521–547.

Bazán (1989). Bernardo Carlos Bazán, "On 'First Averroism' and its Doctrinal Back-ground." In *Of Scholars, Savants, and Their Texts. Studies in Philosophy and Religious Thought. Essays in Honor of Arthur Hyman,* Ruth Link-Salinger (ed.), 9–22. New York: Peter Lang, 1989.

Bazán (1997). Bernardo Carlos Bazán, "The Human Soul: Form *and* Substance? Thomas Aquinas' Critique of Eclectic Aristotelianism." *Archives d'histoire doctrinale et littéraire du Moyen Age* 64 (1997): 95–126.

Bazán (2000). Bernardo Carlos Bazán, "Was There Ever a 'First Averroism'?" in *Geistesle-ben im 13. Jahrhundert,* Jan A. Aertsen and Andreas Speer (eds.). (Miscellanea Medi-aevalia 27), 31–53. Berlin: W. de Gruyter, 2000.

Bazán (2001). Bernardo Carlos Bazán, "Conceptions of the Agent Intellect and the Lim-its of Metaphysics." In *Nach der Verurteilung von 1277: Philosophie und Theologie an der Universität von Paris im letzten Viertel des 13. Jahrhunderts: Studien und Texte (After the Condemnation of 1277: Philosophy and Theology at the University of Paris in the Last Quarter of the Thirteenth Century: Studies and Texts),* Jan A. Aertsen, Kent Emery, Jr., and Andreas Speer (eds.), 178–210. (Miscellanea Mediaevalia 28.) Berlin and New York: W. de Gruyter, 2001.

Bazán (2002). Bernardo Carlos Bazán, "13th Century Commentaries on *De Anima*: From Peter of Spain to Thomas Aquinas." In *In Commento filosófico nell'occidente latino (secoli XIII–XV),* Gianfranco Fioravanti, Claudio Leonardi, and Stephano Perfetti (eds.), 119–184. Turnhout: Brepols, 2002.

Bazán (2003). Bernardo Carlos Bazán, "Siger of Brabant." In *A Companion to Philosophy in the Middle Ages,* Jorge J. E. Gracia and Timothy B. Noone (eds.), 632–640. Oxford: Blackwell, 2003.

Bazán (2005). B. Carlos Bazán. "Radical Aristotelianism in the Faculty of Arts." In *Al-bertus Magnus und die Anfänge der Aristoteles-Rezeption im lateinischen Mittelalter: Von Richardus Rufus bis zu Franciscus de Mayronis=Albertus Magnus and the Beginnings of the Medieval Reception of Aristotle in the Latin West: From Richardus Rufus to Franciscus de Mayronis*, Ludger Honnefelder et al. (eds.), 585–629. Münster: Aschendorff Verlag, 2005.

Benmakhlouf (2000). Ali Benmakhlouf, *Averroès*. Paris: Les Belles Lettres, 2000.

Black (1993). Deborah Louise Black, "Consciousness and Self-Knowledge in Aquinas's Critique of Averroes's Psychology." *Journal of the History of Philosophy* 31 (1993): 349–385.

Black (1996). Deborah Louise Black. "Memory, Individuals, and the Past in Averroes's Psychology." *Medieval Philosophy and Theology* 5 (1996): 161–187.

Black (1997). Deborah Louise Black, "Avicenna on the Ontological and Epistemic Status of Fictional Beings." *Documenti e studi sulla tradizione filosofica medievale* 8 (1997): 425–453.

Black (1999). Deborah Louise Black, "Conjunction and the Identity of Knower and Known in Averroes." *American Catholic Philosophical Quarterly* 73 (1999): 159–184.

Black (2000). Deborah Louise Black. "Imagination and Estimation: Arabic Paradigms and Western Transformations." *Topoi* 19 (2000): 59–75.

Black (2005). Deborah Louise Black, "Psychology: Soul and Intellect." In *Cambridge Companion to Arabic Philosophy*, Peter Adamson and Richard C. Taylor (eds.), 308–326. Cambridge: Cambridge University Press, 2005.

Blaustein (1984). Michael A. Blaustein, *Averroes on Imagination and the Intellect*. PhD dissertation, Harvard University. Ann Arbor, MI: University Microfilms International, 1984.

Blaustein (1986). Michael A. Blaustein, "Aspects of Ibn Bajja's Theory of Apprehension." In *Maimonides and Philosophy: Papers Presented at the Sixth Jerusalem Philosophical Encounter, May 1985*, Shlomo Pines and Yirmiyahu Yovel (eds.), 202–212. Dordrecht: M. Nijhoff, 1986.

Blumenthal (1979). Henry J. Blumenthal, "Themistius, the Last Peripatetic Commentator on Aristotle?" In *Arktouros. Hellenic Studies Presented to Bernard M. W. Knox on the Occasion of His 65th Birthday*, Glen W. Bowersock et al. (eds.), 391–400. Berlin and New York: Walter de Gruyter, 1979.

Bouyges (1922). Maurice Bouyges, "Notes sur les philosophes arabes connus des Latins au Moyen Age; V: Inventaire des textes arabes d'Averroès," *Mélanges de l'Université Saint Joseph* 8 (1922): 3–54.

Bouyges (1923). Maurice Bouyges, "Notes sur les philosophes arabes connus des Latins au Moyen Age; VI: Inventaire des textes arabes d'Averroès (*suite*); Additions et corrections à la Note V; VII: Sur le *De Scientiis* d'Alfarabi, récemment édité en arabe à Saïda, et sur le *De Divisione Philosophiae* de Gundissalinus; VIII: Sur le *De Plantis* d'Aristote-Nicolas, à propos d'un manuscrit arabe de Constantinople." *Mélanges de l'Université Saint Joseph* 9 (1923): 43–94.

Brenet (2003). Jean-Baptiste Brenet, *Transferts du Sujet. La noétique d'Averroès selon Jean de Jandun*. Paris: Librairie Philosophique J. Vrin, 2003.

Browne (1986). Gerald M. Browne, "Ad Themistium Arabum." *Illinois Classical Studies* 11 (1986): 223–245.

Bürgel (1967). J. Christoph Bürgel, *Averroes "contra Galenum." Das Kapitel von der Atmung im Colliget des Averroes als ein Zeugnis mittelalterlich-islamischer Kritik an Galen*. Göttingen: Vandenhoeck and Ruprecht, 1967.

Burnett (1994). Charles Burnett, "Michael Scot and the Transmission of Scientific Culture from Toledo to Bologna via the Court of Frederick II Hohenstaufen." *Micrologus. Natura, scienza e società medievali* 2 (1994): 101–126.

Burnett (1997) Charles Burnett, "Translating from Arabic into Latin in the Middle Ages: Theory, Practice and Criticism." In *Editer, traduire, interpréter: Essais de méthodologie philosophique*, Steve G. Lofts and Philipp W. Rosemann (eds.), 55–78. Louvain-la-Neuve: Editions de l'Institut Supérieur de Philosophie; Louvain and Paris: Editions Peeters, 1997.

Burnett (1999). Charles Burnett, "The 'Sons of Averroes with the Emperor Frederick' and the Transmission of the Philosophical Works by Ibn Rushd." In *Averroes and the Aristotelian Tradition. Sources, Constitution and Reception of the Philosophy of Ibn Rushd (1126–1198). Proceedings of the Fourth Symposium Averroicum* (Cologne, 1996), Gerhard Endress and Jan A. Aertsen with the assistance of Klaus Braun (eds.), 259–299. Leiden: E. J. Brill, 1999.

Burnett (2005). Charles Burnett, "Arabic into Latin: The Reception of Arabic Philosophy into Western Europe." In *The Cambridge Companion to Arabic Philosophy*, Peter Adamson and Richard C. Taylor (eds.), 370–404. Cambridge: Cambridge University Press, 2005.

Burnett and Zonta (2000). Charles Burnett and Mauro Zonta, "Abû Muḥammad 'Abdallâh Ibn Rushd (Averroes junior), *On Whether the Active Intellect Unites with the Material Intellect whilst It Is Clothed with the Body*: A Critical Edition of the Three Extant Medieval Versions, together with an English Translation." *Archives d'histoire doctrinale et littéraire du Moyen Age* 67 (2000): 295–335.

Butterworth (1996). Charles E. Butterworth, "Averroës, Precursor of the Enlightenment?" *Alif. Journal of Comparative Poetics* (American University in Cairo) 16 (1996): 6–18.

Cherniss (1944). H. Cherniss, *Aristotle's Criticism of Plato and the Academy*. Baltimore: Johns Hopkins University Press, 1944.

Cranz (1976). F. Edward Cranz, "Editions of the Latin Aristotle Accompanied by the Commentaries of Averroes" in *Philosophy and Humanism: Renaissance Essays in Honor of Paul Oskar Kristeller*, Edward P. Mahoney (ed.), 116–128. New York: Columbia University Press, 1976.

Cruz Hernández (1978). Miguel Cruz Hernández, "Los límites del Aristotelismo de Ibn Rushd." In *Multiple Averroès. Actes du Colloque International organisé à l'occasion du 850ᵉ anniversaire de la naissance d'Averroès. Paris 20–23 septembre 1976*, Jean Jolivet and Rachel Arié (eds.), 129–153. Paris: Les Belles Lettres, 1978.

Cruz Hernández (1997). Miguel Cruz Hernández, *Abû-l-Walîd Muḥammad Ibn Rushd (Averroes). Vida, obra, pensamiento, influencia*. 2nd ed. Córdoba: Publicaciones de la Obra Social y Cultural Cajasur, 1997. The first edition was published in 1986.

Daiber (1999). Hans Daiber, *Bibliography of Islamic Philosophy*. 2 vols. Leiden and Boston: E. J. Brill, 1999.

D'Ancona and Taylor (2003). Cristina D'Ancona and Richard C. Taylor, "Le Liber de causis." In *Dictionnaire des philosophes antiques. Supplément*, Richard Goulet et al. (eds.), 599–647. Paris: Centre National de la Recherche Scientifique, 2003.

Davidson (1986). Herbert A. Davidson, "Averroes on the Material Intellect." *Viator. Medieval and Renaissance Studies* 17 (1986): 91–137.

Davidson (1988). Herbert A. Davidson, "*Averrois Tractatus de Animae Beatitudine*." In *A Straight Path. Studies in Medieval Philosophy and Culture. Essays in Honor of Arthur Hyman*, Ruth Link-Salinger et al. (eds.), 57–73. Washington, D.C.: Catholic University of America Press, 1988.

Davidson (1992). Herbert A. Davidson, *Alfarabi, Avicenna, and Averroes on Intellect*. Oxford: Oxford University Press, 1992.

Davidson (1997). Herbert A. Davidson, "The Relation between Averroes' Middle and Long Commentaries on the *De Anima*." *Arabic Sciences and Philosophy* 7 (1997): 139–151.

de Libera (1994). Alain de Libera, "Existe-t-il une noétique 'averroiste'?" In *Averroismus im Mittelalter und in der Renaissance*, Friedrich Niewöhner and Loris Sturlese (eds.), 51–80. Zurich: Spur, 1994.

de Libera (2000). Alain de Libera, "Pour Averroès." In *Averroès. L'Islam et la raison. Anthologie des textes juridiques, théologiques et polémiques*, Marc Geoffroy (trans.). Paris: Flammarion, 2000.

Doig (1974). J. C. Doig, "Toward Understanding Aquinas' *Com. in De Anima*. A Comparative Study of Aquinas and Averroes on the Definition of Soul (*De Anima* B, 1–2)." *Rivista di filosofia neo-scolastica* (Milan) 66 (1974): 436–474.

Druart (1994). Thérèse-Anne Druart, "Averroes: The Commentator and the Commentators." In *Aristotle in Late Antiquity*, Lawrence P. Schrenk (ed.), 184–202. Washington, D.C.: Catholic University of America Press, 1994.

Druart (1995). Thérèse-Anne Druart, "Averroes on God's Knowledge of Being Qua Being." In *Studies in Thomistic Theology*, Paul Lockey (ed.), 175–205. Houston: Center for Thomistic Studies, University of St. Thomas, 1995.

Druart (1997a). Thérèse-Anne Druart, "Al-Fârâbî, Ethics, and First Intelligibles." *Documenti e studi sulla tradizione filosofica medievale* 8 (1997): 403–423.

Druart (1997b). Thérèse-Anne Druart, "Medieval Islamic Philosophy and Theology Bibliographical Guide (1994–1996)." *Bulletin de philosophie médiévale* 39 (1997): 175–202.

Druart (2001). Thérèse-Anne Druart, "Medieval Islamic Philosophy and Theology Bibliographical Guide (1996–1998)." *MIDEO* (*Mélanges de l'Institut Dominicain d'Études Orientales du Caire* 24 (2000, but in fact 2001): 381–414.

Druart (2002). Thérèse-Anne Druart, "Brief Bibliographical Guide in Medieval Islamic Philosophy and Theology (1998–2002)." At http://philosophy.cua.edu/faculty/tad/biblio.cfm.

Druart (2004a). "Brief Bibliographical Guide in Medieval Islamic Philosophy and Theology (2002–2004)." At http://philosophy.cua.edu/faculty/tad/Bibliography%2002–04.cfm.

Druart (2004b). Thérèse-Anne Druart, "Metaphysics." In *The Cambridge Companion to Arabic Philosophy*, Peter Adamson and Richard C. Taylor (eds.), 327–348. Cambridge: Cambridge University Press, 2004.

Druart (2006). "Brief Bibliographical Guide in Medieval Islamic Philosophy and Theology (2004–2006)." At http://philosophy.cua.edu/faculty/tad/Bibliography%2004–06.cfm.

Druart and Marmura (1990). Thérèse-Anne Druart and Michael E. Marmura, "Medieval Islamic Philosophy and Theology Bibliographical Guide (1986–1989)." *Bulletin de philosophie médiévale* 32 (1990): 106–135.

Druart and Marmura (1993). Thérèse-Anne Druart and Michael E. Marmura, "Medieval Islamic Philosophy and Theology Bibliographical Guide (1989–1992)." *Bulletin de philosophie médiévale* 35 (1993): 181–219.

Druart and Marmura (1995). Thérèse-Anne Druart and Michael E. Marmura, "Medieval Islamic Philosophy and Theology Bibliographical Guide (1992–1994)." *Bulletin de philosophie médiévale* 37 (1995): 193–232.

Ebbesen (1998). Sten Ebbesen, "Averroism." In *Routledge Encyclopedia of Philosophy*. London: Routledge, 1998. Retrieved July 16, 2004, from http://o–www.rep.routledge.com. libus.csd.mu.edu:80/article/B012.

Elamrani-Jamal (1991). Abdelali Elamrani-Jamal, "Averroès, le *commentateur* d'Aristote?" In *Penser avec Aristote*, Georges Hahn and Mohammed Allal Sinaceur (eds.), 643–651. Toulouse: Editions Erès, 1991.

Elamrani-Jamal (1997). Abdelali Elamrani-Jamal, "Averroès: La doctrine de l'intellect matériel dans le *Commentaire moyen* au *De anima* d'Aristote. Présentation et traduction, suivie d'un lexique-index du chapitre 3, livre III: *De la faculté rationnelle*." In *Langages et philosophie. Hommage à Jean Jolivet*, A. de Libera, A. Elamrani-Jamal, and A. Galonnier (eds.), 281–307. Paris: Librairie Philosophique J. Vrin, 1997.

Elamrani-Jamal (2003). Abdelali Elamrani-Jamal, "*De Anima*. Tradition Arabe." in *Dictionnaire des philosophes antiques. Supplément*, Richard Goulet et al. (eds.), 346–358. Paris: Centre National de la Recherche Scientifique, 2003.

Endress (1995). Gerhard Endress, "Averroes' *De Caelo*, Ibn Rushd's Cosmology in His Commentaries on Aristotle's *On the Heavens*." *Arabic Sciences and Philosophy* 5 (1995): 9–49.

Endress (1999). Gerhard Endress, "Averrois Opera: A Bibliography of Editions and Contributions to the Text." In *Averroes and the Aristotelian Tradition. Sources, Constitution and Reception of the Philosophy of Ibn Rushd (1126–1198). Proceedings of the Fourth Symposium Averroicum* (Cologne, 1996), Gerhard Endress and Jan A. Aertsen with the assistance of Klaus Braun (eds.), 339–381. Leiden: E. J. Brill, 1999.

Endress (2005). Gerhard Endress, "'If God Will Grant Me Life.' Averroes the Philosopher: Studies in the History of His Development." *Documenti e studi sulla tradizione filosofica medievale* 15 (2004): 227–253.

Fakhry (2001). Majid Fakhry, *Averroes (Ibn Rushd). His Life, Works and Influence*. Oxford: Oneworld Publications, 2001.

Falcon (2005). Andrea Falcon, "Commentators on Aristotle." In *The Stanford Encyclopedia of Philosophy* (Winter 2005 Edition), Edward N. Zalta (ed.). URL = http://plato.stanford .edu/archives/win2005/entries/aridestotle-commentators/.

Frank (1958–1959). Richard M. Frank, "Some Fragments of Isḥâq's Translation of the *De Anima*." *Cahiers de Byrsa* 8 (1958–59): 231–251.

Frank (1967). Richard M. Frank, "*Al-maʿnà*: Some Reflections on the Technical Meanings of the Term in the Kalâm and Its Use in the Physics of Muʿammar." *Journal of the American Oriental Society* 87 (1967): 248–259.

Gardet (1971). L. Gardet, "ʿIlm al-Kalâm." In *The Encyclopaedia of Islam. New Edition*, vol. 3, B. Lewis, V. L. Ménage, Ch. Pellat, and J. Schacht (eds.), 1141b–1150b. Leiden: E. J. Brill; London: Luzac, 1971.

Gardet (1978). L. Gardet, "Kalâm." In *The Encyclopaedia of Islam. New Edition*, vol. 4, E. van Donzel, B. Lewis, and Ch. Pellat (eds.), 468b–471a. Leiden: E. J. Brill, 1978.

Gätje (1971). Helmut Gätje, *Studien zur Überlieferung der aristotelischen Psychologie im Islam.* Heidelberg: C. Winter, 1971.

Gauthier (1982a). René Antoine Gauthier, "Le traité *De anima et de potenciis eius* d'un maître ès arts (vers 1225)." *Revue des sciences philosophiques et théologiques* 66 (1982): 3–55.

Gauthier (1982b). René Antoine Gauthier, "Notes sur les débuts (1225–1240) du premier 'Averroïsme.'" *Revue des sciences philosophiques et théologiques* 66 (1982): 321–374.

Gauthier (1983). René Antoine Gauthier, "Notes sur Siger de Brabant. I: Siger en 1265." *Revue des sciences philosophiques et théologiques* 67 (1983): 201–232.

Gauthier (1984). René Antoine Gauthier, "Notes sur Siger de Brabant. II: Siger en 1272–1275. Aubry de Reims et la scission des Normands." *Revue des sciences philosophiques et théologiques* 68 (1984): 3–49.

Geoffroy (1999). Marc Geoffroy, "L'almohadisme théologique d'Averroès (Ibn Rushd)." *Archives d'histoire doctrinale et littéraire du Moyen Age* 66 (1999): 9–47.

Geoffroy (2001). Marc Geoffroy, "Ibn Rushd et la théologie almohadiste. Une version inconnue du Kitâb al-Kashf ʿan manâhij al-adilla dans deux manuscrits d'Istanbul." *Medioevo* 26 (2001): 327–351.

Geoffroy (2002). Marc Geoffroy, "La tradition arabe du Περὶ voῦ d'Alexandre d'Aphrodise et les origines de la théorie farabienne des quatre degrés de l'intellect." In *Aristotele e Alessandro di Afrodisia nella tradizione araba*, Cristina d'Ancona and Giuseppe Serra (eds.), 191–231. (Subsidia Mediaevalia Patavina 3). Padua: Il Poligrafo Casa Editrice, 2002.

Geoffroy (2005). Marc Geoffroy, "Averroè." In *Storia della filosofia nell'Islam medievale*, Cristina d'Ancona (ed.), vol. 2, 722–782. Torino: Giulio Einaudi Editore, 2005.

Geoffroy and Steel (2001). Marc Geoffroy and Carlos Steel (eds. and trans.), *Averroès. La béatitude de l'âme. Editions, traductions et études.* Paris: Librairie Philosophique J. Vrin, 2001. This work contains two short treatises by Averroes, "On Conjunction with the Agent Intellect," translated into French from Hebrew with notes by Marc Geoffroy. These translations are based on Geoffroy's readings of the manuscripts used by J. Hercz (ed. and trans.), *Drei Abhandlungen über die Conjunction des separaten Intellectes mit dem Menschen, von Averroes (Vater und Sohn) aus dem Arabischen übersetzt von Samuel Ibn Tibbon*; Berlin: H. G. Hermann, 1869. Following Hercz and Geoffroy and Steel, I cite these short works as *Epistle 1 On Conjunction* and *Epistle 2 On Conjunction*.

Glasner (2004). Ruth Glasner, "Review of *Averroes. Middle Commentary on Aristotle's De Anima. A Critical Edition of the Arabic Text with English Translation, Notes and Introduction*, Alfred L. Ivry." In *Aestimatio* 1 (2004): 57–61.

Gómez Nogales (1967). Salvador Gómez Nogales, "Problemas alrededor del *Compendio sobre el alma* de Averroes," *Al-Andalus* 32 (1967): 1–36.

Gómez Nogales (1976). Salvador Gómez Nogales, "Saint Thomas, Averroès et l'Averroïsme." In *Aquinas and Problems of His Time*, G. Verbeke and D. Verhelst (eds.), 161–177. Louvain: Leuven University Press, 1976.

Gómez Nogales (1978a). Salvador Gómez Nogales, "En torno a la unidad del enten-
dimiento en Averroes." In *Multiple Averroès. Actes du Colloque International organisé à
l'occasion du 850ᵉ anniversaire de la naissance d'Averroès. Paris 20–23 septembre 1976*, Jean
Jolivet and Rachel Arié (eds.), 251–256. Paris: Les Belles Lettres, 1978.

Gómez Nogales (1978b). Salvador Gómez Nogales, "Bibliografía sobre las obras de
Averroès." In *Multiple Averroès. Actes du Colloque International organisé à l'occasion du
850ᵉ anniversaire de la naissance d'Averroès. Paris 20–23 septembre 1976*, Jean Jolivet and
Rachel Arié (eds.), 351–389. Paris: Les Belles Lettres, 1978.

Gómez Nogales (1993). Salvador Gómez Nogales, "Hacia una nueva interpretación de
Averroes." In *Al encuentro de Averroes*, Andrés Martínez Lorca (ed.), 53–69. Madrid:
Editorial Trotta, 1993.

Gutas (1988). Dimitri Gutas, *Avicenna and the Aristotelian Tradition: Introduction to Reading Avicenna's Philosophical Works*. Leiden and New York: E. J. Brill, 1988.

Gutas (1999a). Dimitri Gutas, "Fârâbî and Greek Philosophy," inside the article "Fârâbî."
In *Encyclopaedia Iranica*, vol. 9, Ehsan Yarshater (ed.), 219a–223b. New York: Bibliotheca
Persica Press, 1999.

Gutas (1999b). Dimitri Gutas, "Averroes on Theophrastus, through Themistius." In *Aver-
roes and the Aristotelian Tradition: Sources, Constitution and Reception of the Philosophy of
Ibn Rushd (1126–1198). Proceedings of the Fourth Symposium Averroicum* (Cologne, 1996),
Gerhard Endress and Jan A. Aertsen (eds.), 125–144. Leiden: E. J. Brill, 1999.

Gutas (2001). Dimitri Gutas, "Intuition and Thinking: The Evolving Structure of Avi-
cenna's Epistemology." In *Aspects of Avicenna*, Robert Wisnovsky (ed.), 1–38. Princeton:
Markus Wiener, 2001. Reprinted from *Princeton Papers: Interdisciplinary Journal of
Middle Eastern Studies,* vol. 9.

Gyekye (1979). Kwame Gyekye (trans.), *Arabic Logic: Ibn al-Ṭayyib's Commentary on Por-
phyry's* Eisagoge. Albany: State University of New York Press, 1979.

Hamesse (2001). Jacqueline Hamesse (ed.), *Les traducteurs au travail: Leurs manuscrits et
leurs méthodes. Actes du Colloque international organisé par le "Ettore Majorana Centre for
Scientific Culture," (Erice, 30 septembre–6 octobre 1999)*. Turnhout, Belgium: Brepols,
2001.

Hamesse and Fattori (1999). Jacqueline Hamesse and Marta Fattori (eds.), *Rencontres de
cultures dans la philosophie médiévale: Traductions et traducteurs de l'antiquité tardive au
XIVe siècle*. Louvain-la-Neuve: Université Catholique de Louvain; Cassino, Italy:
Università degli Studi di Cassino, 1990.

Harvey (1992a). Steven Harvey, "The Place of the Philosopher in the City according to
Ibn Bâjjah." In *The Political Aspects of Islamic Philosophy. Essays in Honor of Muhsin S.
Mahdi*, Charles E. Butterworth (ed.), 199–233. Cambridge, MA: Harvard University
Press, 1992.

Harvey (1992b). Steven Harvey, "Did Maimonides' Letter to Samuel ibn Tibbon Determine Which Philosophers Would Be Studied by Later Jewish Thinkers?" *Jewish
Quarterly Review* 83 (1992): 51–70.

Harvey (1997). Steven Harvey, "Averroes' Use of Examples in His *Middle Commentary*
on the *Prior Analytics* and Some Remarks on his Role as Commentator." *Arabic Sciences and Philosophy* 7 (1997): 91–113.

Harvey (2003). Steven Harvey, "Arabic into Hebrew: The Hebrew Translation Movement and the Influence of Averroes upon Medieval Jewish Thought." In *The Cambridge Companion to Medieval Jewish Philosophy*, Daniel H. Frank and Oliver Leaman (eds.), 258–280. Cambridge: Cambridge University Press, 2003.

Harvey (2005). Steven Harvey, "Islamic Philosophy and Jewish Philosophy." In *The Cambridge Companion to Arabic Philosophy*, Peter Adamson and Richard C. Taylor (eds.), 349–369. Cambridge: Cambridge University Press, 2005.

Harvey (forthcoming). Steven Harvey, "Similarities and Differences among Averroes' Three Commentaries on Aristotle's *Physics*." In *La pensée philosophique et scientifique d'Averroès dans son temps*, J. Puig Montada and A. Hasnaoui (eds.). Paris, forthcoming.

Haskins (1927). Charles Homer Haskins, *Studies in the History of Mediaeval Science*, 2nd ed. Cambridge, MA: Harvard University Press, 1927.

Hasse (1999). Dag Nikolaus Hasse, "Das Lehrstück von den vier Intellekten in der Scholastik: Von den arabischen Quellen bis zu Albertus Magnus." *Recherches de théologie et philosophie médiévales* 66 (1999): 21–77.

Hasse (2000). Dag Nikolaus Hasse, *Avicenna's De Anima in the Latin West. The Formation of a Peripatetic Philosophy of the Soul 1160–1300*. London: Warburg Institute, 2000.

Hasse (2001). Dag Nikolaus Hasse, "Avicenna on Abstraction." In *Aspects of Avicenna*, Robert Wisnovsky (ed.), 39–72. Princeton: Markus Wiener, 2001. Reprinted from *Princeton Papers: Interdisciplinary Journal of Middle Eastern Studies*, vol. 9.

Hasse (2004). Dag Nikolaus Hasse, "The Attraction of Averroism in the Renaissance: Vernia, Achillini, Prassicio." In *Philosophy, Science and Exegesis in Greek, Arabic and Latin Commentaries (Supplement to the Bulletin of the Institute of Classical Studies 83.1–2)*, Peter Adamson, Han Baltussen, and M. W. F. Stone (eds.), v. 2, 131–147. London: ICS, 2004.

Hayoun and de Libera (1991). Maurice-Ruben Hayoun and Alain de Libera, *Averroès et l'averroïsme* (Que sais-je?). Paris: Presses Universitaires de France, 1991.

Huby (1999). Pamela Huby, *Theophrastus of Eresus. Sources for His Life, Writings, Thought and Influence. Commentary Volume 4. Psychology (Texts 265–327) with Contributions on the Arabic Material by Dimitri Gutas*. Leiden: E. J. Brill, 1999.

Hugonnard-Roche (1977). Henri Hugonnard-Roche, "Remarques sur l'évolution doctrinale d'Averroès dans les commentaires au *De caelo*: Le problème du mouvement de la terre." *Mélanges de la casa di Velasquez* 13 (1977): 103–117.

Hugonnard-Roche (1984). Henri Hugonnard-Roche. "L'Epitomé du *De caelo* d'Aristote par Averroès. Questions de méthode et de doctrine." *Archives d'histoire doctrinale et littéraire du Moyen Age* 51 (1984): 7–39.

Hugonnard-Roche (2000). Henri Hugonnard-Roche, "La formulation logique de l'argumentation dans les commentaires d'Averroès au *De caelo*." In *Le commentaire entre tradition et innovation. Actes du Colloque international de l'Institut des traditions textuelles (Paris et Villejuif, 22–25 septembre 1999)*, Marie-Odile Goulet-Cazé et al. (eds.), 387–395. Paris: J. Vrin, 2000.

Hyman (1965). Arthur Hyman, "Aristotle's 'First Matter' and Avicenna's and Averroes' 'Corporeal Form.'" In *Harry A. Wolfson Jubilee Volume*, v. 1, 385–406. Jerusalem: American Academy for Jewish Research, 1965.

Hyman (1981). Arthur Hyman, "Aristotle's Theory of the Intellect and its Interpretation by Averroes." In *Studies in Aristotle*, Dominic J. O'Meara (ed.), 161–191. Washington, D.C.: Catholic University of America Press, 1981.

Hyman (1999). Arthur Hyman, "Averroes' Theory of the Intellect and the Ancient Commentators." In *Averroes and the Aristotelian Tradition. Sources, Constitution and Reception of the Philosophy of Ibn Rushd (1126–1198). Proceedings of the Fourth Symposium Averroicum* (Cologne, 1996), Gerhard Endress and Jan A. Aertsen with the assistance of Klaus Braun (eds.), 188–198. Leiden: E. J. Brill, 1999.

Illuminati (1996). Augusto Illuminati, *Averroè e l'intelletto pubblico. Antologia di scritti di Ibn Rushd sull'anima*. Rome: Manifesto Libri, 1996.

Illuminati (2000). Augusto Illuminati, *Completa beatitudo: L'intelletto felice in tre opuscoli averroisti*. Chiaravalle, Ancona: L'Orecchio di Van Gogh, 2000.

Ivry (1983). Alfred L. Ivry, "Remnants of Jewish Averroism in the Renaissance." In *Jewish Thought in the Sixteenth Century*, B. D. Cooperman (ed.), 243–265. Cambridge, MA: Harvard University Press, 1983.

Ivry (1990). Alfred L. Ivry, "Averroes' Middle Commentary on the *De Anima*." In *Knowledge and the Sciences in Medieval Philosophy. Proceedings of the Eighth International Congress of Medieval Philosophy (SIEPM) Helsinki 24–29 August 1987*, Reijo Työrinoja, Anja Inkeri Lehtinen, and Dagfinn Føllesdal (eds.), v. 3, 79–86. Helsinki: Yliopistopaino, 1990.

Ivry (1991). Alfred L. Ivry, "La logique de la science de l'âme. Etude sur la méthode dans le Commentaire d'Averroès." In *Penser avec Aristote*, Georges Hahn and Mohammed Allal Sinaceur (eds.), 687–700. Toulouse: Editions Erès, 1991.

Ivry (1995). Alfred L. Ivry, "Averroes' Middle and Long Commentaries on the *De Anima*." *Arabic Sciences and Philosophy* 5 (1995): 75–92.

Ivry (1997a). Alfred L. Ivry, "Response [to Davidson (1997)]." *Arabic Sciences and Philosophy* 7 (1997): 153–155.

Ivry (1997b). Alfred L. Ivry, "Averroes' *Short Commentary* on Aristotle's *De Anima*." *Documenti e studi sulla tradizione filosofica medievale* 8 (1997): 511–549.

Ivry (1999). Alfred L. Ivry, "Averroes' Three Commentaries on *De Anima*." In *Averroes and the Aristotelian Tradition. Sources, Constitution and Reception of the Philosophy of Ibn Rushd (1126–1198). Proceedings of the Fourth Symposium Averroicum* (Cologne, 1996), Gerhard Endress and Jan A. Aertsen with the assistance of Klaus Braun (eds.), 199–216. Leiden: E. J. Brill, 1999.

Ivry (2001). Alfred L. Ivry, "The Arabic Text of Aristotle's *De Anima* and Its Translator." *Oriens* 36 (2001): 59–77.

Janssens (1998). Jules Janssens, Review of *Long Commentary. Book 3* (1998) In *Revue philosophique de Louvain* 96 (1998): 720–730.

Jolivet (1991). Jean Jolivet, "Averroès et le décentrement du sujet." *Le choc Averroès. Comment les philosophes arabes ont fait l'Europe. Travaux de l'Université Européenne de la Recherche, Actes du Colloque Averroès 6–8 févier 1991*. In *Internationale de l'Imaginaire* 17–18 (1991): 161–169.

Jolivet (1997). Jean Jolivet. "Etapes dans l'histoire de l'intellect agent." In *Perspectives arabes et médiévales sur la tradition scientifique et philosophique grecque: Actes du colloque de la*

SIHSPAI (Société internationale d'histoire des sciences et de la philosophie arabes et islamiques), Paris, *31 mars–3 avril 1993,* Ahmad Hasnawi, Abdelali Elamrani-Jamal, and Maroun Aouad (eds.), 569–582. Louvain: Peeters; Paris: Institut du Monde Arabe, 1997.

Kassem (1978). Mahmoud Kassem, *Théorie de la connaissance d'après Averroès et son interprétation chez Thomas d'Aquin.* Algiers: Société Nationale d'Edition et de Diffusion, 1978. For the Arabic version of this, see the same author under Qasim (1964).

Kessler (1988). Eckhard Kessler, "The Intellective Soul." In *The Cambridge History of Renaissance Philosophy,* Charles B. Schmitt et al. (eds.), 485–534. Cambridge: Cambridge University Press, 1988.

Khoury (2000). Raif Khoury (ed.), *Averroes (1126–1198), oder der Triumph des Rationalismus: Internationales Symposium anlässlich des 800. Todestages des islamischen Philosophen, Heidelberg, 7.–11. Oktober 1998.* Heidelberg: Universitätsverlag C. Winter, 2002.

Kogan (1981). Barry Kogan, "The Philosophers al-Ghazâlî and Averroes on Necessary Connection and the Problem of the Miraculous." In *Islamic Philosophy and Mysticism,* Parviz Morewedge (ed.), 113–132. Delmar, NY: Caravan Books, 1981.

Kogan (1985). Barry Kogan, *Averroes and the Metaphysics of Causation.* Albany: State University of New York Press, 1985.

Kuksewicz (1968). Zdzislaw Kuksewicz, *De Siger de Brabant à Jacques de Plaisance. La théorie de l'intellect chez les averroïstes latins des XIIIe et XIVe siècles.* Wroclaw: Ossolineum, 1968.

Kuksewicz (1994). Zdzislaw Kuksewicz, "The Latin Averroism of the Late Thirteenth Century." In *Averroismus im Mittelalter und in der Renaissance,* Friedrich Niewöhner and Loris Sturlese (eds.), 101–113. Zurich: Spur, 1994.

Leaman (1994). Oliver Leaman, "Is Averroes an Averroist?" In *Averroismus im Mittelalter und in der Renaissance,* Friedrich Niewöhner and Loris Sturlese (eds.), 9–22. Zurich: Spur, 1994.

Leaman (1996). Oliver Leaman, "Jewish Averroism." In *History of Islamic Philosophy,* Seyyed Hossein Nasr and Oliver Leaman (eds.), 769–780. London and New York: Routledge, 1996.

Leaman (1998a). Oliver Leaman, *Averroes and His Philosophy.* Rev. ed. Richmond, Surrey: Curzon Press, 1998. First edition: Oxford: Clarendon Press; New York: Oxford University Press, 1988.

Leaman (1998b). Oliver Leaman, "Jewish Averroism." In *Routledge Encyclopedia of Philosophy,* E. Craig (ed.). London: Routledge, 1998. Retrieved July 15, 2004, from http://0-www.rep.routledge.com.libus.csd.mu.edu:80/article/J022.

Lyons (1955). M. C. Lyons, "An Arabic Translation of the Commentary of Themistius." *Bulletin of the School of Oriental and African Studies, University of London* 17 (1955): 1–9.

Mahdi (1964). Muhsin Mahdi, "Averroës on Divine Law and Human Wisdom." In *Ancients and Moderns: Essays on the Tradition of Political Philosophy in Honor of Leo Strauss,* Joseph Cropsey (ed.), 114–131. New York: Basic Books, 1964.

Mahoney (1994). Edward P. Mahoney, "Aquinas's Critique of Averroes' Doctrine of the Unity of the Intellect." In *Thomas Aquinas and His Legacy,* David M. Gallagher (ed.), 83–106 (Studies in Philosophy and the History of Philosophy 28). Washington, D. C.: Catholic University of America Press, 1994.

Mahoney and South (1998). Edward P. Mahoney and James B. South, "Renaissance Aristotelianism." In *Routledge Encyclopedia of Philosophy*, E. Craig (ed.). London: Routledge, 1998. Retrieved July 16, 2004, from http://0-www.rep.routledge.com.libus.csd.mu.edu:80/article/C003.

Mandonnet (1899). Pierre Mandonnet, *Siger de Brabant et l'averroïsme latin au XIIIme siècle; étude critique et documents inédits*. Fribourg (Switzerland): Librairie de l'Université, 1899.

al-Marrâkushî (1949). 'Abd al-Wâḥid al-Marrâkushî, *al-Mu'jib fî talkhîs akhbâr al-Maghrib*, M. Sa'îd al-'Uryân and M. al-'Arabî al-'Alamî (eds.). Cairo: Maṭba'at al-Istiqâmah, 1949.

Martínez Lorca (2004). Andrés Martínez Lorca (ed. and trans.), *Sobre el intelecto. Abû-l-Walîd Ibn Rushd (Averroes)*. Madrid: Editorial Trotta, 2004. This work contains Spanish translations of selected texts from the *Short Commentary on the De Anima* (a reprint of the translation of Salvador Gómez Nogales in *Short Commentary on the De Anima* [1987]); from the *Middle Commentary* (a Spanish translation by Martinez Lorca of the French of Abdelali Elamrani-Jamal in Elamrani-Jamal [1997]); and from the *Long Commentary* (translated from the Latin *Long Commentary* [1953] directly into Spanish by Martínez Lorca).

Minio-Paluello (1974). Lorenzo Minio-Paluello, "Michael Scot." In *Dictionary of Scientific Biography*, v. 9, 361–365. New York: Scribner, 1974.

Nardi (1945). Bruno Nardi, *Sigieri di Brabante nel pensiero del Rinascimento Italiano*. Rome: Edizioni Italiane, 1945.

Nardi (1958). Bruno Nardi, *Saggi sull'aristotelismo padovano dal secolo XIV al XVI*. Florence: G. C. Sansoni, 1958.

Niewöhner and Sturlese (1994). Friedrich Niewöhner and Loris Sturlese, (eds.) *Averroismus im Mittelalter und in der Renaissance*. Zurich: Spur, 1994.

Owens (1976). Joseph Owens. "A Note on Aristotle, *De Anima* 3.4, 429b9." *Phoenix* 30 (1976): 107–118.

Oxford Latin Dictionary (1982). Oxford and London: Clarendon Press, 1982.

Park (1988). Katharine Park, "The Organic Soul." In *The Cambridge History of Renaissance Philosophy*, Charles B. Schmitt et al. (eds.), 464–484. Cambridge: Cambridge University Press, 1988.

Peters (1968). F. E. Peters, *Aristoteles Arabus. The Oriental Translations and Commentaries of the Aristotelian Corpus*. Leiden: E. J. Brill, 1968.

Pick (1998). Lucy K. Pick, "Michael Scot in Toledo: *Natura Naturans* and the Hierarchy of Being." *Traditio* 53 (1998): 93–116.

Pick (2004). Lucy K. Pick, *Conflict and Coexistence: Archbishop Rodrigo and the Muslims and Jews of Medieval Spain*. Ann Arbor: University of Michigan Press, 2004.

Pines (1978). Shlomo Pines, "La philosophie dans l'économie du genre humain selon Averroès: Une réponse à al-Farabi?" In *Multiple Averroès. Actes du Colloque International organisé à l'occasion du 850ᵉ anniversaire de la naissance d'Averroès. Paris 20–23 septembre 1976*, Jean Jolivet and Rachel Arié (eds.), 189–207. Paris: Les Belles Lettres, 1978.

Pines (1979). Shlomo Pines, "The Limitations of Human Knowledge according to al-Farabi, Ibn Bajja, and Maimonides." In *Studies in Medieval Jewish History and Literature*,

I. Twersky (ed.), v. 1, 82–109. Cambridge, MA: Harvard University Press, 1979. Re-printed in *Collected Works of Shlomo Pines*, W. Z. Harvey and Moshe Idel (eds.), vol. 5, 404–431. Jerusalem: Magnes Press, 1997.

Pines (1990). Shlomo Pines, "Truth and Falsehood versus Good and Evil. A Study in Jewish and General Philosophy in Connection with the Guide of the Perplexed, I, 2." In *Studies in Maimonides*, I. Twersky (ed.), 95–157. Cambridge, MA: Harvard University Center for Jewish Studies, Harvard University Press 1990.

Poppi (1991). Antonio Poppi, *Introduzione all'Aristotelismo padovano*. 2nd rev. ed. Padua: Editrice Antenore, 1991.

Puig (1992). Josep Puig Montada, "Materials on Averroes's Circle." *Journal of Near Eastern Studies* 51 (1992): 241–260.

Puig (1996). Josep Puig Montada, "Aristotle and Averroes on *Coming-to-be and Passing-Away*." *Oriens* 35 (1996): 1–34.

Puig (1997). Josep Puig Montada, "Les stades de la philosophie naturelle d'Averroès." *Arabic Sciences and Philosophy* 7 (1997): 115–137.

Puig (1998). Josep Puig Montada, *Averroes, juez, médico y filósofo andalusí*. Colección Educación XXI. Seville: Consejería de Educación y Ciencia, 1998.

Puig (2002a). Josep Puig Montada, "Averroes' Commentaries on Aristotle: To Explain and to Interpret." In *In Commento filosofico nell'occidente latino (secoli XIII–XV)*, Gianfranco Fioravanti, Claudio Leonardi, and Stephano Perfetti (eds.), 327–358. Turnhout: Brepols, 2002. Much of what is found here is also in Puig (2002b), but the articles are not completely identical.

Puig (2002b). Josep Puig Montada, "El proyecto vital de Averroes: Explicar e interpretar a Aristoteles." *Al-Qantara* 23 (2002): 11–52.

Puig (2005). Josep Puig Montada, "Averroes: Comentario mahor al libro *Acerca del alma* de Aristóteles. Traducción parcial." *Anales del seminario de historia de la filosofía* 22 (2005): 65–109.

Puig (2007). Josep Puig Montada, "Ibn Bajja." *Stanford Encyclopedia of Philosophy (Fall 2007 Edition)*, Edward N. Zalta (ed.), http://plato.stanford.edu/entries/ibn-bajja/.

Qasim (1964). Mahmoud Qasim, *Naẓarîyah al-maʿrifah ʿinda Ibn Rushd wa-taʾwîli-hâ ladâ Tumâs al-Akwînî* Cairo: Maktabat al-Anglu al-Misriyya, 1964; reprint 1969. For his French version of this, see Kassem (1978).

Ramón Guerrero (1998). Rafael Ramón Guerrero, *Averroes. Sobre filosofía y religión. Introducción y selección de textos*. Pamplona: Universidad de Navarra, 1998.

Renan (1852). Ernest Renan, *Averroès et l'averroïsme. Essai historique*. Paris: Auguste Durand Libraire, 1852. There have been multiple reprints of this work. Among the most recent is *Averroès et l'averroïsme*, with preface by Alain de Libera. Paris: Maisonneuve et Larose, 2002.

Rosemann (1988). Philipp W. Rosemann, "Averroes: A Catalogue of Editions and Scholarly Writings from 1821 Onwards." *Bulletin de philosophie médiévale* 30 (1988): 153–221.

Salman (1937). Dominique Salman, O. P., "Note sur la première influence d'Averroès." *Revue néoscolastique de philosophie* 40 (1937): 203–212.

Schmieja (1999). Horst Schmieja, "*Secundam aliam translationem*—Ein Beitrag zur arabischlateinischen Übersetzung des Grossen Physikkommentars von Averroes." In *Averroes and the Aristotelian Tradition. Sources, Constitution and Reception of the Philosophy of Ibn Rushd (1126–1198). Proceedings of the Fourth Symposium Averroicum* (Cologne, 1996), Gerhard Endress and Jan A. Aertsen (eds.), 316–336. Leiden: E. J. Brill, 1999.

Schmitt (1979). Charles B. Schmitt, "Renaissance Averroism Studied through the Venetian Editions of Aristotle-Averroes (with Particular Reference to the Giunta Edition of 1550–2)." In *Convegno internazionale. L'averroismo in Italia (Roma, 18–20 aprile, 1977)*, 121–142. Rome: Accademia Nazionale dei Lincei, 1979. Reprinted in Charles B. Schmitt, *The Aristotelian Tradition and Renaissance Universities*, v. 7, 121–142. London: Variorum Reprints, 1984.

Schmitt (1983). Charles B. Schmitt, *Aristotle and the Renaissance.* Cambridge, MA: Harvard University Press for Oberlin College, 1983.

Schmitt et al. (1988). Charles B. Schmitt, et al. (eds.), *The Cambridge History of Renaissance Philosophy.* Cambridge and New York: Cambridge University Press, 1988.

Sezgin (2000). Fuat Sezgin et al. (eds.), *Galen in the Arabic Philosophical Tradition. Texts and Studies Collected and Reprinted.* Fuat Sezgin et al. (eds.). Frankfurt am Main: Institute for the History of Arabic-Islamic Science at Johann Wolfgang Goethe University, 2000.

Siegel (1968). Rudolph E. Siegel, *Galen's System of Physiology and Medicine. An Analysis of His Doctrines and Observations on Bloodflow, Respiration, Tumors and Internal Diseases.* Basel and New York: S. Karger, 1968.

Siegel (1970). Rudolph E. Siegel, *Galen on Sense Perception. His Doctrines, Observations and Experiments on Vision, Hearing, Smell, Taste, Touch and Pain, and Their Historical Sources.* Basel and New York: S. Karger, 1970.

South (2003). James B. South, "John of Jandun." In *A Companion to Philosophy in the Middle Ages*, Jorge J. E. Gracia and Timothy B. Noone (eds.), 372–376. Oxford: Blackwell, 2003.

Steinschneider (1893) (1956). Moritz Steinschneider, *Die hebraeischen Übersetzungen des Mittelalters und die Juden als Dolmetscher.* 2 pts. in one vol. Berlin: Kommissionsverlag des Bibliographischen bureaus, 1893. Reprint Graz: Akademische Druck- u. Verlagsanstalt, 1956.

Stone (2000). M. W. F. Stone, "The Soul's Relation to the Body: Thomas Aquinas, Siger of Brabant and the Parisian Debate on Monopsychism." In *History of the Mind-Body Problem*, Tim Crane and Sarah Patterson (eds.), 34–69. London: Routledge, 2000.

Tamani and Zonta (1997). G. Tamani and M. Zonta, *Aristoteles Hebraicus. Versioni, commenti e compendi del Corpus Aristotelicum nei manoscritti ebraici delle biblioteche italiane* (Eurasiatica. Quaderni del Dipartimento di Studi Eurasiatici. Università degli Studi Ca' Foscari di Venice, 46). Venice: Supernova, 1997.

Taylor (1998a) Richard C. Taylor, "Averroes on Psychology and the Principles of Metaphysics." *Journal of the History of Philosophy* 36 (1998): 507–523.

Taylor (1998b). Richard C. Taylor, "Personal Immortality in Averroes' Mature Philosophical Psychology." In *Documenti e studi sulla tradizione filosofica medievale* 9 (1998): 87–110.

Taylor (1998c). Richard C. Taylor, "Averroes' Philosophical Analysis of Religious Propositions." In *Was ist Philosophie im Mittelalter? Qu'est-ce que la philosophie au Moyen Age? What Is Philosophy in the Middle Ages?: Akten des X. Internationalen Kongresses für mittelalterliche Philosophie der Société internationale pour l'étude de la philosophie médiévale, 25. bis 30. August 1997 im Erfurt*, Jan A. Aertsen and Andreas Speer (eds.), 888–894. Miscellanea Mediaevalia 26. Berlin and New York: Walter de Gruyter, 1998.

Taylor (1999a). Richard C. Taylor, "Remarks on Cogitatio in Averroes' *Commentarium Magnum in Aristotelis De Anima Libros*." In *Averroes and the Aristotelian Tradition. Sources, Constitution and Reception of the Philosophy of Ibn Rushd (1126–1198). Proceedings of the Fourth Symposium Averroicum* (Cologne, 1996), Gerhard Endress and Jan A. Aertsen with the assistance of Klaus Braun (eds.), 217–255. Leiden: E. J. Brill, 1999.

Taylor (1999b). Richard C. Taylor. "Averroes' Epistemology and Its Critique by Aquinas." In *Medieval Masters: Essays in Memory of Msgr. E. A. Synan*, R. E. Houser (ed.), 147–177. (Thomistic Papers VII). Houston: Center for Thomistic Studies, University of St. Thomas, 1999.

Taylor (2000a). Richard C. Taylor, "*Cogitatio, Cogitativus* and *Cogitare*: Remarks on the Cogitative Power in Averroes." In *L'élaboration du vocabulaire philosophique au Moyen Age*, Jacqueline Hamesse and Carlos Steel (eds.), 111–146. Louvain-la-Neuve: Peeters, 2000.

Taylor (2000b). Richard C. Taylor, "'Truth does not contradict truth': Averroes and the Unity of Truth." *Topoi* 19.1 (2000): 3–16.

Taylor (2003). Richard C. Taylor, "Averroes." In *A Companion to Philosophy in the Middle Ages*, Jorge J. E. Gracia and Timothy B. Noone (eds.), 182–195. Oxford: Blackwell, 2003.

Taylor (2004a). Richard C. Taylor, "Averroes: Religious Dialectic and Aristotelian Philosophical Thought." In *The Cambridge Companion to Arabic Philosophy*, Peter Adamson and Richard C. Taylor (eds.), 180–200. Cambridge: Cambridge University Press, 2004.

Taylor (2004b). Richard C. Taylor, "Improving on Nature's Exemplar: Averroes' Completion of Aristotle's Psychology of Intellect." In *Philosophy, Science and Exegesis in Greek, Arabic and Latin Commentaries* (Supplement to the Bulletin of the Institute of Classical Studies 83.1–2), Peter Adamson, Han Baltussen, and M. W. F. Stone (eds.), v. 2, 107–130. London: Institute of Classical Studies, 2004.

Taylor (2005). Richard C. Taylor, "The Agent Intellect as 'Form for Us' and Averroes's Critique of al-Fârâbî." *Tópicos* (Universidad Panamericana, Mexico City) 29 (2005): 29–51. Reprinted with corrections in *Proceedings of the Society for Medieval Logic and Metaphysics* 5 (2005): 18–32. http://www.fordham.edu/gsas/phil/klima/SMLM/PSMLM5/PSMLM5.pdf

Taylor (2007). Richard C. Taylor, "Averroes: God and the Noble Lie." In *Laudemus viros gloriosos: Essays in Honor of Armand Augustine Maurer, CSB*, R. E. Houser (ed.), 38–59. Notre Dame, IN: University of Notre Dame Press, 2007.

Taylor (forthcoming). Richard C. Taylor, "Averroes' Philosophical Conception of Separate Intellect and God." In *La pensée philosophique et scientifique d'Averroès dans son temps*, J. Puig Montada and A. Hasnaoui (eds.). Paris, forthcoming.

Teicher (1935). Jacob Teicher, "I commenti di Averroè sul 'De Anima' (Considerazioni generali e successione cronologica." *Giornale della Società Asiatica Italiana* [second series] 3 (1935): 233–256.

Thijssen (2003). Hans Thijssen, "Condemnation of 1277." In *The Stanford Encyclopedia of Philosophy* (Spring 2003 Edition), Edward N. Zalta (ed.). URL = http://plato.stanford. edu/archives/spr2003/entries/condemnation/.

Thorndike (1965). Lynn Thorndike, *Michael Scot*. London: Nelson, 1965.

Twetten (1995). David B. Twetten, "Averroes on the Prime Mover Proved in the Physics." *Viator* 26 (1995): 107–134.

Twetten (2007). David B. Twetten, "Averroes' Prime Mover Argument." In *Averroès et les averroïsmes juif et latin. Actes du Colloque International (Paris, 16–18 juin, 2005)*, J. B. Brenet (ed.), 9–75. Turnhout: Brepols, 2007.

Ullmann (1970). Manfred Ullmann, *Die Medizin im Islam*. Leiden and Cologne: E. J. Brill, 1970.

Urvoy (1991). Dominique Urvoy, *Ibn Rushd (Averroes)*, Olivia Stewart (trans.). London and New York: Routledge, 1991.

Urvoy (1996). Dominique Urvoy, *Ibn Rushd (Averroès)*. Paris: Cariscript, 1996. French version of Urvoy (1991), corrected and augmented.

Urvoy (1998). Dominique Urvoy, *Averroès. Les ambitions d'un intellectuel musulman*. Paris: Flammarion, 1998.

van Oppenraay (1990). Aafke M. I. van Oppenraay, "Quelques particularités de la méthode de traduction de Michel Scot." In *Rencontres de cultures dans la philosophie médiévale: Traductions et traducteurs de l'antiquité tardive au XIVe siècle*, Jacqueline Hamesse and Marta Fattori (eds.), 121–129. Louvain-la-Neuve: Université Catholique de Louvain; Cassino, Italy: Università degli Studi di Cassino, 1990.

Van Steenberghen (1966) (1991). Fernand Van Steenberghen, *La philosophie au XIIIe Siècle*. Paris: Béatrice-Nauwelaerts; Louvain: Publications Universitaires, 1966; 2nd ed. 1991.

Van Steenberghen (1970). Fernand Van Steenberghen, *Aristotle in the West. The Origins of Latin Aristotelianism*. Leonard Johnston (trans.). 2nd ed. Louvain: Nauwelaerts, 1970. Translation of *Aristote en Occident. Les origines de l'aristotélisme parisien*. Louvain: Editions de l'Institut Supérieur de Philosophie, 1946.

Van Steenberghen (1977). Fernand Van Steenberghen, *Maître Siger de Brabant*. Louvain: Publications Universitaires; Paris: Vander-Oyez, 1977.

Vennebusch (1964). Joachim Vennebusch, "Zur Bibliographie des psychologischen Schrifttums des Averroes." *Bulletin de philosophie médiévale* 6 (1964): 92–100.

Vernet (1971). J. Vernet, "Ibn al-Ṭayyib." In *The Encyclopaedia of Islam. New Edition*, B. Lewis, V. L. Ménage, Ch. Pellat, and J. Schacht (eds.), v. 3, 955a. Leiden: E. J. Brill; London: Luzac, 1971.

von Kügelgen (1994). Anke von Kügelgen, *Averroes und die arabische Moderne. Ansätze zu einer Neubegründung des Rationalismus im Islam*. Leiden: E. J. Brill, 1994.

von Kügelgen (1996). Anke von Kügelgen, "A Call for Rationalism: 'Arab Averroists' in the Twentieth Century." *Alif. Journal of Comparative Poetics* (American University in Cairo) 16 (1996): 97–132.

Walzer (1962). Richard Walzer, *Greek into Arabic. Essays on Islamic Philosophy.* Cambridge, MA: Harvard University Press; Oxford: Bruno Cassirer, 1962.

Walzer (1965). Richard Walzer, "Djâlînûs." In *The Encyclopaedia of Islam. New Edition,* v. 2, B. Lewis, Ch. Pellat, and J. Schacht (eds.) 402a–403b. Leiden: E. J. Brill; London: Luzac, 1965.

Wéber (1978). Ed. H. Wéber, "Les apports positifs de la noétique d'Ibn Rushd à celle de Thomas d'Aquin." *Multiple Averroès. Actes du Colloque International organisé à l'occasion du 850ᵉ anniversaire de la naissance d'Averroès. Paris 20–23 septembre 1976,* Jean Jolivet and Rachel Arié (eds.), 210–248. Paris: Les Belles Lettres, 1978.

Wéber (1994). Edouard-Henri Wéber, "Les emprunts majeurs à Averroès chez Albert le Grand et dans son école." In *Averroismus im Mittelalter und in der Renaissance,* Friedrich Niewöhner and Loris Sturlese (eds.), 149–179. Zurich: Spur, 1994.

Wéber (1998) Edouard-Henri Wéber. "L'identité de l'intellect et de l'intelligible selon la version latine d'Averroès et son interprétation par Thomas d'Aquin." *Arabic Sciences and Philosophy* 8 (1998): 233–257.

Wedin (1988). Michael Wedin, *Mind and Imagination in Aristotle.* New Haven: Yale University Press, 1988.

Wippel (1977). John F. Wippel, "The Condemnations of 1270 and 1277 at Paris." *Journal of Medieval and Renaissance Studies* 7 (1977): 169–201.

Wippel (1998). John F. Wippel, "Siger of Brabant." In *Routledge Encyclopedia of Philosophy,* E. Craig (ed.). London: Routledge, 1998. Retrieved July 15, 2004, from http://www.rep.routledge.com/article/B102.

Wippel (2003). John F. Wippel, "The Parisian Condemnations of 1270 and 1277." In *A Companion to Philosophy in the Middle Ages,* J. J. E. Gracia and T. Noone (eds.), 65–73. Oxford: Blackwell, 2003.

Wirmer, Thomas Institut (2006). David Wirmer (project director) *Averroes-Database* at http://www.thomasinst.uni-koeln.de/averroes/index.htm, with comprehensive bibliography to Fall 2006 at http://www.thomasinst.uni-koeln.de/averroes/bibliography.htm.

Wolfson (1931). Harry A. Wolfson, "Plan for the publication of a *Corpus Commentariorum Averrois in Aristotelem.*" *Speculum* 6 (1931): 412–427.

Wolfson (1958). Harry A. Wolfson, "The Plurality of Immovable Movers in Aristotle and Averroes." *Harvard Studies in Classical Philology* 63 (1958): 233–253.

Wolfson (1961). Harry A. Wolfson, "The Twice-Revealed Averroes." *Speculum* 36 (1961): 373–392.

Wolfson (1963). Harry A. Wolfson, "Revised Plan for the Publication of a *Corpus Commentariorum Averrois in Aristotelem.*" *Speculum* 38 (1963): 88–104, with "Corrigendum," 39 (1964): 378. Reprinted in *Studies in the History of Philosophy and Religion. Harry Austryn Wolfson,* Isadore Twersky and George H. Williams (eds.), v. 1, 430–454. Cambridge, MA: Harvard University Press, 1973. My citations are from the 1973 reprint.

Yousif (1997). Ephrem-Isa Yousif, *Les philosophes et traducteurs syriaques.* Paris: L'Harmattan, 1997.

Yousif (2003). Ephrem-Isa Yousif, *La floraison des philosophes syriaques*. Paris: L'Harmattan, 2003.

Zonta (1994). Mauro Zonta, "Osservazioni sulla traduzione ebraica de *Commento Grande* di Averroe al *De Anima* di Aristotele." *Annali di Ca' Foscari. Rivista della Facoltà di Lingue e Letterature Straniere dell' Università di Venezia* 25 (1994): 15–28.

Zonta (1996). Mauro Zonta, *La filosofia antica nel medioevo ebraico: le traduzioni ebraiche medievali dei testi filosofici antichi*. Brescia: Paideia, 1996.

Zonta (2001). Mauro Zonta, "La tradizione guideo-araba ed ebraica del *De Intellectu* di Alessandro di Afrodisia e il testo originale del *Commento* di Averroè." *Annali di Ca' Foscari. Rivista della Facoltà di Lingue e Letterature Straniere dell' Università di Venezia* 40.3 (2001) (Serie orientale 32), 17–35; Arabic text of Averroes' *Commentary on the De Intellectu of Alexander*, 27–34. A Hebrew translation of this work was edited by Herbert Davidson in 1988. See *Commentary on the De Intellectu of Alexander* (2001) above.

Index

General Index of the Translation

essence, 4, 45, 54, 176, 335

establish, 20, 34, 47, 68, 70, 86, 161–62, 398, 400

eternal, 17, 60, 62–63, 78, 128, 143–45, 184, 306, 315, 322–24, 351, 355–57, 360–61, 387, 391, 396–98

eternity, 144

everlasting, 144–45

evil, 267–68, 379–80

exemplar, 345

exist, 5, 7, 10, 11, 14–17, 19, 21, 24, 26, 28–29, 41, 47–48, 50–51, 53–54, 62, 66–67, 71–72, 75, 79, 85, 89–90, 93, 96–100, 102–7, 109–16, 123–25, 127, 129, 131, 133–37, 139–40, 144–46, 153, 158–59, 162, 164–66, 168, 170, 172, 177, 180–81, 184, 188, 192–93, 199, 201, 204, 206, 214, 220–21, 228, 233–35, 237, 239, 242–43, 245–46, 260, 263, 265, 268, 275–76, 283, 288, 293–94, 302, 307, 309–10, 316, 324, 326, 332, 337, 340, 348, 362–68, 373, 379, 381, 383–84, 286–87, 392, 396–400, 402–9, 414, 420–22, 424, 426, 428, 430–33, 435, 441–42

existence, 20, 43, 103–4, 110, 117, 134, 157, 172, 174, 180, 192, 264, 287, 293–94, 306–7, 312, 314, 323, 327, 336, 351–52, 357, 360, 362, 378, 383, 386, 393, 400, 403–4, 433–34

existent, 10, 15, 325, 368, 400, 404

extremities, 233–34, 238

extrinsic, 14, 64, 71, 214, 268, 325, 439–40

eye, 15, 76, 100, 116–19, 131, 186, 199, 210, 218–19, 227, 252, 267, 277, 280–81, 346, 389, 436

eyelids, 218–19

false, 14, 33, 44–45, 67, 91, 152, 156, 276–82, 284–85, 287–89, 314, 326, 344, 363–65, 370–71, 379, 400

falsity, 45, 287–88, 363–65, 370–71, 379–80

fear, 18–19, 23, 75, 411–12

figure, 36, 154, 283, 344, 354, 390, 427–28, 433

figure (noun), 18, 26, 35, 137–40, 151–52, 154, 193, 195–96, 205, 239, 254, 257,

282–83, 332, 344, 354, 390, 410, 427–28, 433

second figure (of the syllogism) 151–52, 282

spherical figure, 193, 195–96

finger, 400, 410

finite, 60–61, 63, 152–53, 407

fire, 24–25, 27, 30, 35–37, 42, 49–50, 88–89, 91, 96, 149–54, 161–63, 184, 188–90, 215, 237, 242, 251–52, 310, 329, 360, 377–78, 439–40

fish, 186, 191, 204, 208, 214

fish scales, 186

flat, 202–3, 227–28

flavor, 135–36, 140, 175, 209–13, 218–26, 228, 233, 242, 245–47, 260, 263–65, 270, 441

flesh, 69–72, 87, 89, 115, 211, 226–34, 236–41, 244, 250–52, 266–67, 335–39, 381

food, 112, 134–36, 142–44, 150, 152–53, 155–56, 159–61, 209, 214–15, 430, 432, 434–35, 442

foot, feet, 45, 215, 221–22, 284

form, 1, 3, 11, 19–23, 26, 31–33, 40, 42, 54, 67–68, 70–72, 87, 89–90, 93, 95–100, 102, 106–7, 109–10, 113–18, 120–21, 127–28, 130–32, 144–48, 152, 155, 158–62, 164, 167, 169, 172, 176, 182–85, 218, 220, 242, 244, 252, 262–63, 265, 270–72, 276–78, 281, 298–308, 310, 312–18, 320–21, 323, 325–32, 335–45, 348, 350–53, 355–56, 358–61, 365, 367–69, 376–78, 383, 386–93, 395, 397–404, 415, 422, 426, 430

final form for us, 387

first form, 107, 338

First Form (God), 326

form for us, 355–56, 383, 387

forms of the imagination, 329, 345, 358–59, 374, 388, 399

imagined form, 176, 308, 320, 323, 325, 365, 426

intelligible form, 304, 313, 343

material form, 19, 32, 302–4, 326–28, 359–60, 386, 398

non-material forms, 360

sensible form, 32, 242, 244, 307, 337, 339, 350